Handbook of Steroids

Handbook of Steroids

Edited by Dwyane Mason

hayle
medical

New York

Hayle Medical,
750 Third Avenue, 9th Floor,
New York, NY 10017, USA

Visit us on the World Wide Web at:
www.haylemedical.com

ISBN: 978-1-63241-789-3

Printed in China.

Cataloging-in-Publication Data

Handbook of steroids / edited by Dwyane Mason.
p. cm.
Includes bibliographical references and index.
ISBN 978-1-63241-789-3
1. Steroids. 2. Steroids--Research. 3. Steroid drugs. I. Mason, Dwyane.
RM297.S74 H36 2019
615.36--dc23

Table of Contents

Preface

Steroids are organic compounds having four rings arranged to their structure in a specific molecular configuration. There are two main functions of a steroid, i.e., to function as an important component of cell membranes which alter membrane fluidity, and to function as a signaling molecule. Most steroids are found in animals, plants, and fungi. The process through which the steroids are generated from cholesterol and changed into other steroids is known as steroidogenesis. The topics included in this book on steroids are of utmost significance and bound to provide incredible insights to readers. It unfolds the innovative aspects of steroids which will be crucial for the detailed study of the subject. For all readers who are interested in the study of steroids, the case studies included in this book will serve as an excellent guide to develop a comprehensive understanding.

This book is a comprehensive compilation of works of different researchers from varied parts of the world. It includes valuable experiences of the researchers with the sole objective of providing the readers (learners) with a proper knowledge of the concerned field. This book will be beneficial in evoking inspiration and enhancing the knowledge of the interested readers.

In the end, I would like to extend my heartiest thanks to the authors who worked with great determination on their chapters. I also appreciate the publisher's support in the course of the book. I would also like to deeply acknowledge my family who stood by me as a source of inspiration during the project.

Editor

A Cohort Historical Analysis of the Relationship between Thyroid Hormone Malady and Alpha-Human Herpesvirus Activation

Shao-Hsuan Hsia[1] **and Victor Hsia S**[2*]

[1]*Department of Pediatrics, Division of Pediatric Critical Care Medicine, Chang Gung Memorial Hospital, College of Medicine, Chang-Gung University, Kweishan, Taiwan*

[2]*School of Pharmacy, University of Maryland Eastern Shore, Princess Anne, MD 21853, USA*

[*]**Corresponding author:** Victor Hsia S, School of Pharmacy, University of Maryland Eastern Shore, Princess Anne, MD 21853, USA, E-mail: vhsia@umes.edu

Abstract

Background: A number of physiological factors have been suggested to participate in the alpha- Human Herpesvirus (αHHV) reactivation, such as hormonal aberration. Thyroid hormone (TH) was shown to play a suppressive role in Herpes Simplex Virus Type-1 (HSV-1) gene expression and replication in cell culture and animal models. We hypothesize that reactivation of αHHV in humans may be due to, at least in part, by TH status.

Methods: Prior to implementing a full-scale population-based prospective inquiry into this hypothesis, a pilot study using a medical claims data base and a case-controlled, retrospective cohort investigation was conducted to develop a hypothetical link between TH complication and αHHV reactivation. Using diagnostic codes for treating thyroid disorders and αHHV infections as proxies for biologic/clinic outcomes, we queried a large, comprehensive hospital data base to construct two patient cohorts: Cohort 1 was comprised of patients receiving TH diagnoses over a twelve-year period, and Cohort 2 was composed of patients not receiving TH diagnoses during this period. Diagnoses of αHHV were recorded for each cohort and the difference in the frequency was examined for statistical significance. Demographic analyses such as age, gender, etc were also performed.

Results: Using 2X2 contingency table analyses and Statistical Analysis Software (SAS), an Odds Ratio (OR) of 2.83 was observed for the total population of 21 years old and above with a chi-square of 61.55 and $p < 0.001$, confirming that a severe significant difference was found between these two cohorts. This result suggested that patients with αHHV diagnosis have higher chances to have TH disorders. Additional investigation revealed that female were at higher/significant probability to have both TH and αHHV diagnosis, indicating a link of αHHV reactivation to a complex hormonal profile difference between genders. Our observation indicated that female patients of 21 years of age and above exhibited a very high incidence (OR of 3.40, $p < 0.001$) compared to the male groups (OR of 1.91, $p < 0.05$), indicating the possibility that hormonal alteration in females maybe transient but robust and can lead to αHHV reactivation more often than the males.

Conclusion: These results indicated that TH dysfunction may have implication in αHHV pathogenesis and females exhibited much higher probability to suffer αHHV reactivation due to TH disruption. Although the results from this pilot study have limitations and require additional controlled clinical examination such as more detailed patient records, lab data, therapeutic outcome, etc, it provides a tool to assess the effects of hormone imbalance on virus reactivation by retrospective analyses using existing large scale data base.

Keywords: αHHV; HSV-1; Thyroid Hormone; Retrospective study; Viral reactivation; Risk ratio; Odds ratio; Medical claims; ICD-9 diagnostic codes

Introduction

Thyroid hormone (TH or T3) is known to have important regulatory functions for normal biological processes. TH produces its physiological effects primarily through its nuclear receptor (TR), which is a transcriptional factor that controls gene expression and the net outcome, is determined by TH level [1]. Hormone imbalances have been suggested to affect viral pathogenesis [2]. Latest literatures proposed that TH participated in the regulation of HSV-1 gene silencing and replication and may have influence during viral latency/ reactivation [3,4].

HSV-1 belongs to the superfamily of alpha Human Herpesvirus (αHHV) and represents one of the most widespread infections [5]. Besides HSV-1, HSV-2 and Varicella Zoster Virus (VZV) are also grouped in the αHHV category sharing close similarity of their genomes [6-9]. These viruses are widespread in US population, evidenced by the sero-prevalence rates of 57.7% [10]. These viruses have a complex infection pattern. Following the lytic assault of epithelial cells, the virus may enter sensory neurons of trigeminal ganglia and establish latency, in which the virus remained dormant without gene expression and replication. The reactivation happened temporarily at different sites connected to the trigeminal nerves such as the mucosa, lips, eyes, or perioral area of the face causing minor lesions such as fever blisters [11]. Encephalitis caused by HSV-1 reactivation accounted for approximately 10% of all viral encephalitis [12]. The molecular mechanisms leading to αHHV reactivation remain ambiguous [13].

Literatures and clinical studies reported that episodes of stress, facial injury, etc. that triggered reactivation of αHHV also showed evidences of decreased level of TH levels [2]. The working hypothesis is that αHHV latency and reactivation may be affected, at least in part, by the TH status. In another word, transient hypothyroidism may alleviate TH-mediated suppression of viral replication and promote viral gene expression and reactivation. However, there is no controlled clinical evidence in human subjects supporting this hypothesis.

Materials and Methods

Study design

To support the working hypothesis from pre-clinical standpoints, a case-control, retrospective investigation querying a hospitalization data base from a large research/teaching hospital was performed using diagnoses codes as a measure of disease status. This type of research approach is considered as a prerequisite step in the further development of prospective clinical investigation to test the hypothesis that anomalous TH level is associated with reactivation of the αHHV.

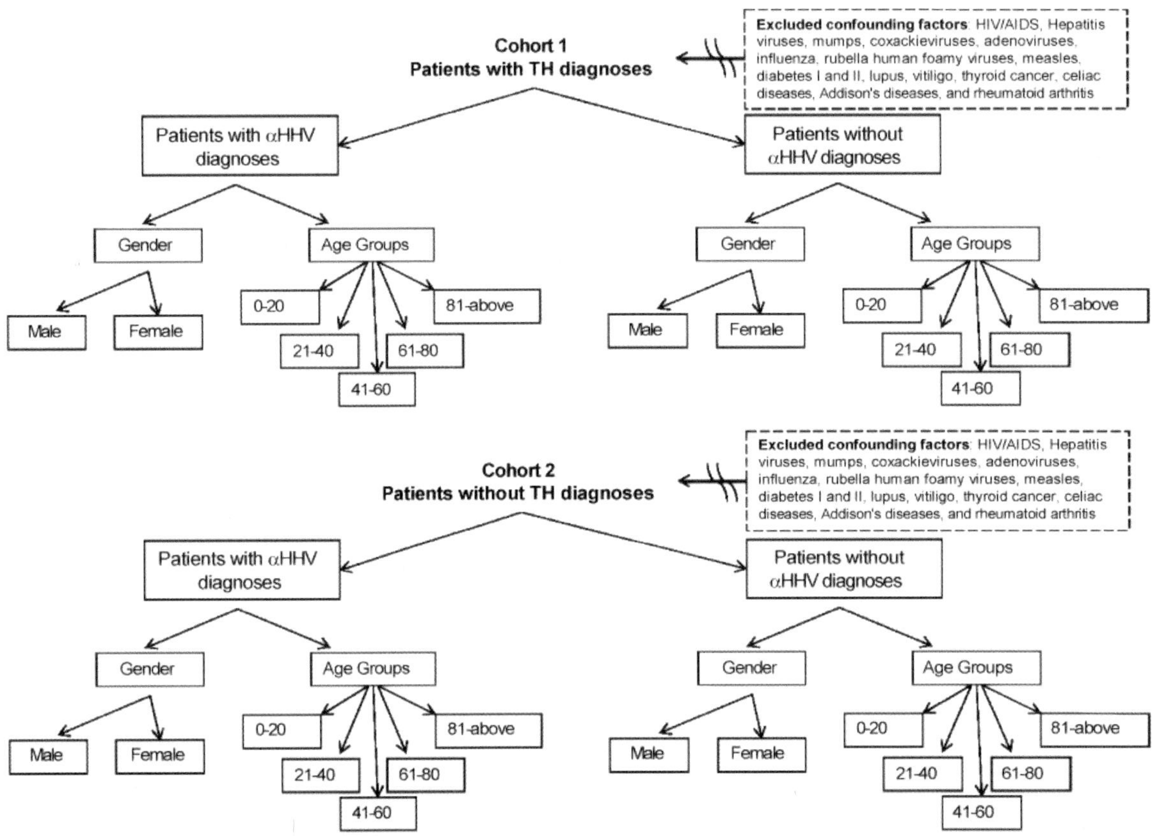

Figure 1: Experimental design of the cohort studies. ICD9 diagnosis codes were collected from 2001-2012 and divided into two groups based on the diagnoses of their TH level. After categorized into two cohorts with or without TH diagnoses, each group was further separated into different units based on their gender and age. To ensure the data validity, confounding factors were cleared.

Study populations

The data of patients who were hospitalized within a twelve-year period (2001-2012) were obtained from Chang Gung Memorial Hospital, a large research/teaching comprehensive hospital in Taiwan. The ICD-9 codes for Disorders of Thyroid Gland (240.xx to 246.xx) and αHHV infections (VZV: 053.xx and HSV: 054.xx) were collected and analyzed. Demographic data such as years, genders, age groups, etc were assessed to comprehend the features of this population. Of all the patients receiving examination within this twelve-year period, the following specific diagnosis data were categorized: 1) total number of patients for all diagnoses within the time period; 2) number of patients without diagnoses of αHHV and thyroid dysfunction; 3) number of patients with diagnoses for thyroid dysfunction; 4) number of patients with diagnoses for thyroid malady and no diagnoses of αHHV; 5) number of patients with diagnoses of αHHV; 6) number of patients receiving diagnoses of αHHV without diagnoses for thyroid dysfunction; and 7) number of patients receiving diagnoses of both αHHV AND thyroid disorders. This analysis was also performed on different genders and age groups to compare the effects of putative sex differences. The strategy was summarized in Figure 1.

Eligibility criteria

Confounding factors were removed to ensure the eligibility and authenticity of the results. Factors excluded are HIV/AIDS, Hepatitis viruses, mumps, coxackieviruses, adenoviruses, influenza, rubella human foamy viruses, measles, diabetes I and II, lupus, vitiligo, thyroid cancer, celiac diseases, Addison's diseases, and rheumatoid arthritis. Specific codes were used for the purposes of exclusions (Figure 1).

Statistical analysis

To examine the hypothetical risk of developing αHHV disease if encountered TH disorders, we performed historic cohort statistical analyses (2X2 contingency table analyses and Statistical Analysis Software (SAS)) to measure an odds ratio or risk ratio for assessment of relative risk. In another word, higher relative risk number represents higher probability of developing a αHHV disease (risk) related to TH disorder (condition). For example, If a virus outbreak is linked to thyroid dysfunction, then a significant difference in the diagnoses should be obvious between the cohorts, evidenced by a calculated Odds Ratio (OR) of >1 and a significant p-value would indicate a correlation between thyroid abnormality and viral infection, as described by the alternative measure of diagnoses. On the contrary, null hypothesis would be presented as no difference between these two cohorts, indicating that thyroid malady is not linked to activation of virus. To analyze these two groups of subjects, each cohort was sorted according to the absence (-) or presence (+) of the correspondent condition, this statistical software then calculated standard measures for Rates, Risk Ratio, Odds, Odds Ratio, etc. Risk Ratio was calculated as Rate (group 1)/Rate (group 2); rate reflects the proportion in group with condition present. Odds Ratio was measured as Odds (group 1)/ Odds (group 2), as Odds (group 1) = present (group 1)/absent (group 1) and Odds (group 2) = present (group 2)/absent (group 2).

Results

Characteristics of the Patients

A total of 1,516,372 patients (male: 759,904; female: 756,468) were hospitalized from 2001 to 2012 and the ICD-9 codes were obtained anonymously.

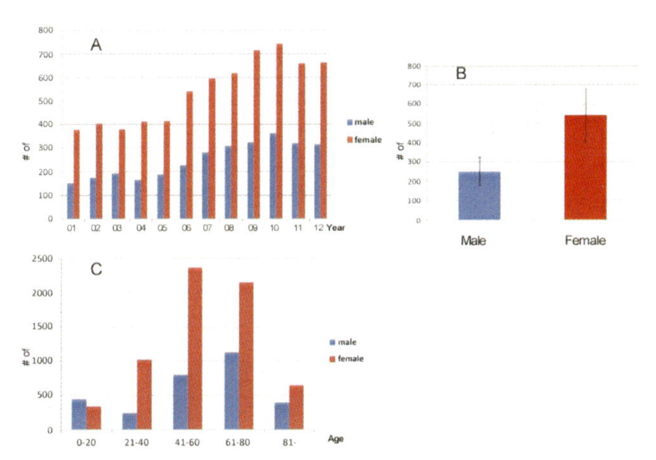

Figure 2: Analyses of patients with TH diagnoses.

A. TH diagnoses between 2001-2012

B. Gender difference of patients suffering TH dysfunction from 2001-2012. The p value is <0.05.

C. TH diagnoses in different age groups

Patients (both male and female) diagnosed with TH disorders increased gradually throughout the years and peaked in 2009-2010 and remained high in 2011 and 2012 (Figure 2A). Based on the existing records from the database (2001-2012), females had twice as much TH disorders than the males (Figure 2B). In addition, there was no gender difference regarding TH abnormality before twenty years of age (Figure 2C). However, TH dysfunction became a prominent issue for females over 21 years old compared to the male counterpart, especially for those who were 21-80 years of age (Figure 2C). As for the αHHV diagnoses, young patients under 20 in both genders had a very high numbers of hospitalization record (Figure 3A and 3B). There was no gender difference in adult αHHV diagnoses but the age group of 61-80 exhibited higher cases of virus-related hospitalization (Figure 3B).

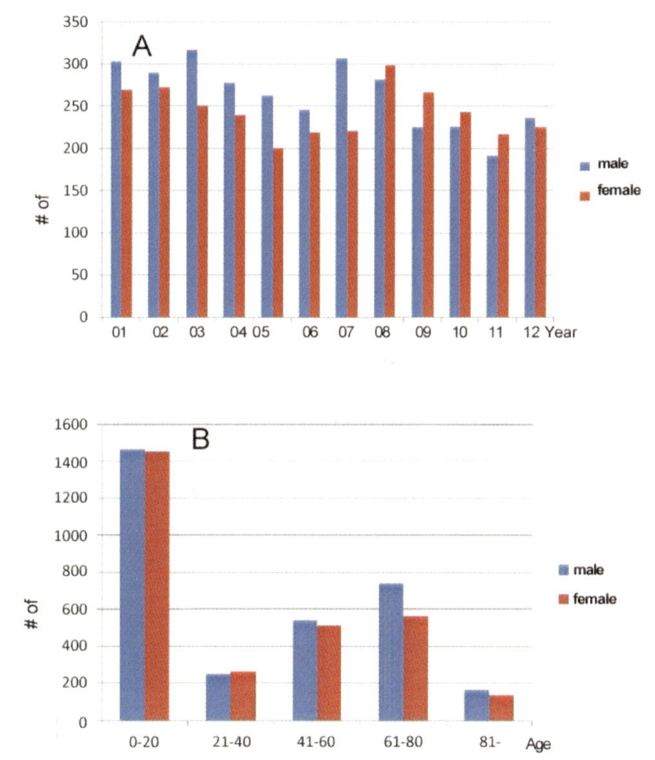

Figure 3: Analyses of patients with αHHV diagnoses.

A. αHHV diagnoses between 2001-2012

B. αHHV diagnoses in different age groups

Association of TH dysfunction and αHHV reactivation

After the screening of confounding factors and removal of unqualified diagnoses, the computer analyses showed that 56 patients possessed both TH and αHHV diagnoses codes, 13 males and 43 females, during 2001-2012 (Figure 4A). Additional investigations analyzing among age groups indicated that female patients between 21-80 years of age exhibited much higher diagnoses than the same age group of males (Figure 4B). This finding probably resulted, at least in part, from the fact that more females in these age groups were diagnosed with TH disorders than the males (Figure 2B).

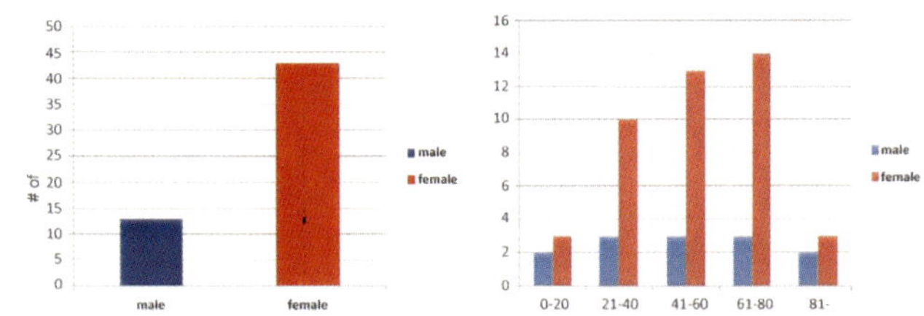

Figure 4: Analyses of patients with both TH and αHHV diagnoses.

A. αHHV+TH+ diagnoses between genders

B. αHHV+TH+ diagnoses among age groups

To address the relative risk of αHHV infection related to a condition of TH dysfunction, OR/RR were measured for assessment. The results showed that the OR/RR was approximately 1.46 for total hospitalized population of all ages between 2001and 2012 with p value less than 0.005 (Table 1A), indicating that patients suffering αHHV infections exhibited increased chance of having TH disorders.

		αHHV		
		-	+	Total
T	+ (group 1)	9484	56	9540
H	- (group 2)	1500799	6033	1506832
	Total	1510283	6089	1516372
			.95 Confidence Intervals	
		Observed	Lower limit	Upper limit
	Risk Ratio	1.4661	1.1272	1.906
	Odds Ratio	1.4689	1.1282	1.9125
		Chi-Square		
	Phi	Yates	Pearson	
		7.8	8.26	
	p	0.00523	0.004053	

Table 1A: Statistical analyses of odds ratio of all age groups; Of total population, p value < 0.005

Further studies revealed that female patients possessed slightly increased relative risk by showing an OR of 1.72 with p value less than 0.005 (Table 1B).

		αHHV		
		-	+	Total
T	+ (group 1)	6484	43	6527
H	- (group 2)	747065	2876	749941
	Total	753549	2919	756468
			.95 Confidence Intervals	
		Observed	Lower limit	Upper limit
	Risk Ratio	1.7179	1.2725	2.3192
	Odds Ratio	1.7226	1.2735	2.3302
		Chi-Square		
	Phi	Yates	Pearson	
		12.05	12.76	
	p	0.000518	0.000354	

Table 1B: Statistical analyses of odds ratio of all age groups; Of all females, p value < 0.001

Male patients, however, showed no significant difference between patients suffering TH disorder or not (Table 1C). Together these observations suggested that TH dysfunction-related αHHV reactivation were more obvious in females than males.

		αHHV		
		-	+	Total
T	+ (group 1)	2999	13	3012
H	- (group 2)	753736	3156	756892
	Total	756735	3169	759904
			.95 Confidence Intervals	
		Observed	Lower limit	Upper limit
	Risk Ratio	1.03	0.6	1.78
	Odds Ratio	1.03	0.6	1.78
		Chi-Square		
	Phi	Yates	Pearson	
		0	0.02	
	p	1	0.88	

Table 1C: Statistical analyses of odds ratio of all age groups; Of all males, p value is 0.88

Our additional analyses displayed the differences of patients diagnosed with αHHV and TH disorders among age groups (Figure 4B). Thus we performed statistical analyses excluding patients under 20 years of age of both genders and focusing on patients of 21 years old and above. The results demonstrated that it is significant with an OR of 2.83 and p value less than 0.001 (Table 2A).

		αHHV		
		-	+	Total
T	+ (group 1)	8787	51	8838

H	- (group 2)	1504000	3200	1507200
	Total	1512787	3251	1516038
			.95 Confidence Intervals	
		Observed	Lower limit	Upper limit
	Risk Ratio	2.82	2.15	3.70
	Odds Ratio	2.83	2.16	3.72
		Chi-Square		
	Phi	Yates	Pearson	
		59.75	61.55	
	p	<.0001	<.0001	

Table 2A: Statistical analyses of odds ratio over 21 years of age; Of total population, p value < 0.001

If concentrated on females over 21 years of age the statistics is even more significant with OR of 3.40 and p value less than 0.0001 (Table 2B), compared to males (OR: 1.91) with p value less than 0.05 (Table 2C). Collectively these data indicated that adult females exhibited very high probability of suffering TH malady-associated αHHV infections than the male counterpart.

		αHHV		
		-	+	Total
TH	+ (group 1)	1434	40	1474
	- (group 2)	750036	6142	751678
	Total	751470	6182	757652
			.95 Confidence Intervals	
		Observed	Lower limit	Upper limit
	Risk Ratio	3.34	2.45	4.54
	Odds Ratio	3.40	2.48	4.67
		Chi-Square		
	Phi	Yates	Pearson	
		63.4	65.72	
	p	<.0001	<.0001	

Table 2B: Statistical analyses of odds ratio over 21 years of age; Of females, p value < 0.001

		αHHV		
		-	+	Total
TH	+ (group 1)	1691	11	1702
	- (group 2)	753895	2559	756454
	Total	755586	2570	758156
			.95 Confidence Intervals	
		Observed	Lower limit	Upper limit
	Risk Ratio	1.91	1.05	3.44
	Odds Ratio	1.91	1.05	3.47
		Chi-Square		
	Phi	Yates	Pearson	
		3.9	4.77	
	p	0.048	0.028	

Table 2C: Statistical analyses of odds ratio over 21 years of age; Of males, p value < 0.05

Discussion

Rationales

The relationship between αHHV reactivation and TH dysfunction were not discussed until 2010 when publications showed that TH can suppress the replication and gene expression of HSV-1, a αHHV, in cultured neuronal cells [3,4]. Bioinformatics revealed several putative TH responsive elements within the HSV-1 regulatory sequences and were identified to produce regulatory effects by molecular biology studies [3,4]. There are rationales to suggest TH level can affect αHHV reactivation and latency. For example, both TH and its nuclear receptors are available in ganglia neurons where HSV-1 established latency [14,15] and can modulate neuronal survival, differentiation, maturation [16], raising the possibility of regulating the HSV-1 latency/reactivation. Recent evidences indicated that TH participated in controlling neurite outgrowth and axonal elongation/transport [17], both are critical for HSV-1 latency, via nerve growth factor (NGF)-TrkA-PI3 Kinase signaling pathway using a unique non-genomic mechanism [18]. It is likely that TH enhances NGF-mediated PI3-Kinase cascade to promote HSV-1 latency and transient low TH may instead increase the chance of reactivation. However, direct clinical or epidemiological studies regarding the effect of TH on HSV-1/VZV reactivation, to our knowledge, are not available at this point.

Clinical significance

Many scenarios that reduce TH levels can trigger HSV-1 reactivation [2]. For instance, a clinical study indicated that a patient with myxedema coma under corticosteroid regime suffered severe herpes simplex encephalitis diagnosed with extremely low thyroxine level less than 5.2 nmol/L (normal range 12-30 nmol/L) [19]. Furthermore, it is well documented that corticosteroid changes have been shown to induce HSV-1 reactivation in animal studies [20,21]. These observations prompted us to perform a large-scale population-based cohort examination to examine this hypothesis using existing hospitalized data.

Disparity of genders and ages

Our analyses confirmed the general opinion that females exhibited more TH dysfunction than males (Figure 2A and 2B). The data also showed that more TH dysfunctions were diagnosed while people age with peak observed at 41-60 years of age (Figure 2C). Although we do not observe the gender/age difference in αHHV diagnoses, the results demonstrated that females had significantly higher odds ratio than males when we linked the relationships of TH malady and αHHV infections, particularly between 21-80 years of age (Figure 4 and Table 2). It is likely due to the complex profiles of hormonal regulation in females or other influence from female dominant hormones. The exact mechanisms are yet clear.

During an independent study, our collaborators queried a regional hospital database in US using similar strategy. The preliminary results showed that the OR of HSV-1 patient's experienced TH dysfunction for total population is 8-time higher (unpublished data). It is likely due to under- diagnoses. However, we do not exclude the possibilities of health disparity and/or cultural/environmental factors.

Thyroid hormone malady/autoimmunity affected adults as well as children significantly [22,23]. The correlation is not significant in young patients especially in children. However, the correlation may be underestimated because many children with primary hypothyroidism are subclinical or asymptomatic and remain under-diagnosed [24-26].

Advantages and Disadvantages

This kind of retrospective design has some marked advantages over prospective studies since the historical investigation characteristically involve shorter period of time to complete since patients suffering disorders have already been identified and diagnosed. This fact would be generally beneficial since it is less expensive to carry on the studies and the resources should be focused on the collection and analyses of data only.

Retrospective studies have several drawbacks such as the bias of data selection and statistical difficulties, etc. that may influence the validity. In addition, the chronological connection of exposures and outcomes are usually challenging for assessment but an accurate record-keeping may be able to resolve the issues.

Conclusion

The present study suggested that TH level may play a critical role in αHHV reactivation and TH levels can become a standard biomarker for recurrent αHHV diagnoses. Furthermore, physicians can be advised of the future relative risk of αHHV occurrence of their patients and appropriate medical TH treatment may be considered while treating patients of HSV-1, HSV-2, and VZV. The results of the pilot study provided justification to the hypothetical link between anomalous TH level and reactivation of the αHHV in humans. It is noted that the number of patients possessed both TH and alpha-HHV diagnoses codes is tremendously low compared to the total number of patients in the database. It is likely due to the number of our confounding factors since a lot of cases were removed to avoid complication from other diseases. Consequently, more investigations from other databases are necessary and additional population- based prospective investigation is of importance to assess more accurate nature of the connection.

Acknowledgements

The editorial assistance from Dr. Robert Freeman is appreciated. We acknowledge the support from the Department of Pediatrics at the Chang Gung Memorial Hospital in Taiwan. SVH is further supported by NINDS/NIH R01NS081109.

References

1. Hsia SC, Shi YB (2002) Chromatin disruption and histone acetylation in regulation of the human immunodeficiency virus type 1 long terminal repeat by thyroid hormone receptor. Mol Cell Biol 22: 4043-4052.
2. Hsia SC, Bedadala GR, Balish MD (2011) Effects of thyroid hormone on HSV-1 gene regulation: implications in the control of viral latency and reactivation. Cell Biosci 1: 24.
3. Bedadala GR, Pinnoji RC, Palem JR, Hsia SC (2010) Thyroid hormone controls the gene expression of HSV-1 LAT and ICP0 in neuronal cells. Cell Res 20: 587-598.
4. Hsia SC, Pinnoji RC, Bedadala GR, Hill JM, Palem JR (2010) Regulation of herpes simplex virus type 1 thymidine kinase gene expression by thyroid hormone receptor in cultured neuronal cells. J Neurovirol 16: 13-24.
5. Taylor TJ, Brockman MA, McNamee EE, Knipe DM (2002) Herpes simplex virus. Front Biosci 7: d752-764.
6. Jiang LF, Gan L, Chen JX, Wang ML (2012) [The genotyping and molecular evolution of varicella-zoster virus]. Bing Du Xue Bao 28: 584-590.
7. Koshizuka T, Suzutani T (2012) [Anti alpha-herpesvirus drugs]. Nihon Rinsho 70: 558-563.
8. Kanai K, Yamada S, Inoue N (2010) [Varicella-zoster virus (VZV)]. Uirusu 60: 197-207.
9. Mori I, Nishiyama Y (2005) Herpes simplex virus and varicella-zoster virus: why do these human alphaherpesviruses behave so differently from one another? Rev Med Virol 15: 393-406.
10. Xu F, Sternberg MR, Kottiri BJ, McQuillan GM, Lee FK, et al. (2006) Trends in herpes simplex virus type 1 and type 2 seroprevalence in the United States. JAMA 296: 964-973.
11. Hill JM, Wen R, Halford WP (1998) Pathogenesis and Molecular Biology of HSV Latency and Ocular Reactivation in the Rabbit. Methods Mol Med 10: 291-315.
12. Martinez PA, Diaz R, Gonzalez D, Oropesa L, Gonzalez R, et al. (2007) The effect of highly active antiretroviral therapy on outcome of central nervous system herpesviruses infection in Cuban human immunodeficiency virus-infected individuals. J Neurovirol 13: 446-451.
13. Goel N, Mao H, Rong Q, Docherty JJ, Zimmerman D, et al. (2002) The ability of an HSV strain to initiate zosteriform spread correlates with its neuroinvasive disease potential. Arch Virol 147: 763-773.
14. Walter IB, Droz B (1995) Nuclear and cytoplasmic triiodothyronine-binding sites in primary sensory neurons and Schwann cells: radioautographic study during development. J Neuroendocrinol 7: 127-136.
15. Glauser L, Barakat Walter I (1997) Differential distribution of thyroid hormone receptor isoform in rat dorsal root ganglia and sciatic nerve in vivo and in vitro. J Neuroendocrinol 9: 217-227.
16. Walter IB (1996) Triiodothyronine exerts a trophic action on rat sensory neuron survival and neurite outgrowth through different pathways. Eur J Neurosci 8: 455-466.
17. Barakat-Walter I, Riederer BM (1996) Triiodothyronine and nerve growth factor are required to induce cytoplasmic dynein expression in rat dorsal root ganglion cultures. Brain Res Dev Brain Res 96: 109-119.
18. Hiroi Y, Kim HH, Ying H, Furuya F, Huang Z, et al. (2006) Rapid nongenomic actions of thyroid hormone. Proc Natl Acad Sci U S A 103: 14104-14109.
19. Doherty MJ, Baxter AB, Longstreth WT Jr (2001) Herpes simplex virus encephalitis complicating myxedema coma treated with corticosteroids. Neurology 56: 1114-1115.
20. Marquart M, Bhattacharjee P, Zheng X, Kaufman H, Thompson H, et al. (2003) Ocular reactivation phenotype of HSV-1 strain F(MP)E, a corticosteroid-sensitive strain. Curr Eye Res 26: 205-209.
21. Higaki S, Gebhardt BM, Lukiw WJ, Thompson HW, Hill JM (2002) Effect of immunosuppression on gene expression in the HSV-1 latently

infected mouse trigeminal ganglion. Invest Ophthalmol Vis Sci 43: 1862-1869.

22. Pueschel SM, Pezzullo JC (1985) Thyroid dysfunction in Down syndrome. Am J Dis Child 139: 636-639.
23. Cassio A, Ricci G, Baronio F, Miniaci A, Bal M, et al. (2010) Long-term clinical significance of thyroid autoimmunity in children with celiac disease. J Pediatr 156: 292-295.
24. Nicoletti A, Bal M, De Marco G, Baldazzi L, Agretti P, et al. (2009) Thyrotropin-stimulating hormone receptor gene analysis in pediatric patients with non-autoimmune subclinical hypothyroidism. J Clin Endocrinol Metab 94: 4187-4194.
25. Calaciura F, Motta RM, Miscio G, Fichera G, Leonardi D, et al. (2002) Subclinical hypothyroidism in early childhood: a frequent outcome of transient neonatal hyperthyrotropinemia. J Clin Endocrinol Metab 87: 3209-3214.
26. Cambiaso P, Orazi C, Digilio MC, Loche S, Capolino R, et al. (2007) Thyroid morphology and subclinical hypothyroidism in children and adolescents with Williams syndrome. J Pediatr 150: 62-65.

2

Heterogeneous Clinical Manifestations of Cushing's Syndrome in a Family with Primary Pigmented Nodular Adrenocortical Disease

Shih-Chen Tung[1*], **Daw-Yang Hwang**[2], **Joseph W. Yang**[3], **Hwee-Yeong Ng**[4] **and Chien-Te Lee**[4]

[1]*Division of Endocrinology and Metabolism, Department of Internal Medicine, Kaohsiung Chang Gung Memorial Hospital and Chang Gung University College of Medicine, Kaohsiung, Taiwan; 123 Ta-Pei Road, Niao-Sung District, Kaohsiung City 83301, Taiwan*

[2]*Division of Nephrology, Department of Internal Medicine, Kaohsiung Medical University Hospital and Kaohsiung Medical University, Kaohsiung, Taiwan; No.100, Tzyou 1st Road, Kaohsiung City 807, Taiwan*

[3]*Division of Urology, Department of Surgery, Kaohsiung Chang Gung Memorial Hospital and Chang Gung University College of Medicine, Kaohsiung, Taiwan; 123 Ta-Pei Road, Niao-Sung District, Kaohsiung City 83301, Taiwan*

[4]*Division of Nephrology, Department of Internal Medicine, Kaohsiung Chang Gung Memorial Hospital and Chang Gung University College of Medicine, Kaohsiung, Taiwan; 123 Ta-Pei Road, Niao-Sung District, Kaohsiung City 83301, Taiwan*

[*]**Corresponding author:** Shih-Chen Tung, Department of Internal Medicine, Kaohsiung Chang Gung Memorial Hospital and Chang Gung University College of Medicine, Kaohsiung, postal address: 123 Ta-Pei Road, Niao-Sung District, Kaohsiung City 83301, Taiwan, E-mail: tungqq44112@yahoo.com.tw

Abstract

Purpose: To evaluate the clinical manifestations of Cushing's Syndrome (CS) and associated genetic mutation in patients with Primary Pigmented Nodular Adrenocortical Disease (PPNAD).

Methods: Seven family members were screened for mutations of the PRKAR1A gene. Gene mutation screening used genomic DNA (from peripheral blood leukocytes and, in some cases, adrenal gland tissue) and subsequent DNA sequencing. The five patients showing genetic mutation were assessed clinically for baseline cortisol and adrenocorticotropic hormone and adrenal imaging studies (abdominal computed tomography and adrenal scintigraphy). Low-dose and high-low dexamethasone suppression tests were performed in these five patients.

Results: *PRKAR1A* gene mutation was detected in five of the seven family members. Four of the five gene mutation-positive patients presented with overt CS due to pathology-proven PPNAD. After unilateral adrenalectomy in these four patients, overt CS persisted for two patients and CS symptoms abated for the other two. The remission period of CS was >11 years in one instance (case III-2) and continues for >12 years in the other (case II-4), with no observable disease of the contralateral non-resected adrenal gland. For each of the two remission patients, one adrenal gland had been larger (by abdominal computed tomography) and had had stronger function (by 131I-6β-iodomethyl-19-norcholesterol scintigraphy) than the other. In one (case III-2) of the two remission patients, one adrenal displayed focal PPNAD while the other displayed diffuse PPNAD. The clinical manifestations of CS did not resolve after unilateral adrenalectomy in case II-2 and III-7. The fifth gene mutation-positive patient (case III-4) is still in the latent stage of CS.

Conclusions: The clinical manifestations of CS and adrenal image features in patients with PPNAD are heterogeneous. Detailed adrenal imaging of these patients is necessary to assist with the decision to perform unilateral adrenalectomy.

Keywords Cushing's syndrome; Primary pigmented nodular adrenocortical disease

Introduction

Primary Pigmented Nodular Adrenocortical Disease (PPNAD) is a rare cause of adrenal Cushing's Syndrome (CS). It occurs sporadically or as part of a familial syndrome called Carney Complex (CNC) [1]. PPNAD was observed in about 26-32% of CNC patients [2,3]. However, histological evidence of PPNAD was found in almost every patient with CNC who underwent an autopsy [2]. In the disease process of PPNAD, both adrenal glands are involved and feature small brown black nodules separated by atrophic adrenal cortex. The adrenal sizes associated with PPNAD range from small to slightly enlarged. The cut surfaces of the adrenal nodules vary in color from yellow-tan to gray, brown, and black [4]. Microscopically, the nodules consist of large cortical cells with lipofuscin pigment and internodular cortical atrophy [1,5].

We present the clinical manifestations of CS and the adrenal imaging and pathological features of family members with PPNAD and a common, single mutation of the PRKAR1A gene.

Subjects and Methods

Subjects

Seven members of a family were screened for mutation of the PRKAR1A gene. The five patients with the mutation were aged 24-45 years and included one female and four males. Four of the five patients presented with clinical features of CS and eventually had an adrenalectomy.

Methods

Plasma and urine cortisol levels were measured by commercial radioimmunoassay kits. Plasma Adrenocorticotropic Hormone (ACTH) levels were measured by immunoradiometric assay. Low-dose and high-dose dexamethasone suppression tests were performed in these five gene mutation patients. Adrenal imaging studies included abdominal Computed Tomography (CT) and adrenal scintigraphy.

Genomic DNA was extracted from peripheral blood leukocytes from each of the seven family members using the QIAamp DNA Blood Mini Kit (Qiagen GmbH, Hilden, Germany) and from paraffin-embedded adrenal gland tissue available for four of the seven family members using the QuickExtract FFPE DNA Extraction Kit (Epicentre Biotechnologies, Madison, WI) according to the manufacturer's protocol.

All 10 exons of the PRKAR1A gene and their intron-exon boundaries were amplified by polymerase chain reaction (PCR) using primers described previously [6]. Semi-nested PCR analysis of exon 2 in the DNA obtained from the paraffin-embedded adrenal tissue was performed using the reverse primer 5′-CAACCTCTCAAAGTATTCCCTGA-3′ for the second PCR cycle. PCR products were separated by electrophoresis on a 1.5% agarose gel and sequenced by ABI 3730 XL DNA Analyzer (Applied Biosystems, Foster City, CA). The study protocol was approved by the institutional review board, and informed consent was obtained from each of the seven family members.

Results

Family member studies Case II-2 (index patient)

The detailed history of this index patient was reported by Tung et al., 2005 [7]. Briefly, a 41-year-old man (Figure 1), born in November 1949, came to our outpatient department in October 1990 with cushingoid appearance. The patient's father also had cushingoid features, but due to his death, his clinical characteristics were not analyzed as part of this study. Endocrine studies of this index patient revealed adrenal CS (Table 1). A paradoxical rise of 24-h urinary free cortisol (UFC) to 2-day high-dose dexamethasone suppression test (HDDST, 2 mg dexamethasone every 6 hours orally for a total of 8 doses) was observed (Table 1). Adrenal scintigraphy with 131I-6β-iodomethyl-19-norcholesterol (NP-59) showed uptake in both adrenal glands on the seventh day after NP-59 injection. Abdominal Magnetic Resonance Imaging (MRI) in July 1991 showed a tiny nodule at the lateral limb of the right adrenal gland [7]. A right total adrenalectomy was performed on October 4, 1991, and diffuse PPNAD was confirmed pathologically [7]. Two weeks after right adrenalectomy, a repeated 2-day Low-Dose Dexamethasone Suppression Test (LDDST, 0.5 mg dexamethasone every 6 hours orally for a total of 8 doses) and 2-day HDDST still could not suppress plasma cortisol or 24-h UFC levels. A repeated CT of the abdomen on October 22, 1991 revealed a left adrenal nodule, 2.0 cm in diameter, which was missed during the reading of a previous abdominal CT because of its unusual location in the left renal hilar region [7]. A left total adrenalectomy was performed in December 1991, and diffuse PPNAD was proved microscopically. Features of CS then resolved gradually.

A left thyroid nodule was palpated in February 2002. Ultrasonography of the thyroid demonstrated two hypoechoic nodules in the left lobe and three in the right lobe [7]. Bilateral total thyroidectomies and excision of left lateral neck lymph nodes were performed in March 2002. Papillary Thyroid Carcinomas (PTC) with metastases to multiple lymph nodes were confirmed pathologically [7]. Analysis of this patient's genomic DNA obtained from peripheral blood leukocytes and paraffin-embedded left adrenal tissue both showed a c.46C>T nucleotide mutation (p.R16X nonsense amino acid mutation) in the PRKAR1A gene.

Case III-1

This woman aged 26 years and 7 months (the eldest daughter of the index patient; born in September 1974) (Figure 1) came to our outpatient department in April 2001 for screening of CS because her father had PPNAD. She was previously diagnosed with PTC based on pathology and underwent bilateral total thyroidectomy at another hospital in August 2000. Her height was 153 cm; weight, 71 kg; and blood pressure, 120/80 mm Hg. Cushingoid features were not present, except for abdominal obesity. Plasma cortisol level was suppressed to 0.56 μg/dL with overnight LDDST (1 mg dexamethasone orally at 2300 h). Analysis of this patient's genomic DNA obtained from peripheral blood leukocytes did not show mutation of the PRKAR1A gene.

Case III-2

The detailed history of this patient was reported by Tung et al., 2012 [8]. Briefly, a 24-year-old woman (the second daughter of the index patient; born in November 1975) (Figure 1) was admitted in May 2000 due to cushingoid appearance for about 6 months and weight gain of 10 kg over the preceding 9 months. Endocrine studies revealed adrenal CS. Paradoxical increase of 24-h UFC to 2-day HDDST was found (Table 1). Abdominal CT revealed a left adrenal nodule (3 x 2 cm diameter) [8] and a normal-sized right adrenal gland. Adrenal scintigraphy using NP-59 showed tracer uptake in the left adrenal gland and non-visualization of the right adrenal gland throughout the examination course. A retroperitoneoscopic left total adrenalectomy was performed in July 2000. The cut surface of the left adrenal nodule was yellow-tan without obvious black pigmentation. Microscopically, non-pigmented adrenocortical adenoma was the major portion and focal PPNAD was the minor portion of this left adrenocortical nodule [8]. The cushingoid features of the patient gradually disappeared thereafter. A very low baseline morning plasma cortisol level (0.97 μg/dL at 0800 h) was measured 1.5 months after left adrenalectomy. Six months later, the baseline plasma cortisol and ACTH levels at 0800 h were normal (8.7 μg/dL and 38.8 pg/mL, respectively). Apparent cushingoid features still had not returned 122 months later, despite non-suppression of the plasma cortisol level (7.12 μg/dL) by overnight LDDST.

In May 2011, the patient was re-admitted because of a 13 kg weight gain during the preceding 6 months. A paradoxical rise of 24-h UFC during the 2-day HDDST was observed [8]. Both abdominal CT and MRI showed a normal-sized right adrenal gland. Subtotal right adrenalectomy (about 80% of the right adrenal gland resected) via the traditional thoracoabdominal approach was performed on May 25, 2011. The cut surface of the right adrenal gland was grossly observed to be brown-black. Diffuse PPNAD was confirmed microscopically [8]. Analysis of this patient's genomic DNA obtained from peripheral blood leukocytes and bilateral adrenal tissues both showed a c.46C>T mutation (p.R16X) in the PRKAR1A gene [8].

Case III-3

This 23-year-old woman (the third daughter of the index patient; born in March 1978) (Figure 1) came to our outpatient department in December 2000 for screening of CS. Her height was 156 cm; weight, 45 kg; and blood pressure, 90/60 mm Hg. Cushingoid features were not found during physical examination. Plasma cortisol level was suppressed to 0.90 μg/dL by overnight LDDST. Analysis of genomic DNA obtained from peripheral blood leukocytes demonstrated no mutation of the PRKAR1A gene.

Case III-4

This man aged 21 years and 5 months (the fourth child of the index patient; born in November 1979) (Figure 1) came to our outpatient department in April 2001 for screening of CS because of his father's PPNAD. His height was 169 cm; weight, 60 kg; and blood pressure, 120/80 mm Hg. Cushingoid features were not observed during physical examination. Baseline plasma cortisol and ACTH levels at 0800 h were 5.32 μg/dL and 42.1 pg/mL, respectively. Plasma cortisol was suppressed to 3.23 μg/dL and 4.57 μg/dL (Table 1) by overnight LDDST in April 2001 and December 2006, respectively. Image studies and adrenalectomy were not performed because of the absence of clinical manifestations of CS. However, analysis of this patient's genomic DNA obtained from peripheral blood leukocytes identified a c.46C>T mutation (p.R16X) in the PRKAR1A gene.

Tests	Case II-2	Case II-4	Case III-2	Case III-7	Case III-4
Baseline plasma cortisol level (μg/dL)					
0800 h (normal range, 9-23)	37.9	26.1	17.5	17.3	5.32
1600-2200 h (normal range, 3-13)	33.8	20.4		14.1	
Baseline 24-h urinary free cortisol level (μg/24-h) (normal range, 34-122)	1008	786	952		
Baseline plasma ACTH level (pg/mL)	5.10	8.29	2.05	14.6	42.1
0800 h (normal range, 9-52)					
Overnight low-dose dexamethasone suppression test*					
Plasma cortisol level at 0800 h	32.3	24.3	20.9	13.8	4.57
Two-day low-dose dexamethasone suppression test**					
Plasma cortisol level at 0800 h	36.9	20.1	17.3		
24-h urinary free cortisol level	1162	762	1066		
Overnight high-dose dexamethasone suppression test					
Plasma cortisol level at 0800 h				18.3	
Two-day high-dose dexamethasone suppression test					
Plasma cortisol level at 0800 h	33.7	20.0	22.9		
24-h urinary free cortisol level	1470	676	1489		

Table 1: Endocrinological studies (before adrenalectomy) in the five patients with primary pigmented nodular adrenocortical disease. *Overnight low-dose dexamethasone suppression test: 1 mg dexamethasone orally at 2300 h and blood sampling for cortisol level the following morning at 0800 h. ** Two-day low-dose dexamethasone suppression test: 0.5 mg dexamethasone orally every 6 h for 2 days and blood sampling for cortisol level at 0800 h on the third day of testing. Collecting 24-h urine for free cortisol level from 0800 h on the second day to 0800 h on the third day after dexamethasone administration. §Overnight high-dose dexamethasone suppression test: 8 mg dexamethasone orally at 2300 h and blood sampling for cortisol level the following morning at 0800 h. §§Two-day high-dose dexamethasone suppression test: 2 mg dexamethasone orally every 6 h for 2 days and blood sampling for cortisol level at 0800 h on the third day of testing. Collecting 24-h urine for free cortisol level from 0800 h on the second day to 0800 h on the third day after dexamethasone administration.

Case II-4

The detailed history of this patient was reported by Tung et al., 2009 [9].Briefly, in October 2001, a 45-year-old man (the younger brother of the index patient; born in June 1956) (Figure 1) presented to our clinic with a cushingoid appearance. His height was 157 cm; weight, 64 kg; and blood pressure, 146/94 mm Hg. The results of endocrine studies revealed adrenal CS (Table 1). An adrenal scintigraphy using NP-59 showed uptake of the tracer in the left adrenal on the second day and in the right adrenal gland on the fourth day after NP-59 injection [9]. CT of the abdomen revealed a nodule (2 cm diameter) on the left adrenal and a normal-appearing right adrenal gland [9]. A laparoscopic left adrenalectomy was performed in November 2001. The cut surface of the excised left adrenal nodule showed multiple small black nodules. Diffuse PPNAD was confirmed microscopically [9].

In December 2001, baseline plasma cortisol levels still demonstrated a loss of normal circadian rhythm. An overnight LDDST failed to suppress plasma cortisol (14.0 μg/dL). In January 2002, a repeated CT of the abdomen revealed a residual nodule (1.5 cm diameter) on the left adrenal gland. Thus, a left total adrenalectomy

Sixty-nine months after the second procedure, cushingoid appearance of the patient was still absent, although his overnight LDDST revealed a non-suppressible plasma cortisol concentration (12.7 μg/dL). The patient reports via a telephone conversation that the remission of cushingoid features continues 12 years after the second procedure. Analysis of genomic DNA obtained from peripheral blood leukocytes and the paraffin-embedded left adrenal tissues both identified a c.46C>T mutation (p.R16X) in the PRKAR1A gene.

Case III-7

A 25-year-old man (the third son of case II-4; born in July 1981) (Figure 1) came to our outpatient department in August 2006 due to a moon-faced appearance for 1year and weight gain of 5-6 kg in the preceding 1.5 years. As noted above, his father had PPNAD. His height was 157 cm; weight, 58 kg; and blood pressure, 128/72 mm Hg. Physical examination revealed moon face with an excess of acne, buffalo hump, and abdominal obesity. An absence of normal circadian plasma cortisol fluctuations was observed (baseline plasma cortisol levels of 17.3 μg/dL at 0800 h and 14.1 μg/dL at 1600 h) (Table 1). Baseline plasma ACTH level was 14.6 pg/mL. In September 2006, an adrenal scintigraphy using NP-59 showed bilateral adrenal uptake of the tracer on the fifth day after NP-59 injection. Abdominal CT did not find any adrenal nodule in September 2006, August 2007, or April 2010. Left total adrenalectomy via a left flank approach was performed in June 2010. Diffuse PPNAD was proved microscopically. The patient refused right adrenalectomy despite persistent manifestations of CS after left total adrenalectomy. Analysis of this patient's genomic DNA from peripheral blood leukocytes identified a c.46C>T mutation (p.R16X) in the PRKAR1A gene.

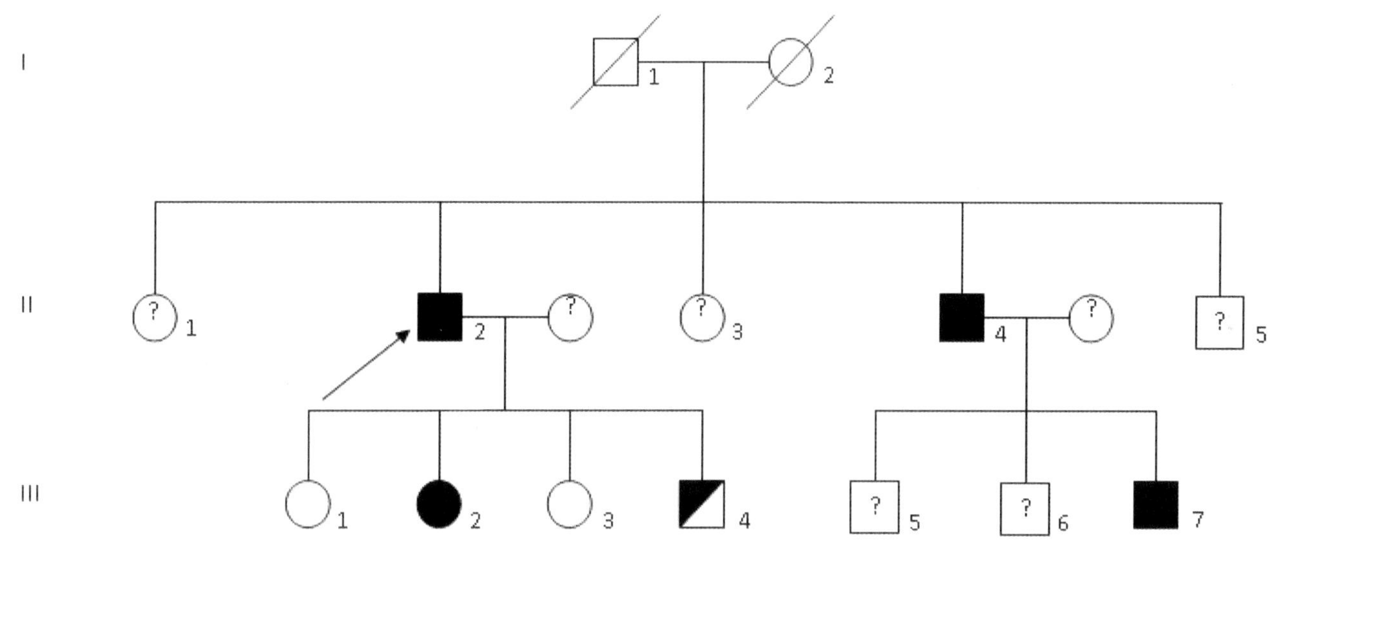

Figure 1: Pedigree of the family. The arrow identifies the index patient (II-2). Squares denote male family members, circles female family members, and a diagonal line a deceased member. Primary pigmented nodular adrenocortical disease with mutation of regulatory subunit R1A of protein kinase A gene and overt Cushing's syndrome. Carrier of gene mutation of regulatory subunit R1A of protein kinase A gene in latent stage of Cushing's syndrome. Unknown for Cushing's syndrome or gene mutation. ? No Cushing's syndrome and no gene mutation

Discussion

Since the first description in 1985 of "the complex of myxomas, spotty pigmentation, and endocrine overactivity" [10], now known as "Carney complex", more than 500 CNC patients have been reported from all ethnicities, and the majority of them (almost 70%) presented with a positive family history [11,12]. CNC is an autosomal dominant disorder featuring skin lesions, cardiac and other myxomas, and different types of endocrine tumors including PPNAD, growth hormone-secreting pituitary tumors, gonadal and thyroid neoplasms, and rarely, benign and malignant psammomatous melanotic schwannomas [13]. The most frequent endocrine manifestation of CNC is PPNAD [14]. There seems to be a bimodal age distribution of PPNAD among CNC patients, a minority present during the first 2-3 years, whereas the majority manifest in the second and third decade of life [2]. Our patients in case II-2, II-4, III-2, and III-7, with PPNAD and mutation of the *PRKAR1A* gene, meet the diagnostic criteria of CNC set by Stratakis et al. [2]. The case III-4 patient has a biological father afflicted with CNC and is a case of PPNAD in the latent phase of CS with mutation of the *PRKAR1A* gene. Therefore, the case III-4 patient is also classified as having CNC.

The clinical manifestations of CS in patients with PPNAD can be divided into three stages: (a) overt (CS present clinically and biochemically), (b) subclinical (no clinical features of CS, but detectable adrenocortical hyperfunction or autonomy or both), or (c) latent (no clinical or laboratory evidence of CS, but the genetic trait is present) [9]. Our index patient (case II-2) still presented overt CS after unilateral total adrenalectomy (Table 2). In case III-2, the patient progressed through all three stages of CS (latent, subclinical, and overt) after unilateral (left) total adrenalectomy, and this progression from latent to overt CS occurred over a period of >11 years in the right PPNAD [8]. For case III-4, the patient remains in the latent CS stage despite carrying the PRKAR1A gene mutation common to his afflicted family members. In case II-4, the first two stages of CS (latent and subclinical) are observed and the remission period of CS persists for >12 years after unilateral total adrenalectomy (Table 2). In case III-7, overt CS persists after unilateral total adrenalectomy (Table 2). Thus, all the five family members with PPNAD displayed various clinical manifestations of CS even though they each had the same mutation (c. 46C>T) in the PRKAR1A gene.

Establishing the diagnosis of PPNAD can be challenging, particularly when PPNAD is the only manifestation of the disease and there are no other afflicted family members. In addition, patients with the disease not only may present atypical forms of CS, such as cyclical or episodic CS, but they may also have normal radiologic imaging or show only subtle nodularity [15,16]. Beyond 18 years of age, a unilateral 2-3 cm diameter adrenal macronodule is common in PPNAD (as in our case II-2, II-4, and III-2) [5,17]. This can make it difficult to distinguish CS due to PPNAD from ACTH-independent unilateral adrenocortical adenoma based on radiological criteria only [9]. A paradoxical increase in 24-h UFC during the Liddle test can be used to identify PPNAD and distinguish it from other causes of adrenal CS [18,19].

The hypercortisolism due to PPNAD resolves after bilateral adrenalectomy [5,15]; however, lifelong glucocorticoid replacement is required after this form of surgery. Mortality and morbidity because of adrenal insufficiency after bilateral total adrenalectomy were reported in patients with PPNAD [20-22]. Carney and Young reported that 6 out of 17 PPNAD patients that underwent unilateral adrenalectomy exhibited remission of their clinical features of CS [15]. Seven other patients had persistence of CS, two died postoperatively, and two were lost to follow-up. These authors also speculate that less than total adrenalectomy may have a place in some selected PPNAD patients who are asymptomatic or only minimally symptomatic [15]. We previously reported a case of PPNAD with remission of CS after unilateral adrenalectomy in 2009 (case II-4) [9]. Here we present additional objective data. For example, from case III-2 and II-4 (Table 2), the observation of larger size (by abdominal CT) and increased function (by adrenal scintigraphy) of the affected left adrenal gland compared to the right may assist in the decision to perform unilateral adrenalectomy as a choice for PPNAD patients to avoid lifelong glucocorticoid replacement therapy. Such a management approach for patients with PPNAD represents a form of patient-centered care.

Case No.	Sex	Age (yr) at first surgery	Manifestations of Cushing's syndrome (CS)	Computed tomography findings	Adrenal scintigraphy*	Adrenalectomy	Pathological findings of adrenal glands	Features of Carney complex	Gene mutation
II-2	Male	42	Overt CS No remission of CS after right total adrenalectomy	Right tiny adrenal nodule, left adrenal nodule (2 cm)	Bilateral adrenal uptake	Bilateral total adrenalectomy	Bilateral diffuse PPNAD	PPNAD, bilateral papillary thyroid carcinoma	PRKAR1A? (c.46 C>T)
III-2	Female	24	Three stages of CS‡ on different dates Remission of CS for >11 years after left total adrenalectomy	Left adrenal nodule (3 x 2 cm), normal-sized right adrenal gland	Left adrenal uptake	Left total adrenalectomy, right subtotal adrenalectomy (80%)	Left focal PPNAD, right diffuse PPNAD	PPNAD, bilateral thyroid cysts	PRKAR1A? (c.46 C>T)
III-4	Male	32§	Latent CS	Not done	Not done	No	Unknown	No screened	PRKAR1A? (c.46 C>T)
II-4	Male	45	Overt CS Persistent remission of CS for >12 years after left total adrenalectomy	Left· adrenal nodule (2 cm), normal-sized right adrenal gland	Earlier uptake of left adrenal than right	Left total adrenalectomy	Left diffuse PPNAD	PPNAD, bilateral thyroid cysts	PRKAR1A? (c.46 C>T)
III-7	Male	29	Overt CS No remission of CS after left total adrenalectomy	Normal-sized bilateral adrenal glands	Bilateral adrenal uptake	Left total adrenalectomy	Left diffuse PPNAD	PPNAD	PRKAR1A? (c.46 C>T)

Table 2: Clinical characteristics in a family with primary pigmented nodular adrenocortical disease (PPNAD). *Adrenal scintigraphy: 131I-6-iodomethyl-19-norcholesterol adrenal scintigraphy. ?PRKAR1A: regulatory subunit R1A of protein kinase A. ‡Three stages of CS: overt, subclinical, and latent Cushing's syndrome. 32: The patient was 32 years old when the gene study was performed in October 2011.

Conclusions

The clinical manifestations of CS and imaging features in our intra-familial PPNAD patients are heterogeneous. The three stages of CS (overt, subclinical, and latent) should be kept in mind in the management of PPNAD. Detailed adrenal imaging of PPNAD patients is necessary to assist with the decision to perform unilateral adrenalectomy.

References

1. Young WF, Carney JA, Musa BU, Wulffraat NM, Lens JW, et al. (1989) Familial Cushing's syndrome due to primary pigmented nodular adrenocortical disease: reinvestigation 50 years later. N Engl J Med 321:1659-1664.
2. Stratakis CA, Kirschner LS, Carney JA (2001) Clinical and molecular features of the Carney complex: diagnostic criteria and recommendations for patient evaluation. J Clin Endocrinol Metab 86: 4041-4046.
3. Stratakis CA, Carney JA, Lin JP, Papanicolaou DA, Karl M, et al. (1996) Carney complex, a familial multiple neoplasia and lentiginosis syndrome. Analysis of 11 kindreds and linkage to the short arm of chromosome 2. J Clin Invest 97: 699-705.
4. Travis WD, Tsokos M, Doppman JL, Nieman L, Chrousos GP, et al. (1989) Primary pigmented nodular adrenocortical disease: a light and electron microscopic study of eight cases. Am J Surg Pathol 13: 921-930.
5. Sarlis NJ, Chrousos GP, Doppman JL, Carney JA, Stratakis CA (1996) Primary pigmented nodular adrenocortical disease: reevaluation of a patient with Carney complex 27 years after unilateral adrenalectomy. J Clin Endocrinol Metab 82: 1274-1278.
6. Kirschner LS, Sandrini F, Monbo J, Lin JP, Carney JA, et al. (2000) Genetic heterogeneity and spectrum of mutations of the PRKAR1A gene in patients with the carney complex. Hum Mol Genet 9: 3037-3046.
7. Tung SC, Wang PW, Huang TL, Yang JW, Chen WJ (2005) Carney complex with primary pigmented nodular adrenocortical disease and bilateral papillary thyroid carcinoma occurring 11 years apart: a case report. Endocrinologist 4: 243-247.
8. Tung SC, Hwang DY, Yang JW, Chen WJ, Lee CT (2012) An unusual presentation of Carney complex with diffuse primary pigmented nodular adrenocortical disease on one adrenal gland and a nonpigmented adrenocortical adenoma and focal primary pigmented nodular adrenocortical disease on the other. Endocr J 59: 823-830.
9. Tung SC, Wang PW, Lee WC (2009) Remission of Cushing's syndrome in a patient with primary pigmented nodular adrenocortical disease with unilateral adrenalectomy: a case study. Endocrinologist 19: 75-78.
10. Carney JA, Gordon H, Carpenter PC, Shenoy BV, Go VL (1985) The complex of myxomas, spotty pigmentation, and endocrine overactivity. (Baltimore) 64: 270-283.
11. Bertherat J, Horvath A, Groussin L, Grabar S, Boikos S, et al. (2009) Mutations in regulatory subunit type 1A of cyclic adenosine 5-monophosphate-dependent protein kinase (PRKAR1A): phenotype analysis in 353 patients and 80 different genotypes. J Clin Endocrinol Metab 94: 2085-2091.
12. Courcoutsakis NA, Tatsi C, Patronas NJ, Lee CC, Prassopoulos PK, et al. (2013) The complex of myxomas, spotty skin pigmentation and endocrine overactivity (Carney complex): imaging findings with clinical and pathological correlation. Insights Imaging 4: 119-133.
13. Horvath A, Bertherat J, Groussin L, Guillaud-Bataille M, Tsang K, et al. (2010) Mutations and polymorphisms in the gene encoding regulatory subunit type 1-alpha of protein kinase A (PRKAR1A): an update. Hum Mutat 31: 369-379.
14. Pereira AM, Hes FJ, Horvath A, Woortman S, Greene E, et al. (2010) Association of the M1V PRKAR1A mutation with primary pigmented nodular adrenocortical disease in two large families. J Clin Endocrinol Metab 95: 338-342.
15. Carney JA, Young WF (1992) Primary pigmented nodular adrenocortical disease and its associated conditions. Endocrinologist 2:6-21.
16. Groussin L, Horvath A, Jullian E, Boikos S, Rene-Corail F, et al. (2006) A PRKAR1A mutation associated with primary pigmented nodular adrenocortical disease in 12 kindreds. J Clin Endocrinol Metab 91: 1943-1949.
17. Doppman JL, Travis WD, Nieman L, Miller DL, Chrousos GP, et al. (1989) Cushing syndrome due to primary pigmented nodular adrenocortical disease: findings at CT and MR imaging. Radiology 172: 415-420.
18. Stratakis CA, Sarlis N, Kirschner LS, Carney JA, Doppman JL, et al. (1999) Paradoxical response to dexamethasone in the diagnosis of primary pigmented nodular adrenocortical disease. Ann Intern Med 131: 585-591.
19. Bourdeau I, Lacroix A, Schürch W, Caron P, Antakly T, et al. (2003) Primary pigmented nodular adrenocortical disease: paradoxical responses of cortisol secretion to dexamethasone occur in vitro and are associated with increased expression of the glucocorticoid receptor. J Clin Endocrinol Metab 88: 3931-3937.
20. Imai T, Funahashi H, Tanaka Y, Tobinaga J, Wada M, et al. (1996) Adrenalectomy for treatment of Cushing syndrome: results in 122 patients and long-term follow-up studies. World J Surg 20: 781-786.
21. Shenoy BV, Carpenter PC, Carney JA (1984) Bilateral primary pigmented nodular adrenocortical disease. Rare cause of the Cushing syndrome. Am J Surg Pathol 8: 335-344.
22. Grant CS, Carney JA, Carpenter PC, van Heerden JA (1986) Primary pigmented nodular adrenocortical disease: diagnosis and management. Surgery 100: 1178-1184.

3

Clomiphene Stimulation Test in Men Abusing Anabolic-Androgenic Steroids for Long Time

Medras M[1,2], Jozkow P[2*], Terpilowski L[3] and Zagocka E[4]

[1]*Department of Endocrinology, Diabetology and Isotope Treatment, Wroclaw Medical University, ul. Pasteura 4, 50-367 Wroclaw, Poland*

[2]*Department of Sports Medicine, University School of Physical Education, ul, Paderewskiego 35, 51-612 Wroclaw, Poland*

[3]*Department of Emergency Medical Services, Wroclaw Medical University, ul. Pasteura 4, 50-367 Wroclaw, Poland*

[4]*Laboratory of Male Infertility, ul. Kosciuszki 108A/18, 50-441 Wroclaw, Poland*

[*]**Corresponding author:** Pawel Jozkow, Department of Sports Medicine, University School of Physical Education, ul. Paderewskiego 35, 51-612 Wroclaw, Poland, E-mail: jozkow@gmail.com

Abstract

Objective: Androgenic-anabolic steroids (AAS) are commonly used by athletes and recreational athletes. In some cases they induce persistent anabolic steroid-induced hypogonadism (ASIH).

Design: In an observational study we assessed the function of the pituitary-gonadal axis in a series of men with suspected ASIH.

Methods: Clomiphene stimulation test (CST) was performed in 13 hypogonadal adult men with previous, prolonged exposure to AAS. We evaluated the response of luteinizing hormone (LH), follicle-stimulating hormone (FSH) and total testosterone (T) to 50 mg of clomiphene daily administered for a week.

Results: Mean concentrations of hormones before and after clomiphene administration were respectively (mean ± SD): 3 ± 1.2 and 8.3 ± 2 mIU/ml for LH; 3 ± 1.1 and 10 ± 14.6 mIU/ml for FSH; and 2.3 ± 0.6 and 7.2 ± 1.7 ng/ml for T ($p<0.001$).

Conclusions: Men with ASIH, after a long-time withdrawal of AAS, present an intact reaction of gonadotropins and testosterone to clomiphene stimulation.

Keywords: Anabolic agents; Hypogonadism; Clomiphene; Diagnostic tests; Gonadotropins; Testosterone

Introduction

Illicit use of AAS is widespread in many parts of the world. Recent surveys show that 2.4% of Australian students report lifetime AAS use [1], while in Sweden between 10 000 and 100 000 subjects may be exposed to AAS every year [2]. In Poland 6.2% of young males and 2.9% of young females admit that they use anabolic agents. Data from other countries and continents suggest that AAS users can be counted in millions [3-5]. The situation is emerging as a public health concern [6].

Side effects of AAS are common and involve diverse body organs and systems [7-9]. One of the most prominent AAS effects is suppression of the hypothalamo-pituitary-gonadal (HPG) axis leading to decreased production of testosterone and spermatozoa. Although the gonadal function usually recovers after withdrawal of AAS, in a growing number of cases there is observed a secondary, functional, often hypogonadotropic, anabolic steroid-induced hypogonadism (ASIH) [10]. Low concentration of testosterone may persist even after several months-long cessations of AAS.

Hypogonadism understood as testosterone deficiency is associated with a broad range of somatic, sexual and psychological symptoms [10-12]. Acquired, hypogonadotropic hypogonadism (AHH) is a consequence of anatomical and functional alterations of the hypothalamus and/or the pituitary. It is found in tumors, infiltrative and vascular disorders of the sellar region. It may be also observed after brain injury, neurosurgery, in the course of anemia, uremia, alcoholism or as a side effect of gonadotropin suppression during endocrinological, psychiatric or urological treatments [13,14]. Data on clinical aspects of ASIH is scarce.

Our aim was to assess the HPG axis with use of the clomiphene stimulation test in adult men with a history of long-term exposure to AAS.

Subjects and Methods

The study had an observational character. It was performed in thirteen adult men (aged 25 ± 4), former AAS users, who were referred to an andrological outpatient clinic because of low testosterone concentration. Studied subjects were informed on the aim of the investigation and the diagnostic procedure to which a written consent was given.

Each athlete had a medical interview with a full andrological check-up. None of the studied cases presented disturbances of sexual differentiation and maturity or physical symptoms of hypogonadism. They did not suffer from any chronic medical conditions and did not receive medications for at least 3 months prior the investigation.

All of the investigated men had total testosterone (T) concentration ≤3.2 ng/ml. Their clinical status was good (normal: body mass index, blood pressure, testicular volume). Four of the studied men fathered children before starting AAS, one – during AAS use.

Our cases derived from the same sport environment and received AAS in a similar manner (3-4 cycles of several weeks duration eg. Deca Durabolin 4000 mg, Omnadren 7000 mg, Metanabol 1200 mg and/or Oxandrolone 5000 mg during a year). They used AAS for 3.9 ± 1.6 years. The drug-free interval before the investigation was 2.1 ± 1.0 years.

Laboratory evaluation consisted of fasting measurements of: luteinizing hormone (LH), follicle-stimulating hormone (FSH), total testosterone (T), estradiol (E2), sex-horrmone binding globulin (SHBG), prolactin (PRL), sperm count assessed after 7-days sexual abstinence. In 7 cases magnetic resonance imaging of the pituitary was performed showing intact anatomy of the sellar region.

After confirmation of hypogonadism a week-long test with 50 mg clomiphene citrate/day, (clomiphene stimulation test, CST) was performed [15,16]. We compared basal and stimulated concentrations of LH, FSH and T.

Blood samples were obtained from the ulnar vein between 7.00 and 9.00 AM. Serum was stored at – 20°C until being used in the certified laboratory. Radioimmunoassay kits were used for measurements of T and E2 (Diagnostic Products Corporation, USA). The intra- and interassay coefficients of variation (CV) were 5.5 % and 5.9% for T and 5.8% and 7.4% for E2. SHBG, FSH and LH were measured using immunoradiometric assay-IRMA kits (Immunotech, Czech Republic). The intra- and interassay CV were 3.8 and 7.0% for SHBG; 5.0% and 3.8% for FSH; 6.7% and 3.7% for LH.

The statistical analysis was performed using the PQ Stat version 1.4.4.126. Concentrations of hormones in the CST test were assessed with the Wilcoxon signed-rank test. Associations among: age, duration of AAS use, duration from AAS withdrawal and results of the CST test were evaluated with U Mann-Whitney test and Spearman's rank correlation coefficient (fold changes of hormones' concentrations). A p-value less than 0.05 were considered significant.

Results

The raw results of the clomiphene stimulation test in the investigated men are presented in table (Table 1).

S.No	Age (years)	Length of AAS use (years)	Length of AAS withdrawal (years)	LH (mIU/ml)	FSH (mIU/ml)	T (nmol/l)
1	22	3	1.5	1.9 8.1	2.7 6.52	2.43 7.3
2	31	5	3	2.8 6.7	3.46 58	2.5 6.92
3	19	3.5	1	1.1 9.9	4.1 6.2	1.37 7.12
4	24	4	2.2	3.72 9.6	3.5 7.46	2.91 7.61
5	22	5	1.2	4.1 9.5	3.53 8.2	3.01 9.9
6	28	7	4	4.48 7.58	3.15 4.2	2.33 7.13
7	27	6	2	1.6 9.1	2.7 7.5	3.2 8.7
8	30	4	3.2	2.2 3.7	1.9 3.0	2.3 10.0
9	32	4.4	2.2	2.1 11.8	0.9 3.2	1.64 6.1
10	29	3.0	1.5	2.68 8.7	1.8 4.1	1.61 6.56
11	25	1.9	1.3	3.2 6.7	2.1 3.3	1.83 3.61
12	21	2	3	4.45 8.8	3.97 7.78	2.2 5.61
13	27	2	1	4.46 7.66	4.73 9.49	2.18 6.74

Table 1: Raw results of the clomiphene stimulation test in the studied subjects. Hormone concentrations before and after (lines below) administration of clomiphene.

Mean concentrations of LH, FSH and T before and after clomiphene administration were respectively (mean±SD): 3 ± 1.2 and 8.3 ± 2 mIU/ml; 3 ± 1.1 and 10 ± 14.6 mIU/ml; 2.3 ± 0.6 and 7.2 ± 1.7 ng/ml ($p<0.001$) (Table 2).

	Descriptive statistics							Wilcoxon signed-rank test P
	Mean	SD	Min	Lower Quartile	Median	Upper Quartile	Max	
LH(mIU/ml)	2.98 8.30	1.17 1.96	1.10 3.70	2.10 7.58	2.80 8.70	4.10 9.50	4.48 11.80	0.0015
FSH(mlU/ml)	2.96 9.92	1.08 14.61	0.90 3.00	2.10 4.10	3.15 6.52	3.53 7.78	4.73 58.00	0.0015
T(ng/ml)	2.27 7.18	0.56 1.71	1.37 3.61	1.83 6.56	2.30 7.12	2.50 7.61	3.20 10.00	0.0015

Table 2: Changes of hormones concentrations in the clomiphene stimulation test. Hormone concentrations before and after clomiphene citrate (lines below).

Neither age of athletes, length of AAS use or length of AAS withdrawal influenced the CST outcomes in our study (Table 3).

	Age (years)	Duration of AAS use(years)	Duration of AAS withdrawal (years)
LH	-0.1735	0.1215	-0.3950
FSH	0.3691	0.2928	0.0083
T	0.2121	0.1768	-0.1878

Table 3: Spearman's rank correlation coefficient between: age of subjects, duration of AAS use and duration of withdrawal and changes of concentration of LH, FSH and T.

Discussion

There is little data on persistent pituitary dysfunction after AAS exposure. Laboratory findings in ASIH usually comprise low/normal levels of gonadotropins and low testosterone. Subjective symptoms do not appear until sometime after the onset of the disorder. Disruption of spermatogenesis may lead to infertility with structural and genetic sperm damage [17,18].

ASIH tends to be temporal. In most cases the androgenic milieu restores within a year after cessation of AAS, however in a number of male athletes low testosterone and sperm production disturbances may persist [19].

ASIH that arises a long time after AAS withdrawal is a poorly recognized condition. The occurrence of ASIH in AAS users is unknown and mechanism leading to hypogonadism and sperm count disturbances remains unexplained. To our knowledge associations between this specific forms of ASIH (eg. duration of AAS abuse, type of AAS used) and alterations of the sperm count have not been addressed in the literature. There is no information on its reversibility as well.

In our experience AAS-induced secondary hypogonadism emerges as an important form of the central nervous system dysfunction. The classical pathways of AAS effects in the brain comprise androgen and estrogen receptors (α, β) which are present in highest concentrations in basal telencephalon and diencephalon. Several enzymes play an important role here: 5α-reductase, aromatase, 3α-HSD, 3β-HSD, and 17β-HSD. AAS are thought to induce transcription and synthesis of new proteins. They may permanently modify activity of sex steroids receptors [20]. Apart from genomic effects, AAS modulate kinase activity, ion channels, and G-protein second-messenger systems. Some of these actions are much quicker than those induced through transcription factors [20]. Testosterone derivatives may act as partial opioid agonists. They may increase beta-endorphin levels in the ventral tegmental area and the thalamus, decrease levels of kappa receptors in the nucleus accumbens and increase: mu, delta and kappa receptor binding in the hypothalamus, striatum and midbrain periaqueductal gray [21,22]. AAS reduce the expression of serotonin receptors in the anterior hypothalamus (1A), globus pallidus (1B) or hippocampus [23,24]. They decrease serotonin concentration in basal forebrain and dorsal striatum [25], but increase in the cerebral cortex [26]. AAS are also likely to influence the brain GABA system and modify the mesolimbic dopamine system by stimulation of dopamine release and synthesis [26].

Clinical application of the clomiphene stimulation test (CST) has a long history with well-understood physiological basis [27]. It is a simple and widely accepted tool to evaluate the hypothalamo-pituitary-gonadal axis in men [15,16]. The CST in healthy subjects leads to doubling of LH, 20-50% increase of FSH and 30-220% increase of testosterone concentration [12]. A similar situation is observed in men with hyperprolactinemia [28] or during aging [29].

In turn organic damage to the CNS or the testicular feminization syndrome are associated with impaired results of the CST [30].

We have to admit that we had no data on the hormonal status of our study cases from before starting AAS doping. However our findings confirm that deregulation of the hypothalamus/the pituitary in men suspected of having ASIH (low LH, FSH and T) is reversible by application of an antiestrogen. Clomiphene stimulation in the studied men induced the same results as in healthy subjects. The mean rise of LH, FSH and T was respectively: 178%, 237% and 215%. Further research is needed to establish the effects of antiestrogens used for longer periods and the influence of this treatment on sperm count. At the moment we have no information on permanence of the antiestrogen effects. There is no doubt that such a pharmacological regimen is more comfortable than gonadotropin therapy. Unlike androgens it has no detrimental effects on gonadal function [31].

We have not observed any differences of gonadotropins or testosterone reactions that would associate with doping course parameters (types of compounds, duration of use, time from withdrawal).

Lack of information on hormonal status (and sperm count) of the investigated subjects before initiation of AAS, missing information on sperm parameters and a small number of cases are major limitations of our observation. All of the studied men declared that clinical symptoms developed after withdrawal of AAS. We can add that five of our cases (38%) fathered children. None of them presented clinical features of congenital hypogonadal hypogonadism.

Future research on antiestrogens application in ASIH should involve monitoring of both: hormonal balance and sperm count.

Conclusions

Long-term AAS users who develop secondary, steroid-induced hypogonadism present an intact reaction of the HPG axis to clomiphene stimulation. Our data support rationale for an antiestrogen application to restore testosterone concentration in such cases.

References

1. Dunn M, White V (2011) The epidemiology of anabolic-androgenic steroid use among Australian secondary school students. J Sci Med Sport 14: 10-14.
2. Lood Y, Eklund A, Garle M, Ahlner J (2012) Anabolic androgenic steroids in police cases in Sweden 1999-2009. Forensic Sci Int 219: 199-204.
3. Galduróz JC, Noto AR, Nappo SA, Carlini EA (2005) Household survey on drug abuse in Brazil: study involving the 107 major cities of the country--2001. Addict Behav 30: 545-556.
4. RachoÅ D, Pokrywka L, Suchecka-RachoÅ„ K (2006) Prevalence and risk factors of anabolic-androgenic steroids (AAS) abuse among adolescents and young adults in Poland. Soz Praventivmed 51: 392-398.
5. Harmer PA (2010) Anabolic-androgenic steroid use among young male and female athletes: is the game to blame? Br J Sports Med 44: 26-31.

6. Kanayama G, Hudson JI, Pope HG Jr (2008) Long-term psychiatric and medical consequences of anabolic-androgenic steroid abuse: a looming public health concern? Drug Alcohol Depend 98: 1-12.
7. Angell P, Chester N, Green D, Somauroo J, Whyte G, et al. (2012) Anabolic steroids and cardiovascular risk. Sports Med 42: 119-134.
8. Turillazzi E, Perilli G, Di Paolo M, Neri M, Riezzo I, et al. (2011) Side effects of AAS abuse: an overview. Mini Rev Med Chem 11: 374-389.
9. Quaglio G, Fornasiero A, Mezzelani P, Moreschini S, Lugoboni F, et al. (2009) Anabolic steroids: dependence and complications of chronic use. Intern Emerg Med 4: 289-296.
10. Tan RS, Scally MC (2009) Anabolic steroid-induced hypogonadism--towards a unified hypothesis of anabolic steroid action. Med Hypotheses 72: 723-728.
11. Traish AM, Miner MM, Morgentaler A, Zitzmann M (2011) Testosterone deficiency. Am J Med 124: 578-587.
12. Brower KJ (2009) Anabolic steroid abuse and dependence in clinical practice. Phys Sportsmed 37: 131-140.
13. Salenave S, Trabado S, Maione L, Brailly-Tabard S, Young J (2012) Male acquired hypogonadotropic hypogonadism: diagnosis and treatment. Ann Endocrinol (Paris) 73: 141-146.
14. Kanayama G, Brower KJ, Wood RI, Hudson JI, Pope HG Jr (2010) Treatment of anabolic-androgenic steroid dependence: Emerging evidence and its implications. Drug Alcohol Depend 109: 6-13.
15. Petak SM, Nankin HR, Spark RF, Swerdloff RS, Rodriguez-Rigau LJ (2002) American Association of Clinical Endocrinologists Medical Guidelines for clinical practice for the evaluation and treatment of hypogonadism in adult male patients--2002 update. Endocr Pract 8: 440-456.
16. Rabijewski M, ZgliczyÅ„ski W (2009) [Pathogenesis, evaluation and treatment of hypogonadism in men]. Endokrynol Pol 60: 222-233.
17. Pope HG, Kanayama G, Ionescu-Pioggia M, Hudson JI (2004) Anabolic steroid users' attitudes towards physicians. Addiction 99: 1189-1194.
18. de Souza GL, Hallak J (2011) Anabolic steroids and male infertility: a comprehensive review. BJU Int 108: 1860-1865.
19. van Breda E, Keizer HA, Kuipers H, Wolffenbuttel BH (2003) Androgenic anabolic steroid use and severe hypothalamic-pituitary dysfunction: a case study. Int J Sports Med 24: 195-196.
20. Wood RI (2008) Anabolic-androgenic steroid dependence? Insights from animals and humans. Front Neuroendocrinol 29: 490-506.
21. Johansson P, Hallberg M, Kindlundh A, Nyberg F (2000) The effect on opioid peptides in the rat brain, after chronic treatment with the anabolic androgenic steroid, nandrolone decanoate. Brain Res Bull 51: 413-418.
22. Johansson P, Lindqvist A, Nyberg F, Fahlke C (2000) Anabolic androgenic steroids affects alcohol intake, defensive behaviors and brain opioid peptides in the rat. Pharmacol Biochem Behav 67: 271-279.
23. Ricci LA, Rasakham K, Grimes JM, Melloni RH, Jr. (2006) Serotonin-1A receptor activity and expression modulate adolescent anabolic/androgenic steroid-induced aggression in hamsters. Pharmacol Biochem Behav 85: 1-11.
24. Kindlundh AM, Lindblom J, Bergström L, Nyberg F (2003) The anabolic-androgenic steroid nandrolone induces alterations in the density of serotonergic 5HT1B and 5HT2 receptors in the male rat brain. Neuroscience 119: 113-120.
25. Lindqvist AS, Johansson-Steensland P, Nyberg F, Fahlke C (2002) Anabolic androgenic steroid affects competitive behaviour, behavioural response to ethanol and brain serotonin levels. Behav Brain Res 133: 21-29.
26. Kurling S, Kankaanpää A, Ellermaa S, Karila T, Seppälä T (2005) The effect of sub-chronic nandrolone decanoate treatment on dopaminergic and serotonergic neuronal systems in the brains of rats. Brain Res 1044: 67-75.
27. Santen RJ, Leonard JM, Sherins RJ, Gandy HM, Paulsen CA (1971) Short- and long-term effects of clomiphene citrate on the pituitary-testicular axis. J Clin Endocrinol Metab 33: 970-979.
28. Ribeiro RS, Abucham J (2009) Recovery of persistent hypogonadism by clomiphene in males with prolactinomas under dopamine agonist treatment. Eur J Endocrinol 161: 163-169.
29. Da Ros CT, Averbeck MA (2012) Twenty-five milligrams of clomiphene citrate presents positive effect on treatment of male testosterone deficiency - a prospective study. Int Braz J Urol 38: 512-518.
30. Medina M, Ulloa-Aguirre A, Fernández MA, Pérez-Palacios G (1980) The role of oestrogens on gonadotrophin secretion in the testicular feminization syndrome. Acta Endocrinol (Copenh) 95: 314-318.
31. MedraÅ› M, Tworowska U (2001) [Treatment strategies of withdrawal from long-term use of anabolic-androgenic steroids]. Pol Merkur Lekarski 11: 535-538.

4

Differential Cytokine Release from Brain Microvascular Endothelial Cells Treated with Dexamethasone and Multiple Sclerosis Patient Sera

Malgorzata Burek[1*], Aiden Haghikia[2], Ralf Gold[2], Norbert Roewer[1], Andrew Chan[2] and Carola Y Förster[1]

[1]*University of Wurzburg, Department of Anaesthesia and Critical Care, Wurzburg, Germany*

[2]*Ruhr University Bochum, Department of Neurology, St. Josef-Hospital, Bochum, Germany*

[*]**Corresponding author:** University of Würzburg, Department of Anaesthesia and Critical care, Oberdüerrbacher str. 6, 97080 Würzburg, Germany, E-mail: Burek_M@ukw.de

Abstract

Objective: Multiple sclerosis (MS) is a neurodegenerative disorder of the central nervous system (CNS). Damage of the blood-brain barrier integrity is a key pathogenic event leading to the migration of lymphocytes into the CNS and subsequent demyelination. This process is tightly regulated by chemokines and cytokines which are target of therapeutic strategies in MS, such as anti-inflammatory glucocorticosteroid treatment. Here, we examine the effects of dexamethasone-treatment and MS patient sera on the expression of cytokines and chemokines in brain microvascular cell line, cEND in vitro.

Methods: We conducted 96-well Mouse Cytokines and Receptors qPCR arrays to quantitatively compare the cytokine and chemokine expression profiles after treatment with dexamethasone. For selected cytokines, we studied the effects of pre-treatment with MS patient sera from active phase of disease (exacerbation) or in relapse (remission) in combination with dexamethasone.

Results: After dexamethasone treatment, colony stimulating factor 3 (Csf3) and interleukin 17F (IL17f) were significantly up-regulated, whereas the chemokine (C-C motif) ligand 12 (CCL12/MCP-5), chemokine (C-X-C motif) receptor 3 (CXCR3) and kit oncogene (Kit) were significantly down-regulated. These results were confirmed in qRT-PCR using gene-specific primers. For Csf3 and CCL12 we analyzed the dexamethasone-mediated changes in protein levels secreted into the cell culture medium. Dexamethasone treatment increased the release of Csf3 into the culture medium and decreased the release of CCL12 by cEND. Additionally, we examined the effects of MS-patient sera on dexamethasone-induced cytokine secretion. Pretreatment with MS-patient serum from exacerbation phase augmented dexamethasone effects on Csf3 and CCL12 release in cEND cells. The expression of Csf3- and CCL12-receptors was demonstrated on protein and mRNA level in cEND cells.

Conclusion: We identified Csf3 (G-Csf) and CCL12 as cytokines differentially regulated by dexamethasone on mRNA and protein level. This effect was even more pronounced after pretreatment with MS patient serum, especially from patients with acute relapses.

Keywords: Multiple sclerosis; Blood-brain barrier; Glucocorticoids; Dexamethasone; Cytokine; Chemokine; Patient sera; Csf3; CCL12

Introduction

Multiple sclerosis (MS) is a neuroinflammatory disorder characterized by the infiltration of pathogenic T cells into the CNS, which react with myelin antigens [1]. The majority of MS patients suffer initially from the relapsing-remitting form of the disease, which is characterized by attacks of neurological dysfunction followed by a gradual improvement. The exacerbations in relapsing-remitting MS are initiated by breakdown of the blood-brain barrier (BBB), which causes infiltration of activated immune effector cells into the brain and subsequent tissue damage [2,3]. Disruption of the BBB integrity is partially caused by Matrix metalloproteinases (MMPs) which are activated by proinflammatory cytokines increased during exacerbations of MS [4,5]. The levels of MMP-9, MMP-2 and tight junction protein claudin-5 and occludin change in different stages of MS [6]. High-dose glucocorticosteroid (GC) "pulse"-therapy is approved as first line therapy of relapses in MS [7]. The therapeutic GC-mediated effects on peripheral T cells in MS are widely studied [8,9]. In endothelial cells of the BBB, GC treatment reduces MMP levels and activity thereby stabilizing the BBB through higher expression of tight and adherens junction proteins [10-12].

Cytokines and chemokines play an important role in CNS neuroinflammatory disorders. The chemokine family is divided into four subfamilies: CC, CXC, CX_3C and XC, based upon the position of the first and second conserved cysteine (C) residues within the mature peptides. Chemokines receptors are named as G protein-coupled receptors for CC, CXC, CX_3C and XC chemokines [13]. Human primary brain endothelial cells as well as the human brain microvascular endothelial cell line hCMEC/D3 showed the constitutive expression of CXCL8 and CXCL2. CXCL10 and CCL5 were undetectable in resting endothelial cells but were secreted in response to proinflammatory cytokines, TNFα and IFN-γ [14]. Exposure of endothelial cell monolayers to dexamethasone is known to increase the expression of tight junction proteins, therefore substantially decreasing endothelial cell permeability [15].

Previously, we demonstrated barrier compromising effects of MS patient sera using an in vitro model of the BBB, a mouse brain microvascular endothelial cell line cEND [10,16]. In this study we further characterized cEND and analyzed their cytokine and chemokine expression in response to dexamethasone or MS patient sera treatment in vitro. We identified Csf3 and CCL12 genes as strong responders to dexamethasone treatment in brain vascular endothelium in vitro.

Methods

Reagents

Dexamethasone was purchased from Sigma. Stock solution was prepared in ethanol and kept at -20°C. Desired dilution was made directly before the experiment in cell culture medium. The final concentration of ethanol in the treatment medium was lower than 0.01% (v/v). Dexamethasone was used at final concentration of 100 nM, which has been chosen according to the previous kinetics studies performed on brain ECs [10]. Control cells were treated with diluted vehicle only.

Patients and patient sera

The study was approved by local ethics committees. MS patient sera were prepared and used in cell culture as previously described [16]. In brief, sera of RR-MS patients with different time points of last GC treatment and three normal control donors, devoid of clinical signs of infections or immunotherapies, were chosen for the following experimental set-ups. Blood was obtained by venipuncture using CPT Vacutainer containing Na-citrate as anticoagulant (Becton Dickinson). Vacutainers were centrifuged for 20 min at 1650g. Serum with lymphocytes was transferred to new Falcon tubes, centrifuged again at 1200 rpm for 10 min and serum supernatant was removed and stored in aliquots until use. For the cell culture, pooled serum samples from healthy controls and MS patients were used.

Endothelial cell culture

Cerebral microvascular ECs were isolated as described [10,17]. Cells were cultivated in Dulbecco's Modified Eagle's Medium (DMEM) (Sigma) supplemented with 10% fetal calf serum (FCS) and 100 IU/ml penicillin/streptomycin on collagen I coated flasks. Cells were maintained in 37°C and 5 % CO2. Cells were grown to confluence and transferred to serum-low medium (2 % FCS) for differentiation.

Mouse cytokines and receptors 96 stellARray™ qPCR array

Mouse Cytokines and Receptors 96 StellARray™ qPCR arrays (Lonza) (n=3 per condition) were conducted to compare the cytokine expression in cEND treated for 24 hours with vehicle only or 100 nM dexamethasone. The qPCR analyses were performed according to manufacturer instructions using the SYBR® Green Master Mix (Life Technologies) and ABI PRISM 7300 system (Life Technologies). The gene expression fold changes and statistical tests were estimated by Global Pattern Recognition™ (GPR) Data Analysis Tool (Lonza).

Real-time PCR

For real-time PCR, RNA was isolated from cells treated or untreated with dexamethasone using NucleoSpin® RNA II Kit (Macherey-Nagel). One microgram of RNA was used for cDNA synthesis with High Capacity cDNA Reverse Transcription Kit (Life Technologies). Real-time PCR was performed using the SYBR® Green Master Mix (Life Technologies). Primers were designed using Primer3 Software and synthesized by Eurofins MWG Operon and tested for PCR efficiency. The primer sequences were as follows: CXCL2: aagtttgccttgaccctgaa (sense), aggcacatcaggtacgatcc (anti-sense); CXCL12: agtagtggctccccaggttt (sense), gagacagtcttgcggacaca (anti-sense); CCL12: gggaagctgtgatcttcagg (sense), gggaacttcaggggggaaata (anti-sense); Il2rb: atgacccctgtgtggaagag (sense), ggatgctagggagggaagtc (anti-sense); Il17f: gtgttcccaatgcctcactt (sense), gtgcttcttccttgccagtc (anti-sense); CCL7: tgaaaaccccaactccaaag (sense), cattccttaggcgtgaccat (anti-sense); Kit: ttatcctttaggccgtgtgg (sense), tgtggccccttaagtacctg (anti-sense); Il23a: gactcagccaactcctccag (sense), gcactaagggctcagtcag (anti-sense); Csf3: ctcaactttctgcccagagg (sense), taggtggcacacaactgctc (anti-sense); Csf3-R: gagctgtggacacatcgaga (sense), aggaaggcctgggtgtagtt (anti-sense); Ccr2: agagagctgcagcaaaaagg (sense), ggaaagaggcagttgcaaag (anti-sense); GAPDH: ttcaccatggagaaggc (sense), ggcatcgactgtggtcatga (anti-sense). All PCR reactions were performed in triplicate for each target. Data were acquired with the ABI PRISM 7300 system (Life Technologies). The ABI PRISM 7300 SDS software (relative quantification study) was used to determine the threshold cycle (C_t) for each reaction and gene expression was normalized to the expression of the endogenous housekeeping gene GAPDH based on the $2^{-\Delta\Delta Ct}$ method.

Western blot analysis

cEND cells were grown to confluence, differentiated and treated with dexamethasone or vehicle only in serum-free medium for 24 hours. For Western blot analyses, cells were lysed in RIPA buffer supplemented with proteases inhibitors cocktail (Roche). Protein contents were quantified by BCA protein Assay Kit (Thermo Fisher Scientific) and 40 µg of protein were loaded on SDS-polyacrylamide gels for Western blot analysis. For immunoblotting, proteins were transferred to Hybond nitrocellulose membranes (Promega) which were blocked with 10% (w/v) low fat milk in PBS and incubated overnight at 4°C with the respective primary antibody in blocking soultion. Rabbit polyclonal antibody against mouse Csf3R (1:200, #sc-694, Santa Cruz Biotechnology) and goat polyclonal anti-mouse Ccr2 (1:1000, #ab25788, Abcam) and mouse monoclonal anti-β-actin antibody (Sigma; 1:5000) were used. Respective horseradish-peroxidase-labelled secondary antibodies (GE Healthcare) diluted 1:3000 were used. For detection, Enhanced Chemiluminescence (ECL) detection kit (Promega) and FluorChem FC2 Multi-imager II (Alpha Innotech) with CD camera were used. Intensity of protein bands was calculated with the software Alpha View (Alpha Innotech).

Detection of secreted proteins

cEND cells were grown to confluence, differentiated and treated with dexamethasone or vehicle only in serum-free medium for 24 hours. For pretreatment with MS-patient sera, the cells were incubated 24 hours with 5% patient sera. Then the cells were washed with phosphate buffer saline (PBS) (PAA Laboratories) and treated for additional 24 hours with 100 nM dexamethasone in serum free medium. The same amounts of cell culture medium were collected, mixed with ice cold acetone in proportion 1 to 6, followed by 2 hours incubation at -80°C. Precipitated proteins were centrifuged at 13000 g for 10 min at 4°C. The resulting pellets were air dried and resuspended in 1.5x Tris-Tricine sample buffer (Tris-HCL pH 6.8, 50% glycerol, 10% SDS, 10 mg Coomassie Blue G-250). The samples were loaded on

16.5% Tris-Tricine Gel (BioRad). For Western blot detection of secreted G-CSF and CCL12 rabbit anti-mouse G-Csf antibody (Lifespan Biosciences #LS-C42075/28157, at 1:500 dilution) and rabbit anti-mouse CCL12 (AbD Serotec #AAM45, at 1:500 dilution) antibodies were used. As secondary antibody the horseradish-peroxidase-labelled donkey anit-rabbit IgGs (GE Healthcare) diluted 1:3000 were used. For detection, Enhanced Chemiluminescence (ECL) detection kit (Promega) and FluorChem FC2 Multi-imager II (Alpha Innotech) with CD camera were used. Optical density values of protein bands were calculated with the software Alpha View (Alpha Innotech). As a loading control, Coomassie stained gels loaded with the same amount of medium-protein sample were used.

Statistical analysis

All data are presented as mean ± standard deviation (SD) from at least three independent experiments. Statistical analysis was performed with SigmaStat 3.1 Software. For statistical comparison of two groups, we used an unpaired 2-tailed Students t-test; for the comparison of multiple groups, we used 2-way ANOVA followed by Tukey post hoc test. Differences were considered significant for *p* values less than 0.05.

Results

Dexamethasone-mediated changes in the expression of cytokines mRNA in cEND

There are several reports in the literature describing the expression of selected cytokines in brain microvascular endothelial cells (ECs) [14,18,19]. We have previously demonstrated that brain microvascular endothelial cell line cEND responds to TNFα treatment in vitro [20,21]. However, the cEND cells were not yet characterized in terms of expression of cytokines and their receptors. We thus amplified mRNA of different cytokines present in differentiated untreated cEND and then analysed the dexamethasone-mediated changes of cytokine expression in these cells. We performed 96-well real-time transcription polymerase chain reaction (qRT-PCR) arrays (Table 1). The obtained results showed significant dexamethasone-mediated changes in the expression of chemokines and cytokines involved in the inflammation and immune response: Csf3 (10.4-fold), CCL12 (-6.7-fold), CXCR3 (-4.2-fold), Il17f (5.3-fold) and Kit (-3.6-fold). The results obtained with StellArray PCR array were reproduced in the qPCR using gene specific primers which confirmed upregulation of respective genes (Csf3, Il17f, CXCL2, CXCL12, Il2rb, Il23a) (Figure 1). Similarly, the three down-regulated genes (CCL7, CCL12 and Kit) were also found to be down-regulated by real time PCR analysis. Levels of expression changes due to dexamethasone treatment were variable, but Csf3 showed the highest-fold up-regulation among gene of the six selected genes by PCR-array analysis, and the CCL12 showed the highest-fold down-regulation. In conclusion, both methods (commercially available qPCR arrays and quantitative real-time PCR) demonstrated similar dexamethasone-mediated changes in the expression of cytokines by cEND. Detection of mRNA for cytokines and chemokines as shown in Table 1 and Figurel suggests local production as well as the ability of brain microvascular endothelial cells to respond in situ to inflammatory stimuli.

Gene Symbol	GenBank Accession Number	Fold change	P Value	Gene Name
Csf3	NC_000077	10.3	0.01327	colony stimulating factor 3 (granulocyte)
CCL12	NM_011331	-6.7	0.03012	chemokine (C-C motif) ligand 12
CXCR3	NM_009910	-4.2	0.03602	chemokine (C-X-C motif) receptor 3
Il17f	NM_145856	5.3	0.03828	interleukin 17F
Kit	NM_001122733	-3.6	0.04448	kit oncogene
CXCL2	NM_009140	9.4	0.05083	chemokine (C-X-C motif) ligand 2
Ccr5	NM_009917	-5.5	0.07481	chemokine (C-C motif) receptor 5
CXCL12	NM_001012477	2.7	0.08845	chemokine (C-X-C motif) ligand 12
Il22ra1	NM_178257	4.8	0.09177	interleukin 22 receptor, alpha 1
Il2rb	NM_008368	2.8	0.09458	interleukin 2 receptor, beta chain (Il2rb)
CCL7	NM_013654	-2.5	0.09807	chemokine (C-C motif) ligand 7
Il23a	NM_031252	2.9	0.10258	interleukin 23, alpha subunit p19

Table 1: Quantitative dexamethasone-mediated changes in cEND mRNA expression obtained with Mouse Cytokines and Receptors 96 StellARray™ qPCR array.

cEND were left untreated or were treated with 100 nM dexamethasone for 24 hours. Mouse Cytokines and Receptors 96 StellARray™ qPCR arrays were conducted according to manufacturers' instruction (n=3 per treatment). The gene expression fold changes and p values were calculated by Global Pattern Recognition™ (GPR) Data Analysis Tool (Lonza).

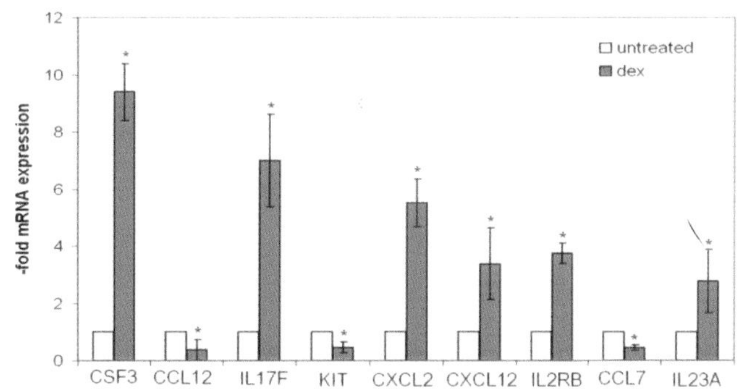

Figure 1: Dexamethasone-mediated changes in mRNA expression of selected cytokines in cEND cells

Confluent and differentiated cEND cells were treated with 100 nM dexamethasone (dex) for 24 hours followed by total RNA extraction and quantitative real-time PCR with gene specific primers described in Methods section. Cytokine expression was normalized to GAPDH and expressed as fold over untreated cells, which was set as 1. The data (mean ± SD) present the results of three independent experiments. Statistical analysis was performed by t-test; *p<0.05.

Differential effects of dexamethasone treatment on G-Csf and CCL12 secretion

To study the influence of dexamethasone treatment on the protein level, we selected Csf3 which was significantly increased on mRNA level. Granulocyte-colony stimulating factor, G-Csf (other names CSF3OS, C17orf33), a key hemopoietic factor of the myeloid lineage is encoded by Csf3 gene [22]. As a second protein, we selected CCL12 (other names MCP-5 and Scya12) [23], whose mRNA was significantly decreased after dexamethasone treatment. Since the cytokines and growth factors are rapidly released from the cells, we used the cell culture medium from cells cultured without serum for Western blot analysis.

While basal G-Csf release in untreated cells was hardly detectable, cells treated with dexamethasone released 2.5- fold (p=0.029) higher amounts of G-Csf into the medium (Figure 2A). CCL12 was highly secreted by untreated cells, whereas the treatment with dexamethasone led to a reduction by 0.7-fold (p=0.002) in the secreted CCL12 protein (Figure 2B). These results agree with those from the mRNA analysis in cEND cells after dexamethasone treatment as shown in Figure 1.

Confluent and differentiated cEND cells were treated for 24 hours with 100 nM dexamethasone (dex) in serum-free medium. Equal amounts of cell culture medium were collected, acetone-precipitated and loaded on 20% Tris-glycine gel, followed by Western blot using anti-Csf3 (A) or anti-CCL12 (B) antibody. As a loading control, a Coomassie stained gel has been used. A representative Western blot is shown. Optical density values of protein bands were calculated with the software Alpha View and data expressed as fold over untreated control, which was set as 1. The data (mean ± SD) present the results of three independent experiments. Statistical analysis was performed by t-test; *p<0.05.

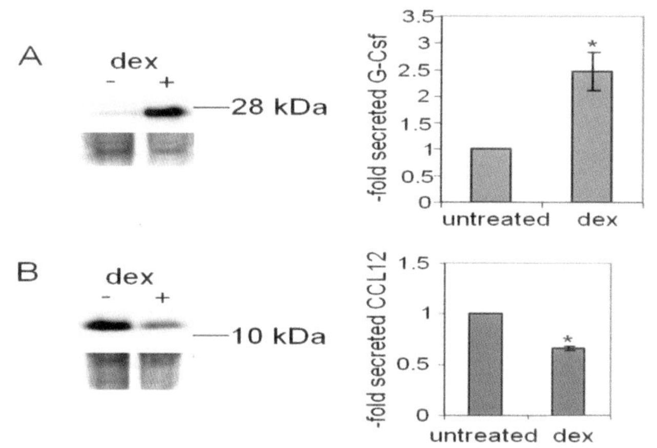

Figure 2: Dexamethasone-treated cEND release different levels of G-Csf and CCL12 into the cell culture medium

Pre-treatment of cEND with MS-patient sera leads to the higher dexamethasone-mediated G-Csf release from cEND treated with exacerbation phase serum

As previously published by us, MS patient sera modify dexamethasone-mediated effects on blood-brain barrier properties [16]. We thus tested, whether pre-treatment of cEND with MS patient sera from different stages of the disease could influence the secretion of G-Csf and CCL12 into the culture medium (Figure 3A and 3B).

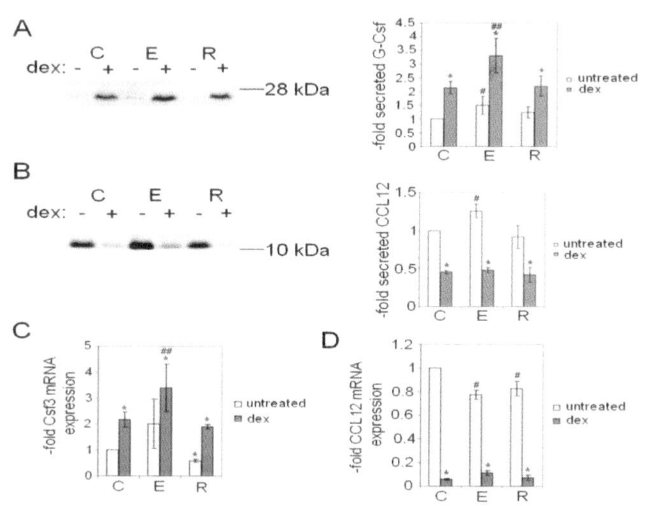

Figure 3: Secretion of G-CSF and CCL12 into the culture medium by cEND pre-treated with MS patient serum with or without dexamethasone treatment

Pre-treatment of cEND with control serum or MS patient serum from exacerbation phase revealed a 1.5-fold (p<0.05) higher release of G-Csf in samples treated with MS patient serum from exacerbation phase, as detected by Western blot (Figure 3A). Interestingly, dexamethasone induction of G-Csf release was also 1.5-fold (p<0.05) higher in exacerbation phase sera pre-treated cells than in control serum pre-treated samples (Figure 3A). CCL12 release into the medium was increased in samples treated with serum from exacerbation phase by 1.3-fold (p<0.05) if compared to the cells treated with control serum (Figure 3B). The changes in G-Csf on the protein level correlated with Csf3 mRNA expression in cEND cells (Figure 3C). Csf3 mRNA expression was 1.6-fold (p<0.05) higher in dexamethasone samples pre-treated with exacerbation serum than in dexamethasone samples pre-treated with the control serum. However, CCL12 mRNA expression (Figure 3D) was decreased in samples pre-treated with both exacerbation (0.77-fold, p<0.05) and remission (0.82-fold, p<0.05) phase patient sera if compared to sample pre-treated with the control patient serum.

cEND cells were treated with MS patient serum (E- exacerbation phase, R- remission phase) or healthy control serum (C) for 24 hours, followed by PBS washing and addition of serum-free medium with or without 100 nM dexamethasone (dex) for additional 24 hours. Equal amounts of the cell culture medium were collected, the proteins were precipitated with acetone and loaded on 20% Tris-glycine gel for electrophoresis followed by Western blot with anti-Csf3 (A) and anti-CCL12 (B) antibody. Densitometric analyses of Western blots are shown at right. The data (mean ± SD) present the results of three independent experiments. Representative Western blots are shown. Statystical analysis was performed by 2-way ANOVA followed by Tukey post hoc test; *p<0.05 for comparisons untreated vs. dexamethasone-treated samples within different serum groups, # p<0.05 for comparisons of dexamethasone-untreated control and patient sera samples, ## p<0.05 for comparisons of dexamethasone-treated control and patient sera samples. (C and D) Messenger RNA expression of Csf3 (C) and CCL12 (D) by cEND pre-treated with MS patient serum with or without dexamethasone treatment. cEND cells were treated with MS patient serum (E- exacerbation phase, R- remission phase) or healthy control serum (C) for 24 hours, followed by PBS washing and addition of serum-free medium with or without 100 nM dexamethasone (dex) for additional 24 hours.

Csf3 and CCL12 expressions were normalized to GAPDH and expressed as fold over with control-serum pre-treated and dexamethasone untreated cells, which was set as 1. The data (mean ± SD) present the results of three independent experiments. Statystical analysis was performed by 2-way ANOVA followed by Tukey post hoc test; *p<0.05 for comparisons untreated vs. dexamethasone-treated samples within different serum groups, # p<0.05 for comparisons of dexamethasone-untreated control and patient sera samples, ## p<0.05 for comparisons of dexamethasone-treated control and patient sera samples.

Mouse brain microvascular endothelial cells express chemokine (C-C motif) receptor 2 and Csf3 receptor mRNA

After showing the dexamethasone-mediated effects on Csf3 and CCL12, we examined whether cEND cells express the receptors for G-Csf and CCL12 (Figure 4). G-Csf binds Csf3R, [24], and CCL12 interact with chemokine (C-C motif) receptor 2 (Ccr2), which also binds CCL2, CCL7, CCL8 and CCL16 [25]. cEND cells express high levels of mRNA for both receptors at a basal level. Analyses of Csf3R mRNA revealed strong dexamethasone-mediated down-regulation by 0.2 -fold (p<0.01), as compared to control untreated cells set as 1 (Figure 4A). No significant changes in Ccr2 mRNA expression were observed in cEND after dexamethasone treatment (Figure 4A). However, both receptors were up-regulated at the protein level in dexamethasone treated cEND (Csf3R by 2-fold and Ccr2 by 1.7-fold, respectively) as shown by Western blot in Figure 4B.

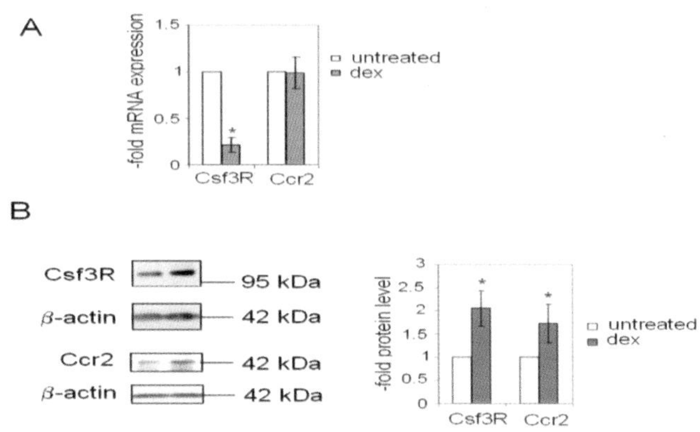

Figure 4: Dexamethasone-mediated changes in Csf3 receptor and Ccr2 mRNA and protein level in cEND

A. cEND cells were treated with 100 nM dexamethasone for 24 hours followed by total RNA extraction and quantitative real-time PCR with gene specific primers. Csf3 receptor (Csf3R) and chemokine (C-C motif) receptor 2 (Ccr2) expression was normalized to GAPDH and expressed as fold over untreated cells, which was set as 1. B. Cell lysates form cEND treated or untreated with 100 nM dexamethasone (dex) were subjected to SDS-PAGE as described in Materials and Methods. Expression of Csf3R and Ccr2 were detected with specific antibodies. A representative Western blot is shown. Optical density values of protein bands were calculated with the software Alpha View and data expressed as fold over untreated control, which was set as 1. The data (mean ± SD) present the results of three independent experiments. Statistical analysis was performed by t-test; * p<0.05.

Discussion

Blood-brain barrier stabilizing effects of GCs have been previously reported [10,16,26]. However, the molecular mechanisms of these effects, especially in different neuroinflammatory disorders, are not completely understood. Cytokines are important mediators which contribute to the immune cell trafficking and functional integrity of different tissues. To further elucidate cytokine regulation in brain microvascular endothelial cells, we designed experiments aiming at providing an expression profile of cytokines in endothelial cells and, subsequently, identifying possible GC targets among cytokines expressed in brain endothelial cells in vitro. In our analysis, we included an in vitro blood-brain barrier model, the immortalized endothelial cells from mouse brain, cEND. This cell line has been previously proven to possess typical endothelial properties [10,20]. GC effects on endothelial barrier functions and the expression of glucocorticoid receptor (GR) have been also previously demonstrated [10,16]. In the present study, we characterized the cytokine mRNA expression profile of cEND cells at a basal level and after dexamethasone treatment. Moreover, we showed the dexamethasone- and MS patient sera mediated regulation of G-Csf and CCL12 in cEND.

First, we analyzed the mRNA products for different cytokines genes constitutively expressed in differentiated cEND without treatment with dexamethasone. Expression of tumor necrosis factor-α (Tnf-α), interleukin 1α and (Il1a, Il1b) and its receptor Ilr1, have been previously described in mouse brain microvascular ECs [27,28]. Also the expression of interleukins known to play a role in the pathogenesis of MS could be detected, e.g. Il6, Il12, Il17, Il25, as well as the receptors Il6ra and Il17ra [29]. Constitutive expression of CCL2 (MCP-1) [30] has been described in brain microvascular ECs and consistently, CCL2 mRNA was detected by us in cEND. The chemokines of CXC and CC subfamilies, which have been described in MS, including CCL2, -3, -4, -5, -7, and CXCL10, were also constitutively expressed by cEND [31]. The detection of gene expression for multiple cytokines and their receptors in cEND make this in vitro model of BBB a valuable tool for studying the leukocyte-endothelial adhesion and motility, as well as BBB properties under inflammatory conditions which are one of the characteristics of MS.

Glucocorticoids are the mainstay in the treatment of MS relapses [1]. We therefore tested dexamethasone-mediated changes in cytokine expression of cEND using qPCR-based arrays. We identified up-regulation of mRNA expression in Csf3, Il17f, CXCL22, CXCL12, Il2rb and Il23a and a down-regulation of mRNA expression in CCL12, CXCR3, Kit and CCL7 after dexamethasone treatment. CXCL2 (MIP-2, macrophage inflammatory protein-2) has been up-regulated by dexamethasone in traumatic brain injury in cells with neuronal morphology [32]. Our results demonstrated that CXCL2 mRNA was highly induced by dexamethasone in brain microvascular EC. CXCL12 (Sdf-1, stromal cell-derived factor-1) was up-regulated by dexamethasone in our system (Table 1 and Figure 2). CXCL12 has been demonstrated to be expressed in healthy adult CNS on neurons and endothelial cells and it was up-regulated in MS lesions [33] suggesting its important role in MS pathology. GC therapy of MS patients reduced CXCR3 (a known receptor for CXCL9, CXCL10 and CXCL11) expression on peripheral blood T cells, thereby diminishing the recruitment of leukocytes into the CNS [34]. We also showed GC-mediated down-regulation of CXCR3 on brain microvascular ECs, which might contribute to beneficial effects of GC in MS. To authors' best knowledge, this is the first report showing dexamethasone-mediated regulation of CCL12 and Il23a. Il23 stimulates the production of interferon gamma and Il10 having an anti-inflammatory function [35,36].

The most prominent changes in the expression were detected for Csf3 and CCL12 mRNA and protein after dexamethasone treatment. CCL12 (Mcp-5) is a proinflammatory chemokine, which was as expected down-regulated by dexamethasone, as already shown for other chemokines from the CC subfamily [30]. CCL12 protein and mRNA expression has been previously demonstrated in mouse brain and mouse endothelial cell of aorta [23]. cEND cells express and secrete high levels of CCL12 constitutively. Pre-treatment of cEND with MS-patient sera changed the levels of CCL12 mRNA and protein in cEND, suggesting an ability of cEND to answer to different components present in MS-patient serum in comparison to serum from healthy donor. CCL12, together with CCL2 have been shown to play a role in the induction of inflammatory response in cyrolesion-EAE (experimental autoimmune encephalomyelitis) as their expression was the highest before the maximum degree of inflammation in the brain was seen [37]. Moreover, multiple sequence polymorphisms resulting in significant amino acid substitutions were identified in CCL12 gene, which was associated with severity of clinical signs and susceptibility to less severe monophasic remitting/nonrelapsing form of EAE [38]. Here, we identified CCL12 as a target gene for GC-action in brain vascular endothelium. Dexamethasone preserves its strong inhibiting effects on CCL12 mRNA and protein in the cells pre-treated with MS patient sera, which might be of interest for MS therapy. Expression of CCL12 receptor, Ccr2 was detected in cEND at the protein and mRNA level. Mice lacking Ccr2 receptors were resistant to the induction of EAE by myelin oligodendrocyte glycoprotein peptide 35-55 [39].

G-Csf is a key hemopoietic factor of the myeloid lineage and has been clinically used in the last decade for treatment of neutropenia and mobilization of bone marrow normal hemopoietic stem cells into the peripheral blood [22]. In microarray study with MS patient samples, G-Csf mRNA was identified as upregulated in acute, but not in chronic MS lesions and treatment of EAE mice with G-Csf ameliorated the disease [40] or reversed ongoing EAE [41]. Here, we demonstrate that mouse brain microvascular endothelial cells secrete high amounts of G-Csf into medium in vitro after stimulation with dexamethasone. Basal G-Csf secretion takes place, although it is hardly detectable. G-Csf is also constitutively secreted by mouse microvascular brain pericytes, which together with endothelial cells and astrocytes are a part of the neurovascular unit [42]. The treatment of cEND cells with MS patient serum from exacerbation phase led to a higher basal G-Csf secretion which was potentiated after treatment with dexamethasone. We demonstrated that cEND cells expressed G-Csf receptor on mRNA and protein level indicating that brain vascular endothelium may play an important role in naturally suppressing acute attacks of MS.

Conclusions

In conclusion, our results as presented here show that cultured mouse brain endothelial cells express high levels of cytokines and chemokines mRNAs and respond to dexamethasone stimulation. Mouse brain endothelial cells express and secrete in vitro CCL12 und Csf3 (G-CSF) and their receptors, thus being able to transduce signals triggered during brain inflammatory or neurodegenerative processes. Additionally, we showed that sera from multiple sclerosis patients influence the mRNA expression and secretion of CCL12 and G-CSF. CCL12 and Csf3 can be assumed as novel dexamethasone targets in brain vascular endothelium.

Acknowledgments

This research was partly supported by the European Union Seventh Framework Programme (FP7/2007-2013) grant under the grant agreement HEALTH-F2-2009-241778 to CYF and MB. The authors are grateful to Elisabeth Wilken for excellent technical assistance.

Authors' contributions

MB designed the study, acquired, analyzed and interpreted the data and wrote the manuscript. AH, RG, AC collected and provided the patient sera and critically revised the manuscript. NR and CYF interpreted the data and critically revised the manuscript. All authors read and approved the final manuscript.

References

1. Tischner D, Reichardt HM (2007) Glucocorticoids in the control of neuroinflammation. Mol Cell Endocrinol 275: 62-70.
2. Steinman L (2001) Multiple sclerosis: a two-stage disease. Nat Immunol 2: 762-764.
3. Engelhardt B (2006) Molecular mechanisms involved in T cell migration across the blood-brain barrier. J Neural Transm 113: 477-485.

4. SzczuciÅ, ski A, Losy J (2007) Chemokines and chemokine receptors in multiple sclerosis. Potential targets for new therapies. Acta Neurol Scand 115: 137-146.
5. Mun-Bryce S, Rosenberg GA (1998) Matrix metalloproteinases in cerebrovascular disease. J Cereb Blood Flow Metab 18: 1163-1172.
6. Benesová Y, Vasku A, Novotná H, Litzman J, Stourac P, et al. (2009) Matrix metalloproteinase-9 and matrix metalloproteinase-2 as biomarkers of various courses in multiple sclerosis. Mult Scler 15: 316-322.
7. Reichardt HM (2004) Immunomodulatory activities of glucocorticoids: insights from transgenesis and gene targeting. Curr Pharm Des 10: 2797-2805.
8. Wüst S, van den Brandt J, Tischner D, Kleiman A, Tuckermann JP, et al. (2008) Peripheral T cells are the therapeutic targets of glucocorticoids in experimental autoimmune encephalomyelitis. J Immunol 180: 8434-8443.
9. Sbiera S, Dexneit T, Reichardt SD, Michel KD, van den Brandt J, et al. (2011) Influence of short-term glucocorticoid therapy on regulatory T cells in vivo. PLoS One 6: e24345.
10. Forster C, Silwedel C, Golenhofen N, Burek M, Kietz S, et al. (2005) Occludin as direct target for glucocorticoid-induced improvement of blood-brain barrier properties in a murine in vitro system. J Physiol 565: 475-486.
11. Rosenberg GA, Dencoff JE, Correa N Jr, Reiners M, Ford CC (1996) Effect of steroids on CSF matrix metalloproteinases in multiple sclerosis: relation to blood-brain barrier injury. Neurology 46: 1626-1632.
12. Lindberg RL, De Groot CJ, Montagne L, Freitag P, van der Valk P, et al. (2001) The expression profile of matrix metalloproteinases (MMPs) and their inhibitors (TIMPs) in lesions and normal appearing white matter of multiple sclerosis. Brain 124: 1743-1753.
13. Murphy PM, Baggiolini M, Charo IF, Hebert CA, Horuk R, et al. (2000) International union of pharmacology. XXII. Nomenclature for chemokine receptors. Pharmacol Rev 52: 145-176.
14. Subileau EA, Rezaie P, Davies HA, Colyer FM, Greenwood J, et al. (2009) Expression of chemokines and their receptors by human brain endothelium: implications for multiple sclerosis. J Neuropathol Exp Neurol 68: 227-240.
15. Förster C, Waschke J, Burek M, Leers J, Drenckhahn D (2006) Glucocorticoid effects on mouse microvascular endothelial barrier permeability are brain specific. J Physiol 573: 413-425.
16. Blecharz KG, Haghikia A, Stasiolek M, Kruse N, Drenckhahn D, et al. (2010) Glucocorticoid effects on endothelial barrier function in the murine brain endothelial cell line cEND incubated with sera from patients with multiple sclerosis. Mult Scler 16: 293-302.
17. Burek M, Salvador E, Förster CY (2012) Generation of an immortalized murine brain microvascular endothelial cell line as an in vitro blood brain barrier model. J Vis Exp : e4022.
18. Berger O, Gan X, Gujuluva C, Burns AR, Sulur G, et al. (1999) CXC and CC chemokine receptors on coronary and brain endothelia. Mol Med 5: 795-805.
19. Hillyer P, Mordelet E, Flynn G, Male D (2003) Chemokines, chemokine receptors and adhesion molecules on different human endothelia: discriminating the tissue-specific functions that affect leucocyte migration. Clin Exp Immunol 134: 431-441.
20. Silwedel C, Forster C (2006) Differential susceptibility of cerebral and cerebellar murine brain microvascular endothelial cells to loss of barrier properties in response to inflammatory stimuli. J Neuroimmunol 179: 37-45.
21. Burek M, Förster CY (2009) Cloning and characterization of the murine claudin-5 promoter. Mol Cell Endocrinol 298: 19-24.
22. Rutella S, Zavala F, Danese S, Kared H, Leone G (2005) Granulocyte colony-stimulating factor: a novel mediator of T cell tolerance. J Immunol 175: 7085-7091.
23. Rodríguez-Sanabria F, Rull A, Beltrán-Debón R, Aragonès G, Camps J, et al. (2010) Tissue distribution and expression of paraoxonases and chemokines in mouse: the ubiquitous and joint localisation suggest a systemic and coordinated role. J Mol Histol 41: 379-386.
24. Germeshausen M, Skokowa J, Ballmaier M, Zeidler C, Welte K (2008) G-CSF receptor mutations in patients with congenital neutropenia. Curr Opin Hematol 15: 332-337.
25. Semple BD, Kossmann T, Morganti-Kossmann MC (2010) Role of chemokines in CNS health and pathology: a focus on the CCL2/CCR2 and CXCL8/CXCR2 networks. J Cereb Blood Flow Metab 30: 459-473.
26. Förster C, Burek M, Romero IA, Weksler B, Couraud PO, et al. (2008) Differential effects of hydrocortisone and TNFalpha on tight junction proteins in an in vitro model of the human blood-brain barrier. J Physiol 586: 1937-1949.
27. Banks WA (1999) Characterization of interleukin-1alpha binding to mouse brain endothelial cells. J Pharmacol Exp Ther 291: 665-670.
28. Zhang W, Smith C, Howlett C, Stanimirovic D (2000) Inflammatory activation of human brain endothelial cells by hypoxic astrocytes in vitro is mediated by IL-1beta. J Cereb Blood Flow Metab 20: 967-978.
29. Codarri L, Fontana A, Becher B (2010) Cytokine networks in multiple sclerosis: lost in translation. Curr Opin Neurol 23: 205-211.
30. Harkness KA, Sussman JD, Davies-Jones GA, Greenwood J, Woodroofe MN (2003) Cytokine regulation of MCP-1 expression in brain and retinal microvascular endothelial cells. J Neuroimmunol 142: 1-9.
31. Trebst C, Ransohoff RM (2001) Investigating chemokines and chemokine receptors in patients with multiple sclerosis: opportunities and challenges. Arch Neurol 58: 1975-1980.
32. Rhodes JK, Sharkey J, Andrews PJ (2009) The temporal expression, cellular localization, and inhibition of the chemokines MIP-2 and MCP-1 after traumatic brain injury in the rat. J Neurotrauma 26: 507-525.
33. Krumbholz M, Theil D, Cepok S, Hemmer B, Kivisäkk P, et al. (2006) Chemokines in multiple sclerosis: CXCL12 and CXCL13 up-regulation is differentially linked to CNS immune cell recruitment. Brain 129: 200-211.
34. Sørensen TL, Trebst C, Kivisäkk P, Klaege KL, Majmudar A, et al. (2002) Multiple sclerosis: a study of CXCL10 and CXCR3 co-localization in the inflamed central nervous system. J Neuroimmunol 127: 59-68.
35. Oppmann B, Lesley R, Blom B, Timans JC, Xu Y, et al. (2000) Novel p19 protein engages IL-12p40 to form a cytokine, IL-23, with biological activities similar as well as distinct from IL-12. Immunity 13: 715-725.
36. de Paus RA, van de Wetering D, van Dissel JT, van de Vosse E (2008) IL-23 and IL-12 responses in activated human T cells retrovirally transduced with IL-23 receptor variants. Mol Immunol 45: 3889-3895.
37. Sun D, Tani M, Newman TA, Krivacic K, Phillips M, et al. (2000) Role of chemokines, neuronal projections, and the blood-brain barrier in the enhancement of cerebral EAE following focal brain damage. J Neuropathol Exp Neurol 59: 1031-1043.
38. Teuscher C, Butterfield RJ, Ma RZ, Zachary JF, Doerge RW, et al. (1999) Sequence polymorphisms in the chemokines Scya1 (TCA-3), Scya2 (monocyte chemoattractant protein (MCP)-1), and Scya12 (MCP-5) are candidates for eae7, a locus controlling susceptibility to monophasic remitting/nonrelapsing experimental allergic encephalomyelitis. J Immunol 163: 2262-2266.
39. Izikson L, Klein RS, Charo IF, Weiner HL, Luster AD (2000) Resistance to experimental autoimmune encephalomyelitis in mice lacking the CC chemokine receptor (CCR)2. J Exp Med 192: 1075-1080.
40. Lock C, Hermans G, Pedotti R, Brendolan A, Schadt E, et al. (2002) Gene-microarray analysis of multiple sclerosis lesions yields new targets validated in autoimmune encephalomyelitis. Nat Med 8: 500-508.
41. Zavala F, Abad S, Ezine S, Taupin V, Masson A, et al. (2002) G-CSF therapy of ongoing experimental allergic encephalomyelitis via chemokine- and cytokine-based immune deviation. J Immunol 168: 2011-2019.
42. Kovac A, Erickson MA, Banks WA (2011) Brain microvascular pericytes are immunoactive in culture: cytokine, chemokine, nitric oxide, and LRP-1 expression in response to lipopolysaccharide. J Neuroinflammation 8: 139.

5

Effects of Prenatal Testosterone Exposure on Sexually Dimorphic Gene Expression in the Neonatal Mouse Cortex and Hippocampus

Chris Armoskus, Thomas Mota, Debbie Moreira and Houng-Wei Tsai*

Department of Biological Sciences, California State University Long Beach, Long Beach, CA 90840, USA

***Corresponding author:** Houng-Wei Tsai, Department of Biological Sciences, California State University Long Beach, 1250 Bellflower Boulevard, Long Beach, CA 90840-3702, USA, E-mail: Houng-Wei.Tsai@csulb.edu

Abstract

Objective: Using gene expression microarrays and reverse transcription with quantitative polymerase chain reaction (RT-qPCR), we have recently identified several novel genes that are differentially expressed in the neonatal male versus female mouse cortex/hippocampus (Armoskus et al.). Since perinatal testosterone (T) secreted by the developing testes masculinizes cortical and hippocampal structures and the behaviors regulated by these brain regions, we hypothesized that sexually dimorphic expression of specific selected genes in these areas might be regulated by T during early development.

Methods: To test our hypothesis, we treated timed pregnant female mice daily with vehicle or testosterone propionate (TP) starting on embryonic day 16 until the day of birth. The cortex/hippocampus was collected from vehicle- and TP-treated, male and female neonatal pups. Total RNA was extracted from these brain tissues, followed by RT-qPCR to measure relative mRNA levels of seven sex chromosome genes and three autosomal genes that have previously showed sex differences.

Results: The effect of prenatal TP was confirmed as it stimulated Dhcr24 expression in the neonatal mouse cortex/hippocampus and increased the anogenital distance in females. We found a significant effect of sex, but not TP, on expression of three Y-linked (*Ddx3y*, *Eif2s3y*, and *Kdm5d*), four X-linked (*Eif2s3x*, *Kdm6a*, *Mid1*, and *Xist*), and one autosomal (*Klk8*) genes in the neonatal mouse cortex/hippocampus.

Conclusion: Although most of the selected genes are not directly regulated by prenatal T, their sexually dimorphic expression might play an important role in the control of sexually differentiated cognitive and social behaviors as well as in the etiology of sex-biased neurological disorders and mental illnesses.

Keywords: Androgenization; Cerebral cortex; Hippocampus; Sex-biased gene; Sex chromosome; Sexual differentiation; Testosterone

Introduction

In many species, including mice and humans, sexual differentiation is essential for the development of distinct brain structure and function between the sexes [1-4]. Besides physiological functions, sex differences are also noted in the prevalence and symptomatology of many neurological diseases and mental illnesses, such as depression, schizophrenia, and autism [5-8]. Therefore, determination of the mechanisms controlling sexual dimorphism in brain structure and function will enhance our understanding of the underlying causes of the sex bias in neurological disorders and assist development of new treatments for these diseases.

Similar to humans, sexual differentiation in mice is determined by the two sex chromosomes: embryos receiving two X chromosomes become females and those with one X and one Y chromosome develop as males. During early embryogenesis, the *Sry* gene in the sex determining region of the Y chromosome encodes a transcription factor expressed in male undifferentiated gonads to induce testicular development [9]. The developing testes secrete testosterone (T) with two perinatal peaks; one occurring around 16-17 days after conception (embryonic days 16 and 17, E16 and E17) and the other peaking a couple of hours after birth [10-12]. The rises in circulating T during the late gestation and immediately after birth are essential for masculinization and/or defeminization of certain behaviors and their underlying neural circuits (organizational effect) [10,13].

To masculinize brain structures and behaviors, T acts directly on androgen receptor (AR) and/or indirectly on estrogen receptors (ERs) via local aromatization of T to estradiol (E2) [3,14,15]. While the effects of estrogens on the developing brain are one of the primary controls of masculinization in rodents, they are less important in human masculinization [16]. ARs and ERs are abundant in the rodent brain, including the cortex and hippocampus [17-20], and functional steroid receptors are important for sex differences in many of the cognitive and social behaviors controlled by these brain regions, such as learning and memory [1,2,21].

Structural differences in male and female cortex and hippocampus are associated with distinct behavioral phenotypes between the sexes. In adult mice, males possess a thicker cortex than females, and this difference depends on circulating hormones, not on sex chromosomes [22]. The rat hippocampus shows increased neurogenesis during the first week of life, which is associated with T exposure [23]. However, the molecular mechanisms underlying the actions of sex steroids on sex differences in expression of downstream target genes remain unclear [24,25].

We have previously observed sex differences in histone modifications in the mouse cortex/hippocampus with more H3 acetylation on K9/14 (H3K9/14Ac) in males around embryonic day 18 (E18) and the day of birth (PN0) and more H3 trimethylation on K9 (H3K9Me3) in males around PN0 and 6 days after birth (PN6) [26]. Sex differences in H3K9/14Ac were regulated by T as a significant increase in H3K9/14Ac, but not H3K9Me3, was found in prenatally T-treated female neonates. Since transcriptional regulation of brain-specific genes by histone modifications is associated with changes in neural function and behavior in mice and rats [27-29], our findings suggest that T might alter gene expression in the mouse brain around the time of birth.

Using gene expression microarrays with reverse transcription quantitative polymerase chain reaction, we have recently identified a group of sex-biased genes expressed in the neonatal mouse cortex/hippocampus [30]. Based on the organizational effect of T on brain sexual differentiation, we hypothesized that some of these sexually dimorphic genes might be regulated by perinatal T, leading to the development of distinct neural functions and behaviors between the sexes. To test our hypothesis, we determined mRNA levels of three Y-linked (*Ddx3y*, *Eif2s3y*, and *Kdm5d*), four X-linked (*Eif2s3x*, *Kdm6a*, *Mid1*, and *Xist*), and four autosomal genes (*Dab2*, *Dhcr24*, *Klk8*, and *Prkdc*) in the cortex/hippocampus of newborn mice prenatally treated with testosterone propionate (TP).

Sex-biased expression of most sex chromosome genes studied here has been previously observed in the whole brain of embryonic, neonatal, and adult mice, and sex differences in their expression might be dependent on the sex chromosomal complement, rather than on gonadal hormones [31-34]. However, no experiment has been conducted in the neonatal cortex/hippocampus to investigate the direct effect of T on their expression, particularly in prenatally androgenized mice. Kumamoto and Oshio (2013) showed that fetal exposure of female mice to bisphenol A (BPA) disrupted X-chromosome inactivation by reducing *Xist* expression in the cerebrum [35]. Based on the weak estrogenic transcriptional activities of BPA, it may be hypothesized that prenatal T, locally converted to E2 by aromatase, alters *Xist* expression to regulate other X-linked gene expression in the neonatal mouse cortex/hippocampus. Therefore, to investigate a possible role of T in the regulation of sexual dimorphism in gene expression, we included seven sex chromosome genes along with four autosomal genes.

Materials and Methods

Animals

Adult male and female C57BL/6J mice were purchased from the Jackson Laboratory (Bar Harbor, ME) and housed in the Animal Care Facility at California State University, Long Beach (CSULB). Mice were kept on a 12:12 light-dark cycle (lights on at 0600). Harlan Teklad LM-485 Mouse/Rat Sterilizable Diet (#7012; Madison, WI) and water were provided ad libitum. Neonatal pups used in these studies were generated by breeding the adult mice. After pairing with a male, the females were examined daily, and the day on which a mating plug was observed was designated as embryonic day 0 (E0). Males were removed during late gestation (E14-E17). All experimental procedures were approved by CSULB Institutional Animal Care and Use Committee in accordance with Association for Assessment and Accreditation of Laboratory Animal Care International (AAALAC) guidelines.

Experimental design

Beginning on E16, pregnant female mice were treated daily with subcutaneous injections of vehicle (0.05 ml sesame oil) or TP (100 μg dissolved in 0.05 ml sesame oil; Sigma-Aldrich, St. Louis, MO). On the day of birth (PN0), neonatal pups (n=11 per sex per treatment) were sacrificed by decapitation. All pups were randomly selected from nine litters produced by seven dams (2-6 pups per litter). Vehicle-treated male and female neonates came from four (two male-dominant and two female-dominant) and five (three female-dominant and two male-dominant) litters, respectively. TP-treated males were collected from four litters (two female-dominant and two male-dominant) while TP-treated females were from three litters (two female-dominant and one male-dominant). The brains were immediately removed and coronally blocked between 2.55 mm and 4.95 mm from the most rostral end based on the Atlas of the Developing Mouse Brain at E17.5, P0, and, P6 [36]. The top half of the block, including the cerebral cortex and hippocampus, was dissected out, frozen on dry ice, and stored at -80°C until processing for RNA extraction. Expression of selected sexually dimorphic genes was quantified by RT-qPCR. The sex of the pups was determined first by examining the presence of pigmentation in the anogenital regions; males showed a pigment spot over the scrotum whereas females lacked pigmentation [37]. Testes were then dissected out from the males to further confirm their sex. In addition, the anogenital distance (AGD) was measured from these neonates to determine masculinization effects of TP on peripheral tissue. Using digital calipers, two measurements were taken under magnification: one from the top of the anus to the bottom of the genitalia (inner distance), and a second from the bottom of anus to the top of the genitalia (outer distance). Measurements were averaged and subjected to statistical analysis.

RNA extraction and cDNA synthesis

Total RNA was extracted from the mouse cortex/hippocampus using the RNeasy® Lipid Tissue Mini kit (Qiagen, Valencia, CA) according to the manufacturer's protocol. Using a Bio-Rad SmartSpec™ Plus spectrophotometer (Hercules, CA), the RNA concentration of each sample (1:50 dilution in 10 mM Tris, pH = 7.5) was determined by measuring the absorbance at 260 nm (A260), and its purity was determined by the ratio of the absorbance measured at 260 nm (A260) and 280 nm (A280). The ratios of A260/A280 between 1.9 and 2.1 were considered acceptable [38]. The cDNA templates were synthesized from 1 μg extracted RNA in 20-μl reactions using the Bio-Rad iScript™ cDNA synthesis kit with a mix of oligo(dT) and random hexamer primers. The reverse transcription was performed at 25°C for 5 min, 42°C for 30 min, and 85°C for 5 min in a Bio-Rad MyCycler™ thermocycler.

PCR primer design and testing

We first looked through the literature and Harvard PrimerBank (http://pga.mgh.harvard.edu/primerbank/) to find PCR primers for selected genes. In the absence of found primers, new primers were designed and checked for their suitability using the Primer3 program (http://primer3.wi.mit.edu/). Primers were checked for specificity using NCBI's Primer-BLAST program (http://www.ncbi.nlm.nih.gov/tools/primer-blast/) against RefSeq RNA to ensure no non-specific matches. When designing primers that could match multiple transcript variants, their sequences were aligned in ClustalW (http://www.genome.jp/tools/clustalw/), and only the primers that amplified a consensus region were used.

Gene Symbol	RefSeq Accession	Forward Primer (5'-3')	Reverse Primer (5'-3')	Product Size (bp)	Annealing Temperature (°C)
Actb*	NM_007393.3	CCAGATCATGTTTGAGACCTTCAA	CCAGAGGCATACAGGGACAGC	78	59
Dab2	NM_001008702.2	TCATTCTCCCTATGGCTTGG	GCTGAGCAGAATCCAGTTCC	83	60
Ddx3y	NM_012008.2	GGGTCTGTGATAAGGACAGTTCA	CACGACCACCAATACCATCATAG	177	60
Dhcr24	NM_053272.2	CTCTGGGTGCGAGTGAAGG	TTCCCGGACCTGTTTCTGGAT	195	60
Eif2s3x	NM_012010.3	GGTGAGGGTGGAGTGACTCT	TTCCCATGAGCTACGTGACCA	152	60
Eif2s3y	NM_012011.1	GGTGCTGTTGGAGCATTACC	TCAACTCGTCGGCTTAGAGC	269	58
Kdm5d	NM_011419.3	CCAGGATCTGACGACTTTCTACC	TTCTCCGCAATGGGTCTGATT	113	58
Kdm6a	NM_009483.1	CGGGCGGACAAAAGAAGAAC	CATAGACTTGCATCAGATCCTCC	203	60
Klk8	NM_008940.2	GATCCTGGAAGGTCGAGAGTG	CTGCTCCGGCTGATCTCTG	193	58
Mid1	NM_183151.1	CTGTGACGGCACCTGTCTC	AAACGGCTGACTGTTGGTCTT	205	58
Prkdc	NM_011159.2	CTGTGACGGCACCTGTCTC	TCTCAATCTGAGGACGAATTGC	203	58
Rpl13a*	NM_009438.5	ATGAGGTCGGGTGGAAGTACC	CAGGAGTCCGTTGGTCTTGAG	179	62
Xist	NR_001570.2	GCTGGTTCGTCTATCTTGTGGG	GGATCCTGCACTGGATGAGT	225	58

Table 1: List of the PCR primer sequences. *indicates a reference/housekeeping gene.

All PCR primers were purchased from Eurofins MWG Operon (Huntsville, AL) and listed in Table 1 with the annealing temperatures and sizes of the resulting PCR products in base pairs (bp).

All primers were tested to ensure suitability for PCR amplification using GoTaq® Hot Start Green Master Mix (Promega, Madison, WI) according to the manufacturers' protocol for 40 cycles. Initial tests used an annealing temperature of 2°C below the lower melting temperature of the two the primers. PCR reactions were conducted on two or three independent samples, with at least one male and one female sample, along with a negative, no template control (NTC). PCR products were run on a 1.5 % agarose gel, visualized by ethidium bromide staining, and compared to a 100bp DNA ladder (Fisher Scientific, Pittsburgh, PA). Primers were rejected as unsuitable for quantification if they featured multiple products, no products, visible product in the NTC, or a product that was not of the size predicted based on RefSeq transcripts.

Four dilution stocks were prepared, two from PN0 male cortex/hippocampus cDNA and two from PN0 females, with 8 serial dilutions ranging from 1:8 to 1:1024, dilution being measured from the output of cDNA synthesis. Reactions include 4 μl of sample at a specific dilution, 1 μl each of forward and reverse primers at 840 nM, and 6 μl of ABsolute™ QPCR SYBR® Green Mix (Waltham, MA). Reactions were run on an Agilent Stratagene® MX3000P™ qPCR system with MxPro QPCR software (Santa Clara, CA) used for determining cycle of threshold (Ct)-values. Reactions were run with an initial 15 min denaturation/polymerase-activation step at 95°C, followed by 40 cycles of 15 s at 95°C, 1 min at the annealing temperature, and 30 s at 72°C; qPCR amplification was followed by a dissociation step with 1 min at 95°C, 30 s at 60°C, and 30 s at 95°C. Results were analyzed by linear regression with log base 2 of the dilution as the predictor and Ct of the reaction as the response. Primers were rejected as unsuitable for quantification if the average R2 of the regression was below 0.95, Ct values at the 1:16 dilution were above 30, or the dissociation curve showed multiple peaks.

RT-qPCR

RT-qPCR was conducted to measure relative mRNA levels under the same conditions as described in the dilution tests, with the sample in the reaction being 4 μl of 1:16 diluted cDNA along with a no-template control which used water in place of cDNA sample. Two replicate reactions for each sample were run and their Ct values averaged before further analysis. For a given sample unnormalized relative quantification (RQ) values for gene expression were calculated using Pfaffl's method against a baseline of vehicle-treated females for all cases except Y chromosome genes; for Y chromosome genes a baseline of vehicle-treated males was used [39,40]. RQ values of the target gene were divided by the geometric mean of the RQ values of the two stable reference genes (*Actb* and *Rpl13a*) to yield normalized relative quantification (NRQ) values [41]. NRQ values more than two standard deviations from their group mean were trimmed to two standard deviations from the group mean in the same direction. NRQ values were used as measurements of gene expression and subjected to statistical testing.

Statistical analyses

The data from individual groups were first tested for normality of the residuals by the Anderson-Darling test and next tested for equality of variances using Levene's test; if significant deviations were detected ($p<0.05$), a log transformation was applied to the data. After showing normality and homogeneity of variances, the data were then analyzed by two-way ANOVA to evaluate the effects of sex, TP treatment, and their interaction. When two-way ANOVA showed significant interactions, Tukey's post-hoc test was used to determine which groups were significantly different. If the variances were not homogeneous after log transformation, Bonferroni corrected t-tests were performed for multiple comparisons. For Y-chromosome genes, due to deviations from normality in female samples, Kruskal-Wallis was run to compare all four groups, followed by a two-tailed, two-sample t-test to compare vehicle-treated and TP-treated males. Analyses were run in Minitab. Data are shown as mean±SEM.

Results

Mouse body weight, tissue weight, and RNA yield

No significant sex differences in mean body weight, tissue weight, or RNA yield were observed among vehicle- and TP-treated, male and female neonatal mice (Table 2). Interestingly, a significant effect of TP treatment was found on brain tissue weight, with greater cortex/hippocampus weight in TP-treated mice than vehicle-treated controls ($p = 0.022$). However, the tissue weight difference was reversed in RNA yields, as total RNA amounts extracted from TP-treated samples tended to be lower than vehicle-treated controls ($p = 0.067$).

Effect of prenatal TP on AGD

Two-way ANOVA of mean AGD of the neonatal mice receiving prenatal treatment of vehicle or TP revealed significant effects of sex ($p<0.001$), treatment ($p = 0.005$), and their interaction ($p = 0.021$) (Figure 1). TP had no effect on AGD in males, but significantly increased AGD (16%) in females, from 1.62 ± 0.02 mm (vehicle, n = 7) to 1.88 ± 0.02 mm (TP, n = 10) ($p<0.001$). Although the AGD of TP-treated females remained significantly shorter than vehicle-treated males ($p<0.001$), prenatal exposure of female mice to TP during late gestation resulted in partial masculinization of their external genitalia.

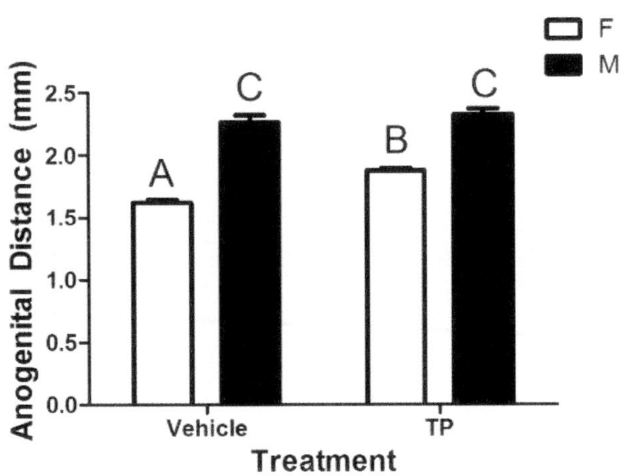

Figure 1: Anogenital distance measurements of neonatal female (F) and male (M) mice prenatally treated with either vehicle or testosterone propionate (TP). Different letters indicate significant differences between two groups based on post-hoc Tukey's test ($p<0.05$). Bars are mean±SEM.

Effect of prenatal TP on Y chromosome gene expression in the neonatal cortex/hippocampus

TP administration had no effect on expression of the three Y chromosome genes, *Ddx3y*, *Eif2s3y*, and *Kdm5d* in the cortex/hippocampus of neonatal mice. Regardless of TP treatment, the three Y-linked genes were exclusively expressed in the cortex/hippocampus of males, not females ($p<0.001$) (Figure 2). In addition, relative mRNA levels of these genes were similar between TP- and vehicle-treated male neonates, indicating that prenatal exposure of male embryos to extra T did not alter Y-linked gene transcription.

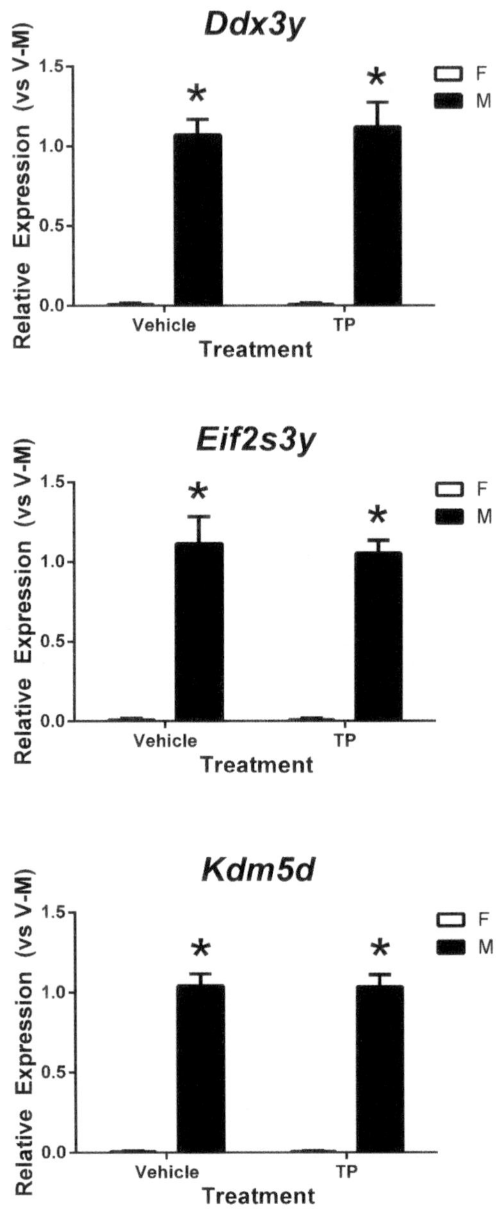

Figure 2: Effects of prenatal testosterone propionate (TP) treatment on relative mRNA levels of three Y chromosome genes in the neonatal female (F) and male (M) mouse cortex/hippocampus measured by RT-qPCR. Gene expression was quantified relative to vehicle-treated male (V-M). * indicates significant difference between females and males ($p<0.05$). Bars are mean±SEM.

Group	N	Mouse Body Weight (g)	Cortex/Hippocampus Weight (mg)	RNA Yield (µg)
Vehicle				
Females	11	1.30 ± 0.04	18.68 ± 1.42	49.73 ± 3.89
Males	11	1.31 ± 0.03	18.38 ± 1.97	39.77 ± 2.23
TP				
Females	11	1.24 ± 0.02	24.09 ± 1.29	36.26 ± 2.50
Males	11	1.25 ± 0.02	22.27 ± 1.70	39.92 ± 5.19

Table 2: Mouse weights, brain tissue weights, and RNA yields in prenatally vehicle- and testosterone propionate (TP)-treated mice. Data are shown as mean±SEM

Effect of prenatal TP on X-linked gene expression in the neonatal mouse cortex/hippocampus

The expression of four X-linked genes (*Xist*, *Eif2s3x*, *Kdm6a*, and *Mid1*) linked or associated with X-chromosome inactivation and with escape from inactivation was greater in the neonatal cortex/hippocampus of females than in males. The greatest difference between the sexes was in expression of *Xist*, which was approximately 2,500-fold higher in female pups regardless of TP treatment ($p<0.001$) (Figure 3, top left panel).

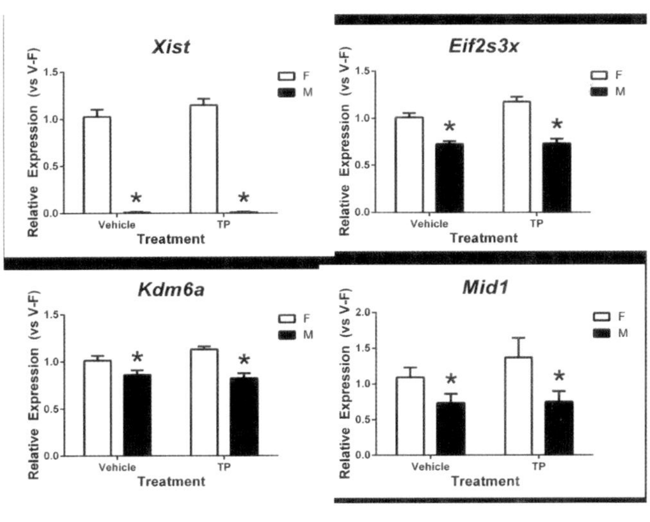

Figure 3: Effects of prenatal testosterone propionate (TP) on expression of four X-linked genes in the neonatal cortex/hippocampus of female (F) and male (M) mice. Gene expression quantified relative to vehicle-treated female (V-F). * indicates significant difference between females and males ($p<0.05$). Bars are mean ± SEM.

In contrast, the other three X-linked genes, *Eif2s3x*, *Kdm6a*, and *Mid1*, were expressed in both sexes, and showed a 1.39-, 1.12- and 1.45-fold higher expression, respectively, in the female cortex/hippocampus compared to that of the male (Figure 3). No significant effect of TP treatment or its interaction with sex on these four X chromosome genes was observed, but interestingly, there was a trend of TP effect on *Eif2s3x* expression ($p = 0.067$) and a 1.25-fold change in *Mid1* mRNA levels of TP-treated females as compared to vehicle-treated controls (1.37 ± 0.29 vs. 1.09 ± 0.14).

Effect of TP on autosomal gene expression in the neonatal mouse cortex/hippocampus

In the neonatal mouse cortex/hippocampus, *Dab2* expression showed no significant effect of sex or TP, but there was a strong interaction ($p = 0.052$) (Figure 4, top panel). In vehicle-treated male mice, *Dab2* mRNA levels (1.19 ± 0.13) increased to 119% of female controls (1.01 ± 0.04); however, this trend was reversed in TP-treated animals with 1.25 times greater expression in females (1.46 ± 0.15) as compared to males (1.16 ± 0.12).

In contrast, *Klk8* expression in the neonatal mouse cortex/hippocampus was sex dependent, and was higher in males than females regardless of treatment ($p = 0.003$) (Figure 4, middle panel). Interestingly, TP treatment seems to enhance the difference in *Klk8* expression between the sexes; TP-treated male pups showed a 1.64-fold increase in *Klk8* expression over TP-treated females while there was only a 1.12-fold change between vehicle-treated male and female mice.

There were no differences in *Prkdc* expression in the neonatal cortex/hippocampus between the sexes ($p = 0.079$), or in response to TP ($p = 0.132$), nor was there an interaction ($p = 0.446$) (Figure 4, bottom panel). Vehicle-treated male mice (1.21 ± 0.10) showed a 1.21-fold increase in *Prkdc* expression as compared to vehicle-treated females (1.01 ± 0.05), and this masculine trend seemed to be dependent on testosterone because increased *Prkdc* mRNA levels were observed in TP-treated females (1.18 ± 0.08).

Unlike the other three autosomal genes shown above, *Dhcr24* showed no hint of sex difference; however, TP treatment significantly increased *Dhcr24* gene expression in the cortex/hippocampus of both male and female pups, with 1.21-fold higher expression in TP-treated mice than in vehicle-treated controls ($p = 0.047$) (Figure 5).

Discussion

AGD is a sexually dimorphic trait that has been used as an anatomical marker of prenatal androgen exposure in both rodents and humans [42-44]. In mice, the AGD is positively correlated with T exposure in utero as it increases and becomes more male-like in female pups when their uterine neighbors are male [45]. In addition, female rats exposed to TP on gestation days 14-18 display increased AGD after birth [46,47]. Further, in utero treatment with flutamide, an androgen receptor antagonist that blocks the action of androgen, decreases the AGD in males on the day of birth [48]. In the current study, the AGD in female pups treated prenatally with TP was intermediate between that of vehicle-treated females and male controls (Figure 1), which is consistent with results obtained in rats [46]. Several factors might contribute to the inability of prenatal TP treatment to fully masculinize the female external genitalia. First, the dose of TP used might increase circulating T to levels intermediate between the low levels characteristic of female fetuses and the higher physiological male levels. Second, TP treatment was initiated 2 days after the testicular development had begun; thus TP-treated female embryos were exposed to T later than males. Last, development of the external genitalia is controlled by a combination of androgen-dependent and -independent mechanisms [49]. Nevertheless, the foregoing results confirm that TP treatment of pregnant dams results in partial masculinization of peripheral genital tissues of their female pups.

The mouse Y chromosome consists of a small pseudoautosomal region (PAR), and the remaining non-recombining region (NRY), which contains 27 protein-coding genes, including *Ddx3y*, *Eif2s3y*, and *Kdm5d* [50]. *Ddx3y* protein is an ATP-dependent RNA helicase with a conserved DEAD (Asp-Glu-Ala-Asp) box motif, and many of the DEAD box proteins are implicated in RNA metabolism, splicing, and translation [51]. *Eif2s3y* encodes subunit 3 of the translation elongation and initiation factor 2 (eIF2), which determines the rate of protein translation [52,53]. *Kdm5d* protein demethylates di- and tri-methylated lysine 4 of histone H3 (H3K4), and di- and tri-methylation of H3K4 are often observed on the active gene promoter associated with increased transcription [54,55]. Since females do not have a Y chromosome, the NRY genes are exclusively expressed in male mouse brains [31-34]. Expression of six NRY genes, including *Ddx3y*, *Eif2s3y*, and *Kdm5d*, was reported to occur exclusively in male embryonic and neonatal brains [31]. This study used the four core genotypes (FCG) mouse model, XX gonadal males (XX*Sry*) and females (XX) as well as XY gonadal males (XY-*Sry*) and females (XY-), thereby demonstrating that neonatal XY− females and XY−*Sry* males both displayed similar mRNA levels of these Y chromosome genes regardless of their gonadal sex. These results indicated that expression of Y-linked genes, such as *Ddx3y*, *Eif2s3y*, and *Kdm5d*, might not be regulated by testicular androgens. The results presented herein not only confirm male-specific expression of *Ddx3y*, *Eif2s3y*, and *Kdm5d* in the neonatal mouse cortex/hippocampus (Figure 2), but also provide direct evidence to support androgen-independent regulation of these Y-linked genes in the male mouse brain.

In contrast to males, that have two distinct sex chromosomes, X and Y, female mammals have two X chromosomes, one of which is transcriptionally silenced by X-inactivation, which equalizes the dosage of X-linked genes between the sexes. Using RNA sequencing in a female diploid Mus musculus×Mus spretus cell line, 13 X-linked genes, including *Eif2s3x*, *Kdm6a*, *Mid1*, and *Xist*, are found to be transcribed from the inactive X chromosome while most genes on the inactive X are silenced [56]. *Eif2s3x*, *Kdm6a*, and *Xist* have also been confirmed as X escape genes in the neonatal mouse brain [57]. The *Xist* gene encodes a large untranslated RNA responsible for mediating X inactivation [58]. Because *Xist* is only transcribed from the inactive X chromosome, it is expressed at much higher levels in female tissues [32,59]. *Eif2s3x* and *Kdm6a* have functional homologues, *Eif2s3y* and Uty, on the Y chromosome, respectively, so female expression of these two X escape genes is believed to balance their gene products between the sexes [31,60,61]. *Eif2s3x* encodes subunit three of eIF2 and is nearly identical to its homologous Y-linked copy, *Eif2s3y* [62]. *Kdm6a* encodes a histone lysine demethylase that removes methylation at lysine 27 of histone H3 (H3K27), an epigenetic mark linked to gene repression [63,64]. In humans, *KDM6A* gene mutations are associated with Kabuki syndrome, a rare genetic disease with developmental delay, mild to moderate intellectual disability, and postnatal growth retardation [65]. The *Mid1* gene was shown to span the PAR boundary of the mouse X and Y chromosomes, with its first three exons in the X-unique region and the remaining 7 exons in the PAR [66]. Since the three most 5' exons are required for its transcription, *Mid1* is only expressed from the X, not the Y, chromosome, yielding female-biased expression of Mid1. In mice, lack of Mid1 disrupts the specification of the midbrain/cerebellar boundary, resulting in an abnormal development of the most anterior cerebellar lobes [67]. In humans, *MID1* mutation has been identified as responsible for the X-linked form of Opitz G/BBB syndrome, characterized by facial anomalies, laryngotracheoesophageal defects, and genitourinary abnormalities [68,69].

The current results confirm female-biased expression of *Xist*, *Eif2s3x*, *Kdm6a*, and *Mid1*, consistent with our previous study [30]. In addition, they demonstrate that their expression is not dependent on prenatal TP levels, indicating that in the neonatal mouse cortex/hippocampus, these four X-linked genes are mainly regulated by X-chromosomal gene dosage, rather than sex steroids (Figure 3). Our results are supported by a recent study using the Y* mouse model with four different genotypes, normal XX females (XX), 1X females, (XY*X), 2X males (XXY*), and 1X males (XY*) [33]. Expression of *Eif2s3x*, *Kdm6a*, and *Xist* in the whole brains of 2X mouse embryos (XX and XXY*) was greater than that in 1X embryos (XY*X and XY*) and was independent of their gonads. In the same study, there was no sexual dimorphism in *Mid1* expression in embryonic mouse brains. Mid1 is located in the PAR of the mouse X and Y chromosomes, and the chromosomal rearrangement of this region in the Y* mouse might disrupt its differential expression between the sexes.

In contrast to the study by Kumamoto and Oshio (2013), prenatal TP treatment had no effect on *Xist* mRNA levels in females, suggesting that AR or ERs may not involve regulation of *Xist* expression and that suppression of *Xist* expression by BPA might be mediated by other receptor systems and molecular targets. In addition, *Eif2s3x*, *Kdm6a*, and *Mid1* are transcribed from both the active and inactive X chromosomes, and based on the <2-fold difference in expression between the sexes, we speculate that there are unequal transcription rates from the two alleles of these X escape genes in the neonatal female cortex/hippocampus. Interestingly, among these three genes, a trend of increased *Eif2s3x* mRNA levels was elicited by prenatal TP (Figure 3), implying that X escape gene expression might be modulated by sex steroids and their receptors during early development. The potential hormonal regulation of *Eif2s3x* expression by sex steroids is in part supported by the presence of a potential estrogen responsive element (ERE) located within a 1 kb region down-stream of its transcription start site (unpublished observation).

The autosomal gene, *Dab2*, encodes a novel phosphoprotein and in the developing CNS, its expression is primarily restricted to secretory cells, immature neuroepithelial cells, endothelial cells, and in populations of mononuclear phagocytes [70]. *Dab2* is up-regulated in degenerated rat ventral prostate by androgen deprivation [71], suggesting that its expression in brain might be dependent on T. The *Klk8* (kallikrein related-peptidase 8) gene, located on mouse chromosome 7, encodes a tryptic serine protease that processes extracellular matrix [72,73]. *Klk8* is highly expressed in the mouse brain and concentrated in the hippocampus, anterior olfactory nucleus, septal nuclei, diagonal band of Broca, amygdala, and limbic cortex [74]. *Klk8* knockout mice show aberrant synapse formation in the hippocampus, suppression of long-term potentiation, and impaired spatial memory [75-77] as well as increased anxiety [78]. *Prkdc* is found on mouse chromosome 16 and encodes the catalytic subunit of the DNA-dependent protein kinase, which is involved in DNA double strand break repair and cell death induced by DNA damage [79,80]. *Prkdc* knockout mice show increased germ cell apoptosis that leads to testicular degeneration [81]. In addition, double knockout of *Prkdc* together with Atm (ataxia telangiectasia mutated homolog) leads to lethality tied to greatly increased apoptosis of postmitotic neurons, suggesting an important role in neurodevelopment [82].

Among the four autosomal genes tested in the present study, we confirmed male-biased expression of *Klk8* in the neonatal mouse cortex/hippocampus (Figure 4).

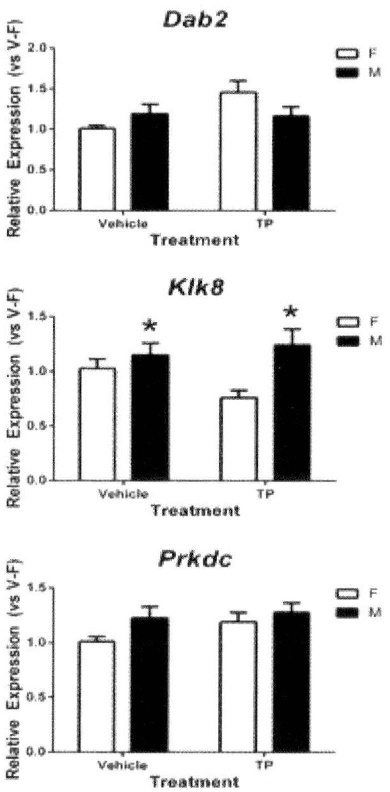

Figure 4: Effects of prenatal testosterone propionate (TP) treatment on expression of three autosomal genes in the neonatal female (F) and male (M) mouse cortex/hippocampus. Gene expression was normalized relative to the average of vehicled-treated female (V-F). *indicates significant difference between females and males ($p<0.05$). Bars are mean ± SEM.

Although sex differences in *Dab2* and *Prkdc* mRNA levels were insignificant, vehicle-treated male mice displayed an approximate 20% increase in their expression as compared to females (18% for *Dab2* and 21% for *Prkdc*), showing a trend toward male bias with the fold changes comparable to those we observed previously [30]. This variability between studies could be due to the sample size as we used fewer animals per group (n=10-11) in the current study than previously (n=16-18) to accommodate the 96-well qPCR platform, which might render our results underpowered to detect the sex difference. In addition, although prenatal TP treatment did not change mRNA levels of these three genes in the neonatal mouse cortex/hippocampus, but the interactions between sex and TP treatment for expression of both *Dab2* ($p = 0.052$) and *Klk8* ($p = 0.051$) approached significance, strongly suggesting that these genes might be partially modulated or influenced by prenatal TP. One possible explanation for this observation is the heterogeneity of cell types in the cortex and hippocampus. Immunoreactivity for intracellular AR is abundant in the adult rat cerebral cortex, but limited to the pyramidal neurons within layers II/III and V/VI [83]. This finding suggests that the action of T on gene expression might occur specifically within sub-populations of cortical or hippocampal cells, rather than globally throughout the entire brain, which may mask the significance of T on expression of the autosomal genes.

To determine whether prenatal TP treatment exerts an effect on brain *Dhcr24*, we assessed mRNA levels of *Dhcr24* in the cortex/hippocampus of vehicle- and TP-treated neonates. *Dhcr24* encodes 3-beta-hydroxysterol delta-24-reductase, which converts desmosterol to cholesterol [84]. *Dhcr24* also mediates anti-apoptotic and anti-oxidative activities by inhibiting the activation of caspase 3, one of the key modulators of apoptosis, and binding to p53 to displace Mdm2, resulting in p53, a tumor suppressor, accumulation [85]. *Dhcr24* gene is activated by ER in neurons and glia cells [86] and by AR in prostate cells [87] and rat glioma C6 cells [88]. The androgen-responsiveness of *Dhcr24* may be mediated by the direct action of AR because an androgen responsive element (ARE) is present in the human *DHCR24* promoter (-4384 to -2892 bp) [87]. In the present study, we found no sex difference in *Dhcr24* mRNA levels of the neonatal mouse cortex/hippocampus, but its expression was increased by prenatal TP treatment in both sexes (Figure 5), confirming that *Dhcr24* is an androgen-regulated gene. The lack of a sex difference in *Dhcr24* mRNA levels might be due to insufficient secretion of endogenous T by the developing testes.

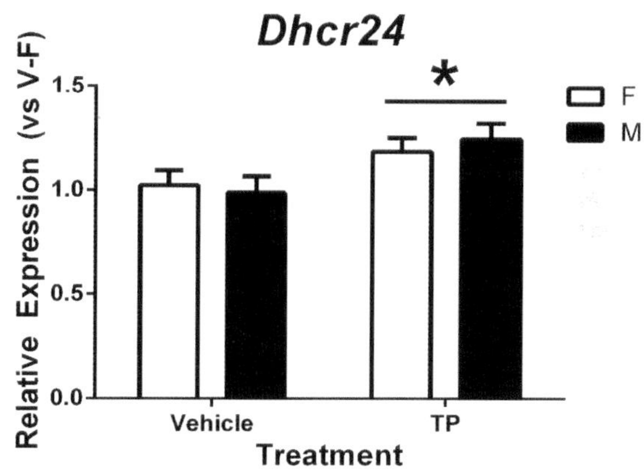

Figure 5: Effects of prenatal testosterone propionate (TP) treatment on relative mRNA levels of *Dhcr24* in the neonatal female (F) and male (M) mouse cortex/hippocampus. Gene expression quantified by RT-qPCR relative to vehicle-treated female (V-F). *indicates significant difference between vehicle and TP treatment ($p<0.05$). Bars are mean ± SEM.

In summary, we have confirmed sex differentiated expression of seven sex chromosome genes (*Ddx3y*, *Eif2s3y*, *Eif2s3x*, *Kdm5d*, *Kdm6a*, *Mid1*, and *Xist*) and one autosomal gene (*Klk8*) in the neonatal mouse cortex/hippocampus, and demonstrated that their expression is not regulated by T during late gestation. Further, our results suggest that expression of these genes is elicited mainly by the actions of the sex chromosomes which thereby genetically program the cortex and hippocampus, ultimately resulting in sexual dimorphism in social and cognitive behaviors as well as in the underlying neural circuits. In addition, based on trends of altered expression in some of the above genes and the presence of steroid receptors in subpopulations of cortical and hippocampal cells, future studies will focus on the roles of these genes in cells expressing AR and/or ERs.

Acknowledgements

We thank Courtney Donovan, Michelle Thai, and Kathy Trang for their technical assistance. The authors are also grateful to Dr. Sandra Legan for her valuable comments and suggestions that help improve this manuscript. This work was supported by California State University Program for Education and Research in Biotechnology (CSUPERB) Faculty-Student Collaborative Research Seed Grant, and National Institutes of Health Grants SC3GM102051 and R25GM0500089.

References

1. Frick KM, Gresack JE (2003) Sex differences in the behavioral response to spatial and object novelty in adult C57BL/6 mice. Behav Neurosci 117: 1283-1291.
2. Sutcliffe JS, Marshall KM, Neill JC (2007) Influence of gender on working and spatial memory in the novel object recognition task in the rat. Behav Brain Res 177: 117-125.
3. Hines M (2006) Prenatal testosterone and gender-related behaviour. Eur J Endocrinol 155 Suppl 1: S115-121.
4. Bonthuis PJ, Cox KH, Searcy BT, Kumar P, Tobet S, et al. (2010) Of mice and rats: key species variations in the sexual differentiation of brain and behavior. Front Neuroendocrinol 31: 341-358.
5. Baron-Cohen S, Knickmeyer RC, Belmonte MK (2005) Sex differences in the brain: implications for explaining autism. Science 310: 819-823.
6. Deng Z, Sobell JL, Knowles JA (2010) Epigenetic alterations in schizophrenia. 8: 358-365.
7. Amenson CS, Lewinsohn PM (1981) An investigation into the observed sex difference in prevalence of unipolar depression. J Abnorm Psychol 90: 1-13.
8. Conley CS, Rudolph KD (2009) The emerging sex difference in adolescent depression: interacting contributions of puberty and peer stress. Dev Psychopathol 21: 593-620.
9. Kopsida E, Stergiakouli E, Lynn PM, Wilkinson LS, Davies W (2009) The Role of the Y Chromosome in Brain Function. Open Neuroendocrinol J 2: 20-30.
10. Motelica-Heino I, Castanier M, Corbier P, Edwards DA, Roffi J (1988) Testosterone levels in plasma and testes of neonatal mice. J Steroid Biochem 31: 283-286.
11. Ward IL, Ward OB, Affuso JD, Long WD 3rd, French JA, et al. (2003) Fetal testosterone surge: specific modulations induced in male rats by maternal stress and/or alcohol consumption. Horm Behav 43: 531-539.
12. Vom Saal FS, Bronson FH (1980) Sexual characteristics of adult female mice are correlated with their blood testosterone levels during prenatal development. Science 208: 597-599.
13. Phoenix CH, Goy RW, Gerall AA, Young WC (1959) Organizing action of prenatally administered testosterone propionate on the tissues mediating mating behavior in the female guinea pig. Endocrinology 65: 369-382.
14. Davis EC, Popper P, Gorski RA (1996) The role of apoptosis in sexual differentiation of the rat sexually dimorphic nucleus of the preoptic area. Brain Res 734: 10-18.
15. Forger NG (2009) Control of cell number in the sexually dimorphic brain and spinal cord. J Neuroendocrinol 21: 393-399.
16. Morris JA, Jordan CL, Breedlove SM (2004) Sexual differentiation of the vertebrate nervous system. Nat Neurosci 7: 1034-1039.
17. Shughrue PJ, Merchenthaler I (2001) Distribution of estrogen receptor beta immunoreactivity in the rat central nervous system. J Comp Neurol 436: 64-81.
18. Lu SF, McKenna SE, Cologer-Clifford A, Nau EA, Simon NG (1998) Androgen receptor in mouse brain: sex differences and similarities in autoregulation. Endocrinology 139: 1594-1601.
19. Shah NM, Pisapia DJ, Maniatis S, Mendelsohn MM, Nemes A, et al. (2004) Visualizing sexual dimorphism in the brain. Neuron 43: 313-319.
20. DonCarlos LL, Sarkey S, Lorenz B, Azcoitia I, Garcia-Ovejero D, et al. (2006) Novel cellular phenotypes and subcellular sites for androgen action in the forebrain. Neuroscience 138: 801-807.
21. Rizk A, Robertson J, Raber J (2005) Behavioral performance of tfm mice supports the beneficial role of androgen receptors in spatial learning and memory. Brain Res 1034: 132-138.
22. Markham JA, Jurgens HA, Auger CJ, De Vries GJ, Arnold AP, et al. (2003) Sex differences in mouse cortical thickness are independent of the complement of sex chromosomes. Neuroscience 116: 71-75.
23. Zhang JM, Konkle AT, Zup SL, McCarthy MM (2008) Impact of sex and hormones on new cells in the developing rat hippocampus: a novel source of sex dimorphism? Eur J Neurosci 27: 791-800.
24. Kerr JE, Allore RJ, Beck SG, Handa RJ (1995) Distribution and hormonal regulation of androgen receptor (AR) and AR messenger ribonucleic acid in the rat hippocampus. Endocrinology 136: 3213-3221.
25. Ivanova T, Beyer C (2000) Ontogenetic expression and sex differences of aromatase and estrogen receptor-alpha/beta mRNA in the mouse hippocampus. Cell Tissue Res 300: 231-237.
26. Tsai HW, Grant PA, Rissman EF (2009) Sex differences in histone modifications in the neonatal mouse brain. Epigenetics 4: 47-53.
27. Forger NG, Rosen GJ, Waters EM, Jacob D, Simerly RB, et al. (2004) Deletion of Bax eliminates sex differences in the mouse forebrain. Proc Natl Acad Sci U S A 101: 13666-13671.
28. McCarthy MM, Auger AP, Bale TL, De Vries GJ, Dunn GA, et al. (2009) The epigenetics of sex differences in the brain. J Neurosci 29: 12815-12823.
29. Murray EK, Hien A, de Vries GJ, Forger NG (2009) Epigenetic control of sexual differentiation of the bed nucleus of the stria terminalis. Endocrinology 150: 4241-4247.
30. Armoskus C, Moreira D, Bollinger K, Jimenez O, Taniguchi S, et al. (2014) Identification of sexually dimorphic genes in the neonatal mouse cortex and hippocampus. Brain Res 1562: 23-38.
31. Xu J, Burgoyne PS, Arnold AP (2002) Sex differences in sex chromosome gene expression in mouse brain. Hum Mol Genet 11: 1409-1419.
32. Dewing P, Shi T, Horvath S, Vilain E (2003) Sexually dimorphic gene expression in mouse brain precedes gonadal differentiation. Brain Res Mol Brain Res 118: 82-90.
33. Wolstenholme JT, Rissman EF, Bekiranov S (2013) Sexual differentiation in the developing mouse brain: contributions of sex chromosome genes. Genes Brain Behav 12: 166-180.
34. Yan HX, Yang W, Zhang R, Chen L, Tang L, et al. (2006) Protein-tyrosine phosphatase PCP-2 inhibits beta-catenin signaling and increases E-cadherin-dependent cell adhesion. J Biol Chem 281: 15423-15433.
35. Kumamoto T, Oshio S (2013) Effect of fetal exposure to bisphenol A on brain mediated by X-chromosome inactivation. J Toxicol Sci 38: 485-494.
36. Paxinos G, Halliday G, Watson C, Koutcherov Y, Wang H (2007) Atlas of the Developing Mouse Brain at E17.5, P0, and P6. Academic Press, Burlington, MA 01803, USA.
37. Wolterink-Donselaar IG, Meerding JM, Fernandes C (2009) A method for gender determination in newborn dark pigmented mice. Lab Anim (NY) 38: 35-38.
38. White P (2004) Evaluating Concentration and Purity of RNA. University of Pennsylvania - Functional Genomics Core: 1-2.
39. Pfaffl MW (2001) A new mathematical model for relative quantification in real-time RT-PCR. Nucleic Acids Res 29: e45.
40. Hellemans J, Mortier G, De Paepe A, Speleman F, Vandesompele J (2007) qBase relative quantification framework and software for management and automated analysis of real-time quantitative PCR data. Genome Biol 8: R19.

41. Vandesompele J, De Preter K, Pattyn F, Poppe B, Van Roy N, et al. (2002) Accurate normalization of real-time quantitative RT-PCR data by geometric averaging of multiple internal control genes. Genome Biol 3: RESEARCH0034.
42. Faber K, Hughes C (1992) Anogenital distance at birth as a predictor of volume of the sexually dimorphic nucleus of the preoptic area of the hypothalamus and pituitary responsiveness in castrated adult rats. Biol Reprod 46: 101-104.
43. Graham S, Gandelman R (1986) The expression of ano-genital distance data in the mouse. Physiol Behav 36: 103-104.
44. Dean A, Sharpe RM (2013) Clinical review: Anogenital distance or digit length ratio as measures of fetal androgen exposure: relationship to male reproductive development and its disorders. J Clin Endocrinol Metab 98: 2230-2238.
45. Hurd PL, Bailey AA, Gongal PA, Yan RH, Greer JJ, et al. (2008) Intrauterine position effects on anogenital distance and digit ratio in male and female mice. Arch Sex Behav 37: 9-18.
46. Hotchkiss AK, Lambright CS, Ostby JS, Parks-Saldutti L, Vandenbergh JG, et al. (2007) Prenatal Testosterone Exposure Permanently Masculinizes Anogenital Distance, Nipple Development, and Reproductive Tract Morphology in Female Sprague-Dawley Rats. Toxicological Sciences 96: 335-345.
47. Wolf CJ, Hotchkiss A, Ostby JS, LeBlanc GA, Gray LE Jr (2002) Effects of prenatal testosterone propionate on the sexual development of male and female rats: a dose-response study. Toxicol Sci 65: 71-86.
48. McIntyre BS, Barlow NJ, Foster PM (2001) Androgen-mediated development in male rat offspring exposed to flutamide in utero: permanence and correlation of early postnatal changes in anogenital distance and nipple retention with malformations in androgen-dependent tissues. Toxicol Sci 62: 236-249.
49. Blaschko SD, Cunha GR, Baskin LS (2012) Molecular mechanisms of external genitalia development. Differentiation 84: 261-268.
50. Skaletsky H, Kuroda-Kawaguchi T, Minx PJ, Cordum HS, Hillier L, et al. (2003) The male-specific region of the human Y chromosome is a mosaic of discrete sequence classes. Nature 423: 825-837.
51. Abdelhaleem M (2005) RNA helicases: regulators of differentiation. Clin Biochem 38: 499-503.
52. Proud CG (2005) eIF2 and the control of cell physiology. Semin Cell Dev Biol 16: 3-12.
53. Gebauer F, Hentze MW (2004) Molecular mechanisms of translational control. Nat Rev Mol Cell Biol 5: 827-835.
54. Bernstein BE, Humphrey EL, Erlich RL, Schneider R, Bouman P, et al. (2002) Methylation of histone H3 Lys 4 in coding regions of active genes. Proc Natl Acad Sci U S A 99: 8695-8700.
55. Santos-Rosa H, Schneider R, Bannister AJ, Sherriff J, Bernstein BE, et al. (2002) Active genes are tri-methylated at K4 of histone H3. Nature 419: 407-411.
56. Yang F, Babak T, Shendure J, Disteche CM (2010) Global survey of escape from X inactivation by RNA-sequencing in mouse. Genome Res 20: 614-622.
57. Wang X, Soloway PD, Clark AG (2010) Paternally biased X inactivation in mouse neonatal brain. Genome Biol 11: R79.
58. Senner CE, Brockdorff N (2009) Xist gene regulation at the onset of X inactivation. Curr Opin Genet Dev 19: 122-126.
59. Yang X, Schadt EE, Wang S, Wang H, Arnold AP, et al. (2006) Tissue-specific expression and regulation of sexually dimorphic genes in mice. Genome Res 16: 995-1004.
60. Xu J, Deng X, Disteche CM (2008) Sex-specific expression of the X-linked histone demethylase gene Jarid1c in brain. PLoS One 3: e2553.
61. Xu J, Watkins R, Arnold AP (2006) Sexually dimorphic expression of the X-linked gene Eif2s3x mRNA but not protein in mouse brain. Gene Expr Patterns 6: 146-155.
62. Ehrmann IE, Ellis PS, Mazeyrat S, Duthie S, Brockdorff N, et al. (1998) Characterization of genes encoding translation initiation factor eIF-2gamma in mouse and human: sex chromosome localization, escape from X-inactivation and evolution. Hum Mol Genet 7: 1725-1737.
63. Xu J, Andreassi M (2011) Reversible histone methylation regulates brain gene expression and behavior. Horm Behav 59: 383-392.
64. Martin C, Zhang Y (2005) The diverse functions of histone lysine methylation. Nat Rev Mol Cell Biol 6: 838-849.
65. Lederer D, Grisart B, Digilio MC, Benoit V, Crespin M, et al. (2012) Deletion of KDM6A, a histone demethylase interacting with MLL2, in three patients with Kabuki syndrome. Am J Hum Genet 90: 119-124.
66. Palmer S, Perry J, Kipling D, Ashworth A (1997) A gene spans the pseudoautosomal boundary in mice. Proc Natl Acad Sci U S A 94: 12030-12035.
67. Lancioni A, Pizzo M, Fontanella B, Ferrentino R, Napolitano LM, et al. (2010) Lack of Mid1, the mouse ortholog of the Opitz syndrome gene, causes abnormal development of the anterior cerebellar vermis. J Neurosci 30: 2880-2887.
68. Dal Zotto L, Quaderi NA, Elliott R, Lingerfelter PA, Carrel L, et al. (1998) The mouse Mid1 gene: implications for the pathogenesis of Opitz syndrome and the evolution of the mammalian pseudoautosomal region. Hum Mol Genet 7: 489-499.
69. Quaderi NA, Schweiger S, Gaudenz K, Franco B, Rugarli EI, et al. (1997) Opitz G/BBB syndrome, a defect of midline development, is due to mutations in a new RING finger gene on Xp22. Nat Genet 17: 285-291.
70. Cheung KK, Mok SC, Rezaie P, Chan WY (2008) Dynamic expression of Dab2 in the mouse embryonic central nervous system. BMC Dev Biol 8: 76.
71. Zhoul J, Hernandez G, Tu SW, Huang CL, Tseng CP, Hsieh JT (2005) The role of DOC-2/DAB2 in modulating androgen receptor-mediated cell growth via the nongenomic c-Src-mediated pathway in normal prostatic epithelium and cancer. Cancer Res 65: 9906-9913.
72. Oka T, Akisada M, Okabe A, Sakurai K, Shiosaka S, et al. (2002) Extracellular serine protease neuropsin (KLK8) modulates neurite outgrowth and fasciculation of mouse hippocampal neurons in culture. Neurosci Lett 321: 141-144.
73. Harada A, Ishikawa Y, Shiosaka S (2004) Regulation of hippocampal neuropsin (KLK8) mRNA by steroid hormones. 43: 552.
74. Suzuki J, Yoshida S, Chen ZL, Momota Y, Kato K, et al. (1995) Ontogeny of neuropsin mRNA expression in the mouse brain. Neurosci Res 23: 345-351.
75. Hirata A, Yoshida S, Inoue N, Matsumoto-Miyai K, Ninomiya A, et al. (2001) Abnormalities of synapses and neurons in the hippocampus of neuropsin-deficient mice. Mol Cell Neurosci 17: 600-610.
76. Terayama R, Bando Y, Murakami K, Kato K, Kishibe M, et al. (2007) Neuropsin promotes oligodendrocyte death, demyelination and axonal degeneration after spinal cord injury. Neuroscience 148: 175-187.
77. Yoshida S (2010) Klk8, a multifunctional protease in the brain and skin: analysis of knockout mice. Biol Chem 391: 375-380.
78. Horii Y, Yamasaki N, Miyakawa T, Shiosaka S (2008) Increased anxiety-like behavior in neuropsin (kallikrein-related peptidase 8) gene-deficient mice. Behav Neurosci 122: 498-504.
79. Burma S, Chen DJ (2004) Role of DNA-PK in the cellular response to DNA double-strand breaks. DNA Repair (Amst) 3: 909-918.
80. Norbury CJ, Zhivotovsky B (2004) DNA damage-induced apoptosis. Oncogene 23: 2797-2808.
81. Maser RS, Wong K, Sahin E, Xia H, Naylor M, et al. (2007) DNA-Dependent Protein Kinase Catalytic Subunit Is Not Required for Dysfunctional Telomere Fusion and Checkpoint Response in the Telomerase-Deficient Mouse. Molecular and Cellular Biology 27: 2253-2265.
82. Gladdy RA, Nutter LMJ, Kunath T, Danska JS, Guidos CJ (2006) p53-Independent Apoptosis Disrupts Early Organogenesis in Embryos Lacking Both Ataxia-Telangiectasia Mutated and Prkdc. Molecular Cancer Research 4: 311-318.
83. Kritzer M (2004) The distribution of immunoreactivity for intracellular androgen receptors in the cerebral cortex of hormonally intact adult male

and female rats: localization in pyramidal neurons making corticocortical connections. Cereb Cortex 14: 268-280.

84. Waterham HR1, Koster J, Romeijn GJ, Hennekam RC, Vreken P, et al. (2001) Mutations in the 3beta-hydroxysterol Delta24-reductase gene cause desmosterolosis, an autosomal recessive disorder of cholesterol biosynthesis. Am J Hum Genet 69: 685-694.

85. Wu C, Miloslavskaya I, Demontis S, Maestro R, Galaktionov K (2004) Regulation of cellular response to oncogenic and oxidative stress by Seladin-1. Nature 432: 640-645.

86. Peri A, Danza G, Serio M (2005) Seladin-1 as a target of estrogen receptor activation in the brain: a new gene for a rather old story? J Endocrinol Invest 28: 285-293.

87. Bonaccorsi L, Luciani P, Nesi G, Mannucci E, Deledda C, et al. (2008) Androgen receptor regulation of the seladin-1/DHCR24 gene: altered expression in prostate cancer. Lab Invest 88: 1049-1056.

88. Zu H, Wu J, Zhang J, Yu M, Hong Z (2012) Testosterone up-regulates seladin-1 expression by iAR and PI3-K/Akt signaling pathway in C6 cells. Neurosci Lett 514: 122-126.

6

An Update on Subclinical Hypopituitarism

Paula Andujar-Plata[1], **Eva Fernandez-Rodriguez**[1] **and Felipe F. Casanueva**[1,2,3*]

[1]*Endocrinology Division, Complejo Hospitalario Universitario de Ourense (CHUO), SERGAS, Ourense, 32005, Spain*

[2]*Departamento de Medicina, Universidad de Santiago de Compostela, Santiago de Compostela, 15706, Spain*

[3]*Centro de InvestigaciónBiomédicaen Red (CIBER) de FisiopatologíaObesidad y Nutrición, InstitutoSalud Carlos III, Santiago de Compostela, 15706, Spain*

***Corresponding author:** Dr. Felipe F. Casanueva, Endocrinology Division, Hospital Clinico Universitario, Travesía da Choupana s/n. Santiago de Compostela, La Coruña, 15706, Spain, E-mail: felipe.casanueva@usc.es

Abstract

Subclinical deficiency of pituitary hormones represents an intermediate situation among normal pituitary secretion and overt hypopituitarism. Clinical hypopituitarism is associated with impaired morbidity and mortality, but there are not many studies on these topics in the subclinical setting. Moreover, clinical manifestations and diagnosis criteria are not well defined, so this entity is probably an underdiagnosed disorder. Long-term controlled studies are needed to establish a correct definition of subclinical hypopituitarism and to know its clinical implications, optimal methods of diagnosis, and indications for substitutive treatment. This review will focus on the evidence related to epidemiology, clinical manifestations, diagnosis, and treatment of subclinical hypopituitarism.

Keywords: Hypopituitarism; Subclinical hypopituitarism; Pituitary insufficiency; Partial growth hormone deficiency; Partial adrenocorticotropic hormone deficiency

Introduction

Hypopituitarism is the insufficient secretion of one or more pituitary hormones caused by pituitary and/or hypothalamic disorders [1]. Hormonal deficiency can be isolated or multiple, with the gonadotropic and somatotropic axes the most frequently affected. Clinical manifestations associated to hypopituitarism are often nonspecific and will depend on the underlying disease, age, rate of onset, and degree of hormonal defect. The clinical importance of hypopituitarism is its association with increased mortality compared with the general population and its association with increased morbidity [2-7]. In fact, changes in body composition, glucose intolerance, hypertension, or altered lipid profile have been detected in these patients [8,9].

In clinical practice, we can observe intermediate situations between established hormone deficiencies and normal pituitary function, which could be considered milder or subclinical forms of hypopituitarism. These conditions, although theoretically would not cause clear symptoms, could be related to the mild impairment of morbidity and mortality as clinical hypopituitarism. However, there is no consensus on the methods of diagnosis and treatment in these subclinical cases.

In this article, we review the epidemiology, clinical manifestations, diagnosis, and treatment of subclinical hormone pituitary deficiencies.

Epidemiology of Subclinical Hypopituitarism

There are few data available about the prevalence and incidence of hypopituitarism in the general population. In a well-defined population in the northwest of Spain, our group reported a prevalence of hypopituitarism of 37.5 cases per 100,000 inhabitants and an incidence of 2.07 cases per 100,000 inhabitants per year over a period of 10 years (2000-2009) [10].

Data about the epidemiology of subclinical hypopituitarism have not been reported in the general population, although there are studies evaluating subclinical pituitary deficiencies in some specific subgroups of patients. For example, subclinical hypopituitarism was detected in 29% of patients evaluated after 6 to 9 months of a traumatic brain injury and in 77% of patients treated with cerebral radiotherapy [11]. There are studies that evaluated some isolated subclinical deficiencies. Subclinical thyroid-stimulating hormone (TSH) deficiency was reported in 20.3% of patients who were previously irradiated because of head and neck tumors [12] and in 38% of patients with type 2 diabetes [13], using the thyrotropic releasing hormone (TRH) test for diagnosis.

As previously mentioned, subclinical hypopituitarism does not produce symptoms that can be seen, and the methods for diagnosis are not well established. These conditions probably make subclinical hypopituitarism an underdiagnosed disorder.

Causes of Subclinical Hypopituitarism

The etiology of subclinical hypopituitarism is the same as that of clinical hypopituitarism [14] (Table 1). In adults, the most common cause is a pituitary adenoma or its treatment (surgery or radiotherapy). Benign pituitary adenomas, which are the most frequent pituitary masses, and particularly macroadenomas (≥ 1 cm) are commonly associated with hormone deficiencies. Probable mechanisms include the compression of normal pituitary tissue, compression of the blood flow, and interruption of hypothalamic–pituitary communication.

Although pituitary surgery is sometimes associated with some degree of recovery in pituitary function, it can be a cause of hormone deficit [15]. Tumor size, tumor infiltration, or surgeon experience are some factors involved in the development of hypopituitarism. Radiotherapy is another cause of hypopituitarism, and its effect is dose-dependent. Newer methods of irradiation can lower the prevalence of subclinical hypopituitarism, although there is still risk involved [16]. Other possible causes of subclinical hypopituitarism include traumatic brain injury, Sheehan's syndrome, infiltrative and immunological diseases, and genetic disorders.

Pituitary tumours	
-	Adenomas
-	Other pituitary tumours
Parasellar tumours	
-	Craniopharyngiomas
-	Chordomas
-	Germinomas
-	Meningiomas
-	Gliomas
-	Metastases
-	Others
Brain injury	
-	Neurosurgery
-	Radiotherapy
-	Traumatic brain injury
Vascular disease	
-	Pituitary apoplexy
-	Sheehan's syndrome
-	Subarachnoid haemorrhage
-	Stroke
Infiltrative and immunological disease	
-	Sarcoidosis
-	Tuberculosis
-	Histiocytosis
-	Haemochromatosis
-	Lymphocytic hypophysitis
Infections	
-	Meningitis
-	Encephalitis
-	Abscess
Genetic causes: mutations in PROP1, PIT1, HESX1, LHX4, LHX3, GH, Kallman syndrome	
Primary empty sella	
Idiopathic	

Table 1: Causes of subclinical hypopituitarism.

Clinical Manifestations of Subclinical Hypopituitarism

Subclinical growth hormone deficiency

Clinical manifestations of subclinical hypopituitarism varied based on the age of onset, although the clinical course is usually insidious and without specific symptoms, especially in adults.

In children, the main feature of growth hormone deficiency (GHD) is decreased growth velocity and short height. However, in adulthood, this deficiency can be unrecognized, because the symptoms can be nonspecific. Adults with severe GHD can show changes in body composition with increased fat mass and decreased muscle mass, reduced bone mineral density, metabolic changes (glucose intolerance and altered lipid profile), cardiac changes with premature atherosclerosis and low energy, and reduced quality of life [17-21].

Patients with subclinical GHD could present some of the clinical manifestations of severe GHD but with less intensity. It has been shown that patients with intermediate values in stimulation tests present changes in body composition at an intermediate degree between healthy subjects and patients with severe GHD. Studies of body composition have demonstrated that subjects with subclinical GHD have increased fat mass, reduced lean body mass, and increased skin-fold thickness [22]. This intermediate state has been also associated with impaired insulin sensitivity, impaired lipid profile, and carotid intima-media thickness [23,24]. These changes seem to be related to IGF-I levels.

Another study found that, compared with healthy people, patients who were insufficient in growth hormone (GH) had higher levels of plasminogen activator inhibitor type-I (PAI-I), suggesting an increased cardiovascular risk [25]. A more recent study showed a correlation among the GH axis, the visceral adiposity index, and cardiometabolic risk; thus, apparently healthy patients could have some degree of visceral adipose dysfunction associated with GH and IGF-I levels, but without overt GHD [26]. However, more investigations are needed to support the association between subclinical GHD and increased cardiovascular risk.

Subclinical gonadotropin deficiency

Symptoms of follicle stimulating hormone/luteinizing hormone (FSH/LH) deficiency depend on the age at onset. Before the age of puberty, males with FSH/LH deficiency have small penises and testes, and women with FSH/LH deficiency have primary amenorrhea with the absence of breast development. In adulthood, males show impaired sexual function, reduction of testicular size, infertility, and weakness, and women have menstrual irregularities or amenorrhoea and infertility.

Subclinical gonadotropin deficiency is difficult to establish in women by clinical features, because normal menstruation would exclude it. However, men with subclinical gonadotropin deficiency can have mild symptoms such as low sexual desire, erectile dysfunction, and poor morning erection or fatigue, in relation with testosterone levels [27].

Subclinical adrenocorticotropic hormone deficiency

Chronic corticotropin deficiency usually causes weight loss and lethargy, although it can be asymptomatic if cortisol production is enough for day-to-day activity. Therefore, patients with subclinical adrenocorticotropic hormone (ACTH) deficiency will probably present symptoms only with concomitant stress or illness, when an increase in cortisol secretion is required. In these situations, patients will present typical symptoms of acute deficiency: nausea, vomiting, weakness, hypotension and fever, abdominal pain, or hypovolemic shock in more severe cases.

Subclinical thyroid-stimulating hormone deficiency

Subclinical hypothyroidism could be associated with similar symptoms of overt deficiency: lack of energy, weakness, cold intolerance, or constipation. In children, undiagnosed hypothyroidism can be associated with mental and growth retardations, but mild congenital TSH deficiency based on one patient diagnosed at 6 years of age did not shown any impact on intellectual status or mental development [28].

Subclinical primary hypothyroidism has been associated with higher frequency of hypercholesterolemia, atherosclerosis, and coronary heart disease, and with increased risk of coronary heart events (especially in those with TSH>10 mUI/L) [29]. Nevertheless, no studies are available as yet that evaluate the influence of milder TSH deficiencies on the cardiovascular or metabolic systems.

Subclinical prolactin deficiency

Clinically, prolactin (PRL) deficiency is only characterized by the impossibility to puerperal lactogenesis [30]. Most likely, subclinical deficiency does not cause any symptoms.

Diagnosis of Subclinical Hypopituitarism

Subclinical growth hormonedeficiency

Diagnosis of GHD usually requires a stimulation test [31], although it is not necessary in situations with known structural pituitary disease, the presence of three other hormones deficiencies, and a low IGF-I level. GHD can be interpreted as a continuum with a GH response to a provocative test range from a normal GH response to severe GHD (Table 2). The insulin tolerance test is the gold standard for diagnosis, and a peak GH response <3 μg/L is indicative of severe deficiency in adults [32], whereas a response over 7 μg/L is considered normal. Peaks of GH response between these values represent intermediate conditions of GHD.

Test	Normal peak of GH response (μg/L)	Severe deficiency (μg/L)	Probably subclinical deficiency (μg/L)
Insulin tolerance test	>7	<3	3-7
GHRH-arginine test	>16.5	<9.1	9.1-16.5
GHRH-GHRP6 test	>20	<10	10-20

Table 2: Stimulation tests for diagnosis of GH deficiency.

The growth hormone releasing hormone (GHRH)-arginine test is also employed for diagnosis with similar sensitivity and specificity than theinsulin tolerance test. A peak of GH below 9.1 μg/L is necessary for GHD diagnosis, and it is excluded when the GH response is >16.5 μg/L. Intermediate values would suggest mild impairment of GH secretion [33,34]. These cutoffs values are dependent on body mass index.

Another provocative test employed in the diagnosis of GHD is the GHRH-GHRP6 test, which confirms diagnosis of GHD if the GH peak is less than 10 μg/L and excludes deficiency if it is >20 μg/L [35]. Again, levels between 10 and 20 μg/L could represent subclinical deficiency.

Besides the stimulation tests, other parameters can reflect GH secretion as stimulated UC (area under curve) GH secretion. Values above 1000 are indicative of normal secretion, and values less than 250 indicate a diagnosis of GHD; results between 250 and 1000 would indicate subclinical secretion [36].

IGF-I levels have not showed utility for subclinical GHD diagnosis, because low levels do not discriminate between normal and impaired secretion [37]. However, a recent study has suggested that IGF-I SDS (standard deviation score) can be used as marker of somatotropin function and of hypopituitary severity [38], although more research is needed specifically in the subclinical setting.

In children, subclinical GHD is more difficult to define, although there is at least one case of a child diagnosed after an insulin tolerance test, in whom growth and development was normal [39].

Subclinical gonadotropin deficiency

Hypogonadotropic hypogonadism is diagnosed with a low serum testosterone and/or estradiol concentration and the absence of increased FSH and LH. However, the diagnosis of subclinical states is difficult to define.

In women, normal menstruation cycles exclude gonadotropin deficiency, and there is not a cutoff that establishes subclinical deficiency in patients with normal menstruation. In men, subclinical deficiency would be defined as normal testosterone levels with FSH or LH below the 5th percentile that may be associated with the initial symptoms previously described [40].

Subclinical adrenocorticotropic hormone deficiency

Low cortisol levels in the morning of <80 nmol/L indicate complete ACTH deficiency, whereas levels >400 nmol/L are completely normal. A subclinical corticotropic deficiency would be characterized by normal basal cortisol and ACTH levels, but with an insufficient response to the stimulation test (<500 nmol/L). The insulin tolerance test is the gold standard for detection of central adrenal failure [41], although the low-dose ACTH stimulation test (1 μg) has demonstrated a strong correlation with the ITT with fewer side effects [42]. The high dose of ACTH, 250 μg, can be also used but it is less sensitive for early diagnosis of chronic ACTH deficiency with normal basal cortisol levels. An optimal threshold for subclinical deficiency with this test has not been established.

In subjects with traumatic brain injury, subclinical ACTH deficiency has been also defined as basal ACTH or cortisol levels below the 5th percentile [39], but without sufficient evidence.

Subclinical thyroid-stimulating hormonedeficiency

In contrast with the other axis, stimulation tests are not used in clinical practice to diagnosis TSH deficiency, so subclinical cases can go unrecognized. The TRH test would be an option to detect intermediate defects. In fact, in patients with diabetes type 2 without pituitary disease and normal basal levels of TSH and free T4 and T3, this test detected impaired TSH secretion in approximately 38% of patients, considered as subclinical hypopituitarism [13].

In patients with traumatic brain damage, subclinical TSH deficiency has been defined as low free-T4 (<5th percentile) with normal total-T4 or vice versa [39].

Subclinical PRL deficiency

The TRH test can be used for PRL diagnosis in patients with low PRL levels. A Turkish study showed that the TRH test was more compatible with postpartum agalactia than with PRL levels to detect lactotroph deficiency, particularly in patients with PRL basal levels between 4 and 7.8 ng/ml [43].

Treatment of subclinical hypopituitarism

There is not much data about GH treatment in subclinical defects. A Brazilian study showed that treatment with recombinant human GH in children with mild GHD (defined as GH peak of 5 to 10 ng/mL after the stimulation test) achieved height gain. Height-SDS after the first year of treatment was higher in children with mild deficiency compared with those with severe deficiency, but no difference was found at the last assessment. Differences in GH doses were not observed [44].

Regarding subclinical ACTH deficiency, there is a study that concludes that conventional replacement with 10 mg twice daily of hydrocortisone in these patients produces hypercortisolemia [45], so treatment should avoid physiological conditions without stress.

There are no data for or against substitutive treatment in patients with subclinical TSH and with gonadotropin deficiency. Long-term randomized studies analyzing the impact of substitutive treatment in subclinical deficiencies are needed.

In conclusion, subclinical hypopituitarism is an entity not well defined and probably underdiagnosed because of the lack of specific symptoms and well-defined criteria for diagnosis. Long-term controlled studies are needed to investigate the main symptoms of these patients, the implications in morbidity and mortality, the best method for diagnosis, and the specific cut-offs and need/benefits of substitutive treatment.

Acknowledgement

This work was supported by grants from the Fondo de Investigacion Sanitaria (PI14/01012), and CIBER Fisiopatologia de la Obesidad y Nutricion (CIBERobn; CB06/003), Instituto de Salud Carlos III (ISCIII)-FEDER, Subdireccion General de Evaluacion y Fomento de la Investigacion, Spain.

References

1. Toogood AA, Stewart PM (2008) Hypopituitarism: clinical features, diagnosis, and management. Endocrinol Metab Clin North Am 37: 235-261.
2. Rosén T, Bengtsson BA (1990) Premature mortality due to cardiovascular disease in hypopituitarism. Lancet 336: 285-288.
3. Bates AS, Van't Hoff W, Jones PJ, Clayton RN (1996) The effect of hypopituitarism on life expectancy. J Clin Endocrinol Metab 81: 1169-1172.
4. Tomlinson JW, Holden N, Hills RK, Wheatley K, Clayton RN, et al. (2001) Association between premature mortality and hypopituitarism. West Midlands Prospective Hypopituitary Study Group. Lancet 357: 425-431.
5. Lindholm J, Nielsen EH, Bjerre P, Christiansen JS, Hagen C, et al. (2006) Hypopituitarism and mortality in pituitary adenoma. Clin Endocrinol (Oxf) 65: 51-58.
6. Bülow B, Hagmar L, Mikoczy Z, Nordström CH, Erfurth EM (1997) Increased cerebrovascular mortality in patients with hypopituitarism. Clin Endocrinol (Oxf) 46: 75-81.
7. Erfurth EM, Bülow B, Hagmar LE (2000) Is vascular mortality increased in hypopituitarism? Pituitary 3: 77-81.
8. Shahi M, Beshyah SA, Hackett D, Sharp PS, Johnston DG, et al. (1992) Myocardial dysfunction in treated adult hypopituitarism: a possible explanation for increased cardiovascular mortality. Br Heart J 67: 92-96.
9. Kaji H, Iida K, Takahashi Y, Okimura Y, Chihara K (2007) Hormone replacement therapy and vascular risk disorders in adult hypopituitarism. Endocr J 54: 239-245.
10. Fernandez-Rodriguez E, Lopez-Raton M, Andujar P, Martinez-Silva IM, Cadarso-Suarez C, et al (2013) Epidemiology, mortality rate and survival in a homogeneous population of hypopituitary patients. Clin Endocrinol (Oxf) 78: 278-284.
11. Taphoorn MJ, Heimans JJ, van der Veen EA, Karim AB (1995) Endocrine functions in long-term survivors of low-grade supratentorial glioma treated with radiation therapy. J Neurooncol 25: 97-102.
12. Bhandare N, Kennedy L, Malyapa RS, Morris CG, Mendenhall WM (2007) Primary and central hypothyroidism after radiotherapy for head-and-neck tumors. Int J Radiat Oncol Biol Phys 68: 1131-1139.
13. Small M, Cohen HN, MacLean JA, Beastall GH, MacCuish AC (1986) Impaired thyrotrophin secretion following the administration of thyrotrophin-releasing hormone in type II diabetes mellitus. Postgrad Med J 62: 445-448.
14. Ascoli P, Cavagnini F (2006) Hypopituitarism. Pituitary 9: 335-342.
15. Nomikos P, Ladar C, Fahlbusch R, Buchfelder M (2004) Impact of primary surgery on pituitary function in patients with non-functioning pituitary adenomas -- a study on 721 patients. Acta Neurochir (Wien) 146: 27-35.
16. Xu Z, Lee Vance M, Schlesinger D, Sheehan JP (2013) Hypopituitarism after stereotactic radiosurgery for pituitary adenomas. Neurosurgery 72: 630-637.
17. De Boer H, Blok GJ, Voerman HJ, De Vries PM, van der Veen EA (1992) Body composition in adult growth hormone-deficient men, assessed by anthropometry and bioimpedance analysis. J Clin Endocrinol Metab 75: 833-837.
18. Beshyah SA, Gelding SV, Andres C, Johnston DG, Gray IP (1995) Beta-cell function in hypopituitary adults before and during growth hormone treatment. Clin Sci (Lond) 89: 321-328.
19. de Boer H, Blok GJ, Voerman HJ, Phillips M, Schouten JA (1994) Serum lipid levels in growth hormone-deficient men. Metabolism 43: 199-203.
20. Markussis V, Beshyah SA, Fisher C, Sharp P, Nicolaides AN, et al. (1992) Detection of premature atherosclerosis by high-resolution ultrasonography in symptom-free hypopituitary adults. Lancet 340: 1188-1192.

21. Merola B, Cittadini A, Colao A, Longobardi S, Fazio S, et al. (1993) Cardiac structural and functional abnormalities in adult patients with growth hormone deficiency. J Clin Endocrinol Metab 77: 1658-1661.
22. Murray RD, Adams JE, Shalet SM (2004) Adults with partial growth hormone deficiency have an adverse body composition. J Clin Endocrinol Metab 89: 1586-1591.
23. Murray RD, Shalet SM (2005) Insulin sensitivity is impaired in adults with varying degrees of GH deficiency. Clin Endocrinol (Oxf) 62: 182-188.
24. Colao A, Di Somma C, Spiezia S, Rota F, Pivonello R, et al. (2006) The natural history of partial growth hormone deficiency in adults: a prospective study on the cardiovascular risk and atherosclerosis. J Clin Endocrinol Metab 91: 2191-2200.
25. Murray RD, Wieringa G, Lawrance JA, Adams JE, Shalet SM (2010) Partial growth hormone deficiency is associated with an adverse cardiovascular risk profile and increased carotid intima-medial thickness. Clin Endocrinol (Oxf) 73: 508-515.
26. Di Somma C, Ciresi A, Amato MC, Savastano S, Savanelli MC, et al. (2015) Alteration of the growth hormone axis, visceral fat dysfunction, and early cardiometabolic risk in adults: the role of the visceral adiposity index. Endocrine 49: 492-502.
27. Wu FC, Tajar A, Beynon JM, Pye SR, Silman AJ, et al. (2010) Identification of late-onset hypogonadism in middle-aged and elderly men. N Engl J Med 363: 123-135.
28. Smail PJ, Isles TE, Ackroyd RS (1979) A boy with low-TSH hypothyroidism. Arch Dis Child 54: 475-477.
29. Rodondi N, den Elzen WP, Bauer DC, Cappola AR, Razvi S, et al. (2010) Subclinical hypothyroidism and the risk of coronary heart disease and mortality. JAMA 304: 1365-1374.
30. Zargar AH, Masoodi SR, Laway BA, Shah NA, Salahudin M (1997) Familial puerperal alactogenesis: possibility of a genetically transmitted isolated prolactin deficiency. Br J Obstet Gynaecol 104: 629-631.
31. Ho KK1; 2007 GH Deficiency Consensus Workshop Participants (2007) Consensus guidelines for the diagnosis and treatment of adults with GH deficiency II: a statement of the GH Research Society in association with the European Society for Pediatric Endocrinology, Lawson Wilkins Society, European Society of Endocrinology, Japan Endocrine Society, and Endocrine Society of Australia. Eur J Endocrinol 157: 695-700.
32. [No authors listed] (1998) Consensus guidelines for the diagnosis and treatment of adults with growth hormone deficiency: summary statement of the Growth Hormone Research Society Workshop on Adult Growth Hormone Deficiency. J Clin Endocrinol Metab 83: 379-381.
33. Colao A, Di Somma C, Pivonello R, Loche S, Aimaretti G, et al. (1999) Bone loss is correlated to the severity of growth hormone deficiency in adult patients with hypopituitarism. J Clin Endocrinol Metab 84: 1919-1924.
34. Colao A, Cerbone G, Pivonello R, Aimaretti G, Loche S, et al. (1999) The growth hormone (GH) response to the arginine plus GH-releasing hormone test is correlated to the severity of lipid profile abnormalities in adult patients with GH deficiency. J Clin Endocrinol Metab 84: 1277-1282.
35. Popovic V, Leal A, Micic D, Koppeschaar HP, Torres E, et al. (2000) GH-releasing hormone and GH-releasing peptide-6 for diagnostic testing in GH-deficient adults. Lancet 356: 1137-1142.
36. Koppeschaar HP, Popovic V, Leal A, Otero XL, Torres E, et al. (2004) Growth hormone (GH) peaks versus areas under the curve in the diagnosis of adult GH deficiency: analysis of the variables provided by the GHRH + GHRP-6 test. Pituitary 7: 15-20.
37. Mitchell H, Dattani MT, Nanduri V, Hindmarsh PC, Preece MA, et al. (1999) Failure of IGF-I and IGFBP-3 to diagnose growth hormone insufficiency. Arch Dis Child 80: 443-447.
38. Tirosh A,2, Toledano Y2,3, Masri-Iraqi H, et al. (2016) IGF-I levels reflect hypopituitarism severity in adults with pituitary dysfunction. Pituitary .
39. Zimmerman TS, White MG, Daughaday WH, Goetz FC (1967) Hypopituitarism with normal or increased height. Report of two cases, with measurement of plasma growth hormone levels. Am J Med 42: 146-150.
40. Bavisetty S, Bavisetty S, McArthur DL, Dusick JR, Wang C, et al. (2008) Chronic hypopituitarism after traumatic brain injury: risk assessment and relationship to outcome. Neurosurgery 62: 1080-1093.
41. Endert E, Ouwehand A, Fliers E, Prummel MF, Wiersinga WM (2005) Establishment of reference values for endocrine tests. Part IV: Adrenal insufficiency. Neth J Med 63: 435-443.
42. Thaler LM, Blevins LS Jr. (1998) The low dose (1-microg) adrenocorticotropin stimulation test in the evaluation of patients with suspected central adrenal insufficiency. J Clin Endocrinol Metab 83: 2726-2729.
43. Diri H, Tanriverdi F, Karaca Z, Senol S, Unluhizarci K, et al. (2014) Extensive investigation of 114 patients with Sheehan's syndrome: a continuing disorder. Eur J Endocrinol 171: 311-318.
44. Cardoso DF, Martinelli CE Jr2, Campos VC, Gomes ES, Rocha IE, et al. (2014) Comparison between the growth response to growth hormone (GH) therapy in children with partial GH insensitivity or mild GH deficiency. Arq Bras Endocrinol Metabol 58: 23-29.
45. Agha A, Liew A, Finucane F, Baker L, O'Kelly P, et al. (2004) Conventional glucocorticoid replacement overtreats adult hypopituitary patients with partial ACTH deficiency. Clin Endocrinol (Oxf) 60: 688-693.

7

Hormones and Nocturia: Guidelines for Medical Treatment?

An-Sofie Goessaert*, Johan Vande Walle, Ayush Kapila and Karel Everaert

Ghent University Hospital, De Pintelaan 185, 9000 Ghent, Belgium

***Corresponding author:** An-Sofie Goessaert, Urology Department, Ghent University Hospital, De Pintelaan 185, 9000 Ghent, Belgium, E-Mail: an-sofie.goessaert@uzgent.be

Abstract

Nocturnal polyuria (NP) is an important cause of nocturia and it is related to an imbalance in water and/or sodium homeostasis. Antidiuretic hormone (ADH) and atrial natriuretic peptide (ANP) are believed to play an important role in this excessive urine production overnight, however, many other hormones are involved. ADH and ANP are both directly and indirectly influenced by the renin-angiotensin-aldosterone system (RAAS), prostaglandins antagonize both ADH and RAAS and sex hormones have a predominantly antidiuretic effect by stimulating ADH and RAAS, meaning that any disturbance can lead to an imbalance in diuresis. Since nocturia is a condition affecting sleep, melatonin secretion can also be affected, leading to a decrease in the antidiuretic effect and to an increase of nocturnal urine production. Depending on the underlying condition affecting any of these hormones, a more specific therapeutic approach might lead to a restoration of the normal diuresis cycle and to a good night's sleep. The characteristics of each of these hormones, the pathophysiology in NP and the therapeutic implications are set out in this review.

Keywords: Nocturnal polyuria; Antidiuretic hormone; Renin-angiotensin-aldosterone; Atrial natriuretic peptide; Pathophysiology; Therapeutic implications

Introduction

Nocturia is the need to get up once or more to void at night. The underlying problem can be reduced bladder capacity, diurnal polyuria and nocturnal polyuria; each of these can be caused by several conditions. In this review we would focus on the problem of nocturnal polyuria [1].

To fully understand this topic, a basic knowledge of water and sodium homeostasis is necessary. Nocturnal polyuria due to disturbances in water handling is usually caused by an impairment of the antidiuretic hormone. If a disturbance in sodium handling seems to be the problem, natriuretic peptides are often involved [2,3]. Both of these hormones affect and are affected by the renin-angiotensin-aldosterone system [4]. But there is also evidence that other hormones, such as melatonin and sex hormones affect these pathways one way or another [5,6].Therefore this article highlights the physiological mechanisms of each of these hormones and discusses how this fits in the pathophysiology of nocturnal polyuria, providing evidence for pharmacotherapeutic options.

Antidiuretic Hormone

Characteristics

ADH is the predominant hormone that regulates the rate of free water excretion. It is a neurohypophyseal polypeptide that is synthesized in the supraoptic and paraventricular nuclei and is secreted after migration to the posterior lobe of the pituitary as a response to the appropriate stimuli [7]. ADH secretion is mainly influenced by the input from the osmotic and volume receptors, with an increase due to hyperosmolality and volume depletion, respectively. But multiple other stimuli play a role such as stress situations, nausea and hypoglycemia. Nicotine and morphine also enhance ADH release [8,9].

There are three receptors for ADH, by binding to the V1 receptor vasoconstriction and prostaglandin release occurs; stimulation of the V1b or V3 receptor facilitates the release of adrenocorticotropic hormone (ACTH) in the pituitary. Activation of the V2 receptor mediates the antidiuretic response by fusing the ADH-sensitive water channels, aquaporin-2, with the luminal membrane of the collecting tubules in the nephrons. This process allows water to be reabsorbed down the osmotic gradient towards the systemic circulation across the basolateral membrane. Once the ADH effect has worn off, the water channels return to the cytoplasm after endocytosis [10].

ADH also appears to affect electrolyte handling by enhancing sodium reabsorption and secretion of potassium in the cortical collecting tubule; however, these effects do not seem to be of major importance in maintaining the electrolyte balance [11,12].

NP pathophysiology

In older people with nocturnal polyuria a decrease in nocturnal ADH secretion seems to be an important factor. Moon et al. and Asplund found this impaired circadian rhythm of plasma ADH levels during night time in small study samples (12 and 23 subjects, respectively) with a mean age of 68 and 71 years old, respectively [13,14].

And although a loss of circadian rhythm of ADH is believed to be a normal aging process, the contribution of an impairment of this hormone is reinforced by the evidence that low nocturnal ADH levels are also found in children with nocturnal enuresis based on nocturnal polyuria [15].

Studies in which the urinary ADH levels were measured show conflicting evidence, Hirayama et al. found a decrease in urinary ADH excretion early in the morning in patients with NP, while Akiyama et al. showed that more than 30% of the older people (>50 years old, mean age 75) with NP present with increased urinary ADH excretion rates. The latter implies that not only an impaired secretion may cause NP, but also an impaired response to ADH, which can be caused for example by drugs and electrolyte abnormalities [16,17].

Therapeutical implications

Desmopressin is a synthetic analogue of ADH and is currently the only drug approved for treatment of nocturia due to nocturnal polyuria. Compared to the endogenous ADH, desmopressin has a pronounced antidiuretic effect and little to no vasopressor effect [18].

Desmopressin has proven to lower nocturnal urine production and to prolong the initial sleep period, thus improving the sleep quality of the patients. Beneficial effects both on short-term and long-term have been confirmed [19,20]. Adverse effects are limited; however, a risk for potentially fatal hyponatriemia has to be taken in account, definitely in an older population and in women who seem to be more prone to this adverse effect [21].

Renin-Angiotensin-Aldosterone System

Characteristics

The renin-angiotensin-aldosterone system is of major importance in maintaining blood pressure and fluid volume. It exerts this function through regulation of renal blood flow and solute reabsorption, thereby affecting the urine production [4].

Renin: The activity of these systems depends on the level of renin gene expression and on conversion of prorenin to active renin by proteolytic removal of a 43 amino acid prosegment. Renin is stored in secretory granules of the juxtaglomerular cells of the kidney and is released in response to various physiological stimuli, such as low blood pressure blockade of Ang II production or decreases in distal tubular sodium. It is an enzyme that triggers the cascade by cleaving the liver-derived angiotensinogen into angiotensin I (Ang I) [22,23].

The major determinant of renin secretion is sodium intake; low intake or fluid loss lowers the extracellular volume and stimulates renin secretion [24]. There are three mechanisms regulating renin release. The first is through afferent arteriolar baroreceptors; in response to low arterial perfusion pressure renin release increases. The second is through sympathetic innervation of the juxtaglomerular cells, stimulation of these neurons leads to norepinephrine release and subsequent stimulation of beta1-adrenergic receptors stimulating renin release. The third is a negative feedback mechanism through binding of Ang II to AT1 and AT2 receptors [25,26].

Angiotensin: Within the lungs, the inactive Ang I is converted by the angiotensin-converting enzyme (ACE) into the active angiotensin II. The effect of Ang II depends on the type of receptor that is stimulated. Binding of AngII to the AT1-receptor results in a variation of effects on vasculature, heart and kidney, such as vasoconstriction, increase of cardiac contractility and aldosterone and ADH secretion. Sodium reabsorption is not only stimulated indirectly through aldosterone, but also directly through stimulation of sodium transport in the early proximal tubule [22,23].

Stimulation of AT2-receptors results in the opposite effect with vasodilation and natriuresis, however, since these receptors are highly expressed in fetal tissues but then substantially regress, they are believed to be of minor importance in adults [27].

Aldosterone: Aldosterone is a mineralocorticoid hormone that is synthesized and secreted by the adrenals in response to Ang II and potassium. It stimulates mineralocorticoid receptors in the distal nephron leading to sodium reabsorption through epithelial sodium channels. The accompanying water retention expands blood and extracellular fluid volumes [28].

In situations of aldosterone overproduction, such as in primary hyperaldosteronism, an 'aldosterone escape' is seen, where the initial sodium retention is counteracted by increased ANP levels and an elevation in systemic blood pressure leading to natriuresis after 1 to 2 days in order to restore plasma volume towards normal [29].

NP pathophysiology

In children with nocturnal enuresis based on nocturnal polyuria a lack of circadian rhythm in plasma angiotensin II levels is found, which correlates with an attenuated rhythm in mean blood pressure [30]. And although evidence is limited, it has also been described that nocturnal angiotensin II levels are lower in adults with NP, together with a decrease in ADH [31]. Besides, a link between a non-dipping pattern in mean arterial blood pressure and nocturia in adults is found, pleading for the same underlying pathophysiologic mechanisms as found in children with nocturnal polyuria [32]. This non-dipping pattern is characterized by diminished renal sodium excretory capability, low plasma renin activity and normal aldosterone levels. The relative aldosterone excess with sodium retention during daytime leads to enhanced sodium excretion during night time [33]. In arterial hypertension higher levels of blood pressure are required to excrete the same amount of sodium, which is called pressure-natriuresis [32]. This pressure natriuresis is accomplished by increased glomerular capillary pressure, as seen in deteriorated renal function and increasing age [34].

The non-dipping pattern is also found in subjects with sodium sensitive hypertension, in whom a significant rise in blood pressure occurs as a response to sodium loading. Many factors seem to play a role in this type of hypertension, salt sensitivity is related to older age, female sex, and is possibly genetically determined. Lower renin and aldosterone levels are found in these subjects, together with a decreased number of beta2-receptors. Atrial natriuretic peptide also seems to play a role, although there is no consensus on lower levels of ANP or a lower response to ANP [35].

Therapeutical implications

In subjects with sodium sensitive hypertension a reduction in sodium intake has been proven to be effective in lowering nocturnal blood pressure and thus affecting the nocturnal sodium excretion. In high sodium load the defect in sodium excretory capability becomes more evident, leading to the above mentioned mechanisms and thus nocturnal polyuria. Sodium restriction is considered one of the most important lifestyle measures to address hypertension and renal diseases and can indirectly affect nocturnal urine production [36].

Angiotensin II type 1 receptor blockers administered in the morning seem to restore the circadian rhythms of blood pressure and natriuresis from nocturnal non-dipping to dipping patterns in patients with chronic kidney disease. This is, however, not only due to inhibition of the RAS itself, but mainly through enhanced renal sodium excretion during daytime [37]. This is similar to the effect of diuretics on nocturnal polyuria as described below [38].

Natriuretic peptide

Characteristics

Atrial natriuretic peptide: Atrial natriuretic peptide (ANP) is the main natriuretic hormone; it is a 28-amino-acid polypeptide that is released from myocardial cells in the atria and in some cases the ventricles. ANP stimulates natriuretic peptide receptors (NPR) in the glomeruli and inner medullary collecting ducts [39].

This peptide functions as a direct vasodilator and also increases urinary sodium and water excretion. The latter effect is mediated by various renal and extra renal changes. The natriuretic action is primarily caused by inhibition of sodium reabsorption in the medullary collecting tubule. There still is controversy about the same effect on the proximal tubule, but in case of high ANP levels glomerular filtration rate is increased, which also leads to natriuresis [40].

But there are other pathways through which ANP exercises its natriuretic and diuretic effects, such as through the effect on the renin-angiotensin-aldosterone system. In the proximal tubule, ANP inhibits the angiotensin-mediated sodium and fluid reabsorption. Besides that, ANP antagonizes the actions of aldosterone and of ADH [41,42].

Brain natriuretic peptide: Brain natriuretic peptide (BNP) is homologous to ANP and is present in both the brain and the heart. Circulating concentration of BNP is less than 20% of that of ANP, but in congestive heart failure patients it can easily exceed these rates [43]. The physiologic role of BNP remains to be determined, but it definitely plays a role in volume status. In ten male volunteers volume loading with an infusion of 15 ml/kg of 0.9% NaCl led to a short-lasting increase of plasma NT-pro-ANP (prohormone of ANP) and a delayed increase in plasma NT-pro-BNP, together with a parallel increase in urine flow, renal excretion of sodium and NT-pro-BNP. The increased urinary NT-pro-BNP excretion during volume loading suggests a possible role of BNP in sodium homeostasis in men [44]. In a study on 74 male subjects aged 50 or older a correlation between increased NT-pro-BNP and leg edema has been found [45]. Furthermore, BNP is used for volume estimation in dialysis patients, since BNP level variations correlate positively with volume status alterations in this specific patient group [46].

NP Pathophysiology

The driving force behind excessive diuresis during night time can be a rise in nocturnal sodium excretion due to increased ANP levels. This is known to be the pathophysiological mechanism of nocturnal polyuria in patients with sleep apnea syndrome [47]. The inspiratory efforts against a closed airway during sleep apnea cause a negative intrathoracic pressure with cardiac distension that leads to the release of ANP with consequential sodium and water excretion and inhibition of both ADH and the renin-angiotensin-aldosterone system [48].

ANP and BNP levels are usually higher in patients with severe heart failure compared to people with normal heart function, so this is also assumed to be the mechanism of NP in patients with congestive heart failure. And although increased ANP levels have been described in the older population with NP, other studies do not observe significant differences in natriuretic peptide levels between NP patients and controls, both without cardiac failure. This suggests that NP might be a sign of undetected cardiac failure in older persons [49,50].

Therapeutical implications

Furosemide is a short-acting loop diuretic often used in the treatment of heart failure or edema. When administered in the afternoon, approximately 6 hours before bedrest, it stimulates an early evening diuresis resulting in a decreased nocturnal voiding frequency [38]. This has been demonstrated in older men with lower urinary tract symptoms (LUTS) and can safely be combined with desmopressin or terazosin [51,52]. In children with desmopressin-resistant nocturnal polyuria increased sodium excretion overnight was found and adding furosemide in the morning to desmopressin treatment led to an increase of diuresis of diluted urine in the morning without affecting the concentrating capacity overnight [53]. As in desmopressin treatment it is important to regularly check electrolyte balance since furosemide affects not only sodium excretion, but also enhances potassium, calcium and magnesium excretion (Table1 and Figure 1).

	Antidiuresis			Diuresis
What?	Arginine-vasopressine or antidiuretic hormone	Angiotensine II	Aldosterone	Atrial natriuretic peptie
Site of synthesis?	Neurohypophysis	Lungs	Adrenal glands	Atria
Site of effect in kidney?	Cortical and medullary collecting tubule	Proximal tubule	Cortical collecting tubule (epithelial sodium channels)	Glomeruli & inner medullary collecting duct
Receptors?	V2-receptor	AT1-receptor	MR-receptor	NPR-A
Main effect in kidney?	Antidiuresis through water reabsorption by fusion of aquaporin-2 channels with luminal membrane	Antidiuresis through: Sodium reabsorption, both directly and indirectly (stimulation of aldosterone secretion)	Antidiuresis through sodium reabsorption	Natriuresis through: inhibition of sodium reabsorption directly and indirectly (inhibition of RAAS) inhibition of water reabsorption indirectly (diminish response to ADH)

		Water reabsorption, indirectly (sodium reabsorption and stimulation of ADH)		
Stimulating factors?	Hyperosmolality Hypovolemia stress e.g. pain hypoglycemia	Increase in renin due to: Low blood volume Low Na+ concentration in distal tubule Drop in blood pressure	Ang II Plasma K+ concentration ACTH	Volume expansion with atrial stretch Aldosterone escape
Role in nocturnal polyuria?	Reduced e.g. in nocturnal enuresis	Reduced e.g. in hypertension	Reduced e.g. sleep apnea syndrome	Increased e.g. in heart failure
V: Vasopressin; AT: Angiotensin; MR: Mineralocorticoid; NPR: Natriuretic Peptide Receptor; ADH: Antidiuretic Hormone; RAAS: Renin-Angiotensin-Aldosteron System; Ang: Angiotensin; ACTH: Adrenocorticotropic Hormone				

Table 1: Main antidiuretic and diuretic hormones and characteristics

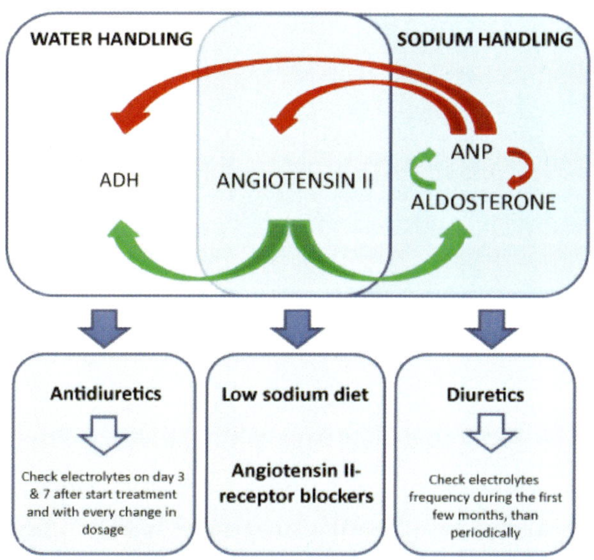

Figure 1: Stimulating and inhibiting effects of hormones involved in water and sodium handling and therapeutical implications

Other hormones

Prostaglandins: Prostaglandins are derivatives from the metabolism of arachidonic acid, catalyzed by the coclooxygenase (COX) enzyme. In the kidney, COX-1 controls renal hemodynamics and glomerular filtration rate, COX-2 plays a role in salt and water excretion [54].

Prostaglandin E2 (PGE2) is synthesized both in the glomeruli and tubules, it lowers the renal vascular resistance and increases renal perfusion through dilatation of the renal vascular bed. The tubular effect of PGE2 is an antagonistic effect of ADH and thus implies local modulation of water and electrolyte transport; however, the major function of the ADH-prostaglandin relationship may be the regulation or renal hemodynamics [55]. ProstaglandinI2 (PGI2) or prostacyclin is synthesized in the glomeruli and mainly affects renal homeostatic mechanisms by antagonizing the vasoconstrictor effects of both norepinephrine and angiotensin II in the vessels [54,55]. The effects of ANP are also influenced by prostaglandins, since the ANP-related natriuresis seems to depend on redistribution of renal blood flow due to an increase in urinary excretion of prostaglandins and a decrease of renin secretion [56].

Since prostaglandins are synthezised through COX-enzymes, a beneficial effect of non-steroidal anti-inflammatory drugs in some patients with nocturia is not surprising. A Japanese study in which men with benign prostate hypertrophy (BPH) were treated with loxoprofen because BPH treatment did not improve nocturia, reported in 74% of the cases an improvement or disappearance of nocturia [57]. Treatment of 26 patients with nocturnal polyuria with diclofenac gave a significant decrease in nocturia episodes from 2.7 to 2.3 and a significant decrease in ratio of night time to 24h urine volume from 44% to 39%, however, clinical relevance of these decreases is doubtful [58]. The effect of NSAIDs on nocturia can be explained through several pathways: reduction of urine production at the kidney, decrease in urinary sensation at the bladder, increase of urinary sensation threshold at the central nervous system or alteration of sleep at the brain. However, PGE2 and PGI2 normally only start playing an important role in maintaining GFR in patients with compromised renal hemodynamics. This means that a good effect of NSAIDs is mainly expected in older patients or patients with congestive heart failure, cirrhosis or nephrosis, but since there is a risk of gastric ulcers and deterioration of kidney function, NSAIDs are not indicated to be used in older or precarious patients. Most common reported adverse events in treatment with NSAIDs for nocturia are gastric discomfort, leg edema and urinary frequency in the morning [57,58].

Melatonin: Melatonin is a pineal hormone that is particularly known for its circadian secretion rhythm with a prominent nocturnal peak as a response to the light-dark rhythm. It also influences the circadian rhythm of other hormones and since the melatonin (MT) receptors are distributed throughout the whole body, it has a large variation in effects [59]. These effects also imply an influence of the above mentioned hormones.

A colocalization of melatonin receptors and ADH neurons in the suprachiasmatic, paraventricular and supraoptic nuclei has been described, suggesting that melatonin might directly modulate the hypothalamic-pituitary-adrenal axis and thus might also have an impact on the antidiuretic effect of ADH [60]. Besides, a renin-angiotensin system in the brain seems to modulate melatonin synthesis. Interaction between locally produced angiotensin II and melatonin in the pineal gland affects the peripheral renin-angiotensin system and thus indirectly urine production [5]. The relation between neuroendocrine functions and the cardiovascular system might also be regulated through ANP, since acute injections of ANP stimulate melatonin secretion, however, administration of oral melatonin does not seem to affect ANP plasma concentrations; the true link between melatonin and ANP remains to be elucidated [61,62].

Only few studies are performed with melatonin as treatment for nocturia. One study examined the effect of 2 mg melatonin on nocturia compared to placebo in patients with benign prostate hyperplasia. A statistically significant difference in nocturia episodes was found, however, a reduction of 0.32 episodes does not seem clinically relevant. Besides, since it was studied in a population with BPH, it is difficult to estimate the influence of BPH on nocturia and on the effect of melatonin treatment [63]. Another study comparing the effect of melatonin and rilmazafone, a hypnotic agent, on nocturia also showed a significant decrease in nocturia episodes, together with an increase in the serum melatonin levels. Before treatment, all patients considered their nocturia problem as bothersome, after 4 weeks of treatment, 70% of the patients considered it to be no longer bothersome.

Although the link between sleep disorders and nocturia has not been elucidated yet, it is certain that there is a relation between both and it is important to counsel about the presence of sleep disturbances when considering treatment for nocturia.

Sex hormones: In women, estrogens and progestogens are the main sex hormones. Estrogens are steroid hormones synthesized from androgens under stimulation of follicle stimulating hormone by the ovaries and in lower concentrations by the liver, adrenal glands, breasts and fat. Action of estrogens is mediated by the estrogen receptor, resulting in various effects on menstrual cycle, sexual characteristics et cetera [64].

Progesterone is also a steroid hormone synthesized from the cholesterol-derived pregnenolone by the ovaries and adrenal glands. It is the precursor of aldosterone and after conversion into 17-hydroxyprogesterone of cortisol and androstenedione, the latter can be converted to testosterone, estrone and estradiol. Progesterone binds to the progesterone receptor and has key effects in the reproductive system and nervous system [65].

Testosterone is in small amounts present in women, but is the main sex hormone in men. Like the other steroid hormones, it is derived from cholesterol. Testosterone exerts its effect through binding to the androgen receptor at one hand and by conversion to estradiol and activation of estrogen receptors at the other hand. It plays a key role in the development of male reproductive tissues such as testes and prostate, it is necessary for normal sperm development and promotes secondary sexual characteristics. Furthermore, testosterone is essential for general well-being [66].

ADH secretion is subjected to circadian rhythms, but also to the menstrual cycle in women. Increased basal and nocturnal ADH concentrations are found in the midfollicular phase of the menstrual cycle; postmenopausal women who take in estrogen will have increased ADH, whereas the combination of estrogen and progesterone lowers the ADH concentrations [67-69].

High estrogen states decrease baseline plasma-osmolality and sodium by resetting of the osmoreceptors for thirst and ADH release. However, in this situation ADH secretion persists and slightly hypotonic plasma is maintained [67]. Another study suggests that 3beta- 17beta-estradiol (E2) augments osmotic ADH secretion with water retention as a consequence, however, the enhanced fluid retention was mainly based on an increase in renal sodium reabsorption [68].

The effects on sodium excretion can be attributed to the relation between estrogens and progestogens and the renin-aldosterone system. High doses of estrogens stimulate the synthesis of angiotensinogen and the consecutive increase in angiotensin II slightly reduces renal blood flow and increases sodium and blood pressure. At the other hand, endogenous or exogenous progesterone promotes sodium loss which leads to a compensatory increase in the activity of the renin-angiotensin-aldosterone system. Combination treatment of ethinylestradiol and progestogens may therefore enhance the estrogen effects on body sodium and blood pressure, also since some synthetic progestogens are weak estrogen receptor agonists [6].

Literature on the link between androgens and the hormones involved in the water and sodium homeostasis is limited. Men seem to have higher plasma concentrations of ADH compared to women and present with a higher sensitivity in ADH response [68]. Gender differences in blood pressure are attributed to the relation between androgens and the renin-aldosterone system. A greater activation of the RAS with higher blood pressure levels in males is partly attributed to these androgens. Castration seems to result in a normalization of blood pressure and downregulation of the intrarenal RAS [70].

Athough some studies do not report an effect, several other studies have shown a beneficial effect of estrogen on the symptom of nocturia [71]. As well oral administration as topical application of estrogen in postmenopausal women leads to a significant decrease in nocturnal frequency within 3 months after the beginning of the therapy [72]. A trial with 2 mg 17 beta-oestradiol combined with 2.5, 5, 10 or 15 mg dydrogesterone led to complete cure of nocturia in 65% of the 26 postmenopausal women with baseline nocturia who completed 6 months of hormonal therapy [73]. A randomized controlled trial studying the effect of oestradiol-releasing rings and oestriol pessaries in postmenopausal women showed a decrease in the number of nocturia episodes of 51% and 54%, respectively [74]. So regardless of the type of estrogen replacement therapy that is used, an effect on nocturia can be seen.

No direct effect of testosterone on nocturia has been described, but drugs that indirectly target testosterone such as 5-alpha-reductase inhibitors seem to have an effect on nocturia, however, the effect is rather small. Doxazosin and combination therapy with finasteride resulted in a larger reduction of nocturia-episodes than placebo, but the net difference was less than 0.20 fewer nocturnal voiding episodes at 1 and 4 years [75] (Table 2).

Hormones	Main effect	Consequence	Therapeutical implication for NP
Prostaglandins: PGE2 PGI2	? antagonizes ADH ? antagonizes RAAS	Diuresis	NSAIDs
Melatonin	stimulates ADH stimulates RAAS	Antidiuresis	Melatonin

Sex hormones: estrogens progesterone testosterone	? stimulates ADH, Renin, Ang II, ANP; inhibits Aldosteron ? stimulates Aldosteron; antagonizes ADH, ANP ? stimulates ADH, Renin, Ang II	Antidiuresis	Replacement therapy if necessary
PGE2: Prostaglandin E2; PGI2: Prostaglandin I2; ADH: Antidiuretic Hormone; RAAS: Renin-Angiotensin-Aldosterone System; ANP: Atrial Natriuretic Peptide; NSAIDs: Non-Steroidal Anti-Inflammatory Drugs			

Table 2: Influence of prostaglandins, melatonin and sex hormones on the antidiuretic and diuretic hormones

Conclusion

Different hormonal pathways are involved in urine production. With increasing age circadian rhythms of these hormones vanish, making older people more susceptible to a large nocturnal urine production. However, at any age, it is an imbalance in this hormonal regulation that can lead to an excessive urine production and thus nocturnal polyuria.

Addressing the underlying pathologies that affect either directly or indirectly water or sodium handling and thus urine production can relieve people from bothersome nocturia or nocturnal urinary incontinence based on nocturnal polyuria and can improve both their sleep quality and quality of life.

References

1. Cornu JN, Abrams P, Chapple CR, Dmochowski RR, Lemack GE, et al. (2012) A contemporary assessment of nocturia: definition, epidemiology, pathophysiology, and management--a systematic review and meta-analysis. Eur Urol 62: 877-890.
2. Herek J, Fitzgerald M, Mohindra M, Wickman C, Leehey J, et al (2010) Solute and Water Excretion Patterns in Patients with Nocturnal Polyuria. International Journal of Nephro-Urology 2: 526-531.
3. Miller M (2000) Nocturnal polyuria in older people: pathophysiology and clinical implications. J Am Geriatr Soc 48: 1321-1329.
4. Carey RM, Siragy HM (2003) Newly recognized components of the renin-angiotensin system: Potential roles in cardiovascular and renal regulation. Endocrine Reviews 24: 261-271.
5. Campos LA, Cipolla-Neto J, Amaral FG, Michelini LC, Bader M, et al. (2013) The Angiotensin-melatonin axis. Int J Hypertens 2013: 521783.
6. Oelkers WK (1996) Effects of estrogens and progestogens on the renin-aldosterone system and blood pressure. Steroids 61: 166-171.
7. Zimmerman EA, Nilaver G, Hou-Yu A, Silverman AJ (1984) Vasopressinergic and oxytocinergic pathways in the central nervous system. Fed Proc 43: 91-96.
8. Sladek CD (1983) Regulation of vasopressin release by neurotransmitters, neuropeptides and osmotic stimuli. Prog Brain Res 60: 71-90.
9. Robertson GL, Athar S (1976) The interaction of blood osmolality and blood volume in regulating plasma vasopressin in man. J Clin Endocrinol Metab 42: 613-620.
10. Birnbaumer M (2000) Vasopressin receptors. Trends Endocrinol Metab 11: 406-410.
11. Lencer WI, Brown D, Ausiello DA, Verkman AS (1990) Endocytosis of water channels in rat kidney: cell specificity and correlation with in vivo antidiuresis. Am J Physiol 259: C920-932.
12. Field MJ, Stanton BA, Giebisch GH (1984) Influence of ADH on renal potassium handling: a micropuncture and microperfusion study. Kidney Int 25: 502-511.
13. Asplund R (2002) Diuresis pattern, plasma vasopressin and blood pressure in healthy elderly persons with nocturia and nocturnal polyuria. Neth J Med 60: 276-280.
14. Moon DG, Jin MH, Lee JG, Kim JJ, Kim MG, et al. (2004) Antidiuretic hormone in elderly male patients with severe nocturia: a circadian study. BJU Int 94: 571-575.
15. AbdelFatah D, Shaker H, Ismail M, Ezzat M (2009) Nocturnal polyuria and nocturnal arginine vasopressin (AVP): a key factor in the pathophysiology of monosymptomatic nocturnal enuresis. Neurourol Urodyn 28: 506-509.
16. Akiyama T, Hirayama A, Fujimoto K, Torimoto K, Yoshida K, et al. (2007) Cutoff value of urinary arginine vasopressin for nocturnal polyuria in elderly men. Urology 69: 98-102.
17. Hirayama A, Fujimoto K, Akiyama T, Hirao Y (2006) Decrease in nocturnal urinary levels of arginine vasopressin in patients with nocturnal polyuria. Urology 68: 19-23.
18. CvetkoviÄ RS, Plosker GL (2005) Desmopressin: in adults with nocturia. Drugs 65: 99-107.
19. Chang YL, Lin AT, Chen KK (2007) Short-term effects of desmopressin on water and electrolyte excretion in adults with nocturnal polyuria. J Urol 177: 2227-2229.
20. Juul KV, Klein BM, Nørgaard JP (2013) Long-term durability of the response to desmopressin in female and male nocturia patients. Neurourol Urodyn 32: 363-370.
21. Juul KV, Klein BM, Sandström R, Erichsen L, Nørgaard JP (2011) Gender difference in antidiuretic response to desmopressin. Am J Physiol Renal Physiol 300: F1116-1122.
22. Griendling KK, Murphy TJ, Alexander RW (1993) Molecular biology of the renin-angiotensin system. Circulation 87: 1816-1828.
23. Paul M, Poyan Mehr A, Kreutz R (2006) Physiology of local renin-angiotensin systems. Physiol Rev 86: 747-803.
24. MacGregor GA, Markandu ND, Roulston JE, Jones JC, Morton JJ (1981) Maintenance of blood pressure by the renin-angiotensin system in normal man. Nature 291: 329-331.
25. Kurtz A (2011) Renin release: sites, mechanisms, and control. Annu Rev Physiol 73: 377-399.
26. Friis UG, Madsen K, Stubbe J, Hansen PB, Svenningsen P, et al. (2013) Regulation of renin secretion by renal juxtaglomerular cells. Pflugers Arch 465: 25-37.
27. Crowley SD, Gurley SB, Oliverio MI, Pazmino AK, Griffiths R, et al. (2005) Distinct roles for the kidney and systemic tissues in blood pressure regulation by the renin-angiotensin system. J Clin Invest 115: 1092-1099.
28. Funder JW, Mihailidou AS (2009) Aldosterone and mineralocorticoid receptors: Clinical studies and basic biology. Mol Cell Endocrinol 301: 2-6.
29. Granger JP, Burnett JC Jr, Romero JC, Opgenorth TJ, Salazar J, et al. (1987) Elevated levels of atrial natriuretic peptide during aldosterone escape. Am J Physiol 252: R878-882.
30. Rittig S, Matthiesen TB, Pedersen EB, Djurhuus JC (2006) Circadian variation of angiotensin II and aldosterone in nocturnal enuresis: relationship to arterial blood pressure and urine output. J Urol 176: 774-780.
31. Matthiesen TB, Rittig S, Nørgaard JP, Pedersen EB, Djurhuus JC (1996) Nocturnal polyuria and natriuresis in male patients with nocturia and lower urinary tract symptoms. J Urol 156: 1292-1299.
32. Feldstein CA (2013) Nocturia in arterial hypertension: a prevalent, underreported, and sometimes underestimated association. J Am Soc Hypertens 7: 75-84.
33. Satoh M, Kikuya M, Ohkubo T, Mori T, Metoki H, et al. (2011) Aldosterone-to-renin ratio and nocturnal blood pressure decline in a general population: the Ohasama study. J Hypertens 29: 1940-1947.
34. Pelayo JC, Harris DC, Shanley PF, Miller GJ, Schrier RW (1988) Glomerular hemodynamic adaptations in remnant nephrons: effects of verapamil. Am J Physiol 254: F425-431.

35. Weinberger MH (1996) Salt sensitivity of blood pressure in humans. Hypertension 27: 481-490.
36. Uzu T, Ishikawa K, Fujii T, Nakamura S, Inenaga T, et al. (1997) Sodium restriction shifts circadian rhythm of blood pressure from nondipper to dipper in essential hypertension. Circulation 96: 1859-1862.
37. Fukuda M, Wakamatsu-Yamanaka T, Mizuno M, Miura T, Tomonari T, et al.(2011) Angiotensin receptor blockers shift the circadian rhythm of blood pressure by suppressing tubular sodium reabsorption. Am J Physiol Renal Physiol 301:953-957.
38. Reynard JM, Cannon A, Yang Q, Abrams P (1998) A novel therapy for nocturnal polyuria: a double-blind randomized trial of frusemide against placebo. Br J Urol 81: 215-218.
39. Cho Y, Somer BG, Amatya A (1999) Natriuretic peptides and their therapeutic potential. Heart Dis 1: 305-328.
40. Chopra S, Cherian D, Verghese PP, Jacob JJ (2013) Physiology and clinical significance of natriuretic hormones. Indian J Endocrinol Metab 17: 83-90.
41. Ganguly A (1992) Atrial natriuretic peptide-induced inhibition of aldosterone secretion: a quest for mediator(s) Am J Physiol 263: E181-194.
42. Nonoguchi H, Sands JM, Knepper MA (1988) Atrial Natriuretic Factor Inhibits Vasopressin-Stimulated Osmotic Water Permeability in Rat Inner Medullary Collecting Duct. J Clin Invest 82:1383-1390.
43. Mukoyama M, Nakao K, Hosoda K, Suga S, Saito Y, et al. (1991) Brain Natriuretic Peptide As A Novel Cardiac Hormone in Humans - Evidence for An Exquisite Dual Natriuretic Peptide System, Atrial-Natriuretic-Peptide and Brain Natriuretic Peptide. J Clin Invest 87:1402-1412.
44. Heringlake M, Heide C, Bahlmann L, Eichler W, Pagel H, et al. (2004) Effects of tilting and volume loading on plasma levels and urinary excretion of relaxin, NT-pro-ANP, and NT-pro-BNP in male volunteers. J Appl Physiol (1985) 97:173-179.
45. Hirayama A, Torimoto K, Yamada A, Tanaka N, Fujimoto K, et al. (2011) Relationship between nocturnal urine volume, leg edema, and urinary antidiuretic hormone in older men. Urology 77: 1426-1431.
46. Roueff S, Martin E, Chauffert ML, Poli I, Kihal K, et al. (2008) Brain natriuretic peptide variations are linked to volume status in hemodialysis patients. Clin Nephrol 70: 508-513.
47. Bing MH, Jennum P, Moller LA, Mortensen S, Lose G (2012) Obstructive sleep apnea in a Danish population of men and women aged 60-80 years with nocturia. J Clin Sleep Med 8: 515-520.
48. Umlauf MG, Chasens ER (2003) Sleep disordered breathing and nocturnal polyuria: nocturia and enuresis. Sleep Med Rev 7: 403-411.
49. Carter PG, Cannon A, McConnell AA, Abrams P (1999) Role of atrial natriuretic peptide in nocturnal polyuria in elderly males. Eur Urol 36: 213-220.
50. Torimoto K, Hirayama A, Samma S, Yoshida K, Fujimoto K, et al. (2009) The relationship between nocturnal polyuria and the distribution of body fluid: assessment by bioelectric impedance analysis. J Urol 181: 219-224.
51. Cho MC, Ku JH, Paick JS (2009) Alpha-Blocker Plus Diuretic Combination Therapy as Second-line Treatment for Nocturia in Men With LUTS: A Pilot Study. Urology 73:549-553.
52. Fu FG, Lavery HJ, Wu DL (2011) Reducing nocturia in the elderly: a randomized placebo-controlled trial of staggered furosemide and desmopressin. Neurourol Urodyn 30: 312-316.
53. De Guchtenaere A, Vande Walle C, Van Sintjan P, Donckerwolcke R, Raes A, et al. (2007) Desmopressin resistant nocturnal polyuria may benefit from furosemide therapy administered in the morning. J Urol 178: 2635-2639.
54. Weir MR (2002) Renal effects of nonselective NSAIDs and coxibs. Cleve Clin J Med 69 Suppl 1: SI53-58.
55. Schlondorff D (1986) Renal prostaglandin synthesis. Sites of production and specific actions of prostaglandins. Am J Med 81: 1-11.
56. Salazar FJ, Bolterman R, Hernandez I, Quesada T, Romero JC (1987) Role of prostaglandin and angiotensin II in ANP-induced natriuresis. Agents Actions Suppl 22: 111-123.
57. Araki T, Yokoyama T, Kumon H (2004) Effectiveness of a nonsteroidal anti-inflammatory drug for nocturia on patients with benign prostatic hyperplasia: a prospective non-randomized study of loxoprofen sodium 60 mg once daily before sleeping. Acta Med Okayama 58: 45-49.
58. Addla SK, Adeyoju AB, Neilson D, O'Reilly P(2006) Diclofenac for treatment of nocturia caused by nocturnal polyuria: A prospective, randomised, double-blind, placebo-controlled crossover study. European Urology 49:720-725.
59. Hardeland R (2012) Neurobiology, pathophysiology, and treatment of melatonin deficiency and dysfunction. ScientificWorldJournal 2012: 640389.
60. Wu YH, Zhou JN, Balesar R, Unmehopa U, Bao AM, et al. (2006) Distribution of MT1 melatonin receptor immunoreactivity in the human hypothalamus and pituitary gland: Colocalization of MT1 with vasopressin, oxytocin, and corticotropin-releasing hormone. J Comp Neurol 499: 897-910.
61. Lissoni P, Pelizzoni F, Perego M, Fondrini G, Grugni G, et al. (1990) A study of heart-pineal interactions: atrial natriuretic peptide response to melatonin administration in healthy humans. J Pineal Res 9: 167-170.
62. Lissoni P, Pelizzoni F, Grugni G, Guzzaloni G, Mauri O, et al. (1990) Melatonin Response to Atrial-Natriuretic-Peptide Administration in Healthy-Volunteers. J Cardiovasc Pharmacol 16:850-852.
63. Drake MJ, Mills IW, Noble JG (2004) Melatonin pharmacotherapy for nocturia in men with benign prostatic enlargement. J Urol 171: 1199-1202.
64. Gruber CJ, Tschugguel W, Schneeberger C, Huber JC (2002) Production and actions of estrogens. N Engl J Med 346: 340-352.
65. Graham JD, Clarke CL (1997) Physiological action of progesterone in target tissues. Endocr Rev 18: 502-519.
66. Shahidi NT (2001) A review of the chemistry, biological action, and clinical applications of anabolic-androgenic steroids. Clin Ther 23: 1355-1390.
67. Graugaard-Jensen C, Hvistendahl GM, Frøkiaer J, Bie P, Djurhuus JC (2008) The influence of high and low levels of estrogen on diurnal urine regulation in young women. BMC Urol 8: 16.
68. Stachenfeld NS, DiPietro L, Palter SF, Nadel ER (1998) Estrogen influences osmotic secretion of AVP and body water balance in postmenopausal women. Am J Physiol 274:187-195.
69. Vokes TJ, Weiss NM, Schreiber J, Gaskill MB, Robertson GL (1988) Osmoregulation of thirst and vasopressin during normal menstrual cycle. Am J Physiol 254: R641-647.
70. Maric-Bilkan C, Manigrasso MB (2012) Sex differences in hypertension: contribution of the renin-angiotensin system. Gend Med 9: 287-291.
71. Moehrer B, Hextall A, Jackson S (2003). Oestrogens for urinary incontinence in women. Cochrane Database Syst Rev 2: CD001405.
72. Long CY, Liu CM, Hsu SC, Chen YH, Wu CH, et al. (2006) A randomized comparative study of the effects of oral and topical estrogen therapy on the lower urinary tract of hysterectomized postmenopausal women. Fertil Steril 85: 155-160.
73. Kok AL, Burger CW, van de Weijer PH, Voetberg GA, Peters-Muller ER, et al. (1999) Micturition complaints in postmenopausal women treated with continuously combined hormone replacement therapy: a prospective study. Maturitas 31: 143-149.
74. Lose G, Englev E (2000) Oestradiol-releasing vaginal ring versus oestriol vaginal pessaries in the treatment of bothersome lower urinary tract symptoms. BJOG 107: 1029-1034.
75. Johnson TM 2nd, Burrows PK, Kusek JW, Nyberg LM, Tenover JL, et al. (2007) The effect of doxazosin, finasteride and combination therapy on nocturia in men with benign prostatic hyperplasia. J Urol 178: 2045-2050.

Effect of Coeliac Disease on Gastrointestinal Tract and Immunity

Fikry Elbossaty W*

Department of Chemistry, Biochemistry Division, Faculty of Science, Damietta University, Damietta, Egypt

***Corresponding author:** Fikry Elbossaty W, Department of Chemistry, Biochemistry Division, Faculty of Science, Damietta University, Damietta-34517, Egypt, E-mail: walaafikry1985@gmail.com

Abstract

Coeliac disease (CD) is an inflammatory genetic auto immune disease in which the patient have sensitivity against gluten which a protein present in wheat and some food. Once gluten enter the body, this induce immune system to make innate and acquired immune response in which the immune system produce autoantibodies which migrate in to small intestine and induced inflammation which effect on the function of small intestine not only but also the body secreted some mediators which increase the permeability of tissue to these antibodies and maybe cause damage in other organs. No medication for CD, the only treatment method is diet which gluten free in addition to the patients must be take some supplementation as a result of deficiency consequence since mal absorption. If this disease not diagnosis early it may be developed to produce different type of malignancy.

Keywords: Coeliac disease; Autoimmune disease; HLADQ2; HLADQ8; IgA deficiency

Introduction

Through all the diseases in our world, there are two different categories of immune diseases, the autoimmune and auto inflammatory disease. Autoimmune disorders are conditions that occur when the immune system mistakenly attacks and destroys healthy body tissue. Medline Plus suggests that there are "more than 80 different types of autoimmune disorders". Antigens include bacteria, viruses, cancer cells, toxins and blood or tissues from another person or species. The immune system produces antibodies that destroy these harmful substances [1].

Auto inflammatory diseases arise from disorders with the innate immune system. We have the adaptive immune system which selectively targets and fights infectious agents using antibodies. Then we have the innate immune system which fights anything in the body that it recognizes as foreign or non-self with a general and immediate response. Autoimmune and inflammatory both involve the adaptive immune system. "Autoimmune and Auto inflammatory diseases share common characteristics in that both groups of disorders result from the immune system attacking the body's own tissues, and also result in increased inflammation. Physicians and scientists should focus on disrupting these gut-immune pathways to understand the impact of gut flora activity on activity of autoimmune and auto inflammatory conditions" [2].

Celiac disease (CD) is a serious genetic autoimmune disease which affecting primarily the small intestine that happens in people who are genetically predisposed. CD is an autoimmune mediated enteropathy caused by a permanent intolerance to gluten in genetically predisposed individuals [3].

Gluten is the storage protein which present in wheat, rye, and barley that gives the dough its preferred baking properties. Celiac Disease is not a food allergy-it is an autoimmune disease [4].

Prevalence of Celiac Disease

CD is estimated to affect 1 in 100 people worldwide. Two and one-half million Americans are undiagnosed and are at risk for long-term health complications. Due to variable signs and symptoms it is assumed that about 85% of people affected are undiagnosed. The rate amongst adult blood donors in USA, Iran, Israel, Syria and Turkey is 1.2%, 0.60%, 0.64%, 1.61% and 1.15%, respectively (Figure 1a) [5].

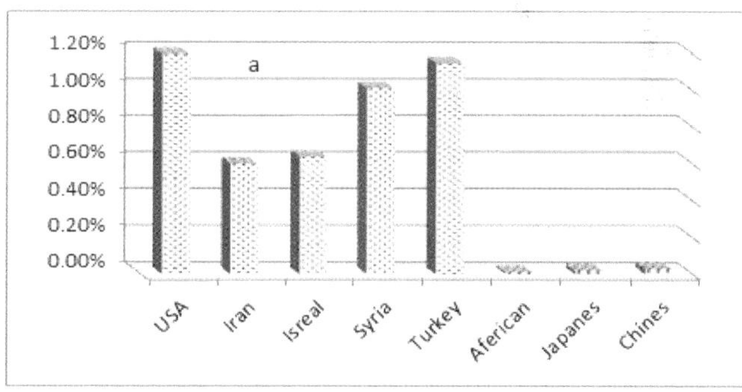

Figure 1a: Prevalence of Celiac disease (Statistical representation).

People of African, Japanese and Chinese descent are rarely diagnosed; this may be due to lower prevalence of the genetic risk factors, such as HLA-DQ8. People of Indian ancestry seem to have a similar risk to those of Western Caucasian ancestry. Coeliac disease is slightly more common in women than in men. Celiac disease is hereditary, meaning that it runs in families. A large multicenter study in the U.S. found a prevalence of 0.75% in not-at-risk groups, rising to 1.8% in symptomatic people, 2.6% in second-degree relatives (like grandparents, aunt or uncle, grandchildren, etc.) of a person with coeliac disease and 4.5% in first-degree relatives (siblings, parents or children).

This profile is similar to the prevalence in Europe. Other populations at increased risk for coeliac disease, with prevalence rates ranging from 5% to 10%, include individuals with Down and Turner syndromes, Type 1 diabetes, and autoimmune thyroid disease (Figure 1b) [6].

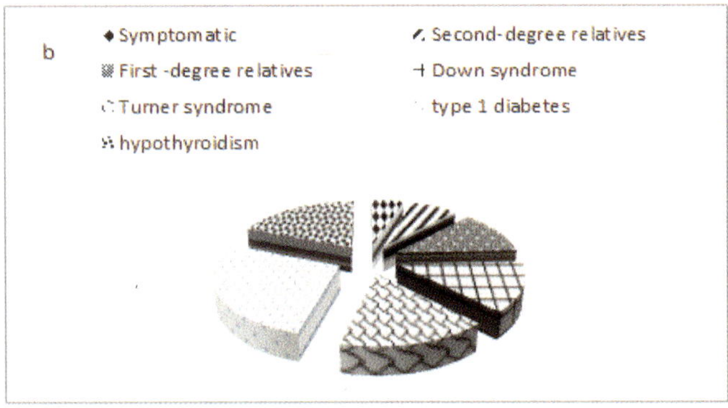

Figure 1b: Prevalence of Celiac disease.

Signs and Symptoms of CD

A new US Preventive Services Task Force found that insufficient evidence on the effectiveness of screening for celiac disease in asymptomatic adults, adolescents, and children with regard to morbidity, mortality, or quality of life [7].

There were different symptoms for celiac disease which can be different from person to other according to age, gender, country, and disease severity. Sign and symptoms of CD were summarized in Table 1 [8].

Sign	Causes
Gastrointestinal symptoms	
Chronic diarrhea	An inflammatory reaction in the small-bowel may produce shortening of the villi lining the small intestine
Abdominal distention	
Malabsorption	
Loss of appetite	
Malignant disease	
Small-bowel adenocarcinoma	Malignant diseases are more frequent in patients with long-term untreated classical CD
Esophageal and oropharyngeal squamous-cell carcinoma	
Non-Hodgkin's lymphoma	
Autoimmune disorders	
Insulin-dependent type 1 diabetes	CD is an inflammatory disorder which associate with other secondary autoimmune reactions
HLA-based autoimmune thyroiditis (e.g., Hashimoto's disease)	
Sjögren's syndrome	
Neurological disorders	

Table 1: Signs and symptoms of CD.

Classification of CD

Recognition of the different clinical presentations of CD is important in order to accurately early diagnose and decrease the risk of long-term complications.CD can be classified in to 4 groups according to clinical manifestation [9].

- Classical CD is accompanied with symptoms of gastrointestinal malabsorption.
- Atypical CD is characterized by non-prominent gastrointestinal manifestations with little or no symptoms. This may be the most common form of CD. Patients may present with chronic fatigue, anemia, dental enamel hypoplasia, reflux, bloating, migraines, osteoporosis, short stature, constipation, infertility, muscle weakness and/or depression.
- Silent CD is pronounced as asymptomatic patients with positive serological tests and villous atrophy on biopsy.
- Latent CD is characterized by positive serological tests, but with a normal small bowel biopsy. Patients are asymptomatic, but often develop symptoms and/or histological changes at late stage.

Mechanism Action of CD

CD appears to be multifactorial, there were different reasons for induce CD disease, CD is inflammatory autoimmune disease in which once the diet rich with gluten enter the body this stimulate the body to produce enzymes called trans-glutamines which responsible for protein sequence change, this alteration lead to activation of immune system, and in response to immune response more autoantibodies were produced which responsible for inflammation of small intestine and effect on absorption of different nutrients and caused malabsorption [3].

Also, there was another reason for induced CD which known as genetic factors. Almost all people (95%) with coeliac disease have either the variant HLA-DQ2 (major) allele or the HLA-DQ8 (minor) allele. The massive of people with CD have one of two types of the HLA-DQ protein. HLA-DQ is part of the MHC class II antigen-presenting receptor system and distinguishes cells between self and non-self for the purposes of the immune system. The two subunits of the HLA-DQ protein are encoded by the *HLA-DQA1* and *HLA-DQB1* genes, which located on the short arm of the sixth chromosome. Membrane leaking permits peptides of gliadin that stimulate two levels of immune response, the innate response and the adaptive (T-helper cell mediated) response.

One protease-resistant peptide from α-gliadin contains a region that stimulates lymphocytes and results in the release of interleukin-15. This innate response to gliadin results in immune-system signaling that attracts inflammatory cells and increases the release of inflammatory chemicals [10]. There are several pathways including cellular signals that may be involved in the mucosal damage in CD. Deamidation of gluten peptides by tissue tTG reinforces presentation of gluten peptides by HLA-DQ2 or HLA-DQ8 molecules of plasmacytoid dendritic cells (pDCs) to T cells, which activate gluten-reactive Th1 cells and produce high levels of proinflammatory cytokines. IL-21 is overproduced in the mucosa of CD patients, where it helps sustain T-bet expression and IFN-γ production. Th1 cytokines promote increased cytotoxicity of IELs and natural killer (NK) T cells which cause apoptotic death of enterocytes by the Fas/Fas ligand system, or IL-15-induced perforin/granzyme and NKG2D-MICA signaling pathways. IFN-α released by activated pDCs perpetuates the inflammatory reaction by inducing Th1 cells to produce IFN-γ. IL-21 and IL-15 produced by DCs and intraepithelial cells also inhibit transforming growth factor beta signaling and regulatory T cells (Tregs) function. Additionally, the production of Th2 cytokines, Th2 cells drives the activation and clonal expansion and differentiate of B cells into plasma cells secreting anti-gliadin and anti-tissue transglutaminase antibodies, which interact with extracellular tTG, and may induce epithelial damage [11].

Hence in CD, there is impaired suppressor activity of Tregs. This defect in Tregs function could play a role in the pathogenesis of CD and in CD autoimmunity [12].

How CD was Diagnosed

The early disease diagnosis, the early recovery from disease and inhibit the disease compliments. Diagnosis of many disease depend on the different signs, but in case of CD disease there were some people suffer from CD but without and signs or symptoms. So, it is very important to discover new tools for early diagnosis of CD, not only but also accurate diagnosis due to the similarity between CD and other gastrointestinal symptoms.

Guidelines for CD diagnosis from the European Society for Paediatric Gastroenterology, Hepatology, and Nutrition (ESPGHAN) propose the option to omit the duodenal biopsy in the diagnosis of CD if all 4 of the following criteria are met in children and adolescents [13]

- Signs and symptoms suggestive of CD
- Anti-transglutaminase type 2 antibody (anti-TG2) levels more than 10 times the upper limit of normal
- Positive confirmation tests of anti-endomysium-IgA antibodies (EMA)
- At-risk HLA-DQ2 or HLA-DQ8

According to Nevoral et al., intestinal biopsies for CD could be omitted in 28% of patients when ESPGHAN guidelines (European Society for Pediatric Gastroenterology, Hepatology and Nutrition) are applied. The authors found that because of the high accuracy of serologic tests and clinical symptoms of CD, the new guidelines seem applicable even without HLA testing. Of the 345 biopsied children, 213 (62%) had anti-TG titers greater than 10 times the upper limit of normal and positive EMA antibodies. Ninety-nine (29%) of the patients also had symptoms suggestive of CD in addition to EMA positivity and elevated titers of anti-TG greater than 10 times the upper limit of normal [14].

The diagnosis methods for CD were mentioned below [15].

Blood tests

Serological blood tests are the first-line exploration necessary to make a diagnosis of CD. Its sensitivity draws a parallel with the degree of histological lesions. People who present minor damage of the small intestine may have seronegative results so many patients with CD often are neglected. Serological blood tests were included autoantibodies which secreted according to the entrance of gluten in to small intestine as:

- IgA endomysial antibody (IgA EMA; highest diagnostic accuracy) with a sensitivity and specificity of 90% and 99%, respectively [16].

a. IgA tissue transglutaminase antibody (IgA tTG)

b. IgA antigliadin antibody (IgA AGA)

c. IgG antigliadin antibody (IgG AGA)

Serologic studies for CD can be divided into two groups, according to the target antigens [15].

- Anti-tTG antibody tests with higher sensitivity (99%) and specificity (>90%).
- Antigliadin antibody tests were there no longer routinely recommended, because of their lower sensitivity and specificity.

For the reason that the major implications of a diagnosis of CD, certified strategies recommend that a positive blood test is still followed by an endoscopy and biopsy. A negative serology test may still be followed by a recommendation for endoscopy and duodenal biopsy if clinical suspicion remains high.

Antibody testing may well be combined with HLA testing if the diagnosis is vague. TGA and EMA testing are the most sensitive serum antibody tests, but as a negative HLA-DQ type omits the diagnosis of CD, testing also for HLA-DQ2 or DQ8 maximizes sensitivity and negative predictive values [17].

Endoscopy

Most people with CD have a small intestine that seems to be normal on endoscopy before the biopsies are examined. However, five findings have been associated with a high specificity for CD: scalloping of the small bowel folds, paucity in the folds, a mosaic pattern to the mucosa, prominence of the sub mucosa blood vessels, and a nodular pattern to the mucosa. European recommendations suggest that in children and adolescents with symptoms which are compatible with CD, the diagnosis can be made without the need for intestinal biopsy if anti-tTG antibodies titres are very high (10 times the upper limit of normal) [18].

Differentiating between Confirmed Celiac Disease and Unconfirmed Celiac Disease

Gastroenterologists are already familiar with the association of CD with several immune and non-immune based diseases in the digestive system, including ulcerative colitis, Crohn's disease, microscopic colitis, autoimmune liver diseases, fatty liver and elevated liver transaminase levels. However, many diseases outside the digestive system have also been linked with CD, both in its overt and silent forms [19].

The association of dermatitis herpetiformis with gluten sensitive enteropathy is widely recognized. Diseases most typically associated with silent CD are immune-based disorders, such as type 1 diabetes mellitus, autoimmune thyroid diseases, Sjögren's syndrome and Addison's disease. An association with atopy has also been described, but this has been disputed. Other disease associations of uncertain pathogenesis include dental enamel defects, epilepsy with cerebral calcification, neuropathy, cerebellar ataxia, chorea and infertility [20].

Treatment of CD

At this time, the only treatment for celiac disease is lifelong adherence to a strict gluten-free diet. Individuals suffer from CD must be avoid foods containing wheat, rye and barley, or its derivatives such as bread and beer. Consumption insignificant quantities of gluten, can initiate abdominal destruction. Until now there is no medication which will avoid destruction or protect the body from attacking the gut as soon as gluten is taken. The food which are allowed or not allowed for CD patients are summarized in Table 2 [21].

Diet allowed in CD		Diet not allowed in CD
Corn	Nuts	Wheat
Sorghum	Meat	
Millet	Fish	
Kasha	Egg	
Beans/Peas	Rye	
Quinoa	Barley	
Potato	Breads	
Soybean	Pasta	
Tapioca	Kamut	
Triticale	Einkorn	

Table 2: List of diet in CD patients.

There was new trend in the future to try solving the problem of coeliac disease, this trend can be used as new strategy to treatment of CD by using different pathways such as [22]:

- Gluten detoxification by using genetic engineering technique on wheat species and this improve the structure of these species and allow consumption by the CD patients without any problems.
- Modulation of the intestinal permeability, which responsible for increase the permeability of gluten into gut not only but also increase the mobilization of autoantibodies into intestine and this encourage the immune response reaction and caused inflammation in intestine. this may be occur by the inhibition of zonulin, which act as an endogenous signaling protein linked to increased permeability of the bowel wall and hence increased presentation of gliadin to the immune system by using larazotide acetate [23].
- Modulation of the immune response Coeliac disease represents as inflammatory autoimmune disease, so one of the reason of induce CD is disturbance in immune system so, one of the problem solving is control of immune system work by using some agents like CCX282-B.

Coeliac disease patients must be visit physician to take some supplementation to protect their selves from infection, fatigue, anemia due to deficiency of iron, calcium, zinc which result from malabsorption due to small intestine inflammation [24].

References

1. Abbas A, Lichtman AH, Pillai S (2015) Properties and overview of immune responses. In: Abbas AK, Lichtman AH, Pillai S (8th edn.) Cellular and Molecular Immunology. Elsevier Saunders, Philadelphia, USA.
2. Firestein GS (2016) Mechanisms of inflammation and tissue repair. In: Goldman L, Schafer AI (25th edn.) Goldman's Cecil Medicine, Elsevier Saunders, Philadelphia, USA.
3. Lundin K, Wijmenga C (2015) Coeliac disease and autoimmune disease-genetic overlap and screening. Nat Rev Gastroenterol Hepatol 12: 507-215.
4. Penagini F, Dilillo D, Meneghin F, Mameli C, Fabiano V (2013) Gluten-free diet in children: an approach to a nutritionally adequate and balanced diet. Nutrients 5: 4553-4565.
5. Vivas S, Vaquero L, Martin LR, Caminero A (2015) Age-related differences in celiac disease: Specific characteristics of adult presentation. World J Gastrointest Pharmacol Ther 6: 207-212.
6. Husby S, Koletzko S, Szabo IK, Mearin M, Phillips A (2012) European society for pediatric gastroenterology, hepatology, and nutrition guidelines for the diagnosis of coeliac disease. J Pediatr Gastroenterol Nutr 54: 136-160.
7. Domingo KB, Grossman D, Susan J, Michael J, KarinaW, et al. (2017) USPSTF recommendation: Screening for celiac disease. JAMA 317: 1251-1257.
8. Leffler D, Green P, Fasano A (2015) Extra intestinal manifestations of coeliac disease. Nat Rev Gastroenterol Hepatol 12: 561-571.
9. Tonutti E, Bizzaro N (2014) Diagnosis and classification of celiac disease and gluten sensitivity. Autoimmun Rev 13: 472-476.
10. Jores R, Frau F, Cucca F, Grazia M (2007) HLA-DQB1*0201 homozygosis predisposes to severe intestinal damage in celiac disease. Scand J Gastroenterol 42: 48-53.
11. Berni R, Pezzella V, Amoroso A, Cozzolino T (2016) Diagnosing and treating intolerance to carbohydrates in children. Nutrients 8: 157-166.
12. Fina D, Sarra M, Caruso R, Pallone F, MacDonald TT, et al. (2008) Interleukin 21 contributes to the mucosal T helper cell type 1 response in coeliac disease. Gut 57: 887-892.
13. Granzotto M, Bo SD, Quaglia S, Tommasini A, Piscianz E, et al. (2009) Regulatory T-cell function is impaired in celiac disease. Dig Dis Sci 54: 1513-1519.
14. Schirru E, Jores RD, Congia M (2014) Prudence is necessary in the application of the new ESPGHAN criteria for celiac disease omitting duodenal biopsy: A case report. Eur J Gastroenterol Hepatol 26: 679-680.
15. Nevoral J, Kotalova R, Hradsky O, Valtrova V, Zarubova K, et al. (2013) Symptom positivity is essential for omitting biopsy in children with suspected celiac disease according to the new ESPGHAN guidelines. Eur J Pediatr 173: 497-502.
16. Tovoli F, Masi C, Guidetti E, Negrini G (2015) Clinical and diagnostic aspects of gluten related disorders. World J Clin Cases 3: 275-284.
17. Lionetti E, Castellaneta S, Francavilla R, Pulvirenti A (2014) Introduction of gluten, HLA status, and the risk of celiac disease in children. NEJM 371: 1295-1303.
18. Cerezo ER, Capilla AS, La PD, Teresa JD (2014) Wireless capsule endoscopy: Perspectives beyond gastrointestinal bleeding. World J Gastroenterol 20: 15664-15673.
19. Bardella MT, Valenti L, Pagliari C, Peracchi M, Fare M, et al. (2004) Searching for coeliac disease in patients with non-alcoholic fatty liver disease. Dig Liver Dis 36: 333-336.
20. Pereira AC, Edwards MJ, Buttery PC, Hawkes CH, Quinn NP, et al. (2004) Choreic syndrome and coeliac disease: A hitherto unrecognised association. Mov Disord 19: 478-482.
21. Mulder C, van Wanrooij R, Bakker S, Wierdsma N (2013) Gluten-free diet in gluten-related disorders. Dig Dis 31: 57-62.
22. Castillo N, Theethira T, Leffler DELTA (2015) The present and the future in the diagnosis and management of celiac disease. Gastroenterol Rep 3: 3-11.
23. Woodward J (2016) Improving outcomes of refractory celiac disease-current and emerging treatment strategies. Clin Exp Gastroenterol 9: 225-236.
24. Levy J, Bernstein L, Silber N (2014) Celiac disease: An immune dysregulation syndrome. Curr Probl Pediatr Adolesc Health Care 44: 324-327.

Kaempferol Exhibits Progestogenic Effects in Ovariectomized Rats

May Fern Toh, Emma Mendonca, Sharon L. Eddie, Michael P. Endsley, Daniel D. Lantvit, Pavel A. Petukhov, and Joanna E. Burdette*

Department of Medicinal Chemistry and Pharmacognosy, College of Pharmacy, University of Illinois at Chicago, Chicago, IL 60607, USA

***Corresponding author:** Joanna E. Burdette, 900 S. Ashland Street (M/C 870) Chicago, IL 60607, USA, E-mail: joannab@uic.edu

Abstract

Objective: Progesterone (P_4) plays a central role in women's health. Synthetic progestins are used clinically in hormone replacement therapy (HRT), oral contraceptives, and for the treatment of endometriosis and infertility. Unfortunately, synthetic progestins are associated with side effects, including cardiovascular disease and breast cancer. Botanical dietary supplements are widely consumed for the alleviation of a variety of gynecological issues, but very few studies have characterized natural compounds in terms of their ability to bind to and activate progesterone receptors (PR). Kaempferol is a flavonoid that functions as a non-steroidal selective progesterone receptor modulator (SPRM) *in vitro*. This study investigated the molecular and physiological effects of kaempferol in the ovariectomized rat uteri.

Methods: Since genistein is a phytoestrogen that was previously demonstrated to increase uterine weight and proliferation, the ability of kaempferol to block genistein action in the uterus was investigated. Analyses of proliferation, steroid receptor expression, and induction of well-established PR-regulated targets *Areg* and *Hand2* were completed using histological analysis and qPCR gene induction experiments. In addition, kaempferol *in silico* binding analysis was completed for PR. The activation of estrogen and androgen receptor signalling was determined *in vitro*.

Results: Molecular docking analysis confirmed that kaempferol adopts poses that are consistent with occupying the ligand-binding pocket of PRA. Kaempferol induced expression of PR regulated transcriptional targets in the ovariectomized rat uteri, including *Hand2* and *Areg*. Consistent with progesterone-like activity, kaempferol attenuated genistein-induced uterine luminal epithelial proliferation without increasing uterine weight. Kaempferol signalled without down regulating PR expression *in vitro* and *in vivo* and without activating estrogen and androgen receptors.

Conclusion: Taken together, these data suggest that kaempferol is a unique natural PR modulator that activates PR signaling *in vitro* and *in vivo* without triggering PR degradation.

Keywords: Kaempferol; Progestin; Progesterone receptor; Genistein; Hormone replacement therapy; Botanicals

Introduction

Progesterone (P_4) plays an essential role in female health. The importance of P_4 has led to the continued development of synthetic progesterone receptor (PR) ligands for a variety of women's health issues [1,2]. For example, oral contraceptives, combination hormone replacement therapy (HRT) for the treatment of menopausal symptoms, and to reduce the risk of endometrial hyperplasia and cancer associated with unopposed E_2 therapy [3-5]. These common treatments contain synthetic progestins, such as medroxyprogesterone acetate (MPA), which are associated with deleterious side effects including cardiovascular disease, heart attack, stroke, and breast cancer [6,7]. Side effects are thought to occur primarily due to the promiscuous binding of synthetic progestins to other nuclear receptors such as the androgen receptor (AR), glucocorticoid receptor (GR), and mineralocorticoid receptor (MR) [8]. Therefore, the identification of progestins that have tissue and receptor specificity with minimal side effects is important.

Due to the side effects associated with HRT and the perceived safety of natural remedies, millions of menopausal women are seeking alternative therapies in the form of botanical extracts and dietary supplements [9]. Most of the formulas used to treat menopausal symptoms contain estrogenic compounds, such as genistein and 8-prenyl-naringenin that bind and activate estrogen receptors. Unopposed estrogen signaling in the uterus is associated with hyperplasia and cancer [10]. P_4 when combined with E_2 protects against proliferation and hyperplasia of endometrial cells [11]. Therefore, botanical formulations containing both a phytoestrogen and a phytoprogestin should be safer in the uterus. Some botanicals have been identified that contain progestogenic compounds as demonstrated by *in vitro* and *in vivo* assays [12-17].

Selective PR modulators (SPRMs) are a class of PR ligands that function as an agonist, antagonist, or mixed agonist/antagonist and have clinically relevant tissue selectivity [4]. Previous studies demonstrated kaempferol is a non-steroidal phytoprogestin that functions in a cell-specific manner *in vitro* [13]. Kaempferol is a widely distributed dietary flavonoid found in fruits and vegetables that also has anti-oxidant and anti-inflammatory properties [18]. The anti-inflammatory properties of kaempferol appear to be meditated by nuclear factor-κB (NFκB) [19,20]. In animal studies, kaempferol inhibited ovarian cancer tumorigenesis and angiogenesis [21,22]. Moreover, in human epidemiological studies, kaempferol intake significantly decreased (40%) ovarian cancer incidence [21]. The biological activities demonstrated by kaempferol in these previous studies are consistent with kaempferol functioning as a progestin, especially considering progestins are known to inhibit NFκB and are well known to protect against ovarian cancer [23-25].

The objective of this study was to investigate if kaempferol exerts progesterone-like effects *in vivo* using the ovariectomized Sprague-Dawley rat model. Since genistein is a phytoestrogen that was previously demonstrated to increase uterine weight and proliferation [3], the ability of kaempferol to block genistein action in the uterus was investigated. Analyses of proliferation, steroid receptor expression, and induction of well-established PR-regulated targets *Areg* and *Hand2* were completed. In addition, kaempferol *in silico* binding analysis was completed for PR, as was the activation of ER and AR signaling *in vitro* in order to determine receptor specificity. The data from this study suggest that kaempferol interacts with PR, activates the receptor without stimulating its degradation, antagonizes genistein-induced endometrial proliferation, and induces known PR target genes *in vivo*.

Materials and Methods

Reagents

All chemicals and reagents were purchased from Fisher (Hanover Park, IL) or Sigma-Aldrich (St. Louis, MO) unless otherwise indicated. All media for cell culture were purchased from Life Technologies, Inc (Carlsbad, CA). Fetal bovine serum (FBS) and charcoal stripped serum was purchased from Atlanta Biologicals (Norcross, GA). Genistein and kaempferol were purchased form Indofine Chemical Co. (Belle Mead, NJ) and Sigma-Aldrich (St. Louis, MO). Desmethylarzoxifen (DMA) was provided by Dr. Gregory Thatcher (Department of Medicinal Chemistry, University of Illinois at Chicago).

Molecular modeling

The crystal structure of the human PR in complex with the agonist P_4 (PDB: 1A28; 1.8 Å) was used in the docking procedure [26]. The protein model was analyzed using the protein structure preparation module in MOE [27]. All ligands and water molecules were removed and hydrogen atoms were added using Protonate3D. This structure was saved as a PDB file. The 3D structures of the ligands were built and inspected with VIDA and AM1-BCC [28] partial atomic charges were calculated with Molcharge [27] and minimized using OMEGA [27]. All ligands were docked into the binding pocket of PR using GOLD (version 5.1, CCDC, Cambridge, UK) [29]. The active site was defined as all protein atoms within 6 Å of P_4. The scoring function used to rank the docked poses was Chem-PLP. A maximum of twenty docking solutions were generated for each structure, with early termination of the process if the respective RMSDs of the three highest ranked docking solutions were within 1.5 Å RMSD of one another (GOLD default 1 setting: 100,000 Genetic Algorithm (GA) Operations, 5 islands). Flipping of ring free corners, amide bonds, protonated carboxylic acids and planar or pyramidal nitrogen atoms were allowed. MOE was also used to analyze the docking results and generate figures. The top-ranked poses were further co-minimized using MOE LigX module utilizing AMBER12HT force field for optimization and calculation of affinity score [30].

Cell culture and cell lines

Human endometrial stromal cells (HESCs) were provided by Dr. Asgerally Fazleabas (Department of Obstetrics, Gynecology, and Reproductive Biology, Michigan State University, Grand Rapids, MI). HESCs were cultured according to a previous study [29].

Luciferase assay

HESCs were grown in 12-well plates until 80% confluent. MDA-231 were grown in 12-well plates at 100,000 cells per well. Progesterone responsive element (PRE), estrogen responsive element (ERE), or prostate specific antigen (PSA) was performed as previously described and the transfection efficiency and cell viability was normalized to a co-transfected beta-galactosidase plasmid (β-gal) [13]. Transfections preceded treatment for 24 or 48 hours. Cell lysates (50 μL) were placed in 96-well plate. The luciferase activity was quantified as previously described [29]. The results are presented as the average fold induction of treated over untreated cells (DMSO) after correcting for transfection efficiency from triplicate experiments.

Western Blot Analysis

HESC cells were incubated in serum free media with various agents for 48 hours. Cells were lysed in 1X RIPA buffer (50 mM Tris, pH 7.6, 150 mM NaCl, 1% (v/v) Triton X-100, 0.1% (w/v) SDS) and Roche protease inhibitor (Roche, Madison, WI). Protein concentrations were measured using BCA protein assay reagent (BioRad, Hercules, CA). Protein was separated by 7% SDS-PAGE and transferred onto nitrocellulose membrane. Membranes were blocked in 5% non-fat milk in Tris-buffered saline-Tween (TBS-T-1%). PR-A/B proteins were probed for with antibody (Santa Cruz Biotechnology, Santa Cruz, CA) in 5% milk in TBS-T. Membranes were re-probed for actin (Cell Signaling, Danvers, MA) as loading control. Signals were detected using chemiluminescence SuperSignal West Femto Chemiluminescent Kit, (Thermo Scientific, Hanover Park, IL) according to the manufacturer's protocol on Protein Simple FluorChem E (Santa Clara, CA).

Rat study

All animal studies were approved by the UIC Animal Care and Use Committee. Sprague-Dawley ovariectomized (OVX) rats were utilized for this study to eliminate endogenous hormone production. Twenty-four animals weighing 160-180 g were purchased for the study (n=8/group) (Harlan Laboratories, Madison, WI). All rats were housed at 21°C in 12 h light:12 h dark cycles and were fed 7% corn diet (Harlan Laboratories, Madison, WI) devoid of phytoestrogens. Two weeks post ovariectomy, 5.625 mg kaempferol or genistein was dissolved in a DMSO/corn oil mixture and given via oral gavage daily for 8 days based on a previous study demonstrating estrogenic action of genistein at this dose and duration [3]. Control animals were given DMSO/corn oil only. Animals were sacrificed 24 h after the last injection.

Immunohistochemistry

Uteri were carefully excised, weighed, and fixed in 4% paraformaldehyde overnight. Histological analyses were performed according to a previously published study [31]. Primary antibodies utilized in this study included Ki67 (Abcam, Cambridge, MA), PR, ERα and Hand2 (Santa Cruz Biotechnology, Santa Cruz, CA) [32]. For PR, ERα and Ki67, a biotinylated horseradish peroxidase-conjugated anti-rabbit IgG was used as the secondary antibody (1:200, Vector, Burlingame, CA). For Hand2 detection a biotinylated horseradish peroxidase-conjugated anti-goat IgG was used as the secondary antibody (1:200, Vector, Burlingame, CA). Secondary antibody incubation was followed by ABC peroxidase detection enhancement (Vector, Burlingame, CA) and detected by DAB as the chromogen (Vector, Burlingame, CA). Slides were counterstained with haemotoxylin and photomicrographs of sections were obtained using Nikon Eclipse E600 microscope. To assess proliferation in the luminal epithelial cells, a minimum of 300 cells were quantified (2 sections per animal) and the average taken. Data are represented as percentage of positive cells. In the stroma, the entire endometrial section was examined, and the number of proliferating stromal cells was categorized as 0, no staining; fewer than 5, low; and more than 5, high. High, low and absent Ki67 expression was classified in endometrial stroma for all four groups.

qPCR

Uterine RNA was isolated using Trizol (Invitrogen, Carlsbad, CA) reagent as per manufacturer's instructions. The quality of total RNA was determined spectrophotometrically. Complementary DNA was made using RevertAid first strand cDNA synthesis kit (Fermentes, Glen Burnie, MD) in a total volume of 20 μl. Each real-time PCR consisted of 100 ng cDNA, 10 μl FastStart SYBR Green PCR Master Mix (Roche, Madison, WI), and 0.5 μM forward and reverse primers (IDT, San Jose, CA). PCR analyses were conducted using the following set of primers; *Gapdh* 5'- CATGGCCTTCCGTGTTCCTA-3' (forward) and 5'-CCTGCTTCACCACCTTCTTGAT-3' (reverse), *Rpl1* 5'- CTGTGAGGGCATCAACATTTC-3' (forward) and 5'-GTTGGTGTTCATCCGCTTTC-3' (reverse), *ERα* 5'-AATTCTGACAATCGACGCCAG-3' (forward) and 5'-GTGCTTCAACATTCTCCCTCCTC-3' (reverse), *PR* 5'-CCCGACACTTCCAGCTCTTT-3' (forward) and 5'-TGTGGGATTTGCCACATGGT-3' (reverse), *Hand2* 5'-AAGAGGAAGAAAGAGCTGAATGAGAT-3' (forward) and 5'-CGTTGCTGCTCACTGTGCTT-3' (reverse), *Areg* 5'-AACTGAACTTCTGGAGCCTTC-3' (forward) and 5'-CATGCCATAGCCTAGCTGAT-3' (reverse). Fold change in mRNA expression was determined via the ΔΔCt method, with *Gapdh* as an internal control for *Areg and Rlp1* for *Hand2, PR* and *ERa.* Data reported are the mean fold change ± SEM for three replicates compared to vehicle control.

Statistical analysis

All data were analyzed using one-way ANOVA, followed by Tukey's test for multiple comparisons. Statistical significance was defined as #$p < 0.05$ between groups, *$p < 0.05$ compared to control, groups not marked were not statistically different from each other.

Results

Molecular modeling of kaempferol, MPA and P_4 in PR Ligand Binding Domain (LBD)

Kaempferol was previously reported to bind to PR, activate PRE-luciferase in a concentration-dependent manner, and it was antagonized by RU486 in T47D and human endometrial stromal cells (HESC) [13]. In order to further characterize the ability of kaempferol to bind the PR, a molecular docking study was used to highlight and compare the binding interactions of kaempferol with those of RU486, P_4, and MPA at active site residues. Kaempferol fits into the ligand binding domain (LBD) and has an affinity score comparable to those of RU486, P_4, and MPA (Table 1). Consistent with previous reports, RU486 is a stronger PR binder as compared to P_4 and demonstrated the highest affinity score [33]. Top poses of MPA and kaempferol are shown in Figure 1. The 4'-, 5-, and 7-hydroxyl groups of kaempferol form hydrogen bonds with Gln725, Thr894, Asn719, respectively. The binding pose of MPA is very similar to P_4 and RU486. In addition to the hydrogen bond between the 3-keto group and the side chain amide moiety of Gln725, the acetate group in kaempferol extends into the pocket formed by Leu715, Leu718 and Phe794, which is occupied by the 17α-propynyl group in RU486. Kaempferol's interaction with the LBD of PR is driven by a combination of hydrogen bonding and hydrophobic contacts commonly observed for all PR ligands.

Ligand	Affinity (kcal/mol)
Kaempferol	-8.88
P_4	-11.76
MPA	-14.36
RU486	-15.22

Table 1: Known progesterone receptor ligands used in this study and affinity scores for the best docking poses after co-minimization in the binding site

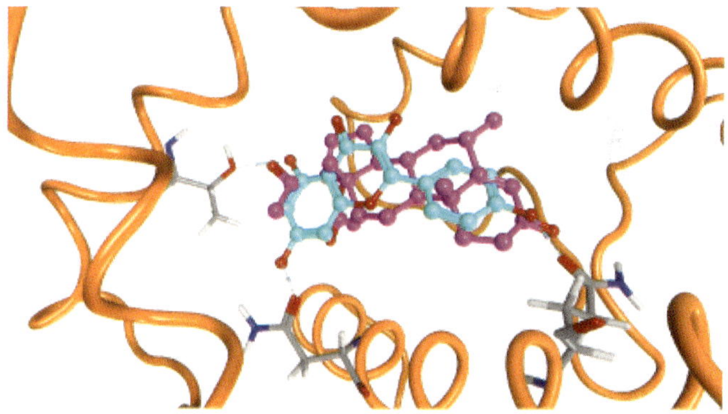

Figure 1: Kaempferol (cyan) and MPA (magenta) bound to the ligand binding domain of PR.

The interactions of the aromatic rings of kaempferol and MPA are similar to P_4 in the ligand binding domain of the receptor. The 4'-hydroxyl group of kaempferol anchors to Gln725 analogous to the keto group of P_4 or MPA. Additionally, the 7-hydroxyl moiety on the phenyl ring forms a hydrogen bond with Asn719 and the 5-hydroxyl group interacts with Thr894. MPA gains more interactions through its ester linked arm that extends into the cavity formed by Leu715, Leu718 and Phe794.

Kaempferol does not increase uterine weight of OVX rats

Since botanicals are mixtures and are often consumed as multi-botanical formulations, the ability of kaempferol to oppose genistein action in the uterus was investigated [34-36]. Genistein is a phytoestrogen found in commonly used botanical supplements soy and red clover that activates ER and increases uterine weight and cell proliferation similar to E_2 [3]. Based on a previous study, Sprague-Dawley rats (200 g) fed 375 µg genistein/g of food/day demonstrated significant uterine weight gain and proliferation [3].

The dose of genistein and the length of treatment in this study were calculated based on the average amount of food consumed per day (15 g/animal/day), indicating that genistein at 5.625 mg/animal/day for 8 days should significantly induce uterine proliferation. Kaempferol's ability to block genistein-induced proliferation in OVX rats after 8 days of oral treatment was investigated (Table 2). As expected, the uterine wet weights of genistein-treated animals were significantly higher than control rats (Table 2). Oral administration of an equal dose of kaempferol (5.625 mg/animal/day) did not significantly increase uterine wet weight compared to control group, indicating that kaempferol did not induce an estrogenic response in the uterus (Table 2), consistent with previous reports [37,38]. Additive effects were not observed on uterine weight in animals co-treated with kaempferol and genistein.

Treatment (5.625mg/animal/day)	Uterine Weight (mg)
Vehicle (control)	63.3 ± 24
Genistein	90.0 ± 17*
Kaempferol	52.0 ± 25
Genistein + Kaempferol	95.7 ± 22*

Table 2: Genistein induced uterine wet weight increase in OVX Sprague-Dawley rats. Animals were administered with vehicle control, genistein, kaempferol and geninstein+kaempferol for 8 days via oral gavage. Data are uterine wet weights (mg) 24 h after last treatment (n = 8 per group). Mean ± SEM (*$p < 0.05$) as determined by one-way ANOVA test.

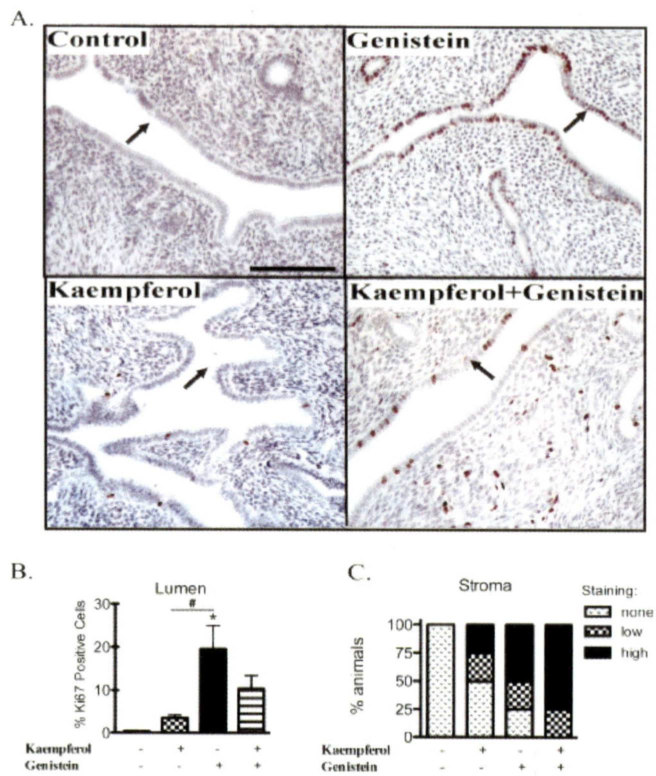

Figure 2: Cell proliferation in response to oral treatment with vehicle (control), genistein, kaempferol and genistein+kaempferol in OVX rat uteri. Representative sections of uterus immunostained for Ki67 (A). Results are represented as percentage of Ki67 positive cells in the luminal epithelium (B). In the stroma, Ki67 staining was categorized as low, medium or high, and shown as percentage of animals from each category (C). Data represented as mean ± SEM of Ki67 positive cells (n = 4 per group). *$p < 0.05$, significantly different from control, #$p < 0.05$, significantly different between groups. Scale bar=100 µm.

Kaempferol inhibits uterine epithelial cell proliferation

P_4 opposes ER-mediated proliferation in the uterine luminal epithelium, while also preparing the uterine stroma to respond to E_2 by inducing stromal proliferation [39-41]. Therefore, the effect of kaempferol, genistein, and the combination on proliferation of rat uterine epithelial cells was investigated. Ki67 staining was utilized to quantify proliferation. Genistein significantly increased luminal epithelial proliferation as compared to control (Figure 2A).

These results are in agreement with previously conducted studies [14]. Kaempferol alone did not increase luminal epithelial proliferation. Importantly, kaempferol when given in combination with genistein decreased proliferation of the uterine luminal epithelial as compared to genistein alone (Figure 2A and 2B). Due to minimal proliferation in the stroma, a semi-quantitative assessment method was used to investigate Ki67 expression. Co-administration of kaempferol and genistein stimulated proliferation of uterine stromal cells when compared to the individual treatments and vehicle control (Figure 2C). These changes in luminal and stromal proliferation from co-administration of kaempferol and genistein are consistent with similar studies which assessed actions of P_4 in the presence of E_2 [11,42].

Kaempferol induces *Areg* mRNA expression and *Hand2* protein levels in the uterus

The anti-proliferative action of P_4 in the uterine epithelial cells is mediated by Hand2 induction [4,32]. Immunohistochemistry and qPCR analyses were used to investigate if Hand2 induction correlated with the anti-proliferative effects of kaempferol.

As predicted, an increase in Hand2 expression was observed in uterine stromal cells after kaempferol treatment (Figure 3A). Hand2 protein expression was not induced by genistein, and a slight increase was observed in rats treated with both genistein and kaempferol (Figure 3A). *Hand2* mRNA changes were not observed in any of the treated animals (Figure 3B). The observed discrepancy between Hand2 protein and mRNA expression is likely based on the technique, as immunohistochemistry allows for analysis of specific uterine cell types, whereas the mRNA analyzed was a heterogeneous mixture of all uterine cell types.

Amphiregulin (Areg) is a secreted protein that is induced by P_4 in the uterus [43]. Kaempferol treatment significantly induced (5-fold)

Areg mRNA compared to vehicle treated animals, suggesting that it can function to increase PR-regulated targets *in vivo* (Figure 3C). Genistein blocked kaempferol-induced *Areg* expression, consistent with the antagonistic effects of E_2 on P_4-mediated induction of *Areg* [43]. Since Areg is a secreted protein, it was not investigated via immunohistochemistry [43].

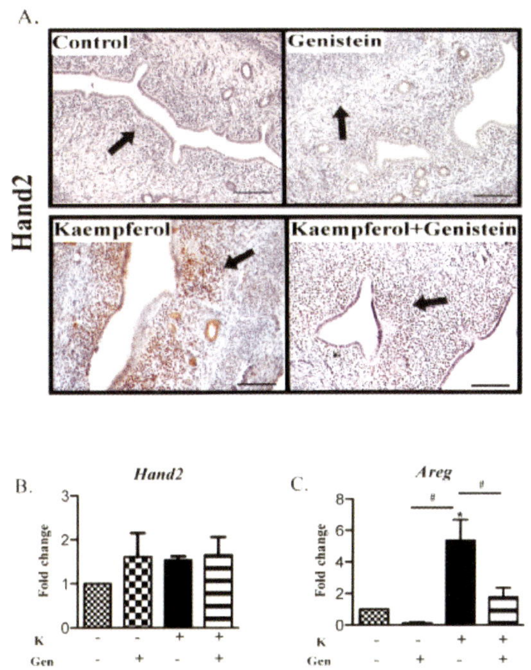

Figure 3: Immunohistochemistry and mRNA expression of P_4 targets (*Hand2* and *Areg*) in the rat uterus after treatment with vehicle control, genistein, kaempferol, and genistein+kaempferol for 8 days. Kaempferol induced expression of *Hand2* protein (A) but not mRNA (B), and induced *Areg* mRNA (C) in the ovariectomized rat uterus. Arrows indicate the uterine stromal compartment. Bar=100μm. qPCR analyses were performed using SYBR technologies. Results were normalized to *Rpl1* for *Hand2* or Gapdh for *Areg*. Mean ± SEM, $*p < 0.05$, significantly different from control, $\#p < 0.05$, significantly different between groups. Scale bar=100 μm.

Genistein and kaempferol treatment modulated uterine PR and ERα protein and mRNA expression

Steroid receptor mRNA and protein levels can be influenced by several physiological factors, including exposure to E_2 and P_4 [44]. To investigate the effects of genistein and kaempferol on steroid receptor expression in the uterus (the myometrium, endometrial stroma, luminal and glandular epithelium), mRNA levels of ER and PRA were measured. To establish cell type specific PR and ER regulation of steroid receptor expression, protein levels were compared using immunohistochemistry.

ERα bound to E_2 triggers its proteasome-dependent protein degradation [4,45]. In order to study ERα regulation, first qPCR for the receptor was performed. *ERa* mRNA levels in whole uterus were not affected by genistein treatment, but was significantly induced by kaempferol and kaempferol combined with genistein (Figure 4A). To investigate ERα protein expression in the different uterine cell types, immunohistochemical analyses were performed. As expected, genistein downregulated ERα protein expression (Figure 4B).

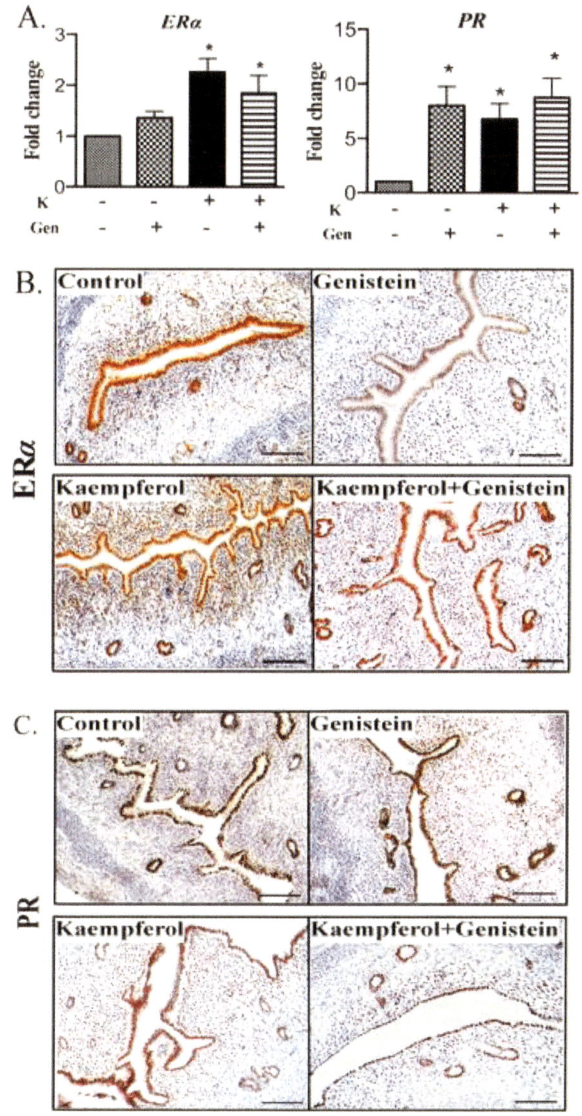

Figure 4: Immunohistochemistry and mRNA expression of ERα and PR in the rat uterus after treatment with vehicle control, genistein, kaempferol, and genistein+kaempferol for 8 days. Kaempferol and genistein differentially regulate *PR* and *ERa* mRNA, protein expression, and localization in the uterus. qPCR analyses were performed using SYBR technologies (A) and uterine sections were stained for ERα (B) and PR (C) expression, n=8 per group. Bar=100 μm. All results were normalized to RPL1. Mean ± SEM. $*p < 0.05$, significantly different from control. Groups unmarked were not statistically different from each other.

Interestingly, the induction of *ERa* mRNA in animals treated with kaempferol alone and in combination group (genistein and kaempferol) was significant and paralleled protein levels (Figure 4A). The lack of uterine weight gain and ERα expression in kaempferol-treated rats confirmed that kaempferol did not function as an estrogenic compound.

PR is an ER-regulated target [44]. Genistein treatment significantly increased PR mRNA and protein expression, confirming that genistein acts as a phytoestrogen in rat uteri [46]. Interestingly, kaempferol and kaempferol combined with genistein also significantly upregulated PR mRNA (Figure 4A). PR immunostaining in the vehicle-treated rat uteri was intense and localized to the nucleus throughout the luminal and glandular epithelial cells, but exposure to genistein and kaempferol increased PR expression in the stroma (Figure 4C). Therefore, kaempferol blocked genistein-induced proliferation and induced expression of PR target genes (*Areg* mRNA and *Hand2*), which is consistent with kaempferol functioning as a progestin. However, kaempferol acted without stimulating the degradation and loss of PR protein or mRNA expression, which typically occurs when PR binds a ligand (Figure 4C).

Kaempferol, E_2 and genistein regulation of PR expression in human endometrial stromal cells (HESC)

Upon P_4 binding, PR is targeted for proteasomal degradation, which could be partially responsible for the resistance to progestin therapy observed in endometriotic patients consuming progestins chronically [47].

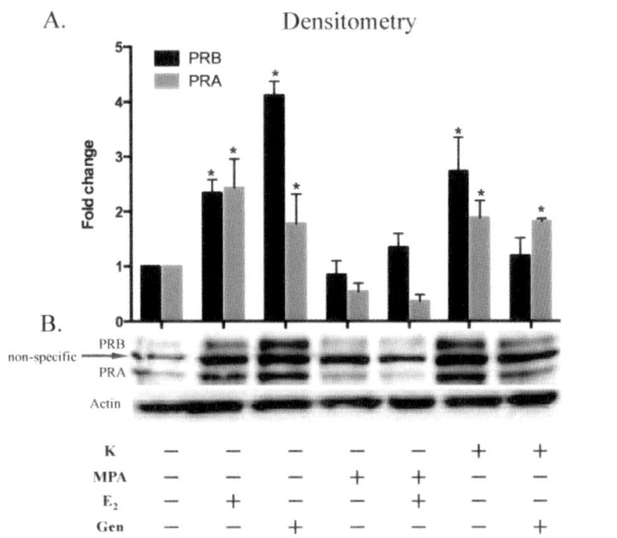

Figure 5: Regulation of PR protein expression in human endometrial stromal cells. Cells were incubated with pure compound for 48 hours. PRA and PRB were induced by E_2 (1 μM), genistein (5 μM) and kaempferol (20 μM) as determined by densitometry (A). PR fold change was analyzed using Image-J in triplicate experiments. $^*p < 0.05$, indicates significant fold change of PR compared to basal DMSO. MPA (20 μM) did not induce PRA and PRB. Membranes were blotted for actin as a loading control (B). Image is a representative blot, experiment repeated in triplicate.

Increased PR expression is mediated by the interaction between ligand-occupied ER with ERE in the PR gene promoter [44]. Since PR mRNA and protein was not reduced in the uteri of kaempferol-stimulated rats and instead actually increased, the regulation of the PR was investigated *in vitro*. PRA and PRB protein expression was analyzed in HESCs treated with MPA, P_4, kaempferol, E_2, and genistein (Figure 5). As expected, after a 48-hr treatment with MPA, HESCs had reduced PR protein expression (Figure 5A). HESCs exposed to E_2 or genistein had increased PR protein expression (Figure 5B). The combination treatment of MPA and E_2 maintained PR expression at basal levels. Similar to the *in vivo* results in rat uteri, kaempferol increased PR protein expression (Figure 5A and 5B). When combined with genistein treatment, kaempferol decreased genistein-induced PR expression, similar to MPA when combined with E_2.

Kaempferol does not induce ERE-luciferase in HESCs

Enhanced PR protein expression in the uterine stroma from kaempferol treatment *in vivo* could be due to activation of ER, which in turn transcriptionally induces PR [44]. Although kaempferol was previously reported to function as an ER modulator in HeLa cells, rat primary osteoblasts and human breast cancer MCF-7 cells in a concentration range of 10-70 μM [48-52], the ability of kaempferol to activate the ER in HESCs has not been reported. Therefore, HESCs were treated with a vehicle control, genistein, kaempferol, and genistein combined with kaempferol and ER activation was monitored by ERE-luciferase transcription (Figure 6). E_2 and genistein, but not kaempferol significantly induced ERE-luciferase expression in HESCs (Figure 6). In agreement with PR protein expression (Figure 5), genistein (5 μM) was as active as E_2 at inducing ERE-luciferase transcription (Figure 6). The ER antagonist desmethylarzoxifen (DMA) (100 nM) significantly inhibited E_2-induced signaling suggesting that these activities are mediated through ER. Despite increased PR protein expression after kaempferol treatment, ERE transcription was not significantly activated (Figure 6).

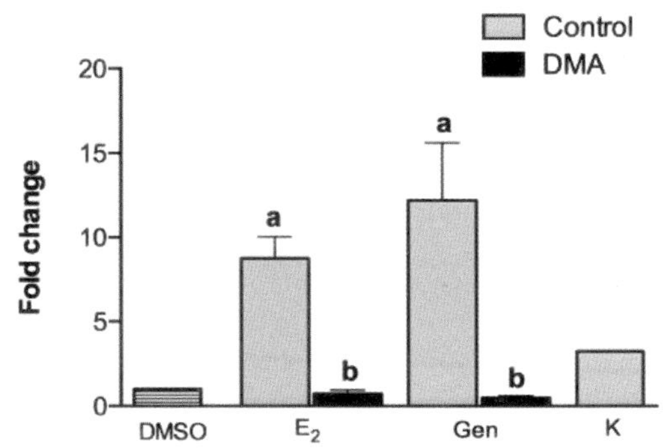

Figure 6: ERE-luciferase induction in human endometrial stromal cells. Endometrial stromal cells were transiently transfected with ERE-luciferase and ERα and treated with pure compounds E_2 (1 μM), genistein (5 μM), and kaempferol (20 μM) with and without the ER antagonist DMA (100 nM) for 48 hours. Data represent mean fold change ± SEM of relative light units normalized to β-gal in triplicate experiments. (a) indicates significant luciferase induction compared to basal DMSO; (b) indicates significant reduction of luciferase induction by DMA as determined by Student's t-Test, n=3, $^*p < 0.05$.

Kaempferol does not induce PSA-luciferase in MDA-MB-231 cells

MPA is one of the most commonly used synthetic progestins [8,53]. Although MPA signals through PR, it also activates other nuclear receptors such as AR, thereby increasing side effects and the risk of breast cancer and cardiovascular disorders [8,54,55]. Thus, it was important to evaluate if kaempferol also activates AR signaling. As PRE and ARE have similar consensus sequences, it is difficult to accurately determine androgen-specific activity when both PR and AR are expressed in a cell [34,56]. Therefore, in this experiment, MDA-MB-231 breast cancer cells, which express AR but not PR, were used. Prostate specific antigen (PSA) is an AR-regulated gene and its proximal promoter is highly responsive to androgens [56,57]. Thus, PSA-luciferase activity was measured in MDA-MB-231 cells to monitor AR activation. As expected, MPA activated PSA-luciferase in MDA-MB-231 cells, verifying that MPA stimulates AR-mediated transcription (Figure 7). In the presence of RU486 (1 μM), an AR antagonist, MPA-induced AR signaling was completely inhibited, further demonstrating MPA activation of AR-mediated transcription (Figure 7). Although there was a trend for increased activation with kaempferol, this was not statistically significant.

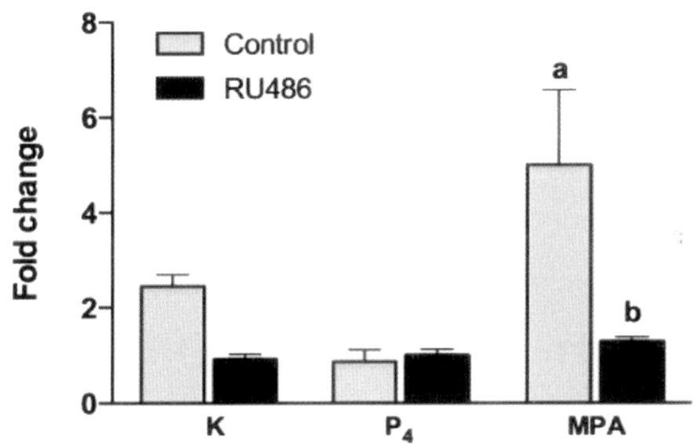

Figure 7: PSA-luciferase induction in MDA-MB-231 cells. MDA-MB-231 cells were transiently transfected with PSA-luciferase and treated with pure compounds kaempferol (20 μM), P_4 (1 μM), and MPA (1 μM)) with and without AR antagonist RU486 (1 μM) for 48 hours. MPA activates PSA-luciferase and can be antagonized by RU486. Kaempferol and P_4 did not significantly activate AR signaling. Data represent mean fold change ± SEM of relative light units normalized to β-gal in triplicate experiments. (a) indicates significant luciferase induction compared to basal DMSO; (b) indicates significant reduction of luciferase induction by RU486 as determined by Student's t-Test, $^{*}p < 0.05$.

Discussion

Many studies have provided evidence that kaempferol may function as progestin, including (i) activation of PR signaling *in vitro* [13], (ii) antagonistic effects when a potent PR agonist is present [13], (iii) similar anti-inflammatory mechanisms when compared to P_4 [18,20] and (iv) protection against ovarian cancer [22,58,59]. To date, there are no reports regarding the progestogenic effects of kaempferol *in vivo*. Therefore, this study investigated the effects of kaempferol on P_4 signaling in the uteri of OVX Sprague-Dawley rats and steroid receptor activation *in vitro*. In this study, the kaempferol treatment of cultured cells and animals were within the range used in previous studies (10-70 μM and 1-100 mg/kg, respectively) [3,13,18,60,61]. These findings, together with previous data, collectively suggest that kaempferol may have the potential to provide progestogenic biological activity *in vivo*, particularly in the uterus.

Computational analysis demonstrated that kaempferol adopts binding poses, which closely mimic the binding conformation and the interactions commonly observed between the LBD of PR and established ligands. The hydrophobic and hydrogen bond interactions of kaempferol are highly analogous to those of the steroid scaffold of P_4. In addition to the interactions expected for the steroid-based backbone of MPA, it gains additional interactions with the binding site through its ester-linked appendage, which may be associated with its agonistic effects. Molecular modeling data are consistent with previous *in vitro* binding analysis performed with kaempferol and the PR ligand binding domain [13]. Future investigations using additional molecular modeling techniques to study the recruitment of coregulatory proteins are warranted to elucidate the molecular mechanisms of kaempferol as a selective progesterone receptor modulator.

One well-established function of P_4 is the inhibition of E_2-induced uterine cell proliferation [1,11]. As a result, progestins are used therapeutically to reduce the proliferation of E_2-dependent endometrial cancers and in endometriosis [62]. Kaempferol reduced genistein-induced proliferation in luminal epithelial cells, while preparing the uterine stroma to respond to genistein, leading to stromal cell proliferation. *Hand2* mediates the anti-proliferative effects of P_4 in the uterus [32]. Although kaempferol treatment stimulated Hand2 protein expression in the uterine stroma, there was no change in *Hand2* mRNA expression. *Hand2* mRNA and protein expression in kaempferol treated uteri likely do not correlate completely because Hand2 is expressed in a discrete area within the uterine stroma, easily detectable by immunohistochemistry, but constituting only a small portion of the total uterine mRNA. Previous *in vivo* studies have reported that P_4 treatment completely abolished E_2-induced proliferation in the uterine epithelium [39,40]. Although kaempferol significantly reduced genistein-mediated proliferation in the uterus, it did not completely eliminate proliferation. However, it is important to note that the differences between P_4 and kaempferol could be due to different routes of treatment administration (oral vs. subcutaneous), potency, and duration. P_4 is poorly orally bioavailable driving the administration of synthetic progestins, like MPA. Since genistein and kaempferol are biologically active in the uterus after oral administration, botanicals (or combination therapies) containing both estrogenic and progestogenic compounds might provide the desired benefits for mitigating menopausal symptoms while also preventing E_2-induced uterine hyperplasia.

Reduced PR protein following progestin administration occurs in P_4 responsive cell types, and may be used to study progestogenic action within a target tissue [13,63,64]. Unexpectedly, the uteri of kaempferol-treated rats maintained expression of PR *in vivo* and in HESCs. This finding was especially intriguing because PR induction is linked to estrogenic signaling [32,35,66], which was not observed with kaempferol treatment, *in vitro* or *in vivo* as demonstrated by no change in ERE-luciferase expression and a lack of increased uterine weight. While kaempferol has been described as a partial ER agonist in human breast cancer cells and cervical cells [49,50], multiple studies investigating the estrogenic actions of kaempferol *in vivo* detected no uterotrophic estrogenic effects [37,60], which is further corroborated in this study. Progestin therapy resistance occurs in some populations of patients with endometrial cancer and endometriosis due to reduced or loss of PR protein expression after prolonged treatment [51,67,68]. Endometrial cancer is the most common gynecological malignancy in the United States and the fifth most common cancer among women in the world [47,53,69]. The anti-proliferative effects of kaempferol, without simultaneously downregulating PR expression raises an interesting possibility that a novel therapeutic approach could be attempted using kaempferol as an alternative for longer-term management of endometriotic symptoms.

The mechanism of progestin action is complex and may exert effects other than those traditionally expected from progestogenic activity [47,70]. Progestins currently available for prescription, such as MPA, interact with other steroidal receptors, including the AR, mineralocorticoid receptor (MR) and glucocorticoid receptor (GR) [8,71]. It has been proposed that AR, GR and MR activity enhance the proliferation of mammary epithelial cells, increasing breast cancer risk [8,72,73]. The androgenic nature of MPA has been suggested to be one mechanism through which it may give rise to blot clots, heart attacks and hypertension [6]. Therefore, an ideal progestin would be devoid of non-specific GR, MR, and AR activity [8,53,74]. Contrary to MPA, kaempferol did not significantly activate AR *in vitro*. However, further studies are needed to confirm kaempferol's action on GR and MR.

Taken together, the results from this study demonstrate that kaempferol functions as a progestin *in vivo* to mediate anti-proliferative effects of genistein in the uterus and modulate steroid receptor expression, without activating AR and ER signaling. The notion that phytoprogestins can be identified provides a new type of endocrine modulator, which could interact with and change endocrine signaling. Endocrine disruption is a critical issue as women are already consuming botanical-based therapies for a variety of conditions, such as infertility, menopause, and premenstrual symptoms [9,75]. Identification and characterization of progesterone-like molecules from natural sources might allow for informed decisions regarding their use as part of complicated multi-botanical formulations or as an alternative to current progestin therapies.

Acknowledgements

This work was supported by NIH R21 AT005377-01A1 to (J.E.B.) from the National Center for Complementary and Alternative Medicine (NCCAM) and the Office for Research in Women's Health, UIC University Graduate Fellowship (M.F.T.), and NIH T32 AT007533-01 to (M.P.E.) from the National Center for Complementary and Alternative Medicine (NCCAM) and the Office of the Director. We appreciate the support from the P50 AT00155 UIC/NIH Center for Botanical Dietary Supplements Research sponsored by the Office of Dietary Supplements and the NCCAM for pilot funding.

References

1. Kim JJ, Sefton EC, Bulun SE (2009) Progesterone receptor action in leiomyoma and endometrial cancer. Prog Mol Biol Transl Sci 87: 53-85.
2. Scarpin KM, Graham JD, Mote PA, Clarke CL (2009) Progesterone action in human tissues: regulation by progesterone receptor (PR) isoform expression, nuclear positioning and coregulator expression. Nucl Recept Signal 7: e009.
3. Santell RC, Chang YC, Nair MG, Helferich WG (1997) Dietary genistein exerts estrogenic effects upon the uterus, mammary gland and the hypothalamic/pituitary axis in rats. J Nutr 127: 263-269.
4. Chwalisz K, Perez MC, Demanno D, Winkel C, Schubert G, et al. (2005) Selective progesterone receptor modulator development and use in the treatment of leiomyomata and endometriosis. Endocr Rev 26: 423-438.
5. Pike MC, Ross RK (2000) Progestins and menopause: epidemiological studies of risks of endometrial and breast cancer. Steroids 65: 659-664.
6. M Meendering JR, Torgrimson BN, Miller NP, Kaplan PF, Minson CT. (2008) Estrogen, medroxyprogesterone acetate, endothelial function, and biomarkers of cardiovascular risk in young women. Am J Physiol Heart Circ Physiol 294: H1630-1637.
7. Li CI, Beaber EF, Tang MT, Porter PL, Daling JR, et al. (2012) Effect of depo-medroxyprogesterone acetate on breast cancer risk among women 20 to 44 years of age. Cancer Res 72: 2028-2035.
8. Ghatge RP, Jacobsen BM, Schittone SA, Horwitz KB (2005) The progestational and androgenic properties of medroxyprogesterone acetate: gene regulatory overlap with dihydrotestosterone in breast cancer cells. Breast Cancer Res 7: R1036-1050.
9. Geller SE, Studee L (2005) Botanical and dietary supplements for menopausal symptoms: what works, what does not. J Womens Health (Larchmt) 14: 634-649.
10. Lee E, Hsu C, Haiman CA, Razavi P, Horn-Ross PL, et al. (2010) Genetic variation in the progesterone receptor gene and risk of endometrial cancer: a haplotype-based approach. Carcinogenesis 31: 1392-1399.
11. Chen B, Pan H, Zhu L, Deng Y, Pollard JW (2005) Progesterone inhibits the estrogen-induced phosphoinositide 3-kinase-->AKT-->GSK-3beta-->cyclin D1-->pRB pathway to block uterine epithelial cell proliferation. Mol Endocrinol 19: 1978-1990.
12. Zava DT, Dollbaum CM, Blen M (1998) Estrogen and progestin bioactivity of foods, herbs, and spices. Proc Soc Exp Biol Med 217: 369-378.
13. Toh MF, Sohn J, Chen SN, Yao P, Bolton JL, et al. (2012) Biological characterization of non-steroidal progestins from botanicals used for women's health. Steroids 77: 765-773.
14. Zava DT, Duwe G (1997) Estrogenic and antiproliferative properties of genistein and other flavonoids in human breast cancer cells in vitro. Nutr Cancer 27: 31-40.
15. Zand RS, Jenkins DJ, Diamandis EP (2000) Steroid hormone activity of flavonoids and related compounds. Breast Cancer Res Treat 62: 35-49.
16. Overk CR, Guo J, Chadwick LR, Lantvit DD, Minassi A, et al. (2008) In vivo estrogenic comparisons of Trifolium pratense (red clover) Humulus lupulus (hops), and the pure compounds isoxanthohumol and 8-prenylnaringenin. Chem Biol Interact 176: 30-39.
17. Burdette JE, Liu J, Lantvit D, Lim E, Booth N, et al. (2002) Trifolium pratense (red clover) exhibits estrogenic effects in vivo in ovariectomized Sprague-Dawley rats. J Nutr 132: 27-30.
18. Calderón-Montaño JM, Burgos-Morón E, Pérez-Guerrero C, López-Lázaro M (2011) A review on the dietary flavonoid kaempferol. Mini Rev Med Chem 11: 298-344.
19. Kim SK, Kim HJ, Choi SE, Park KH, Choi HK, et al. (2008) Anti-oxidative and inhibitory activities on nitric oxide (NO) and prostaglandin E2 (COX-2) production of flavonoids from seeds of Prunus tomentosa Thunberg. Arch Pharm Res 31: 424-428.
20. Hämäläinen M, Nieminen R, Vuorela P, Heinonen M, Moilanen E (2007) Anti-inflammatory effects of flavonoids: genistein, kaempferol, quercetin, and daidzein inhibit STAT-1 and NF-kappaB activations, whereas flavone, isorhamnetin, naringenin, and pelargonidin inhibit only NF-kappaB activation along with their inhibitory effect on iNOS expression and NO production in activated macrophages. Mediators Inflamm 2007: 45673.
21. McCann SE, Freudenheim JL, Marshall JR, Graham S (2003) Risk of human ovarian cancer is related to dietary intake of selected nutrients, phytochemicals and food groups. J Nutr 133: 1937-1942.
22. Luo H, Jiang BH, King SM, Chen YC (2008) Inhibition of cell growth and VEGF expression in ovarian cancer cells by flavonoids. Nutr Cancer 60: 800-809.

23. Lukanova A, Kaaks R (2005) Endogenous hormones and ovarian cancer: epidemiology and current hypotheses. Cancer Epidemiol Biomarkers Prev 14: 98-107.
24. Risch HA (1998) Hormonal etiology of epithelial ovarian cancer, with a hypothesis concerning the role of androgens and progesterone. J Natl Cancer Inst 90: 1774-1786.
25. Lee JY, Shin JY, Kim HS, Heo JI, Kho YJ, et al. (2012) Effect of combined treatment with progesterone and tamoxifen on the growth and apoptosis of human ovarian cancer cells. Oncol Rep 27: 87-93.
26. Williams SP, Sigler PB (1998) Atomic structure of progesterone complexed with its receptor. Nature 393: 392-396.
27. Stawart DTC (2012) Openeye Scientific Software.
28. Jakalian A, Jack DB, Bayly CI (2002) Fast, efficient generation of high-quality atomic charges. AM1-BCC model: II. Parameterization and validation. J Comput Chem 23: 1623-1641.
29. Jones G, Willett P, Glen RC (1995) Molecular recognition of receptor sites using a genetic algorithm with a description of desolvation. J Mol Biol 245: 43-53.
30. Corbeil CR, Williams CI, Labute P (2012) Variability in docking success rates due to dataset preparation. J Comput Aided Mol Des 26: 775-786.
31. King SM, Modi DA, Eddie SL, Burdette JE (2013) Insulin and insulin-like growth factor signaling increases proliferation and hyperplasia of the ovarian surface epithelium and decreases follicular integrity through upregulation of the PI3-kinase pathway. J Ovarian Res 6: 12.
32. Li Q, Kannan A, DeMayo FJ, Lydon JP, Cooke PS, et al. (2011) The antiproliferative action of progesterone in uterine epithelium is mediated by Hand2. Science 331: 912-916.
33. Leonhardt SA, Boonyaratanakornkit V, Edwards DP (2003) Progesterone receptor transcription and non-transcription signaling mechanisms. Steroids 68: 761-770.
34. Petz LN, Ziegler YS, Schultz JR, Kim H, Kemper JK, et al. (2004) Differential regulation of the human progesterone receptor gene through an estrogen response element half site and Sp1 sites. J Steroid Biochem Mol Biol 88: 113-122.
35. Kolodziejczyk-Czepas J (2012) Trifolium species-derived substances and extracts--biological activity and prospects for medicinal applications. J Ethnopharmacol 143: 14-23.
36. Classen-Linke I, Alfer J, Krusche CA, Chwalisz K, Rath W, et al. (2000) Progestins, progesterone receptor modulators, and progesterone antagonists change VEGF release of endometrial cells in culture. Steroids 65: 763-771.
37. Trivedi R, Kumar S, Kumar A, Siddiqui JA, Swarnkar G, et al. (2008) Kaempferol has osteogenic effect in ovariectomized adult Sprague-Dawley rats. Mol Cell Endocrinol 289: 85-93.
38. Stroheker T, Chagnon MC, Pinnert MF, Berges R, Canivenc-Lavier MC (2003) Estrogenic effects of food wrap packaging xenoestrogens and flavonoids in female Wistar rats: a comparative study. Reprod Toxicol 17: 421-432.
39. Martin L, Das RM, Finn CA (1973) The inhibition by progesterone of uterine epithelial proliferation in the mouse. J Endocrinol 57: 549-554.
40. Das RM, Martin L (1973) Progesterone inhibition of mouse uterine epithelial proliferation. J Endocrinol 59: 205-206.
41. Martin L, Finn CA (1970) Interactions of oestradiol and progestins in the mouse uterus. J Endocrinol 48: 109-115.
42. Franco HL, Jeong JW, Tsai SY, Lydon JP, DeMayo FJ (2008) In vivo analysis of progesterone receptor action in the uterus during embryo implantation. Semin Cell Dev Biol 19: 178-186.
43. Das SK, Chakraborty I, Paria BC, Wang XN, Plowman G, et al. (1995) Amphiregulin is an implantation-specific and progesterone-regulated gene in the mouse uterus. Mol Endocrinol 9: 691-705.
44. Kastner P, Krust A, Turcotte B, Stropp U, Tora L, et al. (1990) Two distinct estrogen-regulated promoters generate transcripts encoding the two functionally different human progesterone receptor forms A and B. EMBO J 9: 1603-1614.
45. Nephew KP, Long X, Osborne E, Burke KA, Ahluwalia A, et al. (2000) Effect of estradiol on estrogen receptor expression in rat uterine cell types. Biol Reprod 62: 168-177.
46. Overk CR, Yao P, Chadwick LR, Nikolic D, Sun Y, et al. (2005) Comparison of the in vitro estrogenic activities of compounds from hops (Humulus lupulus) and red clover (Trifolium pratense). J Agric Food Chem 53: 6246-6253.
47. Bulun SE, Cheng YH, Yin P, Imir G, Utsunomiya H, et al. (2006) Progesterone resistance in endometriosis: link to failure to metabolize estradiol. Mol Cell Endocrinol 248: 94-103.
48. Mulac-Jericevic B, Conneely OM (2005) Reproductive tissue-selective actions of progesterone receptors. Ernst Schering Res Found Workshop : 19-37.
49. Oh SM, Kim YP, Chung KH (2006) Biphasic effects of kaempferol on the estrogenicity in human breast cancer cells. Arch Pharm Res 29: 354-362.
50. Wang J, Fang F, Huang Z, Wang Y, Wong C (2009) Kaempferol is an estrogen-related receptor alpha and gamma inverse agonist. FEBS Lett 583: 643-647.
51. Mulac-Jericevic B, Conneely OM (2004) Reproductive tissue selective actions of progesterone receptors. Reproduction 128: 139-146.
52. Guo AJ, Choi RC, Zheng KY, Chen VP, Dong TT, et al. (2012) Kaempferol as a flavonoid induces osteoblastic differentiation via estrogen receptor signaling. Chin Med 7: 10.
53. Madauss KP, Grygielko ET, Deng SJ, Sulpizio AC, Stanley TB, et al. (2007) A structural and in vitro characterization of asoprisnil: a selective progesterone receptor modulator. Mol Endocrinol 21: 1066-1081.
54. Whitehead MI, Townsend PT, Gill DK, Collins WP, Campbell S (1980) Absorption and metabolism of oral progesterone. Br Med J 280: 825-827.
55. DuPont MS, Day AJ, Bennett RN, Mellon FA, Kroon PA (2004) Absorption of kaempferol from endive, a source of kaempferol-3-glucuronide, in humans. Eur J Clin Nutr 58: 947-954.
56. Cleutjens KB, van Eekelen CC, van der Korput HA, Brinkmann AO, Trapman J (1996) Two androgen response regions cooperate in steroid hormone regulated activity of the prostate-specific antigen promoter. J Biol Chem 271: 6379-6388.
57. Shenk JL, Fisher CJ, Chen SY, Zhou XF, Tillman K, et al. (2001) p53 represses androgen-induced transactivation of prostate-specific antigen by disrupting hAR amino- to carboxyl-terminal interaction. J Biol Chem 276: 38472-38479.
58. Gates MA, Tworoger SS, Hecht JL, De Vivo I, Rosner B, et al. (2007) A prospective study of dietary flavonoid intake and incidence of epithelial ovarian cancer. Int J Cancer 121: 2225-2232.
59. Luo H, Rankin GO, Li Z, Depriest L, Chen YC (2011) Kaempferol induces apoptosis in ovarian cancer cells through activating p53 in the intrinsic pathway. Food Chem 128: 513-519.
60. Breinholt V, Hossaini A, Svendsen GW, Brouwer C, Nielsen E (2000) Estrogenic activity of flavonoids in mice. The importance of estrogen receptor distribution, metabolism and bioavailability. Food Chem Toxicol 38: 555-564.
61. Zhang Q, Zhang Y, Zhang Z, Lu Z (2009) Sensitive determination of kaempferol in rat plasma by high-performance liquid chromatography with chemiluminescence detection and application to a pharmacokinetic study. J Chromatogr B Analyt Technol Biomed Life Sci 877: 3595-3600.
62. Kim JJ, Kurita T, Bulun SE (2013) Progesterone action in endometrial cancer, endometriosis, uterine fibroids, and breast cancer. Endocr Rev 34: 130-162.
63. Sheridan PLP, Evans RMR, Horwitz KBK (1989) Phosphotryptic peptide analysis of human progesterone receptor. New phosphorylated sites formed in nuclei after hormone treatment. J Biol Chem 264: 6520-6528.
64. Lange CA, Shen T, Horwitz KB (2000) Phosphorylation of human progesterone receptors at serine-294 by mitogen-activated protein kinase signals their degradation by the 26S proteasome. Proc Natl Acad Sci U S A 97: 1032-1037.

65. Hong SH, Nah HY, Lee JY, Gye MC, Kim CH, et al. (2004) Analysis of estrogen-regulated genes in mouse uterus using cDNA microarray and laser capture microdissection. J Endocrinol 181: 157-167.

66. Tibbetts TA, Mendoza-Meneses M, O'Malley BW, Conneely OM (1998) Mutual and intercompartmental regulation of estrogen receptor and progesterone receptor expression in the mouse uterus. Biol Reprod 59: 1143-1152.

67. Zhao SJ, Chen XJ, Feng YJ (2007) [Influence of long-term treatment with MPA on the biological character of endometrial carcinoma Ishikawa cell]. Fen Zi Xi Bao Sheng Wu Xue Bao 40: 103-112.

68. Zhao S, Li G, Yang L, Li H (2013) Response-specific progestin resistance in a newly characterized Ishikawa human endometrial cancer subcell line resulting from long-term exposure to medroxyprogesterone acetate. Oncology letters 5: 139-144.

69. Wang Y, Hanifi-Moghaddam P, Hanekamp EE, Kloosterboer HJ, Franken P, et al. (2009) Progesterone inhibition of Wnt/beta-catenin signaling in normal endometrium and endometrial cancer. Clin Cancer Res 15: 5784-5793.

70. Druckmann R (2003) Progestins and their effects on the breast. Maturitas 46 Suppl 1: S59-69.

71. Gompel A (2012) Micronized progesterone and its impact on the endometrium and breast vs. progestogens. Climacteric 15 Suppl 1: 18-25.

72. Sørensen GV, Cronin-Fenton DP, Sørensen HT, Ulrichsen SP, Pedersen L, et al. (2012) Use of glucocorticoids and risk of breast cancer: a Danish population-based case-control study. Breast Cancer Res 14: R21.

73. Leo JC, Guo C, Woon CT, Aw SE, Lin VC (2004) Glucocorticoid and mineralocorticoid cross-talk with progesterone receptor to induce focal adhesion and growth inhibition in breast cancer cells. Endocrinology 145: 1314-1321.

74. Sitruk-Ware R (2004) New progestogens: a review of their effects in perimenopausal and postmenopausal women. Drugs Aging 21: 865-883.

75. Kelly JP, Kaufman DW, Kelley K, Rosenberg L, Anderson TE, et al. (2005) Recent trends in use of herbal and other natural products. Arch Intern Med 165: 281-286.

Comparative Studies on Performance of CCC and Preparative RP-HPLC in Separation and Purification of Steroid Saponins from Dioscorea Zingiberensis C.H.Wright

Xinxin Zhang[1], **Jianli Liu**[1], **Wenji Sun**[1] **and Yoichiro Ito**[2*]

[1]*Biomedicine Key Laboratory of Shaanxi Province, Northwest University, 229 Taibai North Road, Xi'an, Shaanxi 710069, China*

[2]*Laboratory of Bioseparation Technology, Biochemistry and Biophysics Center, National Heart, Lung, and Blood Institute, National Institutes of Health, Bethesda, Maryland, USA*

[*]**Corresponding author:** Yoichiro Ito, Laboratory of Bioseparation Technology, Biochemistry and Biophysics Center, National Heart, Lung, and Blood Institute, National Institutes of Health, Bethesda, Maryland, USA, E-mail: zhangxinxin360@126.com

Abstract

Steroid Saponins from Dioscorea zingiberensis C.H.Wright were separated for the first time using two chromatographic methods for comparison: counter-current chromatography (CCC) coupled with evaporative light scattering detector (ELSD) and preparative reversed phase high-performance liquid chromatography (RP-HPLC) with an ultraviolet detector. Ethyl acetate-n-butanol-methanol-water (4:1:2:4, v/v) was chosen as the two-phase solvent system for CCC, while the acetonitrile-water (25:75 for the first step and15:85 for the second step, v/v) was used as the mobile phase in the preparative RP-HPLC. The following five steroid Saponins were purified by these two chromatographic methods, in one-step operation by CCC and by two-step operation in preparative RP-HPLC:

1) 26-O-β-D-glucopyranosyl-(25R)-furost-△5(6)-en-3β,22ζ,26-triol-3-O-β-D-glucopyranosyl-(1→3)-β-D-glucopyranosyl-(1→4)-α-L-rhamnopyranosyl-(1→2)-β-D-glucopyranoside (compound A), 2) 26-O-β-D-glucopyranosyl-(25R)-furost-△5(6)-en-3β,22ζ,26-triol-3-O-β-D-glucopyranosyl-(1→3)-α-L-rhamnopyranosyl-(1→2)-β-D-glucopyranoside (compound B), 3) 26-O-β-D-glucopyranosyl-(25R)-furost-△5(6)-en-3β,22ζ,26-triol-3-O-α-L-rhamnopyranosyl-(1→4)-β-D-glucopyranoside (compound C), 4) 26-O-β-D-glucopyranosyl-(25R)-furost-△5(6), 20(22)-diene-3β,26-diol-3-O-α-L-rhamnopyranosyl-(1→4)-[β-D-glucopyranosyl-(1→3)-β-D-glucopyranosyl-(1→2)]-β-D-glucopyranoside (compound D) and 5) 26-O-β-D-glucopyranosyl-(25R)-furost-△5(6), 20(22)-diene-3β,26-diol-3-O-β-D-glucopyranosyl-(1→4)-α-L-rhamnopyranosy-(1→2)-β-D-glucopyranoside (compound E). The purities of these five steroid saponins separated by both methods were over 95%, and structural identification of these compounds was performed by ESI-MS, and 13C NMR. Comparison of these two established approaches revealed that CCC required a longer separation time but with less solvent consumption, whereas preparative RP-HPLC gave a shorter separation time but with higher solvent consumption. These results demonstrated that either of these two methods of different separation mechanism is feasible, economical and efficient for rapid preparative isolation and purification of steroid saponins from Dioscorea zingiberensis C.H.Wright.

Keywords: CCC; Preparative RP-HPLC; Steroid saponins; Dioscorea zingiberensis C.H.Wright

Introduction

Dioscorea zingiberensis C.H.Wright, a unique plant native in China, is one of the most commonly used raw materials for Chinese Traditional Medicine (CTM) [1]. The steroid saponins, primarily contained in the rhizomes of this plant, are the main bioactive components, and have been applied as a folk treatment for cough, anthrax, rheumarthritis, tumefaction, sprain as well as various cardiac diseases in the TCM for a long time [2-6]. Total steroid saponins extracted from other plants of the Dioscoreaceae family are also widely used in clinic for the treatment of coronary heart disease. For example, Di'aoxinxuekang capsules, containing 35% of total steroid saponins of Dioscorea nipponica Makino, have been used for the treatment of coronary heart disease for more than 10 years in China [7]. Owing to their diverse bioactivities, much attention has been paid to the separation and purification of steroid saponins in recent years. It is known that typical steroid saponins such as diosgenin contain one or more carbohydrate residues [8]. Due to their similar structures and relatively higher polarity, separation and purification often become difficult by means of the conventional chromatographic methods. In addition, the conventional method, such as column chromatography, needs repeated steps which are tedious, time-consuming, and may lead to contamination problem. Furthermore, the overall yield of these methods is usually lower, because some of these compounds are irreversibly adsorbed onto the solid support during the separation [9,10]. Therefore, finding much faster and more efficient methods is of great importance.

With the development of modern separation techniques, counter-current chromatography (CCC) and preparative reversed-phase high-performance liquid chromatography (RP-HPLC) have been used for isolation and purification of active components from traditional Chinese herbs and other natural products. CCC is a support-free liquid-liquid partition method which eliminates irreversible adsorption of samples onto the solid support, providing a wider range of selection of two-phase solvent systems and yielding high purity and recovery [11-15]. Being an amplification mode of analytic HPLC, preparative RP-HPLC has become a powerful tool due to its shorter isolation time, excellent efficiency and high recovery [16-19]. Because of these remarkable characteristics, these two chromatographic methods play an important role in current biochemical researches.

In this paper we report for the first time the separation of five steroid saponins from Dioscorea zingiberensis C.H.Wright using two different chromatographic methods, CCC and preparative RP-HPLC.

Experimental

Apparatus

Preparative CCC instrument employed in this study was a TBE-300A CCC centrifuge (Tauto Biotech Co., Shanghai, China) equipped with a set of three-multilayer coil separation columns and a 20-ml sample loop. The columns were made of polytetrafluoroethylene (PTFE) tubing of 1.5 mm I.D. with a total capacity of 300 ml. The β values (β = r/R, where r is the revolution radius or the distance from the coil to the holder shaft, and R is the revolution radius or the distances between the holder axis and central axis of the centrifuge) ranged from 0.5 at the internal layer to 0.8 at the external layer. The revolution speed of the apparatus was regulated by a speed controller from 0 to 1000 rpm, and 850 rpm was used in this study. The solvent was pumped into the column with a model TBP5002 constant flow pump (Tauto Biotech Co. Ltd, Shanghai, China), and continuous effluent was monitored online with an Alltech 800 evaporative light scattering detector. The effluent was collected by the DBS-100 automatic fraction collector (Huxi Analysis Instrument Factory Co. Ltd, Shanghai, China). This software N2000 workstation (Zhejiang University, Hangzhou, China) was used to record the chromatogram.

Preparative RP-HPLC separation was performed on the Alltech equipment system (Alltech Co. Ltd, California, USA) with a high pressure binary 627 HPLC pump, a manual 2 ml sample loop, and a preparative mode Model 500 UV (Chen Airlines Tech Instrument, Tianjin, China) single wavelength absorbance detector (4.5 μm cell). The separation of steroid saponins was carried out on the GRACE Adsorbosphere (Alltech Co. Ltd, California, USA) C18 column (250 x 22 mm, 10 μm). Evaluation was made on an Allchrom Plus Sever Workstation, and sample fraction was collected by the DBS-100 automatic fraction collector (Huxi Analysis Instrument Factory Co. Ltd, Shanghai, China).

Analytical HPLC separation was performed using the Waters Alliance 2695 equipment (Waters, Milford, MA, USA) with a vacuum degasser, a high pressure quaternary pump, an autosampler, and an Alltech 2000 evaporative light scattering detector. The analytical chromatogram of steroid saponins was obtained with a Welchrom C18 column (250 x 4.6 mm, 5 μm). Evaluation and quantification were made on an Empower Workstation.

Nuclear magnetic resonance (NMR) data were recorded on a Bruker Advance 500 spectrometer (Bruker BioSpin, Rheinstetten, Germany). ESI-MS was performed with Thermo LTQ-XL ion trap mass spectrometer (Thermo Scientific, USA).

Materials

All organic solvents used for CCC and preparative RP-HPLC were of analytical grade and purchased from Tianjin Chemical Factory (Tianjin, China). Acetonitrile used for HPLC was of HPLC-grade, and water purified in a Milli-Q plus system (Millipore, Madrid, Spain) was double distilled water. The rhizomes of Dioscorea zingiberensis C.H.Wright were provided by Yangtze River Pharmaceutical Industry Co., Ltd (Jiangsu, China).

Preparation of total Steroid Saponins

Dried raw rhizomes of Dioscorea zingiberensis C.H.Wright (7 Kg) were powdered and extracted with 70% ethanol for three times. The pooled ethanol extract was evaporated to dryness by a rotary evaporator under reduced pressure, and the residues were redissolved in water and subjected to centrifugation. Then, the supernatant was separated on a D-101 macroporous resin column by eluting with 60% ethanol. The 60% ethanol effluent was collected, and concentrated under reduced pressure to provide a syrup which was redissolved in 2 L of water again and extracted with an equal volume of n-butanol six times successively [20]. The pooled n-butanol extract was concentrated yielding 265 g of residues. In order to further enrich the target components and remove impurities, the residues of n-butanol extract were separated on the silica gel column (100-160 mesh) by eluting with dichloromethane-methanol-water (70:30:10). The effluent was collected according to the Rf value between 0.2~0.5 on thin layer chromatography (TLC) which was developed with a solvent composed of dichloromethane-methanol-water (65:35:10) and then evaporated at 100 °C under reduced pressure. Finally, about 40 g of residues were obtained for subsequent CCC and preparative RP-HPLC separations.

Selection and preparation of two-phase solvent system for CCC

The two-phase solvent system was selected according to the partition coefficient (K) of each target component. Several kinds of solvent systems were prepared each at different volumes and equilibrated in a separation funnel at room temperature. The K values were determined by HPLC analysis as follows: a suitable amount of total steroid saponins (10 mg) was added to 4.0 ml of the pre-equilibrated two-phase solvent system consisted of 2 ml of the upper phase and 2 ml of the lower phase in a 10 ml test tube. The capped test tube was shaken vigorously to thoroughly equilibrate the sample between the two phases. After the equilibration was established, an equal volume (1.5 ml) of each phase was separately transferred into another test tube and evaporated. The residues of each phase were dissolved in an equal volume (2 ml) of methanol and analyzed by HPLC. The K values were calculated according to the equation: $K = A_U/A_L$, while A_U and A_L were the peak area of each compound in the upper and the lower phases, respectively. Ethyl acetate-n-butanol-methanol-water (4:1:2:4, v/v) was finally chosen as the two-phase solvent system. The solvent system was mixed and shaken vigorously to thoroughly equilibrate in a separatory funnel at room temperature, and left over night. Then, the two phases were separated and degassed by sonication for 30 min before use.

Selection of chromatographic conditions in preparative RP-HPLC

The preparative conditions for the RP-HPLC, including separation factor, cycling time and sample loadability, were obtained according to the analytical HPLC chromatographic data. From the suitable analytical HPLC condition, the optimum chromatographic condition for the preparative RP-HPLC was determined by adjusting the sample loads. After testing several kinds of solvent systems, acetonitrile-water with the volumes of 25:75 (v/v) and 15:85 (v/v) were selected as the mobile phase for the first step separation and the second step separation, respectively, while the column packed with the C18 (10 μm, 100 Å) particles based on the previous reference was used as the stationary phase. The mobile phase was degassed by sonication for 30 min before use.

Preparation of sample solution

A 100 mg amount of steroid saponins dissolved in 10 ml of lower phase was used as the sample solution for CCC separation. For RP-HPLC separation, 100 mg of steroid saponins dissolved in 2 ml of acetonitrile-water (25:75, v/v) was used as sample solution for the first step separation, while 80 mg of total steroid saponin sub-fraction collected from the first step separation was dissolved in 2 ml of acetonitrile-water (15:85, v/v) and used as the sample solution for the second step separation.

CCC and preparative RP-HPLC separation procedures

In the CCC experiment, the head-tail elution mode was adopted. A set of three multilayer coil separation columns with a total capacity of 300 ml was first completely filled with the upper stationary phase at a flow rate of 25 ml min^{-1}. Then the apparatus was rotated at 850 rpm while the lower mobile phase was pumped into the head inlet of the column at a flow rate of 2.0 ml min^{-1} in an isocratic elution mode. The sample solution was injected through the injection valve, after a mobile phase emerged at the tail outlet which indicated that a steady state hydrodynamic equilibrium was established in the column. By applying a flow splitter, a small fraction of the effluent from the outlet of the column was continuously monitored with an Alltech 800 ELSD detector (the drift tube temperature was 55°C, and the gas flow rate was 3.0 L min^{-1}), while the rest of the effluent was collected with an automatic fraction collector set at 5 min for each test tube. During the experiment, the separation temperature was controlled at 25°C. After peak fractions A-D were eluted, the centrifuge run was stopped, and the column contents were blown out by nitrogen gas to collect fraction E that was still remained in the column.

In the preparative RP-HPLC experiment, the entire work was performed on the Alltech equipment system. The GRACE Adsorbosphere C18 column (250 x 22 mm, 10 μm) was first entirely equilibrated by the appropriate mobile phase at a flow rate of 16 ml min^{-1}. Then, the sample solution was injected through the 2 ml injection valve, after a stable baseline was recorded by the Allchrom Plus Sever Workstation indicating that a steady state hydrodynamic equilibrium was established in the column. The effluent from the outlet of the column was continuously monitored by the Model 500 UV at 203nm, and collected with an automatic fraction collector at 3 min for each test tube. Throughout this experiment, the separation temperature was kept at room temperature. Peak fractions I were obtained in the first step, while fraction I was further separated by the second step yielding fractions A-C.

Peak fractions of CCC and preparative RP-HPLC were each concentrated under reduced pressure and their residues were ready for subsequent analysis.

HPLC analysis of peak fractions from CCC and preparative RP-HPLC

Purity of each peak fraction from CCC and preparative RP-HPLC separation was determined by analytic HPLC. The analyses were performed with a Welchrom C18 column (250 x 4.6 mm, 5 μm) at 25°C. The mobile phase composed of acetonitrile-water (30:70, v/v) was isocratically eluted at a flow rate of 1.0 ml min^{-1}, and continuously monitored by an Alltech 2000 evaporative light scattering detector (the drift tube temperature at 104°C, and the gas flow rate of 2.8 L min^{-1}. The purity of CCC and preparative RP-HPLC fractions was calculated using the area normalization.

Identification of peak fractions from CCC and preparative RP-HPLC

Identification of the structure of each peak fraction was performed by means of ESI-MS and 13C NMR. The spectra of ESI-MS were obtained by the Thermo LTQ-XL ion trap mass spectrometer, and the spectra of 13C NMR were obtained by the Bruker Advance 500 spectrometer.

Results and Discussion

CCC and preparative RP-HPLC separation and HPLC analysis

In CCC, five steroid saponins were obtained with the two-phase solvent system composed of ethyl acetate-n-butanol-methanol-water (4:1:2:4, v/v) in less than 3.5 h with the total elution volume of 420 ml in one step separation. This separation yielded 18.2 mg of compound A (fraction was collected during 100-120 min), 22.4 mg of compound B (fraction was collected during 130-148 min), 15.7 mg of compound C (fraction was collected during 160-180 min), 10.9 mg of compound D (fraction was collected during 190-205 min), and 10.2 mg of compound E (from the column contents) from 100 mg of the crude extract (Figure 1). The retention of the stationary phase was 42% of the total column capacity after the separation was completed.

In preparative RP-HPLC, the same five steroid saponins were also obtained with the mobile phase of acetonitrile-water (25:75, and 15:85, v/v) in 1h with the total elution volume of 960 ml in two-step separation. Three fractions, I, D and E were obtained in the first step with the mobile phase composed of acetonitrile-water at a volume of 25:75 (v/v). Among those fractions, I was concentrated under reduced pressure and dissolved in suitable solvent which was loaded on the preparative RP-HPLC column and eluted with acetonitrile-water at a volume of 15:85 (v/v). This two-step process yielded 15.7 mg of compound A, 20.5 mg of compound B, 14.2 mg of compound C, 8.5 mg of compound D and 8.8 mg of compound E from 100 mg of the crude extract (Figure 2).

In these two methods both in the reversed elution mode all compounds were eluted in the order of polarity: the most polar compound was eluted first followed by the rest in the order of decreasing polarity. The purities of these five target compounds obtained by these two methods were over 95%. The analytical HPLC chromatogram is shown in Figure 3.

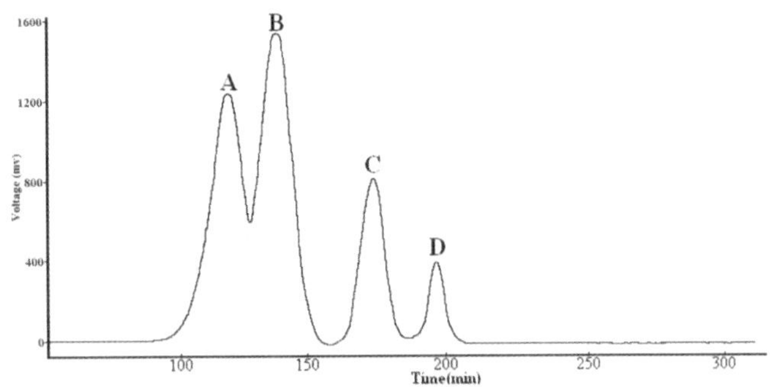

Figure 1: CCC chromatogram of total steroid saponins. Solvent system: ethyl acetate-n-butanol-methanol-water (4:1:2:4, v/v); stationary phase: upper organic phase; mobile phase: lower aqueous phase; flow-rate: 2.0 ml min^{-1}; revolution speed: 850 rpm; sample: 100 mg dissolved in 10 ml lower phase; retention of the stationary phase: 42%; Alltech 800 ELSD condition: drift tube temperature: 55°C; gas flow rate 3.0 L min^{-1}.

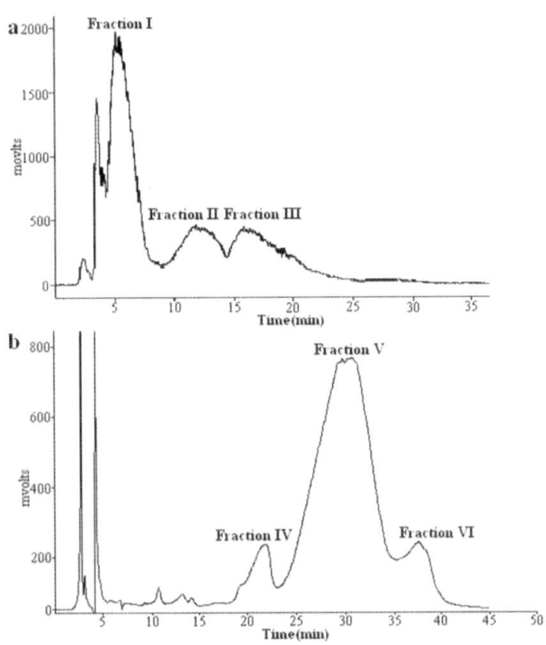

Figure 2: The preparative HPLC chromatograms of total steroid saponins and fraction I. Conditions: The GRACE Adsorbosphere C18 column (250 mm x 22 mm, 10 μm); Flow rate: 16 ml min^{-1}; Injection volume: 2 ml; Model 500 UV detector wavelength monitoring: 203 nm. (a): Mobile phase: acetonitrile-water (25:75, v/v) in separation total steroid saponins; (b): Mobile phase: acetonitrile-water (15:85, v/v) in separation fraction I.

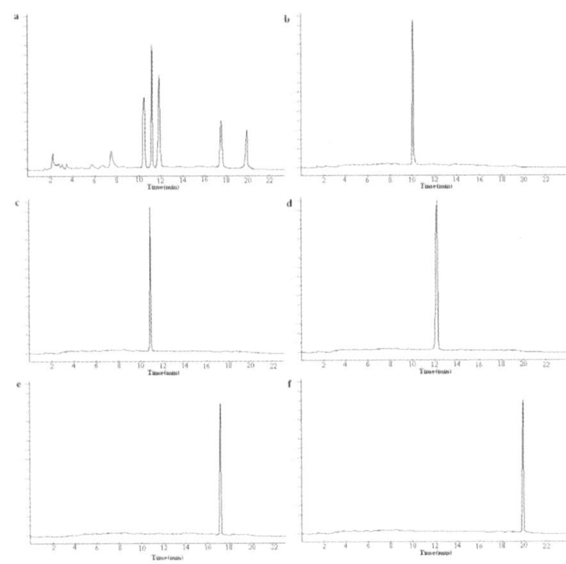

Figure 3: HPLC chromatograms of total saponins, CCC and pre-HPLC peak fractions. Conditions: column: Welchrom C18 column (250x4.6 mm, 5 μm); mobile phase: acetonitrile-water (30:70, v/v); flow rate: 1 ml min-1; Alltech 2000 ELSD condition: drift tube temperature: 104°C; gas flow rate 2.8 L min-1; column temperature: 25°C; injection volume: 10 μL. (a): Total steroid saponins; (b): Compounds A; (c): Compounds B; (d): Compounds C; (e): Compounds D; (f): Compounds E.

Structure Identification of purified compounds.

The structures of five target compounds were confirmed as the steroid saponins shown in Figure 4 by means of the modern spectroscopic techniques, including ESI-MS shown in Figure 5 and 13C NMR in Table 1.

Data of compound A: ESI-MS(m/z): 1249 ([M+Na]+), molecular formula: $C_{57}H_{94}O_{28}$. Compared with Ref [21], compound A was identified as 26-O-β-D-glucopyranosyl-(25R)-furost-Δ5(6)-en-3β,22ζ, 26-triol-3-O-β-D-glucopyranosyl-(1→3)-β-D-glucopyranosyl-(1→4)-α-L-rhamnopyranosyl-(1→2)-β-D-glucopyranoside.

Data of compound B: ESI-MS(m/z): 1087 ([M+Na]+), molecular formula: $C_{51}H_{84}O_{23}$. Compared with Ref [11,21], compound B was identified as 26-O-β-D-glucopyranosyl-(25R)-furost-Δ5(6)-en-3β,22ζ, 26-triol-3-O-β-D-glucopyranosyl-(1→3)-α-L-rhamnopyranosyl-(1→2)-β-D-glucopyranoside.

Data of compound C: ESI-MS(m/z): 925 ([M+Na]+), molecular formula: $C_{45}H_{74}O_{18}$. Compared with Ref [22], compound C was identified as 26-O-β-D-glucopyranosyl-(25R)-furost-Δ5(6)-en-3β,22ζ, 26-triol-3-O-α-L-rhamnopyranosyl-(1→4)-β-D-glucopyranoside.

Data of compound D: ESI-MS(m/z): 1231.67 ([M+Na]+), molecular formula: $C_{57}H_{92}O_{27}$. Compared with Ref [22], compound D was identified as 26-O-β-D-glucopyranosyl-(25R)-furost-Δ5(6),20(22)-diene-3β,26-diol-3-O-α-L-rhamnopyranosyl-(1→4)-[β-D-glucopyranosyl-(1→3)-β-D-glucopyranosyl-(1→2)]-β-D-glucopyranoside.

Data of compound E: ESI-MS(m/z): 1069.33([M+Na]+), molecular formula: C51H82O22; compound E was identified as 26-O-β-D-glucopyranosyl-(25R)-furost-△5(6),20(22)-diene-3β,26-diol-3-O-β-D-glucopyranosyl-(1→4)-α-L-rhamnopyranosy-(1→2)-β-D-glucopyranoside.

Compounds									
Compound A		**Compound B**		**Compound C**		**Compound D**		**Compound E**	
1249 [M+Na]+		1087 [M+Na]+		925 [M+Na]+		1231.67 [M+Na]+		1069.33 [M+Na]+	
Aglycone	Sugar Moiety	Aglycone	Sugar Moiety	Aglycone	Sugar Moiety	Aglycone	Sugar Moiety	Aglycone	Sugar Moiety
(ppm)	(ppm)	(ppm)	(ppm)	(ppm)	(ppm)	(ppm)	(ppm)	(ppm)	(ppm)
37.4 (C-1)	100.9 (Glu'-1)	37.2 (C-1)	100.1 (Glu'-1)	37.8 (C-1)	102.3 (Glu'-1)	37.0 (C-1)	100.3 (Glu'-1)	37.5 (C-1)	99.9 (Glu'-1)
30.5 (C-2)	77.2 (Glu'-2)	31.5 (C-2)	77.3 (Glu'-2)	30.2 (C-2)	73.1 (Glu'-2)	31.4 (C-2)	81.5 (Glu'-2)	30.1 (C-2)	77.2 (Glu'-2)
78.6 (C-3)	77.0 (Glu'-3)	71.7 (C-3)	88.7 (Glu'-3)	78.6 (C-3)	73.5 (Glu'-3)	71.6 (C-3)	76.2 (Glu'-3)	78.0 (C-3)	77.7 (Glu'-3)
38.8 (C-4)	82.1 (Glu'-4)	42.5 (C-4)	69.9 (Glu'-4)	39.9 (C-4)	72.2 (Glu'-4)	42.5 (C-4)	78.6 (Glu'-4)	38.9 (C-4)	82.1 (Glu'-4)
141.3 (C-5)	78.4 (Glu'-5)	140.2 (C-5)	78.0 (Glu'-5)	141.4 (C-5)	74.6 (Glu'-5)	140.5 (C-5)	77.4 (Glu'-5)	140.7 (C-5)	76.2 (Glu'-5)
122.5 (C-6)	62.9 (Glu'-6)	121.9 (C-6)	62.1 (Glu'-6)	121.5 (C-6)	69.2 (Glu'-6)	121.0 (C-6)	61.6 (Glu'-6)	121.8 (C-6)	62.5 (Glu'-6)
32.4 (C-7)	102.0 (Rha'-1)	32.1 (C-7)	101.1 (Rha'-1)	32.4 (C-7)	105.2 (Glu''-1)	32.0 (C-7)	101.7 (Rha'-1)	32.4 (C-7)	101.8 (Rha'-1)
30.9 (C-8)	72.4 (Rha'-2)	31.7 (C-8)	72.0 (Rha'-2)	31.2 (C-8)	75.7 (Glu''-2)	31.2 (C-8)	72.8 (Rha'-2)	31.4 (C-8)	72.5 (Rha'-2)
49.9 (C-9)	72.1 (Rha'-3)	49.5 (C-9)	72.2 (Rha'-3)	50.7 (C-9)	78.5 (Glu''-3)	50.3 (C-9)	72.7 (Rha'-3)	50.3 (C-9)	72.7 (Rha'-3)
37.5 (C-10)	74.2 (Rha'-4)	36.1 (C-10)	73.5 (Rha'-4)	37.2 (C-10)	71.2 (Glu''-4)	36.4 (C-10)	74.1 (Rha'-4)	37.1 (C-10)	74.1 (Rha'-4)
21.2 (C-11)	69.6 (Rha'-5)	20.5 (C-11)	69.8 (Rha'-5)	21.2 (C-11)	78.3 (Glu''-5)	20.7 (C-11)	69.4 (Rha'-5)	21.2 (C-11)	69.5 (Rha'-5)
40.8 (C-12)	18.2 (Rha'-6)	39.4 (C-12)	18.8 (Rha'-6)	40.9 (C-12)	63.5 (Glu''-6)	39.7 (C-12)	18.9 (Rha'-6)	39.6 (C-12)	18.7 (Rha'-6)
41.5 (C-13)	105.7 (Glu''-1)	41.9 (C-13)	103.1 (Glu''-1)	40.5 (C-13)	100.3 (Rha'-1)	40.0 (C-13)	104.3 (Glu''-1)	43.4 (C-13)	104.9 (Glu''-1)
56.8 (C-14)	88.1 (Glu''-2)	56.1 (C-14)	74.0 (Glu''-2)	56.7 (C-14)	78.7 (Rha'-2)	56.6 (C-14)	73.5 (Glu''-2)	54.9 (C-14)	78.6 (Glu''-2)
32.1 (C-15)	74.6 (Glu''-3)	31.2 (C-15)	77.5 (Glu''-3)	32.7 (C-15)	78.9 (Rha'-3)	31.6 (C-15)	88.2 (Glu''-3)	34.5 (C-15)	71.7 (Glu''-3)
81.2 (C-16)	69.2 (Glu''-4)	81.0 (C-16)	71.9 (Glu''-4)	81.4 (C-16)	62.5 (Rha'-4)	80.8 (C-16)	69.7 (Glu''-4)	84.4 (C-16)	78.5 (Glu''-4)
63.8 (C-17)	78.9 (Glu''-5)	62.5 (C-17)	78.3 (Glu''-5)	64.2 (C-17)	79.1 (Rha'-5)	62.3 (C-17)	77.6 (Glu''-5)	64.5 (C-17)	62.8 (Glu''-5)
16.7 (C-18)	61.1 (Glu''-6)	16.4 (C-18)	60.3 (Glu''-6)	16.8 (C-18)	18.2 (Rha'-6)	16.5 (C-18)	61.8 (Glu''-6)	14.1 (C-18)	61.8 (Glu''-6)
20.0 (C-19)	105.2 (Glu'''-1)	19.1 (C-19)	100.2 (Glu'''-1)	19.9 (C-19)		19.7 (C-19)	105.2 (Glu'''-1)	19.4 (C-19)	105.2 (Glu'''-1)
40.9 (C-20)	75.4 (Glu'''-2)	41.4 (C-20)	78.4 (Glu'''-2)	41.5 (C-20)		41.6 (C-20)	75.4 (Glu'''-2)	104.9 (C-20)	75.0 (Glu'''-2)
16.6 (C-21)	78.3 (Glu'''-3)	14.8 (C-21)	91.3 (Glu'''-3)	16.2 (C-21)		14.3 (C-21)	78.3 (Glu'''-3)	11.8 (C-21)	78.6 (Glu'''-3)
110.7 (C-22)	71.1 (Glu'''-4)	108.9 (C-22)	69.2 (Glu'''-4)	110.7 (C-22)		109.3 (C-22)	71.8 (Glu'''-4)	152.5 (C-22)	71.2 (Glu'''-4)
36.8 (C-23)	62.3 (Glu'''-5)	31.3 (C-23)	62.6 (Glu'''-5)	37.1 (C-23)		31.6 (C-23)	78.4 (Glu'''-5)	23.7 (C-23)	78.5 (Glu'''-5)
28.5 (C-24)	78.5 (Glu'''-6)	28.4 (C-24)	61.7 (Glu'''-6)	28.4 (C-24)		28.6 (C-24)	63.3 (Glu'''-6)	31.4 (C-24)	61.9 (Glu'''-6)
34.7 (C-25)	105 (Glu''''-1)	30.1 (C-25)		34.1 (C-25)		30.1 (C-25)	106.3 (Glu''''-1)	33.5 (C-25)	
75.6 (C-26)	75.1 (Glu''''-2)	66.9 (C-26)		75.2 (C-26)		66.8 (C-26)	75.7 (Glu''''-2)	74.9 (C-26)	
	78.2 (Glu''''-3)						78.6 (Glu''''-3)		
17.8 (C-27)	71.7 (Glu''''-4)	18.4 (C-27)		17.8 (C-27)		17.2 (C-27)	71.9 (Glu''''-4)	17.3 (C-27)	
	78.4 (Glu''''-5)						78.7 (Glu''''-5)		

	62.4 (Glu''''-6)						62.6 (Glu''''-6)		

Table 1: The corresponding MS and carbon data of five compounds by 13C NMR method.

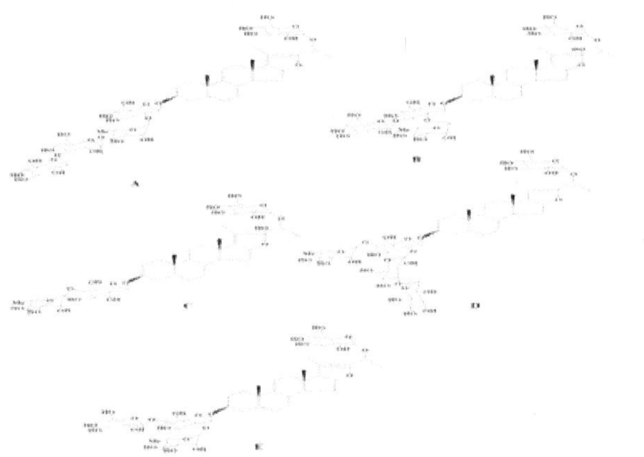

Figure 4: Chemical structures of compounds from Dioscorea zingiberensis C.H.Wright. (A): Compound A; (B): Compound B; (C): Compound C; (D): Compound D; (E): Compound E.

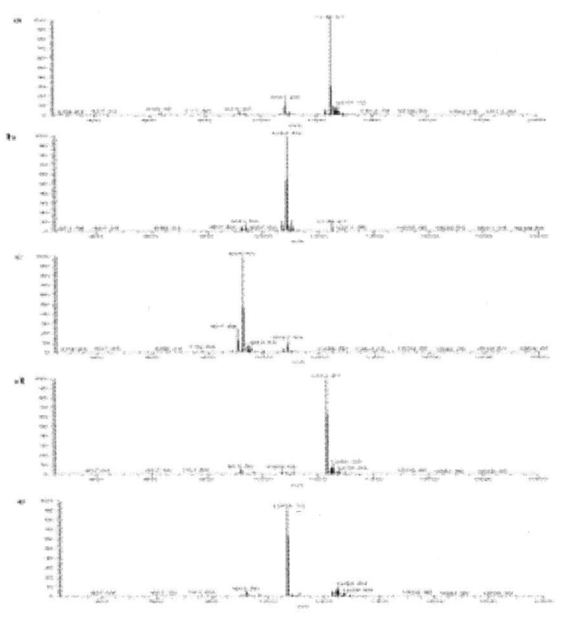

Figure 5: ESI-MS chromatograms of five compounds. (a): Compound A; (b): Compound B; (c): Compound C; (d): Compound D; (e): Compound E.

Optimization of the conditions of CCC and preparative RP-HPLC

In the CCC separation, the first step for selecting a suitable two-phase solvent system requires almost 90% of the entire process of separation. The suitable K values for CCC are in a range of 0.5-2 which gives an efficient separation within a reasonable run time. A smaller K value would elute the solute peaks near the solvent front with low resolution, while a larger K value tends to give better resolution but with broader and more dilute peaks due to a longer elution time [23,24]. Since the steroid saponins in the rhizomes of Dioscorea zingiberensis C.H.Wright contain some carbohydrates, these saponins have comparatively high polarity and satisfactory solubility in hydrophilic solvents. In order to distribute the target compounds between the two phases, both phases must have certain polarity. In the present experiment, various two-phase solvent systems each at different volumes were tested, and the K values of the target compounds in these solvent systems are summarized in Table 2. Finally, the two phase solvent system composed of ethyl acetate-n-butanol-methanol-water at a volume of 4:1:2:4 (v/v/v/v) was selected as the two-phase solvent system for CCC separation. Although the same solvent system at the ratio of 4:2:2:4 (v/v/v/v) exhibited a better retention of stationary phase of 45% than the former one, it looked like inappropriate when considered the K value of compound E, which led to a long separation and dilute as well as broad peak with much solvent waste according to the gold's rules [24]. Therefore, the solvent in the current study was used.

In a preparative RP-HPLC separation, finding suitable lab-scale preparative conditions from the analytical HPLC chromatographic data is the most challenging work in the whole experiment [25]. The preparative chromatographic data should be optimized for faster production rate and higher purity. The production rate depends mainly on the cycling time, whereas the purity is determined by the following two factors, i.e., the resolution and the sample saturation capacity on the column. The cycling time and the resolution can be calculated from the analytical scale chromatographic data, while the sample saturation capacity is only determined by performing overloading experiments or by measuring the equilibrium adsorption isotherms when there is no reference available. The cycling time should be neither too long nor too short. Longer cycling time would result in lower efficiency and consumption of abundant solvent while shorter cycling time couldn't give enough peak resolution of the target compounds. The sample loading capacity should be tested according to the peak resolution where separation factor of approximately 1.5 will produce complete resolution between the two peaks. Based on the previous reference, the column packed with reversed-phase silica gel C18 particle was used as stationary phase, and the mobile phase consisted of acetonitrile-water with thesis of 25:75 (v/v) and 15:85 (v/v) were used in preparative RP-HPLC.

Two-phase solvent systems	Ratio(v/v)	The final retention of stationary phase			K		
			A	B	C	D	E
Chloroform-methanol-water	4:03:02	-	22.2	132.89	25.45	35.1	37.2
Chloroform-n-butanol-methanol-water	4:0.2:3:2	-	136.4	27.5	14.2	33.1	35.9
n-hexane-ethyl acetate-methanol-water	1:1:1:1	-	-	-	-	-	-
Ethyl acetate-n-butanol-water	4:01:05	-	0.16	0.02	0.08	0.32	0.41
Ethyl acetate-n-butanol-methanol-water	4:1:0.5:6	-	0.21	0.04	0.14	0.41	0.53
Ethyl acetate-n-butanol-methanol-water	8:0.5:2:4	28%	0.28	0.1	0.19	0.55	0.72
Ethyl acetate-n-butanol-methanol-water	7:0.5:2:4	30%	0.32	0.14	0.24	0.84	1.03
Ethyl acetate-n-butanol-methanol-water	6:0.5:2:4	32%	0.4	0.21	0.54	1.03	1.52
Ethyl acetate-n-butanol-methanol-water	4:1:2:4	42%	0.49	0.98	1.23	1.58	1.97
Ethyl acetate-n-butanol-methanol-water	4:2:2:4	45%	0.53	1.15	1.74	1.98	2.35

Table 2: Comparison of CCC and preparative RP-HPLC.

Comparison of CCC and preparative RP-HPLC separations

CCC is a recently developed liquid-liquid partition chromatography without solid support giving a choice of various two-phase solvent systems, while the preparative RP-HPLC is a traditional liquid-solid chromatography with high efficiency and high recovery with a column containing a wide range of high efficiency packing material. Therefore, there are a number of differences in their performance between them as described in Table 3. Some performance parameters of these two different approaches are summarized in Table 4, among which some differ greatly. These differences are mainly derived from the different volumes of active stationary phase available in each separation method. The stationary phase in CCC is a liquid which typically comprises 75% or more of the column volume, and the lack of a solid support means that this entire volume is accessible to solute. This contrasts with the relatively low active stationary phase volume of RP-HPLC supports and CCC allows the injection of up to 10% of the column volume without chromatographic disturbance.

It is generally recognized that steroid saponins with few chromophores in their structures have very weak UV absorption. Therefore, the UV detector which is the most popular detector among these detection methods, was not adopted in CCC for separation of steroid saponins. Therefore, the evaporative light scattering detector (ELSD), a universal and non-specific detector, was used for CCC for the present study. However, the UV detector could be used in preparative RP-HPLC for the same purpose where the sensitivity was satisfactory at the wavelength of 203 nm, because the mobile phase was transparent at this wavelength. A small volume of effluent from the outlet of the column was lost in CCC due to a flow splitter used in ELSD, whereas there was no sample wastage in preparative RP-HPLC. In addition, the cycle time was 3.5 h in CCC, while it was 1 h in preparative RP-HPLC. Considering these reasons described above, the latter approach was better than the former one.

The crude extract of total steroid saponins could directly be loaded on the CCC column, and pure compounds could be obtained in one step with the total elution volume of 400 ml. Preparative RP-HPLC separation, on the other hand, required two-step operation and pure compounds were obtained with the total elution volume of 960 ml. This clearly indicates that preparative RP-HPLC approach consumed over double amount of solvent compared to CCC. Therefore, CCC was more cost-effective than preparative RP-HPLC.

The separation efficiency was a little different, if their various aspects were compared just as the pre-paragraph mentioned. Abundant solvent with little water were used, however the mobile phrase composed water at higher in reverse preparative HPLC were applied. Therefore, so many reagents should be condensed at higher temperature and recovered, which was a time-consuming procedure. What's more, the quality of the five compounds would be loss when they were condensed and transferred from this process to another one in the two-step HPLC. At the same time, some quality of separated compounds were absorbed on the solid phrase in HPLC. Therefore, it seemed the separation efficiency in CCC method was a little higher than that in pre-HPLC. Of course, the recoveries of these five compounds revealed the similar results as less quality was lost in CCC.

As stated above, CCC and preparative RP-HPLC each have its own specific advantages: CCC can separate a large amount of crude extracts usually without pre-purification, whereas preparative HPLC produces efficient separation in a short elution time. Recently, combined use of these two methods to isolate and purify some minor and unknown components in crude samples from natural products is becoming a new and superior separation mode over other chromatographic methods due to the complementary action between these two methods [26]. In order to efficiently separate the steroid saponins with high polarity, there is an urgent need for adopting combinational method: with initial preparation preformed by CCC to enrich certain polarity bands containing the chosen targets, followed by further purification using high resolution prep-HPLC procedures with small **particle size**

ODS column, such as 5 μm or 10 μm, the highly pure saponins could be obtained from natural products. Its most significant advantage is that almost quantitative mass balance of components and better resolution were achieved simultaneously within short separation time. Thus, it would facilitate the establishment of optimum separation conditions for almost all kinds of steroid saponins by CCC, prep-HPLC, or with their combination.

Various aspects	CCC	preparative RP-HPLC
Separation mechanism	Liquid-liquid mode	Liquid-solid mode
Irreversible adsorption	None	Some
Cycle time of each separation	Long	Short
Choice of solvent system	Many	Few
Solid phase types	None	Many
Elution mode	Few	Several
Sample preparation	Simple	Complex
Optimizing the chromatographic condition	Complex	Complex
Sample loading capacity	Large	Small
Effluent monitoring method	Few	Many
Selecting solvent system	Time-consuming	Relatively simple
Solvent consumption	Low	High
Amplification from the analytical mode	Relatively simple	Time-consuming
Separation efficiency	A little better	A little worse
Recoveries	higher	Lower

Table 3: Comparison of CCC and preparative RP-HPLC.

Parameters	CCC	RP-HPLC	Ratio CCC/RP-HPLC
Run time/injection (min)	210	60	3.5
Mobile phase flow rate (ml min-1)	2	16	0.125
Operating pressure (Mpa)	2	19.97	0.1
Column volumes (ml)	300	60	5
Sample loading/run (mg)	100	100	1
Injection volume (ml)	10	2	5
Total solvent used	420	960	0.437
Purity of five compounds	Over 95%	Over 95%	Close 1
Detector	ELSD	UV	-

Table 4: Comparison of performance parameters between CCC and RP-HPLC chromatography for 100 mg steroid saponins separation campaigns.

Conclusions

Two approaches including CCC and preparative RP-HPLC were each successfully established for the separation and purification of steroid saponins from the same crude extract of Dioscorea zingiberensis C.H.Wright for the first time. Through comparison of the separation time and solvent consumption between these two approaches, it was found that CCC required a longer separation time with much less solvent consumption, while preparative RP-HPLC gave a much shorter separation time but with higher solvent consumption. Five steroid saponins were successfully isolated and purified from the crude extract at high purity of over 95%. These methods can be further applied to isolate other steroid saponins, especially minor and unknown ones from the crude extracts of natural products.

Acknowledgement

The authors thank Prof. Zhongfu Wang of the Key Laboratory of Resource Biology and Biotechnology in western China for assistance in ESI-MS experiments, and Prof. Yong Sun of the Analysis Test Center for assistance in NMR experiments.

References

1. Li H, Ni JR (2011) Treatment of waste water from Dioscorea zingiberensis tubers used for producing steroid hormones in a microbial fuel cell. Bioresour Technol 102: 2731-2735.
2. Li H, Huang W, Wen YQ, Gong GH, Zhao QB et al. (2010) Anti-thrombotic activity and chemical characterization of steroidal saponins from Dioscorea zingiberensis C.H. Wright. Fitoterapia 81: 1147-1156.
3. Wang YX, Liu H, Bao JG, Hong Y, Yang ZH, et al. (2008) The saccharification-emembrane retrieval-hydrolysis (SMRH) process: a novel approach for cleaner production of diosgenin derived from Dioscorea zingiberensis. J Cleaner Production 16: 1133-1137.
4. Dong YS, Teng H, Qi SS, Liu L, Wang H, et al. (2010) Pathways and kinetics analysis of biotransformation of Dioscorea zingiberensis by Aspergillus oryzae. Biochem Eng J 52: 123-130.
5. Huang W, Zhao HZ, Ni JR., Zuo H, Qiu LL, et al. (2008) The best utilization of D. zingiberensis C.H. Wright by an eco-friendly process. Bioresour Technol 99: 7407-7411.
6. Zhang YQ, Tang LR, An X, Fu E, Ma CF (2009) Modification of cellulase and its application to extraction of diosgenin from Dioscorea zingiberensis C.H. Wright. Biochem Eng J 47: 80-86.
7. Qin Y, Wu XH, Huang W, Gong GH, Li D, et al. (2009) Acute toxicity and sub-chronic toxicity of steroidal saponins from Dioscorea zingiberensis C.H.Wright in rodents. J Ethnopharmacol 126: 543-550.
8. Qiu L, Niu H, Huang W (2011) Ultrasonic and fermented pretreatment technology for diosgenin production from Diosorea zingiberensis C.H. Wright. Chem Eng Res Des 89: 239-247.
9. Cui HY, Jia XY, Zhang X, Zhang J, Zhang ZQ (2011) Optimization of counter-current chromatography for separation of polyphenols from the extract of hawthorn (Crataegus laevigata) with response surface methodology. Sep Purif Technol 77: 269-274.
10. Xiao XH, Guo ZN, Deng JC, Li GK (2009) Separation and purification of isofraxidin from Sarcandra glabra by microwave-assisted extraction coupled with high-speed counter-current chromatography. Sep Purif Technol 68: 250-254.
11. Zhu JB, Guo XJ, Fu SP, Zhang XL, Liang XM, et al. (2010) Characterization of steroidal saponins in crude extracts from Dioscorea zingiberensis C. H. Wright by ultra-performance liquid chromatography/ electrospray ionization quadrupole time-of-flight tandem mass spectrometry. J Pharm Biomed Anal 53: 462-474.

12. Du QZ, Jerz G, Waibel R, Winterhalter P (2003) Isolation of dammarane saponins from Panax notoginseng by high-speed counter-current chromatography. J Chromatogr A 1008: 173-180.
13. Xin XL, Yang Y, Zhong J, Aisa HJA, Wang HQ (2009) Preparative isolation and purification of isobenzofuranone derivatives and saponins from seeds of Nigella glandulifera Freyn by high-speed counter-current chromatography combined with gel filtration. J Chromatogr A 1216: 4258-4262.
14. Shi SP, Jiang D, Zhao MB, Tu PF (2007) Preparative isolation and purification of triterpene saponins from Clematis Mandshurica by high-speed counter-current chromatography coupled with evaporative light scattering detection. J Chromatogr B 852: 679-683.
15. Chen QQ, Hu XF, Li JM, Liu P, Yang Y, et al. (2011) Preparative isolation and purification of cuminaldehyde and p-menta-1,4-dien-7-al from the essential oil of Cuminum cyminuml. by high-speed counter-current chromatography. Anal Chim Acta 689: 149-154.
16. Goetzinger W, Zhang X, Bi G, Towle M, Cherrak D, et al. (2004) High throughput HPLC/MS purification in support of drug discovery. Int J Mass spectrom 238: 153-162.
17. Chtner FF, Angelberger P, Kvaternik H, Hammerschmidt F, Simovc BP (2002) Aspects of 6-[18F]fluoro-L-DOPA preparation: precursor synthesis, preparative HPLC purification and determination of radiochemical purity. J Steinbach Nucl Med Biol 29: 477-481.
18. Vailaya A, Sajonz P, Sudah O, Capodanno V, Helmy R, et al. (2005) Exploiting pH mismatch in preparative high-performance liquid chromatographic recovery of ertapenem from mother liquor streams. J Chromatogr A 1079: 80-91.
19. Sajonz P, Vailaya A, Sudah O, McPherson L, Capodanno V, et al. (2006) Development of a gradient elution preparative high performance liquid chromatography method for the recovery of the antibiotic ertapenem from crystallization process streams. J Chromatogr A 1126: 365-372.
20. Yang RT, Xu DP, Tang SR, Pan FS, Zhao AM, et al. (2008) Isolation and identification of steroidal saponins from fresh rhizome of Dioscorea zingiberensis. Chinese Traditional and Herb Drugs. 4: 493-496.
21. Tang SR, Yang RT, Pan FS, Zhao AM, Pang ZJ (2007) Steroidal saponin and steroidal sapogenin in Chinese Dioscorea L. J Pla Rea Envir. 16: 64-72.
22. Yang RT, Xu DP, Tang SR, Pan FS, Zhao AM, et al. (2008) Isolation and identification of steroidal saponins from fresh rhizome of Dioscorea zingiberensis. Chin Tradition Herbal Drugs 39: 493-496.
23. Yang RT, Tong HY (2010) Research of Steroidal Saponins from the Fresh Rhizomes of Dioscorea zingiberensis. J Chin. Medicinal Materials. 33: 62-64.
24. Yang RT, Tong HY (2010) Ito Y (2005) Golden rules and pitfalls in selecting optimum conditions for high-speed counter-current chromatography. J. Chromatogr. A. 1065: 145-168.
25. Sajonz P, Natishan TK, Antia FD, Frenette R (2005) Optimization of the preparative separation of a chiral pharmaceutical intermediate by high performance liquid chromatography. J. Chromatogr. A 1089: 135-141.
26. Yao S, Luo JG, Huang XF, Kong LY (2008) Application of preparative high-speed counter-current chromatography/preparative high-performance liquid chromatography mode in rapid separation of saponins. J Chromatogr B 864: 69-77.

11

Administration of Anastrozole to Ovariectomized Rats Impairs Working Memory in Association with Plastic Changes to Dendritic Spines on Prefrontal Third-layer Pyramidal Neurons

Dulce A. Velázquez-Zamora[1,2], Nestor I. Martínez-Torres[2], Miguel Cervantes[3] and Ignacio González-Burgos[2*]

[1]*Universidad Politécnica de la Zona Metropolitana de Guadalajara, Tlajomulco de Zúñiga, Jal., México*

[2]*Laboratorio de Psicobiología, División de Neurociencias, Centro de Investigación Biomédica de Occidente, IMSS, Guadalajara, Jal., México*

[3]*Laboratorio de Neurociencias, División de Estudios de Posgrado, Facultad de Ciencias Médicas y Biológicas "Dr Ignacio Chávez", UMSNH, Morelia, Mich., México*

[*]**Corresponding author:** Ignacio González-Burgos PhD, Laboratorio de Psicobiología, División de Neurociencias, Centro de Investigación Biomédica de Occidente, Instituto Mexicano del Seguro Social, Sierra Mojada #800, Col. Independencia, C.P. 44340 Guadalajara, Jal, México,
E-mail: igonbur@hotmail.com

Abstract

Gonadal estrogens influence several neurobiological events related to synaptic plasticity underlying cognitive behavior. Likewise, estradiol synthesized in neurons affects aspects of brain organization associated with cognition. Here, plastic changes to dendritic spines on third-layer pyramidal neurons from the prefrontal cortex of ovariectomized, anastrozole-treated female rats were studied. Anastrozole treatment dampened the efficiency of rats in resolving a spatial working memory test in the "Y" maze when compared with ovariectomized control and proestrus female rats. In addition, the administration of Anastrozole led to an increase in dendritic spines and filopodia on the pyramidal cells studied. The thin, mushroom, stubby and wide spines remained unchanged. Since filopodia are considered to be the precursors of novel spines, the increase in dendritic spines is consistent with the increase in filopodia. However, this was clearly insufficient to drive proper working memory performance, despite the apparent stability in the translation of synaptic information suggested by the similar spine types evident in the ovariectomized controls and the increases observed. These findings show that brain-derived estradiol is necessary for prefrontal activity to account for working memory performance. Further studies will be needed to elucidate the mechanisms underlying such spine enhancement in the absence of estradiol-mediated modulation of plasticity.

Keywords: Anastrozole; Estrogen; Dendritic spines; Plasticity; Working memory; Prefrontal cortex

Introduction

Estrogens, mainly 17β estradiol (E2), have recognized trophic and regulatory roles on the cytoarchitecture, connectivity and function of brain structures. Their activity not only influences events related to sexual behavior and reproductive in adult females but also, neural structures and processes that support other important brain activities like neuroprotection, or learning and memory [1-4]. These effects on neural tissue may be exerted by estrogens synthesized in the ovary, although E2 synthesized in several cerebral structures may also account for some estrogenic actions in the brain [1,5,6]. Thus, both endocrine and paracrine pathways supplying E2 may be involved in its regulatory activity in specific neural structures.

The pathway of steroidogenesis that ends in the synthesis of testosterone is active in neural and glial populations within specific brain structures, driving its metabolic conversion to 5α-dihydrotestosterone by 5α-reductase or to estradiol through the activity of aromatase. Thus, it is likely that these "neurosteroids" can modify neural structure and function in these domains [7-12]. Indeed, testosterone aromatase activity has been shown to drive E2 synthesis in both the hippocampus and the prefrontal cortex of male and female rats, even in the absence of gonadal steroidogenesis [13-16]. These brain structures are mainly involved in different modalities of cognition in the brain and therefore, the estrogenic activity exerted by the E2 produced through ovarian and/or brain steroid synthesis can modify the structural and biochemical neural substrates of cognitive functions [17-20]. Cytoarchitectonic characteristics can be modified by estrogen-related phenomena, including: changes in dendritic spine density and in the proportion of the different spine types on the dendritic branches of pyramidal neurons; synaptic connectivity, activity and strength in hippocampal and prefrontal cortex neuronal circuits. Thus, hippocampal- and prefrontal cortex-dependent cognitive functions are likely to be susceptible to variations in E2 concentration and activity [17,21,22].

Indeed, there is experimental evidence that supports an important role of the estrogen E2 synthesized through testosterone aromatization in these brain structures and its involvement in cognitive functions. Accordingly, inhibition of brain aromatase activity provokes structural and functional alterations to the neural substrate involved in hippocampal- and prefrontal cortex-dependent cognitive functions, leading to deficient performance of both experimental animals and humans in modality-specific learning/memory tests [19,23-30].

In the light of these findings, this study was designed to evaluate the effect of inhibiting aromatase activity in ovariectomized rats. Specifically, the effect on dendritic spine density and on the relative proportions of the different spine types was evaluated in pyramidal neurons located in the layer III of the prefrontal cortex. These changes were correlated with the performance of the experimental animals in an allocentric working memory test.

Materials and Methods

Subjects

Female Sprague-Dawley rats (n=48) weighing 250-300 gm were used in this study. The rats were housed at 25°C under a regular 12/12 h light/dark cycle, and with ad libitum access to water and food, and they were verified to complete three regular estrous cycles lasting 5 days.

Experimental design

The animals were assigned to one of four study groups: 1) a control group of bilaterally ovariectomized rats (Ovx; n=12); 2) another control group of bilaterally ovariectomized rats to which 1 ml of dimethylsulfoxide (DMSO) diluted 3% in saline solution was administered intraperitoneally (i.p., Ovx+Veh; n=12); 3) a further control group of rats studied in the proestrus stage (14:00 h) of their estrous cycle (Proestrus; n=12); and 4) an experimental group of bilaterally ovariectomized rats i.p. administered 1 mg/kg of Anastrozole [31,32] in 20 mg/ml DMSO diluted to 3% in saline solution (Ovx+Ans; n=12). The ovariectomized rats were first anesthetized with ketamine (60 mg/kg, i.m.) followed by 25 mg/kg of sodium pentobarbital (i.p.). The pharmacological treatments to the Ovx, Ovx+Veh and Ovx+Ans rats were applied on day 6 after ovariectomy.

From the first-to-seventh day after ovariectomy, the animals were all handled daily for 15 minutes in order to minimize the effects of stress. Furthermore, prior to the behavioral studies the animals had their food supply restricted to 85% of the daily intake to ensure their motivation for a food reward. In addition, they were not allowed any food for 24 h before behavioral testing. Access to water was always ad libitum. Six animals per group were used for behavioral testing, whilst morphological studies were performed by using the other six rats in each group (Figure 1).

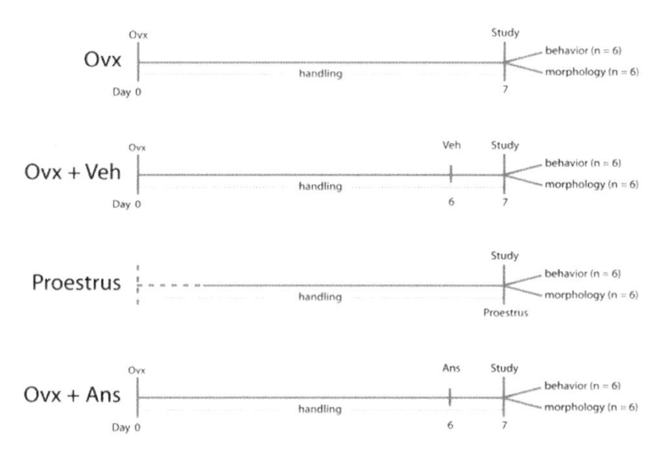

Figure 1: Diagram of the experimental design used in this study.

Behavioral testing

The six animals from each of the study groups were challenged to resolve an allocentric working memory paradigm in a white, opaque acrylic "Y" maze that was situated in an illuminated room with differential visuo-spatial signals. Each of the three arms of the maze could be closed with a sliding door, which were used in function of the test's needs. At the end of the adjacent arms of the Y, a food well below floor level contained cereal as a reward.

Before starting of the behavioral test, the animals were habituated to the maze by allowing them to explore the three arms of the maze freely for ten minutes. The rats were then withdrawn from the maze and immediately reintroduced into it, having placed several pieces of cereal on the floor of each of the three arms and within the wells. When the rat had eaten all the cereal or after a further ten minutes, the animal was returned to its home cage. Twelve trials were then carried out according to a delayed match-to-sample procedure in a single one-day session.

In each trial the rat was introduced into the Y maze, and a study phase was then followed by a delay period and a test phase. The rat was placed in the vertical arm of the Y maze for thirty seconds (introduction) before the starting arm was opened, and it was only allowed to enter the open arm and eat the cereal from the well (study phase). It was then returned to the starting arm for a period of ten seconds (delay period) before the sliding door of the starting arm was opened again, allowing entry into both of the upper arms of the Y maze so that the rat could choose either. However, only the arm that was baited during the study phase contained the reward. If the rat turned to the same arm as in the study phase then a "correct response" was registered in the trial (test phase: Figure 2). Each trial was separated by a thirty-second delay (interval period). To avoid egocentric tendencies in the resolution of the trials, a random design was used such that the rat had to turn to the right in six trials and it had to turn to the left in the other six trials.

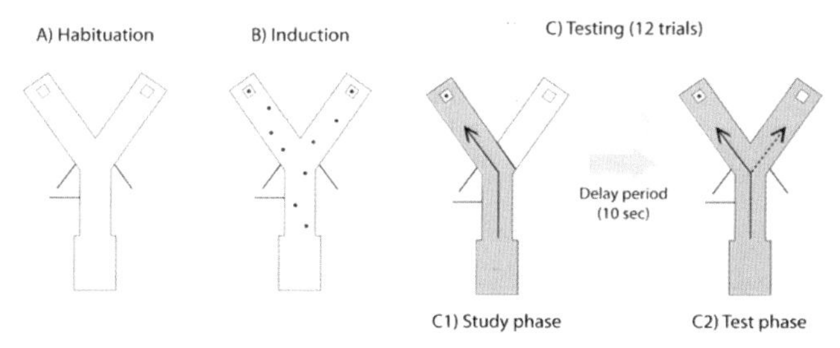

Figure 2: Experimental paradigm designed to evaluate allocentric working memory.

Morphological studies

Rats from each group were anesthetized with ketamine (30 mg/kg, i.m.) and sodium pentobarbital (50 mg/kg, i.p.), and they were then perfused with 200 ml of a phosphate-buffered solution (pH 7.4, 0.01 M) containing sodium heparin (1000 IU/l) as an anticoagulant and procaine hydrochloride (1 g/l) as a vasodilator [33]. The rats were then perfused with 200 ml of a phosphate-buffered 4% formaldehyde fixative solution. Both solutions were perfused at a rate of 11.5 ml/min. The rat's brain was then removed and maintained for at least 48 h in 100 ml of fresh fixative solution. The bilateral blocks of prefrontal tissue were subsequently dissected out according to plates 7-11 of a brain atlas [34] and they were impregnated using a modified version of the Golgi technique [35]. Coronal slices (75 μm thick) were mounted on one slide per animal, and six third-layer pyramidal neurons of the pre-limbic/infralimbic prefrontal cortex from each of the six rats in every group were analyzed. Pyramidal neurons were selected for spine counting based on three morphological criteria: (a) neurons had to be well impregnated; (b) neurons in which the bodies or branches selected for counting were obstructed by blood vessels, glia or heavy clusters of dendrites from neighboring impregnated cells were excluded; and (c) the apical arborization had to be fully impregnated and mainly intact. The dendritic spines were counted along a 50 μm segment on each neuron in the middle section of a secondary dendrite protruding from the apical one (Figure 3, left panel). Sampling of the dendritic spines followed three morphological criteria: (a) belonging to a clearly distinguishable neuron found in layer three of the prefrontal cortex; (b) located on a secondary dendrite protruding from the middle third of the apical dendrite; (c) the dendritic segment selected for counting had to be in a homogenous plane of focus.

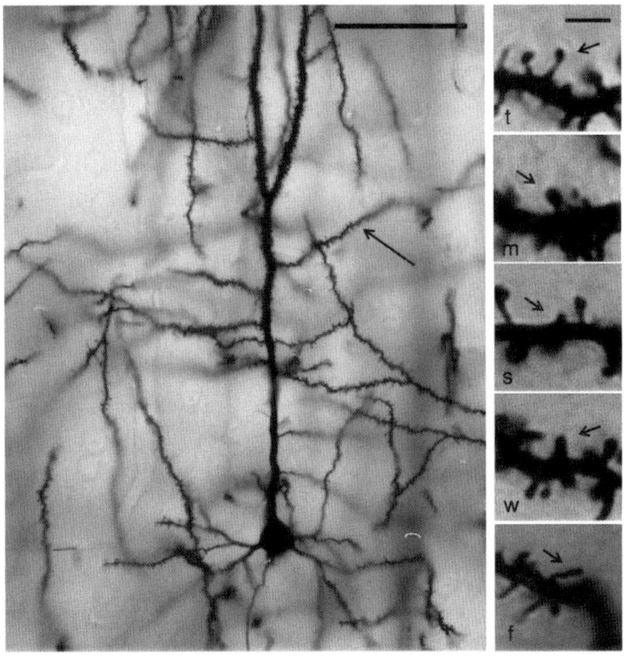

Figure 3: Left panel: photomicrograph of a representative layer III pyramidal neuron from the prelimbic/infralimbic prefrontal cortex, showing a secondary dendrite (arrow) from where the spines were counted. Scale bar=100 μm. Right panel: photomicrographs of thin (t), stubby (s), mushroom (m) and wide (w) spines (arrows), such as those counted in this study. Scale bar=2 μm.

A reliability index was determined for dendritic spine counting in an initial double-blind study: number of agreements-number of disagreements/number of agreements. Once a minimum reliability of 0.95 was reached, dendritic spines from each of the groups were quantified using a "blind" procedure. The density and proportion of thin, mushroom, stubby and wide spines were determined according to previously established criteria [36-38]: thin spines were defined as those in which the neck diameter was less than the total spine length and the head diameter was only slightly greater than the neck diameter; stubby spines were defined as those in which the neck diameter was more than or equal to the spine length; mushroom spines were defined as those in which both the diameter and length of the neck was much smaller than the head diameter, and the neck was shorter than that of thin spines; wide spines, which closely resemble stubby spines, were defined as those in which the total spine length was longer than the neck diameter (Figure 3, right panel). Spine counting was performed at 2,000X using a magnification changer in a light microscope coupled to an image analyzer (LAS 4.0).

Statistics

Behavioral data and spine density were analyzed by one-way ANOVA followed by the Tukey post hoc test, and the relative proportional density of each spine type was analyzed using one-way ANOVA followed by Bonferroni correction post hoc test.

Ethical considerations

All experimental procedures were designed to minimize the pain and discomfort of the experimental animals. The experimental protocol was approved by the Committee for Research Ethics of the Instituto Mexicano del Seguro Social (Mexico), and the experimental procedures were performed according to the NIH guidelines for the Care and Use of Laboratory Animals (NIH Publications No. 80-23, 1996 revision).

Results

Allocentric working memory

The behavioral evaluation of allocentric working memory reflected significant variation between the four groups of animals studied ($F=27.546$, $p<0.0001$). The number of correct responses by the Proestrus rats in the Y maze was more than those recorded by the Ovx ($p<0.0001$), Ovx+Veh ($p<0.0001$) and Ovx+Ans ($p<0.0001$) animals. In addition, the Ovx+Ans rats made fewer correct responses than both the Ovx ($p<0.01$) and Ovx+Veh ($p<0.008$) animals. As expected, no significant differences were observed between the Ovx and Ovx+Veh groups (Figure 4).

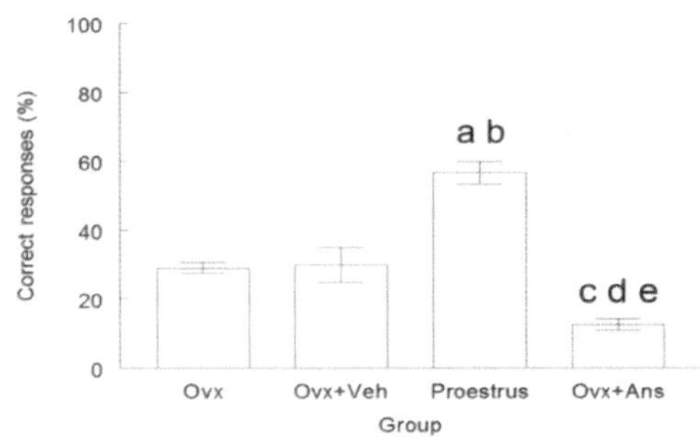

Figure 4: Percentage of the correct responses in the Y maze by ovariectomized rats (Ovx), ovariectomized rats administered the vehicle alone (Ovx+Veh), rats in proestrus (Proestrus) and ovariectomized rats administered Anastrozole (Ovx+Ans). The data are represented as the mean ± SEM: a, *Vs.* Ovx; b, *Vs.* Ovx+Veh; c, *Vs.* Ovx; d, *Vs.* Ovx+Veh; e, *Vs.* Proestrus.

Spine density

When the dendritic spine density was analyzed, significant differences were found between the groups studied (F=16.893, p<0.0001). Pyramidal neurons from layer III of the prefrontal cortex of Proestrus rats had a greater density of dendritic spines than Ovx (p<0.0001), Ovx+Veh (p<0.0001) and Ovx+Ans rats (p<0.04). Similarly, there was a greater density of spines on neurons from Ovx +Ans animals than on those from the Ovx (p<0.01) and Ovx+Veh (p<0.04) groups. Again, there was no difference in spine density between the Ovx and Ovx+Veh rats (Figure 5).

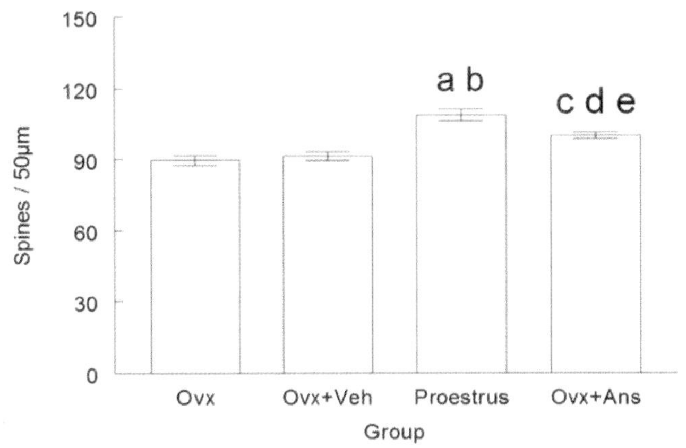

Figure 5: Density of dendritic spines on pyramidal neurons in the prelimbic/infralimbic prefrontal cortex of ovariectomized rats (Ovx), ovariectomized rats administered the vehicle alone (Ovx +Veh), rats in proestrus (Proestrus) and ovariectomized rats administered Anastrozole (Ovx+Ans). The data are represented as the mean ± SEM: A, Vs. Ovx; b, *Vs.* Ovx+Veh; c, *Vs.* Ovx; d, *Vs.* Ovx+Veh; e, *Vs.* Proestrus.

Spine types

The proportion of thin spines (F=4.632, p<0.01), mushroom spines (F=12.989, p<0.0001) and filopodia (F=66.042, p<0.0001) varied between the distinct experimental groups of rats. The density of thin spines was greater in the Proestrus rats than in both the Ovx (p<0.03) and Ov+Ans (p<0.02) groups, while there were no statistical differences between the Ovx, Ovx+Veh and Ovx+Ans rats. Similarly, a higher density of mushroom spines was evident in the Proestrus group when compared to the Ovx (p<0.0001), Ovx+Veh (p<0.0001) and Ovx +Ans rats (p<0.001) and again, there were no differences in the density of mushroom spines between the Ovx, Ovx+Veh and Ovx+Ans groups. The proportions of stubby and wide spines did not vary significantly between the four groups studied. By contrast, there was a significantly higher proportion of filopodial structures in the Ovx+Ans animals than in the three other control groups: the Ovx (p<0.0001), Ovx+Veh (p<0.0001) and Proestrus animals (p<0.0001: Table 1).

Spine type	Ovx	Ovx+Veh	Proestrus	Ovx+Ans
Thin	36.9 ± 1.8	37.8 ± 0.6	44.5 ± 1.4 ^{a}	38.8 ± 2.4 ^{c}
Mushroom	26.1 ± 0.7	26.1 ± 1.8	33.0 ± 1.1 $^{a\,b}$	28.2 ± 0.8 ^{c}
Stubby	22.2 ± 0.7	20.4 ± 1.0	24.0 ± 1.2	24.5 ± 0.4
Wide	6.4 ± 1.1	5.3 ± 0.4	5.3 ± 0.3	6.2 ± 0.2
Filopodia	1.0 ± 0.2	0.2 ± 0.09	0.8 ± 0.2	5.9 ± 0.5 $^{a\,b\,c}$
Mean ± SEM; ANOVA, Bonferroni; p<0.05; a: *vs.* Ovx; b: *vs.* Ovx+Veh; c: *vs.* Proestrus				

Table 1: Density of the different spine types counted in pyramidal neurons from the layer III of the prefrontal cortex of female rats.

Discussion

Clinical [39,40] and experimental [23,41] studies have demonstrated an important regulatory role of estradiol on the morphological and functional characteristics of the neural substrate in the prefrontal cortex involved in the expression of verbal and spatial working memory [42,43]. In particular, the inhibition of estradiol synthesis dampens the ability to solve spatial working memory tests. Such an effect can be produced by interfering with testosterone aromatase activity, a phenomenon observed in women that receive anastrozole as a part of breast cancer therapy [28,44,45].

Anastrozole, as well as letrozole, are nonsteroidal testosterone aromatase inhibitors that bind reversibly to the aromatase enzyme, impeding the synthesis of estradiol otherwise resulting from testosterone aromatization [46,47]. Thus, besides breast cancer therapy, anastrozole has also been used as a clinical pharmacological approach aimed to counteract, trough testosterone aromatase inhibition, other phathophysiological conditions in human beings, such as low-testosterone hypogonadism in elderly men [48]. In addition, anastrozole treatment has resulted in an experimental model of brain-syntetized estrogen insufficiency for different, *in vitro* [49,50] and *in vivo* [51-53], experimental designs.

On the other hand, changes in plasma estradiol levels during the estrus cycles may affect certain characteristics of learning and working memory [54,55] brain processes that require the processing and updating of information to produce short-term memory responses [56,57]. It is well known that peripheral plasma levels of estradiol, resulting from cyclic ovary steroid synthesis and secretion vary from basal values (less than 10 pg/ml) during estrus, and progressively increase trough metaestrus and diestrus to achieve their maximal values on late proestrus (near around 40 pg/ml) [58]. When plasma levels of estradiol are higher, the performance of female rats in resolving spatial working memory tests is preferentially based on allocentric strategies rather than egocentric strategies [59], a result of a switching activity in the prefrontal cortex that foments either allocentric or egocentric performance [60].

Moreover, estradiol therapy improves the deficient performance of ovariectomized rats in prefrontal cortex dependent allocentric working memory tests, as well as eliciting plastic changes and an increase in dendritic spine density, mainly due to the higher proportion of thin dendritic spines in layer III pyramidal neurons of the prefrontal cortex [61,62]. These neurons are involved in determining whether allocentric or egocentric strategies are employed to solve working memory tests, as well as in processing the sensory/motor memory information required for the memory fields to adopt the adequate working memory strategy [63-65] Here, ovariectomized rats resolved the working memory task inefficiently and they did so at a probabilistic level of chance (50%). However, ovariectomized rats that received anastrozole performed below 50% efficiency and they were even less efficient than the control ovariectomized rats. These findings of significantly fewer correct responses when ovariectomized rats received anastrozole in the allocentric spatial working memory test, suggests that the estradiol synthesized in brain structures, including the prefrontal cortex, may fulfill a relevant role in the neural substrates involved in cognitive functions. Indeed, estrogenic activity has been proposed to affect synaptic plasticity and the proportions of dendritic spines, thereby influencing cognitive performance. Such a phenomenon may be particularly relevant if driven by estradiol synthesized locally in specific brain structures rather than being supplied from that synthesized in the ovary [24,66].

There is evidence that the plasticity of dendritic spine synapses driven by the estrogen produced through brain aromatase activity may have different functional characteristics depending on the specific brain structures where they were synthetized, in female rats [19,67,68]. In addition, the effects of aromatase inhibition on dendritic spine plasticity may change in different experimental conditions. Thus, while inhibiting aromatase with letrozole in cycling rats did not affect synaptic spine density on prefrontal cortex pyramidal neurons such treatment did significantly reduce the number of dendritic spine-mediated synapses. Moreover, aromatase inhibition down-regulated synaptophysin and spinophilin expression in the hippocampus of both cycling and ovariectomized rats [30], and in hippocampal cell cultures [68].

In the present work, dendritic spine density on layer III pyramidal neurons in the prefrontal cortex increased significantly as a result of anastrozole-induced inhibition of brain aromatase activity in the absence of a gonadal source of estrogen in the brain. This increase was associated with a higher proportion of filopodia. According to earlier pioneering studies [69], increased dendritic spine density would lead to better synaptic efficiency. Thus, the higher proportion of filopodia may reflect the initial steps of neuronal activation and the development of neural processes during de novo dendritic spine formation [70-73]. However, recent studies suggested that although mature spines could develop from filopodial structures in adult rodents, these might be inactive [74]. The formation of inactive spines would be consistent with our findings, as despite the increase in dendritic spine density in ovariectomized females that received anastrozole, they performed worse in the working memory task. Thus, while the increase in dendritic spines observed would suggests a compensatory response, our behavioral findings show that these morphological changes seem not to provoke functional compensation on neural substrates in the prefrontal cortex when the modulatory activity of estradiol is absent.

Thin spines have been associated with learning capabilities whilst mushroom spines have been related with memory storage [75,76]. Synaptic stimulation through both stubby and wide spines has been suggested to regulate neuron excitability [36,77]. It is noteworthy that the proportional density of any spine type was unaltered by anastrozole administration to the ovariectomized animals. This is particularly relevant given the increase in dendritic spine density and the enhanced working memory impairment. On the one hand, the homogenous increase in spine types would account for the "stable" postsynaptic translation of synaptic information and on the other hand, the non-predominance of a specific type of spine suggests that the lack of E2 has a homogeneous impact on spine dynamics.

Thus, neural processes appear to be altered by the loss of the estrogenic activity resulting from estradiol synthesis by the neural substrates in the prefrontal cortex that drives cognitive activity, a phenomenon that merits further research.

Funding statement

This work received support from the Coordinación de la Investigación Científica, Universidad Michoacana de San Nicolás de Hidalgo (Reg. 108907).

References

1. McEwen BS, Milner TA (2007) Hippocampal formation: Shedding light on the influence of sex and stress on the brain. Brain Res Rev 55: 343-355.
2. McEwen BS, Akama KT, Spencer-Segal JL, MilnervTA, Waters EM (2012) Estrogen effects on the brain: actions beyond the hypothalamus via novel mechanisms. Behav Neurosci 126: 4-16.
3. Sharma K, Mehra RD (2008) Long-term administration of estrogen or tamoxifen to ovariectomized rats affords neuroprotection to hippocampal neurons by modulating the expression of Bcl-2 and Bax. Brain Res 1204: 1-15.
4. Xu X, Zhang Z (2006) Effects of estradiol benzoate on learning-memory behavior and synaptic structure in ovariectomized mice. Life Sci 79: 1553-1560.
5. Compagnone NA, Mellon SH (2000) Neurosteroids: biosynthesis and function of these novel neuromodulators. Front Neuroendocrinol 21: 1-56.
6. Shibuya K, Takata N, Hojo Y, Furukawa A, Yasumatsu N, et al. (2003) Hippocampal cytochrome P450s synthesize brain neurosteroids which are paracrine neuromodulators of synaptic signal transduction. Biochem Biophys Acta 1619: 301-316.
7. Do-Rego JL, Seong JY, Burel D, Leprince J, Luu-The V, et al. (2009) Neurosteroid biosynthesis: enzymatic pathways and neuroendocrine regulation by neurotransmitters and neuropeptides. Front Neuroendocrinol 30: 259-301.
8. Mellon SH, Vaudry H (2001) Biosynthesis of neurosteroids and regulation of their synthesis. Int Rev Neurobiol 46: 33-78.
9. Pelletier G (2010) Steroidogenic enzymes in the brain: morphological aspects. Prog Brain Res 181: 193-207.
10. Plassart-Schiess E, Baulieu EE (2001) Neurosteroids: recent findings. Brain Res Rev 37: 133-140.
11. Stoffel-Wagner B (2001) Neurosteroid metabolism in the human brain. Eur J Endocrinol 145: 669-679.
12. Tabatadze N, Sato SM, Woolley CS (2014) Quantitative Analysis of Long-Form Aromatase mRNA in the Male and Female Rat Brain. Plos One 9: 1-9.
13. Barker JM, Galea LAM (2009) Sex and regional differences in estradiol content in the prefrontal cortex, amygdala and hippocampus of adult male and female rats. Gen Comp Endocrinol 164: 77-84.
14. Hojo Y, Hattori TA, Enami T, Furukawa A, Suzuki K, et al. (2004) Adult male rat hippocampus synthesizes estradiol from pregnenolone by cytochromes P45017alpha and P450 aromatase localized in neurons. Proc Natl Acad Sci 101: 865-870.
15. Roselli CE, Abdelgadir SE, Ronnekleiv OK, Klosterman SA (1998) Anatomic distribution and regulation of aromatase gene expression in the rat brain. Biol Reprod 58: 79-87.
16. Wei J, Yuen EY, Liu W, Li X, Zhong P, et al. (2014) Estrogen protects against the detrimental effects of repeated stress on glutamatergic transmission and cognition. Mol Psychiatry 19: 588-598.
17. Arevalo MA, Azcoitia I, Gonzalez-Burgos I, Garcia-Segura LM (2015) Signaling mechanisms mediating the regulation of synaptic plasticity and memory by estradiol. Horm Behav 74: 19-27.
18. Velázquez-Zamora DA, González-Tapia D, González-Ramírez MM, Flores-Soto ME, Vázquez-Valls E, et al. (2012) Plastic changes in dendritic spines of hippocampal CA1 pyramidal neurons from ovariectomized rats after estradiol treatment. Brain Res 1470: 1-10.
19. Vierk R, Brandt N, Rune GM (2014) Hippocampal estradiol synthesis and its significance for hippocampal synaptic stability in male and female animals. Neuroscience 22: 24-32.

20. Vierk R, Bayer J, Freitag S, Muhia M, Kutsche T, et al. (2015) Structure–function–behavior relationship in estrogen-induced synaptic plasticity. Horm Behav 74: 139-148.
21. Frankfurt M, Luine V (2015) The evolving role of dendritic spines and memory: Interaction(s) with estradiol. Horm Behav 74: 28-36.
22. Velázquez-Zamora DA, González-Tapia D, Feria-Velasco A, González-Burgos I (2014) Estrogenic modulation of memory-associated neuroplasticity. In: González-Burgos I Editor. Estrogens and cognition. Psychobiological and clinical aspects. Research Signpost 1-23.
23. Bayer J, Rune G, Schultz H, Tobia MJ, Mebes I, et al. (2015) The effect of estrogen synthesis inhibition on hippocampal memory. Psychoneuroendocrinology 56: 213-225.
24. Bian C, Zhu H, Zhao Y, Cai W, Zhang J (2014) Intriguing roles of hippocampus-synthesized 17β-estradiol in the modulation of hippocampal synaptic plasticity. J Mol Neurosci 54: 271-281.
25. Galvin C, Ninan I (2014) Regulation of the mouse medial prefrontal cortical synapses by endogenous estradiol. Neuropsychopharmacology 39: 2086-2094.
26. Garcia-Segura LM (2008) Aromatase in the brain: not just for reproduction anymore. J Neuroendocrinol 20: 705-712.
27. Hojo Y, Murakami G, Mukai H, Higo S, Hatanaka Y, et al. (2008) Estrogen synthesis in the brain—Role in synaptic plasticity and memory. Mol Cell Endocrinol 290: 31-43.
28. Phillips KA, Ribi K, Fisher R (2011) Do aromatase inhibitors have adverse effects on cognitive function? Breast Cancer Res 13: 1-7.
29. Rune GM, Frostcher M (2005) Neurosteroid synthesis in the hippocampus: role in synaptic plasticity. Neuroscience 136: 833-842.
30. Zhou L, Fester L, von Blittersdorff B, Hassu B, Nogens H, et al. (2010) Aromatase inhibitors induce spine synapse loss in the hippocampus of ovariectomized mice. Endocrinology 151: 1153-1160.
31. Buzdar AU, Robertson JF, Eiermann W, Nabholtz JM (2002) An overview of the pharmacology and pharmacokinetics of the newer generation aromatase inhibitors anastrozole, letrozole, and exemestane Cancer 95: 2006-2016.
32. Sanford M, Plosker GL (2008) Anastrozole: a review of its use in postmenopausal women with early-stage breast cancer. Drugs 68: 1319-1340.
33. Feria-Velasco A, Karnovsky MJ, (1970) Optimal central nervous system preservation with glutaraldehyde perfusion for ultrastructural study. Arch Invest Med 1: 201-220.
34. Paxinos G, Watson C (1986) The rat brain in stereotaxic coordinates (2nd edn.), Academic Press.
35. González-Burgos I, Tapia-Arizmendi G, Feria-Velasco A (1992) Golgi method without osmium tetroxide for the study of the central nervous system. Biotech Histochem 67: 288-296.
36. González-Burgos I (2009) Dendritic spines plasticity and learning/memory processes: Theory, evidence and perspectives. In: Baylog LR Editor. Dendritic spines. Biochemistry, modelling and properties. Nova Science Publishers pp: 163-186.
37. González-Burgos I (2012) From synaptic transmission to cognition: an intermediary role for dendritic spines. Brain Cogn 80: 177-183.
38. Harris KM, Jensen FE, Tsao BH (1989) Ultraestructure, development and plasticity of dendritic spine synapses in area CA1 of the rat hippocampus: extending our vision with serial electron microscopy and three-dimensional analyses. In: Chan-Palay V and Kôhler CH Editors. The Hippocampus, New Vistas pp: 33-52.
39. Berent-Spillson A, Persad CC, Love T, Sowers M, Randolph JF, et al. (2012) Hormonal environment affects cognition independent of age during the menopause transition. J Clin Endocrinol Metab 97: 1686-1694.
40. Hampson E, Morley EE (2013) Estradiol concentrations and working memory performance in women of reproductive age. Psychoneuroendocrinology 38: 2897-2904.
41. Hara Y, Yuk F, Puri R, Janssen WG, Rapp PR, et al. (2014) Presynaptic mitochondrial morphology in monkey prefrontal cortex correlates with working memory and is improved with estrogen treatment. Proc Natl Acad Sci 7: 486-491.
42. Dumitriu D, Rapp PR, McEwen BS, Morrison JH (2010) Estrogen and the aging brain: an elixir for the weary cortical network. Ann NY Acad Sci 1204: 104-112.
43. León-Domínguez U, Martín-Rodríguez JF, León-Carrión J (2015) Executive n-back tasks for the neuropsychological assessment of working memory. Behav Brain Res 292: 167-173.
44. Bender CM, Merriman JD, Gentry AL, Ahrendt GM, Berga SL, et al. (2015) Patterns of change in cognitive function with anastrozole therapy. Cancer 121: 2627-2636.
45. Shilling V, Jenkins V, Fallowfield L, Howell T (2003) The effects of hormone therapy on cognition in breast cancer. J Steroid Biochem Mol Biol 86: 405-412.
46. Aman U, Buzdar AU, John FR, Robertson JFR, Eiermann W, Nabholtz J-M (2002) An overview of the pharmacology and pharmacokinetics of the newer generation aromatase inhibitors anastrozole, letrozole, and exemestane. Cancer 95: 2006-2016.
47. Dukes M, Edwards PN, Large M, Smith IK, Boyle T (1996) The preclinical pharmacology of "Arimidex" (anastrozole: ZD1033)-a potent, selective aromatase inhibitor. J Steroid Biochem Mol Biol 58: 4796-4805.
48. Leder BZ (2007) Testosterone, estradiol and aromatase inhibitor therapy in elderly men. J Steroid Biochem Mol Biol 106: 162-167.
49. Chamniansawat S, Chongthammakun SA (2012) Priming role of local estrogen on exogenous estrogen-mediated synaptic plasticity and neuroprotection. Exp Mol Med 44: 403-411.
50. Liu M, Hurn PD, Roselli CE, Alkayed NJ (2007) Role of P450 aromatase in sex-specific astrocytic cell death. J Cereb Blood Flow Metab 27: 135-141.
51. Hodosy J, Celec P, Ostatníková D, Cagánová M, Putz Z, et al. (2009) The effect of anastrozol on spatial memory in adult rats. Cent Eur J Biol 4: 186-189.
52. Moradpour F, Naghdi N, Fathollahi Y (2006) Anastrozole improved testosterone-induced impairment acquisition of spatial learning and memory in the hippocampal CA1 region in adult male rats. Behav Brain Res 175: 223-232.
53. Turner KJ, Morley M, Atanassova N, Swantson D, Sharpe RM (2000) Effect of chronic administration of an aromatase inhibitor to adult male rats on pituitary and testicular function and fertility. J Endocrinol 164: 225-238.
54. Hussain D, Hoehne A, Woodside B, Brake WG (2013) Reproductive experience modifies the effects of estradiol on learning and memory bias in female rats. Horm Behav 63: 418-423.
55. Korol DL (2004) Role of estrogen in balancing contributions from multiple memory systems. Neurobiol Learn Mem 82: 309-323.
56. Fuster JM (1999) Synopsis of function and dysfunction of the frontal lobe. Acta Psychiatr Scand Suppl 395: 51-57.
57. Baddeley A (2003) Working memory: looking back and looking forward. Nat Rev Neurosci 4: 829-839.
58. Freeman ME (2006) Neuroendocrine control of ovarian cycle of the rat. In: Neill JD Editor. Knobil and Neill's Physiology of Reproduction Vol 2, Chapter 43, (3rd edn.), Elsevier, pp 2327-2388.
59. Korol DL, Kolo LL (2002) Estrogen-induced changes in place and response learning in young adult female rats. Behav Neurosci 116: 411-420.
60. White NM, McDonald RJ (2002) Multiple parallel memory systems in the brain of the rat. Neurobiol Learn Mem 77: 125-184.
61. Khan MM, Dhandapani KM, Zhang QG, Brann DW (2013) Estrogen regulation of spine density and excitatory synapses in rat prefrontal and somatosensory cerebral cortex. Steroids 78: 614-623.
62. Velázquez-Zamora DA, García-Segura LM, González-Burgos I (2012) Effects of selective estrogen receptor modulators on allocentric working memory performance and on dendritic spines in medial prefrontal cortex pyramidal neurons of ovariectomized rats. Horm Behav 61: 512-517.

63. Fuster JM (1997) The prefrontal cortex: Anatomy, physiology, and neuropsychology of the frontal lobe. (3rd edn.), Lippincott-Raven.
64. Goldman-Rakic PS (1999) The "Psychic" neuron of the cerebral cortex. Ann N Y Acad Sci 868: 13-26.
65. Rich EL, Shapiro M (2009) Rat prefrontal cortical neurons selectively code strategy switches. J Neurosci 29: 7208-7219.
66. González-Flores O, Domínguez-Ordóñez R, González-Burgos I (2015) The celular and molecular mechanisms driving the estrogenic modulation of synaptic activity in mnemonic information processing: Synaptic fundamentals in memory performance. Nova Science Publishers.
67. Kato A, Hojo Y, Higo S, Komatsuzaki Y, Murakami G, et al. (2013) Female hippocampal estrogens have a significant correlation with cyclic fluctuation of hippocampal spines. Front Neu Cir 18: 149.
68. Kretz O, Fester L, Wehrenberg U, Zhou L, Brauckmann S, et al. (2004) Hippocampal synapses depend on hippocampal estrogen synthesis. J Neurosci 24: 5913-5921.
69. Harris KM, Kater SB (1994) Dendritic spines: cellular specializations imparting both stability and flexibility to synaptic function. Ann Rev Neurosci 17: 341-371.
70. Chen CC, Bajnath A, Brumberg JC (2015) The impact of development and sensory deprivation on dendritic protrusions in the mouse barrel cortex. Cereb Cortex 25: 1638-1653.
71. Harris KM (1999) Structure, development, and plasticity of dendritic spines. Curr Opin Neurobiol 9: 343-348.
72. Velázquez-Zamora DA, Martínez-Degollado M, González-Burgos I (2011) Morphological development of dendritic spines on rat cerebellar Purkinje cells. Int J Dev Neurosci 29: 515-520.
73. Yuste R (2010) Dendritic spines. (1st edn.), The MIT Press.
74. Caffino L, Giannotti G, Malpighi C, Racagni G, Fumagalli F (2015) Short-term withdrawal from developmental exposure to cocaine activates the glucocorticoid receptor and alters spine dynamics. Eur Neuropsychopharmacology 25: 1832-1841.
75. Kasai H, Matsuzaki M, Noguchi J, Yasumatsu N, Nakahara H (2003) Structure-stability-function relationships of dendritic spines. Trends Neurosci 26: 360-368.
76. Matsuzaki M, Honkura N, Ellis-Davies GCR, Kasai H (2004) Structural basis of long-term potentiation in single dendritic spines. Nature 429: 761-766.
77. Harris KM, Jensen FE, Tsao B (1992) Three-dimensional structure of dendritic spines and synapses in rat hippocampus (CA1) at postnatal day 15 and adult ages: implications for the maturation of synaptic physiology and long-term potentiation. J Neurosci 12: 2685-2705.

Men's Exposure to Women's Odors: The Effect of Women's Waist to Hip Ratio and Steroid Hormones

Ana Lilia Cerda-Molina[1*], **Leonor Hernández-López**[1], **Javier Iván Borráz-León**[1], **Claudio De la O-Rodríguez**[1] **and Roberto Chavira-Ramírez**[2]

[1]*Departament of Ethology, National Institute of Psychiatry, Mexico*

[2]*Departament Reproductive Biology, National Institute of Medical Sciences and Nutrition, Mexico*

[*]**Corresponding author:** Ana Lilia Cerda-Molina, Departament of Ethology, National Institute of Psychiatry, Mexico-Xochimilco 101, Col. San Lorenzo Huipulco, Tlalpan 14370. Mexico, E-mail: alcm@imp.edu.mx

Abstract

Previous research has shown that axillar and vaginal odors from ovulating women are recognized by men, but no research has been done exploring whether body odors signal other physical attributes of women such as waist-to-hip ratio (WHR) or endocrine status. Our goal was to investigate whether testosterone increased in men after smelling axillary odors of women with different WHR and with low or high levels of steroid hormones. We measured men's testosterone before and after 30 min of being exposed to fresh axillar odors collected from young women or a neutral odor as control situation. Men had to rate the attractiveness and intensity of the scent. We compared the response of men according to women's WHR and salivary testosterone, estradiol and progesterone. Although the main literature commonly reports that men judge a WHR around 0.7 to be more visually attractive, our results showed that men rated samples of high WHR (0.75-0.84) and high estradiol women as more attractive. In addition, men's testosterone increased after smelling the odors of high WHR, high estradiol and high testosterone women. High WHR women exhibited the highest testosterone and estradiol levels compared to the other WHR categories (0.66-0.74). We concluded that scents are cues that not only signal fertility but also physical attributes related to reproductive health.

Keywords: Axillar odors; Waist-to-hip ratio; Testosterone; Estradiol

Introduction

In humans, there are many attractive physical and non-physical traits that might influence mate selection, e.g., facial symmetry [1], body shape [2], body fat [3], or body scent [4-6]. Most research has claimed that humans, similar to other mammals, produce scents that influence not only sexual attraction, but emotions, moods, behaviors, and endocrine function in both sexes [7]. In humans, odor production is primarily concentrated in the apocrine glands of the axillae and is a process linked to the presence of microorganisms (e.g., bacteria). Axillary glands develop around puberty, suggesting a dependence on reproductive hormone fluctuations [8]. Glandular secretions are composed of different fatty acids and steroids, which, in conjunction with the metabolism of bacteria, promote strong odors. Some authors have reported specific androgen-related steroids (i.e., 16-androstenes) as the main component of human axillary odors of both sexes [9]. In women, some of these components have been implicated in the modulation of LH secretion and menstrual synchronization [10].

Different studies have indicated that men can perceive feminine axillary odors as a potential cue to ovulation [6,11-14]. Gildersleeve et al. [6] demonstrated that men accurately discriminated between scent samples from women with high or low fertility and they rated high fertility samples as more attractive than the low fertility ones. In addition, Miller and Maner [13] found that men exposed to T-shirts used by ovulating woman displayed higher levels of testosterone (T) 15 minutes after the exposure, than men exposed to the scent of a non-ovulating woman or to a control scent. However, there has been some recent debate about whether this can occur, because Roney and Simmons [15] did not support Miller and Maner's findings.

On the other hand, Rikowski and Grammer [4] proposed that humans use multiple signals to choose a partner in order to reduce the probability of error when assessing mate quality, suggesting the existence of some concordance of the information people perceive from others. For instance, Cornwell et al. [16] described that women prefer body odors collected from men with a high degree of body symmetry. Both, odors and symmetry are signals conveying individual reproductive information, indicating whether the individual is in good health condition [17], nevertheless the perception of those signals could be modulated by the environment and a learning process [1]. Another parameter signaling good reproductive health during human mate selection is the waist-to-hip ratio (WHR) of women, a measurement that compares the circumference of the waist to that of the hips [2]. According to Singh [18] in women of reproductive age, a gynoid body fat distribution is a reliable indicator of their sex hormone profile, greater success in pregnancy and less risk for major diseases [19-21]. As demonstrated by an extensive literature, men judge a WHR of around 0.7 to be the most appealing shape [1,18,22,23]. In addition, higher WHR (>0.80) has been considered an index of upper body obesity and abdominal fat accumulation; therefore, women in this condition are more susceptible to major diseases such as diabetes, cardiovascular disorders and ovarian cancers than women with a WHR between 0.7 and 0.79 [2,20,24]. Singh [2,23] has indicated that the distribution of body fat, as measured by waist and hip circumference, rather than the overall body fat mass, is correlated with the onset of pubertal endocrinological activity and is a more accurate predictor of many diseases and sex hormones disturbances. Based on this information, we hypothesized that body shape, measured by WHR could be related to the attractiveness of women odors. The existing literature about the reactions of men to feminine scents implies that masculine testosterone could be influenced by the changes of odors during the menstrual cycle [13,14], although Roney and Simmons [15] claimed the contrary. In addition, it is possible that women differ in the degree of odor secretion according to their endocrine state or body fat distribution.

The purpose of this research was to determine whether testosterone levels change in men after smelling freshly collected axillary scents of women but analyzing the influence of the donor's hormonal concentrations and WHR, as we previously analyzed the cycle phase [14]. According to the aforementioned evidence, we expected an increase in the concentration of testosterone in men when: 1) axillary odors came from women with a WHR around 0.7; 2) axillary odors came from women with the highest hormonal concentrations: estradiol (E) and progesterone (P) but not testosterone (T) because fat accumulation in the abdominal region is inhibited by estrogens, but stimulated by testosterone [18,23,24]. In addition, we expected that men rated as more attractive the odors of women with a WHR around 0.7 or with the highest hormonal concentration.

Methods

Participants

We recruited heterosexual undergraduate students. All the participants were paid $15 U.S.D for their collaboration. We discarded the following samples: two males who recognized to be homosexuals, one male whose saliva sample was contaminated with blood, one male whose sample was contaminated with nicotine, one of a depressed man and one of a man because who at the end of the experiment recognized having hormonal situations. In total, there were 115 men participants (age: mean ± SD=23.04 ± 5.5). We designed a standardized interview with women and considered them eligible if: 1) they did not take oral contraceptives or any medication 2) menstrual bleeding occurred every 28-30 days during the last six months 3) they had not received any hormone replacement therapy, 4) they were free of chronic or acute diseases, or any anovulatory symptoms.

Forty-five young women (age: mean ± SD=22 ± 2.8 years) were carefully informed about the purpose of the study and signed a consent form. Men were told they were to participate in an olfactory perception test, in order to avoid a predisposition to search for particular scents; but upon finishing the experiment all the participants were informed what they smelled and the purpose for it. After that, no one disagreed to have their hormones measured.

Collection of women body secretion, saliva samples and WHR

The procedure of the axillary secretion collection was described in Cerda-Molina et al. [14]. We asked women to wear a sterilized cotton pad under both armpits (taped with Micropore TM tape) before they went to bed and after washing the axillary zone with a neutral soap. We instructed volunteers to wear the cotton pad without using any kind of scent (deodorant or perfume) during a whole night and to refrain from engaging in sexual activities with another person the night they had to use the pad. The following morning, the women placed the pads in sterilized plastic containers and delivered them to the laboratory (around 8.00-11.00 h). In the lab women provided a saliva sample (6 ml), they were weighted and had their hips and waists circumferences measured. Immediately after being brought to the laboratory, the cotton pad samples were placed on a covered plastic container connected to an air pump (see below). Male volunteers, chosen at random, were instructed to participate in the test on the days when women brought samples; therefore, they smelled freshly collected material.

Women wore the cotton pads on two different days: one around mid-cycle (when steroid hormones are high) and the other around late luteal phase (when steroid hormones are low); as we did not use any vehicle to dissolve the body secretions, air was used as control situation. Based on previous research, we assumed that ovulation occurs on average 14 days prior to the onset of menstruation [25]. To minimize the variance of the cycle phase duration and of hormone concentrations, we asked all women to start the collection of samples at approximately the 12th-14th days (around ovulation) and 26th -28th days (late luteal phase) of their menstrual cycle, counting forward from the first day of menstruation. We weren't able to corroborate ovulation by means of serum hormone levels, but we obtained saliva samples every time a woman brought cotton pads to the lab. We calculated the waist-to-hip ratio (WHR) by dividing waist circumference/hip circumference in cm [24]. This body measurement was taken by a professional anthropologist, in order to avoid errors. Based on the mean and median value of the WHR of the 41 women (mean and median=0.74), we decided to create two categories of WHR: 0.66-0.74 (n=19) and 0.75-0.84 (n=22), this means that minimum-maximum WHR values were 0.66 and 0.84.

Experimental procedure

All the experiments were performed in two clean, ambient-temperature rooms. Each male participated only once because almost all preferred not to participate again. Every woman participated more than once in different consecutive cycles, and they donated a saliva sample every time they brought axillary samples. All the experiments were done around 9:00 and 14:00 h in order to avoid diurnal variations of hormones. On the day a woman attended the lab to gather the cotton pad, men were contacted and asked to present to the lab; they were also instructed not to have sexual relations for 24 h before presenting to the experiment. After explaining the purpose of the experiment, a male experimenter took the volunteers to the experimental room. The subjects answered a general information questionnaire: age, sexual orientation and use of any medication.

We used a double-blind experimental design where participants did not know what they smelled and male experimenters (who attended male volunteers) were unaware of the odor condition being tested. Volunteers were asked to provide one saliva sample (6 ml, pre-smell sample) at the time when they answered the questionnaire. They were then left alone to start the procedure, as all the steps were explained on the instruction sheets. We used a nebulizer air pump and a surgical face mask to deliver the odor. The body scent was placed on a covered plastic container connected to the air pump. Participants were instructed to use the mask and to turn on the pump according to the following pattern: on for 5 seconds and off for 10 seconds, 10 consecutive times. After sniffing the compounds, the subjects had to evaluate the odor according to intensity and attractiveness on a 0-6 point scale, with 1 corresponding to not at all and 6 corresponding to very strongly. Next, volunteers had to collect the second saliva sample 30 minutes after sniffing the body odors (they were provided with a chronometer). During this time, men watched a BBC video about ocean life, a commonly used technique due to its sexually neutral content [26].

Saliva hormone assays

Immediately after finishing the experimental procedure, saliva samples were frozen using acetone and dry ice, maintained at -70°C during two weeks and freed from mucopolysaccarides by three subsequent freeze-thaw cycles and centrifugation (3000 rpm x 30 min). We measured total testosterone (using chemiluminescence in the IMMULITE® 1000 Siemens counter). Chemiluminescence requires the addition of 500 microliters of standards, control and samples and 1 ml of tracer. The lower limit of sensitivity was 0.15 ng/dl. The interassay coefficient was 8.95% and the intraassay coefficient 8.02%. For estradiol and progesterone, we used solid-phase Coat-A-Count 125 I radioimmunoassays (DPC, Los Angeles, CA) in duplicate, after mixing, 3 hours incubation, and decanting. We diluted the hormone standards as follows: estradiol was diluted 1:30 and progesterone 1:10 by using 4% albumin buffer at a 7.2 pH. The lower limit of sensitivity for each hormone was 0.40 pg/ml for E and 0.093 ng/ml for P. Interassay and intraassay values for E were 7.84% and 7.01%, and 8.01% and 7.56% for P, respectively. The mean (±s.e.m.) of hormones during the ovulatory period were: estradiol, 35.08 ± 2.22 pg/ml; progesterone, 2.157 ± 0.11 ng/ml; testosterone, 1.04 ± 0.0170 ng/dl. The mean during the late luteal (±s.e.m.): estradiol, 3.903 ± 1.61; progesterone, 0.25 ± 0.006; testosterone, 0.68 ± 0.01.

Statistics

The analysis of testosterone concentration in men showed that the values were normally distributed (Kolmogorov-Smirnov Z=0.364, N=130, P=0.456), but scores of the odors were not (Intensity Z=1.426, N=78, P=0.034; Attractiveness Z=2.024, N=78, P=0.001), hence we standardized the data by transforming rates into z-scores.

Female hormone concentrations were assigned to the low or the high categories based on descriptive analysis; we considered as high all concentrations up to the median value, and as low all values below the median. We performed a Generalized Estimating Equations analysis (SPSS version 17) followed by Bonferroni post hoc contrast to compare the ratings of odor perception. The subject variables were men volunteers and women the within-subject variable (repeated variable); hormone levels (high or low) and WHR categories were used as predictors. The scores of attractiveness and intensity of the odor were the dependent variables.

The changes of testosterone in men before and after smelling a female odor were analyzed using factorial repeated-measures ANOVAs. The within-subject factor was T concentration in men before and after smelling the female odor (variable named Time). The between-subjects factors were the stimulation sessions: control air, high or low steroid hormone sample, and WHR categories. We compared pre-smell vs. post-smell concentrations of testosterone by means of a paired sample T test. We included the statistical observed power. We performed a one way ANOVA analyzes to search for differences in estradiol and testosterone that depended on the waist to hip ratio categories. Finally, in order to study the correlation between WHR and hormone levels, we performed Bivariate Partial correlations controlling for the effect of the cycle phase. All data are reported as means (± s.e.m.). Significance in all cases was set at $P \leq 0.05$.

Ethical note

The Bioethics Committee of the Institution approved this research. We followed the Declaration of Helsinki for human research. All participants signed a consent form and were assigned a code number in order to preserve confidentiality.

Results

Changes in men's T according to WHR

The interaction time x WHR showed significant differences (F1,109=3.60, P=0.018, observed power=0.769). Post hoc comparisons (pre-smell vs. post-smell T) indicated that neither air (control situation) nor the odors of women with WHR of 0.66-0.74 promoted changes in T concentration. On the contrary, T increased in those men who perceived odors from women with a WHR of 0.75-0.84 (P=0.034). These results are represented in Figure 1.

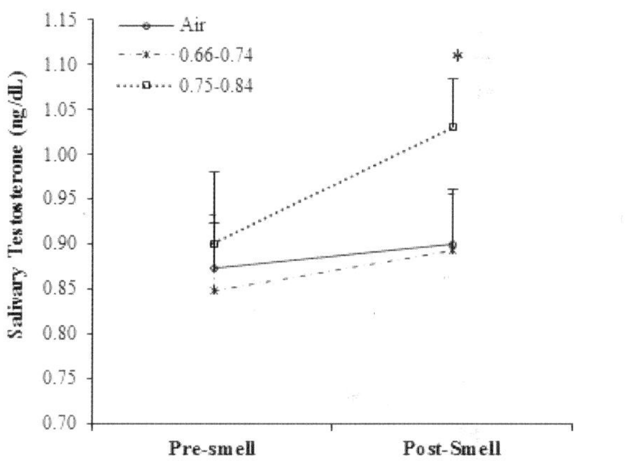

Figure 1: Mean ± s.e.m. of salivary testosterone levels in men before (pre-smell) and after 30 min (post-smell) of being exposed to axillary odors from young women with different WHR categories. *P=0.034 vs. pre-smell condition. T increased after smelling the odor of women with 0.75-0.84 WHR.

Changes in men's T according to women's hormone concentration

Statistical analysis revealed two significant interactions: time x testosterone (F2, 104=5.09, P=0.027, observed power=0.604) and time x estradiol (F2,104=3.70, P=0.03, observed power=0.655). The interaction time x progesterone was not significant (F2, 104=2.878, P=0.098, observed power=0.380). Figure 2 indicates that after exposure to high T women odors, T concentration increased in men (compared to the pre-smell concentration P=0.01). Samples of low T women and control air did not promote changes in men's T (P=0.876 and P=0.674, respectively). The same Figure 2 shows that after exposure to high E women odors, T concentration increased in men (compared to the pre-smell concentration P=0.008). Samples of low E women did not promote changes in men's T (P=0.2).

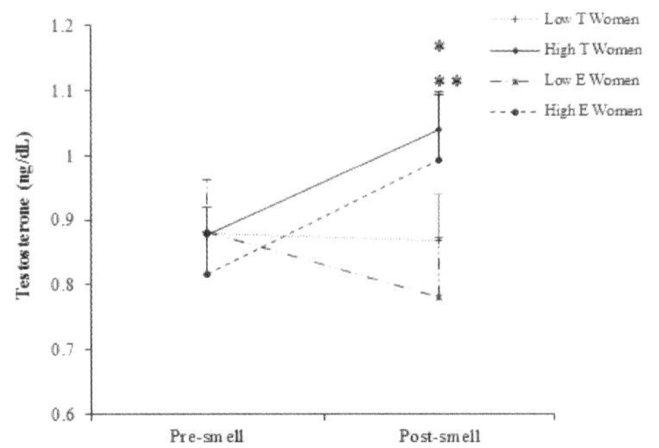

Figure 2: Mean ± s.e.m. of salivary testosterone levels in men before (pre-smell) and after 30 min (post-smell) of being exposed to axillary odors from women with high or low testosterone (T) and high or low Estradiol (E). High T women: * P=0.01 vs. pre-smell condition. High E women: **P=0.008 vs. pre-smell condition.

WHR and hormone concentrations

We found that estradiol and testosterone were significantly different according to WHR (Estradiol: F=7.27, d.f.=1, 80, P=009; Testosterone F=6.242, d.f.=1, 83, P=0.01). Post hoc contrast indicated that both steroid hormones were highest in women in the 0.75-0.84 WHR category compared to those in the 0.66-0.74 category. As Figure 3 shows, testosterone and estradiol were correlated, when controlling for the effect of the cycle phase (T: r= 0.607, n=83, P<0.001; E: r=0.342, N=80, P=0.002).

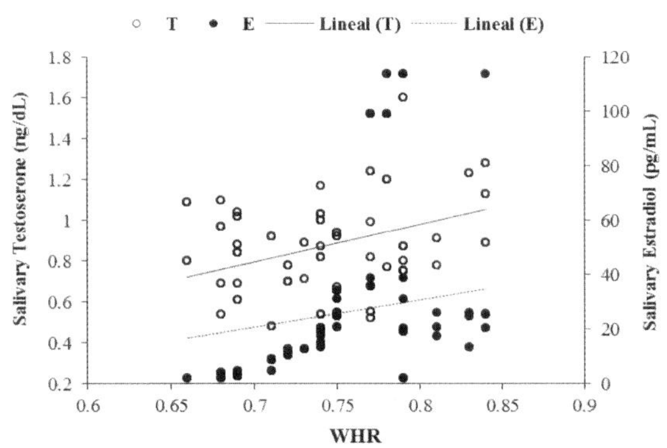

Figure 3: Salivary estradiol and testosterone of 41 women according to their WHR category

Ratings of odor perception

The reliability (Cronbach's alpha) of the odor perception ratings was 0.69. The intensity rating did not change according to WHR (Wald Chi-square=3.112, d.f.=1, P=0.211), but attractiveness did (Wald Chi-square=5.727, d.f.=1, P=0.05). Men rated as more attractive the odors from women in the WHR category of 0.75-0.84 compared to those in the 0.66-0.74 category (0.16 ± 0.05 vs. -0.32 ± 0.02). Men did not judge the odors as more intense according to hormonal levels (E: Wald Chi-square=0.14, d.f.=1, P=0.7; T: Wald Chi-square=0.25, d.f.=1, P=0.61; P: Wald Chi-square=0.8, d.f.=1, P=0.9). Men described as more attractive the odors of women with high levels of estradiol compared to low levels (0.49 ± 0.25 vs. -0.21 ± 0.2), but not those of women with high levels of testosterone or progesterone (E: Wald Chi-square=4.76, d.f.=1, P=0.029; T: Wald Chi-square=0.15, d.f.=1, P=0.69; P: Wald Chi-square=2.1, d.f.=1, P=0.14).

Discussion

We presented evidence that axillary odors from women with different WHR and hormone levels influence men's testosterone. We found a significant increase in men's T after smelling the odors of women with WHR of more than 0.75 and high testosterone and estradiol concentrations. Women odors with the highest concentration of estradiol and those within the WHR category of 0.75-0.84 were rated by men as the most attractive. These findings indicate that hormone concentrations and body shape are factors that play a role in the secretion of women odors. However, these results contradict our prediction that odors from women of around 0.7 WHR would promote changes in men's testosterone, because most literature suggests that men find a female of 0.7 the most visually attractive [2,23,27,28]. However, most of the reports about rating of WHR have been based on modified pictures, models or play boy models, but not on real women; in fact some authors have pointed out that WHR preferences may depend on ethnic, racial, geographical and ecological parameters [29,30]. For instance, Westman and Marlowe [29] studied a population of Hadza men in Tanzania and found that men chose women with higher WHRs (>0.8) as more attractive. The authors suggested that physical attractiveness elements could vary with life conditions, because women in that population do not have a real risk of obesity. Marlowe et al. [30] replicated the study of Hadza preferences but using both frontal and buttocks pictures, and they described the similar preferences (WHRs >0.8 as attractive). The same authors remarked the importance of geographical and ethnical variations in body shape when studying evaluations of attractiveness.

Similarly, Rozmus-Wrzesinska and Pawlowski [31] argue about the importance of WHR preferences in societies with better life conditions. The authors suggested that, in western societies, a low WHR can be valuable for a low fertility-rate population (e.g., one child), but those Latin American countries with a higher fertility rate (e.g., 6 children) and less quality of life should prefer a high WHR in order to secure reproductive success. We reported a mean WHR of 0.74 (range 0.66-0.84), a value similar to other studies of WHR in young Latin American students, 0.73 (range 0.65-0.86) [32,33] and Poland women, 0.73 (range 0.64-0.86); see Marlowe et al., [30] to appreciate a complete comparison of population data. Then, the fat deposits storage on hip and waist might be adaptive as energy reserves when the life in a harsh environment, in which nutritional constraints during pregnancy and lactation are considerable [34].

In this research, we selected those women who reported to have had regular cycles during the last six months (28-30 days) before the experiment, and discarded the women who reported irregular menstruations. It is important to note that selecting regularly cycling women forced us to reduce our sample size.

On the other hand, we found that WHR was correlated with estradiol and testosterone, regardless of the cycle phase. Although some authors have pointed out that fat accumulation in the abdominal region is inhibited by estrogens and stimulated by testosterone [18,24], some other authors have described a different relationship. Kirschner et al. [35] found that the production rates of testosterone, dihydrotestosterone and androstenedione in upper body obese women with WHR >0.85 was higher than in lower body obese women with WHR <0.75. In addition, the increased production of testosterone raised the aromatization of androgens to estrogens, because women with upper body obesity (WHR >0.85) had higher estradiol levels.

Our findings were similar to that described by Kirschner et al. [35] and indicated that women with WHR >0.75 had higher T and E salivary concentrations than women with WHR <0.75. The elevated hormone concentration could indirectly contribute to the synthesis of some kind of chemosignal in the apocrine glands of the armpits as we found that the rise of T in men depended on women's testosterone and estradiol levels. Some authors have suggested that specific reproductive processes could be mediated by the olfactory perception of androgens and estradiol metabolites (e.g., androstenol and estratetraenol [26,36-38]. Preti et al. [39] described cyclic variations of axillary 3α-androstenol in women and found the highest concentrations prior to ovulation. On the other hand, Shinohara et al. [36], showed that menstrual synchrony among women, is the result of the 3α-androstenol capacity to regulate LH secretion after its olfactory perception. If our findings are the result of the perception of an androgen or estrogen compound, then we might assume that female odors could stimulate LH secretion in men, and consequently T secretion. These chemical compounds could be related to the function of signal ovulation, as we collected cotton pads on two different times, one around ovulation and the other few days before menstruation in order to have high and low hormonal concentrations. We did not analyzed cycle phase in this study, as we previously reported this effect [14]; but we performed correlation of WHR with hormones, controlling for cycle phase's effects.

In general, our results indicate that men are able to perceive axillary odors of >0.75 WHR women with the highest levels of E and T, and in response to that odors, increase T concentration. We found support to the hypothesis that odors convey some information about women's physical attractiveness and endocrine condition; therefore we concluded that although humans rely mostly on vision, olfactory information plays an important role in the mate selection process.

Acknowledgments

This study was funded by a grant given to Drs Cerda- Molina AL, Hernández-López L, by "The Comisión de Estudios de Género" of the Cámara Nacional de Diputados de los Estados Unidos Mexicanos (The Mexican House of Representatives). We thank two anonymous reviewers for its corrections and suggestions to improve the manuscript. We also thank Vladimir Barberena for correcting the English.

References

1. Gangestad SW, Thornhill R, Yeo RA (1994) Facial attractiveness, developmental stability, and fluctuating asymmetry. Ethol Sociobiol 15: 73–85.
2. Singh D (1993) Body shape and women's attractiveness : The critical role of waist-to-hip ratio. Hum Nat 4: 297-321.
3. Faries MD, Bartholomew JB (2012) The role of body fat in female attractiveness. Evol Hum Behav 33: 672–681.
4. Rikowski A, Grammer K (1999) Human body odour, symmetry and attractiveness. Proc Biol Sci 266: 869-874.
5. Kuukasjärvi S, Eriksson CJP, Koskela E, Mappes T, Nissinen K, et al. (2004) Attractiveness of women's body odors over the menstrual cycle: the role of oral contraceptives and receiver sex. Behav Ecol 15: 579–584.
6. Gildersleeve KA, Haselton MG, Larson CM, Pillsworth EG (2012) Body odor attractiveness as a cue of impending ovulation in women: evidence from a study using hormone-confirmed ovulation. Horm Behav 61: 157-166.
7. Preti G, Wysocki CJ, Barnhart KT, Sondheimer SJ, Leyden JJ (2003) Male axillary extracts contain pheromones that affect pulsatile secretion of luteinizing hormone and mood in women recipients. Biol Reprod 68: 2107-2113.
8. Rothardt G, Beier K (2001) Peroxisomes in the apocrine sweat glands of the human axilla and their putative role in pheromone production. Cell Mol Life Sci 58: 1344-1349.
9. Berliner DL, Jennings-White C, Lavker RM (1991) The human skin: fragrances and pheromones. J Steroid Biochem Mol Biol 39: 671-679.
10. Shinohara K, Morofushi M, Funabashi T, Mitsushima D, Kimura F (2000) Effects of 5alpha-androst-16-en-3alpha-ol on the pulsatile secretion of luteinizing hormone in human females. Chem Senses 25: 465-467.
11. Singh D, Bronstad PM (2001) Female body odour is a potential cue to ovulation. Proc Biol Sci 268: 797-801.
12. Havlícek J, Dvoráková R, Bartoš L, Flegr§ J (2006) Non-advertized does not mean concealed: body odour changes across the human menstrual cycle. Ethology 112: 81–90.
13. Miller SL, Maner JK (2010) Scent of a woman: men's testosterone responses to olfactory ovulation cues. Psychol Sci 21: 276-283.
14. Cerda-Molina AL, Hernández-López L, De la O-Rodríguez C, Chavira-Ramírez R, Mondragón-Ceballos R (2013) Changes in men's salivary testosterone and cortisol levels, and in sexual desire after smelling female axillary and vulvar scents. Front Endocrinol 4: 1–9.
15. Roney JR, Simmons ZL (2012) Men smelling women: null effects of exposure to ovulatory sweat on men's testosterone. Evol Psychol 10: 703-713.
16. Cornwell RE, Boothroyd L, Burt DM, Feinberg DR, Jones BC, et al. (2004) Concordant preferences for opposite-sex signals? Human pheromones and facial characteristics. Proc Biol Sci 271: 635-640.
17. Gangestad SW, Thornhill R (1998) Menstrual cycle variation in women's preferences for the scent of symmetrical men. Proc Biol Sci 265: 927-933.
18. Singh D (2002) Female mate value at a glance: relationship of waist-to-hip ratio to health, fecundity and attractiveness. Neuro Endocrinol Lett 23 Suppl 4: 81-91.
19. Wass P, Waldenström U, Rössner S, Hellberg D (1997) An android body fat distribution in females impairs the pregnancy rate of in-vitro fertilization-embryo transfer. Hum Reprod 12: 2057-2060.
20. Deurenberg-Yap M, Yian TB, Kai CS, Deurenberg P, VAN Staveren WA (1999) Manifestation of cardiovascular risk factors at low levels of body mass index and waist-to-hip ratio in Singaporean Chinese. Asia Pac J Clin Nutr 8: 177-183.
21. Price GM, Uauy R, Breeze E, Bulpitt CJ, Fletcher AE (2006) Weight, shape, and mortality risk in older persons: elevated waist-hip ratio, not high body mass index, is associated with a greater risk of death. Am J Clin Nutr 84: 449-460.
22. Henss R (2000) Waist-to-hip ratio and female attractiveness. Evidence from photographic stimuli and methodological considerations. Pers Indiv Dif 28: 501–513.
23. Singh D (1993) Adaptive significance of female physical attractiveness: role of waist-to-hip ratio. J Pers Soc Psychol 65: 293-307.
24. Van Anders SM, Hampson E (2005) Waist-to-hip ratio is positively associated with bioavailable testosterone but negatively associated with sexual desire in healthy premenopausal women. Psychosom Med 67: 246–250.
25. Wilcox AJ, Dunson D, Baird DD (2000) The timing of the "fertile window" in the menstrual cycle: day specific estimates from a prospective study. BMJ 321: 1259-1262.
26. Bensafi M, Brown WM, Tsutsui T, Mainland JD, Johnson BN, et al. (2003) Sex-steroid derived compounds induce sex-specific effects on

autonomic nervous system function in humans. Behav Neurosci 117: 1125-1134.

27. Henss R (1995) Waist-to-hip ratio and attractiveness: replication and extension. Pers Indiv Dif 19: 479–488.
28. Streeter SA, McBurney DH (2003) Waist–hip ratio and attractiveness: New evidence and a critique of "a critical test". Evol Hum Behav 24: 88–98.
29. Wetsman A, Marlowe F (1999) How universal are preferences for female waist-to-hip ratios evidence from the Hadza of Tanzania? Evol Hum Behav 20: 219–228.
30. Marlowe F, Apicella C, Reed D (2005) Men's preferences for women's profile waist-to-hip ratio in two societies. Evol Hum Behav 26: 458–468.
31. Rozmus-Wrzesinska M, Pawlowski B (2005) Men's ratings of female attractiveness are influenced more by changes in female waist size compared with changes in hip size. Biol Psychol 68: 299-308.
32. Acuña V, Gómez J, Velázquez A, Chiappa P, Ortíz V (2005) Estudio de Selección de Pareja en Población de Distrito Federal. Conaculta-INAH, México. 159–174.
33. Ramos-Ibáñez N, Ortiz-Hernández L, Ferreyra-Corona L (2011) Exactitud de las mediciones de adiposidad para identificar síndrome metabólico y sus componentes. Medicina Interna de México 27: 244–252.
34. Dixson AF (1998) Primate Sexuality. Oxford, Oxford University Press.
35. Kirschner MA, Samojlik E, Drejka M, Szmal E, Schneider G, et al. (1990) Androgen-estrogen metabolism in women with upper body versus lower body obesity. J Clin Endocrinol Metab 70: 473-479.
36. Shinohara K, Morofushi M, Funabashi T, Kimura F (2001) Axillary pheromones modulate pulsatile LH secretion in humans. Neuroreport 12: 893-895.
37. Jennings-White C (1984) Human primary odors. Perfumer and Flavorist 9: 45–58.
38. Savic I, Berglund H, Gulyas B, Roland P (2001) Smelling of odorous sex hormone-like compounds causes sex-differentiated hypothalamic activations in humans. Neuron 31: 661-668.
39. Preti G, Cutler WB, Christensen CM, Lawley H, Huggins GR, et al. (1987) Human axillary extracts: Analysis of compounds from samples which influence menstrual timing. J Chem Ecol 13: 717-731.

Decrease in Aryl Hydrocarbon Receptor and 17β-Estradiol Receptor (A&B) Gene Expression in The Hypothalamus and The Pineal Gland, After Administration of Dimethylbenz (A) Anthracene, A Mammary Carcinogen, To Sprague-Dawley Female Rats.

Thomas Cadoudal[1,4], Véronique Lenoir[2,4], Graziella Penot[1,4], Indika SH Sathish[3], Yueqin Zhao[3], Xavier Coumoul[1,4], Claude Forest[1,4] and Bernard Kerdelhue[2,4*]

[1]*INSERM UMR-S 747, Université Paris Descartes, Pharmacologie Toxicologie et Signalisation Cellulaire, UFR Biomédicale, 45 Rue des Saints Pères, 75006 Paris, France*

[2]*Chemistry and Biology, Nucleo(s)tides and Immunology for Therapy (CBNIT), CNRS UMR 8601, Université Paris Descartes, PRES Sorbonne Paris Cité, UFR Biomédicale, 45 Rue des Saints-Pères, 75270 Paris Cedex 06, France*

[3]*Epidemiology and Biostatistics CORE, Eastern Virginia Medical School, Norfolk, USA*

[4]*Université Paris Descartes, Sorbonne Paris Cité, Paris, France*

***Corresponding author:** Bernard Kerdelhue, Université Paris Descartes, Neuroendocrinologie, Chemistry and Biology, Nucleo(s)tides and Immunology for Therapy (CBNIT), CNRS UMR 8601, Université Paris Descartes, PRES Sorbonne Paris Cité, UFR Biomédicale, 45 Rue des Saints-Pères, 75270 Paris Cedex 06, France,
E- mail: bernard.kerdelhue@parisdescartes.fr

Abstract

Purpose: The promotion of mammary adenocarcinoma induced by Dimethyl benz (a) Anthracene (DMBA) is preceded by disruptions of the Hypothalamo-Pituitary-Gonadal and Hypothalamo-Pituitary-Adrenal axes and by a reduction of the secretion of Melatonin. We hypothesized that these disruptions might be induced by changes, in neuroendocrine structures of the brain, in the gene expression of receptors for Aryl Hydrocarbon (AHR) and17β-Estradiol (ERS1 and ERS2).

Methods: Sprague Dawley female rats received one single administration of DMBA (75 mg/kg) at 52-55 days of age and were ovariectomized 5 days later. Then, one month later, RNAs from the Pineal Gland, the Hippocampus and the Hypothalamus were prepared and analyzed by real-time PCR for the presence of the transcripts encoding receptors for AHR and 17β-Estradiol (ERS1 and ERS2) together with those encoding Gonadotropin Releasing Hormone (GNRH1),Corticotropin Releasing Hormone (CRH) and Hydroxy-Indol-O-Methyl-Transferase (ASMT),the rate limiting enzyme for the synthesis of Melatonin.

Results: There was a long lasting and almost identical decrease in the expression of AHR, ERS1 and ERS2 in the Hypothalamus and the Pineal Gland. Also, there was an increase in the expression of ASMT and GNRH1 genes in the Pineal Gland, and of the GNRH1 gene in the Hypothalamus.However and, very interestingly, no effect was seen for the expression of any investigated gene in the Hippocampus, a structure of the brain implicated in cognition.

Conclusion: DMBA reduces the brain expression of AHR, ERS1 and ERS2, key transcriptional factors, but only in brain structures involved in the control of neuroendocrine systems.

Keywords: AHR; ERS1; ERS2; Gene expression; DMBA; Brain; Mammary Cancer; Female Rat

Introduction

Female Sprague-Dawley (SD) rats develop mammary adenocarcinoma in response to a single intragastric dose of 7, 12-dimethylbenz (a) Anthracene (DMBA), a polycyclic aromatic hydrocarbon (PHA) [1]. The mechanisms by which DMBA induces mammary tumours in rats have been well characterized. The carcinogen interacts with rapidly proliferating cells in the terminal end buds, forming DNA adducts, which in turn play a role in transforming normal terminal end bud cells into malignant cells [2-4]. The susceptibility of SD rats to DMBA peaks at 55-60 days of age and is eliminated by ovariectomy, suggesting that the inducible action of the carcinogen depends on ovarian hormones [5].

Furthermore, the development of DMBA-induced adenocarcinoma is preceded by a series of disturbances of the Hypothalamo-Pituitary-Gonadal (HPG) axis and the Hypothalamo-Pituitary-Adrenal axis (HPA) axes during the latency period. Along the HPG axis, a blunting of pre-ovulatory surges of plasma Luteinizing Hormone (LH) and Follicle-Stimulating Hormone (FSH) [6] together with an increase in the pre-ovulatory surge of plasma 17β-Estradiol (E_2) [7] were observed in response to DMBA. Also, female rats treated with DMBA displayed a reduction in GNRH1 release associated with a blunted LH release [8]. In addition, disturbances of the expression of the hypothalamic Gonadotropin-Releasing Hormone (GNRH1) and its pituitary receptor genes occur throughout the oestrus cycle [9]. In the HPA axis, a long-term deregulation of circadian and E2-induced corticosterone secretion was observed in DMBA-treated rats [10]. Also, DMBA induces a reduction of the secretion of melatonin from the Pineal Gland [11].

DMBA is a ligand for the Aryl Hydrocarbon Receptor (AHR) which is expressed in the central nervous system, including the Hypothalamus and the Hippocampus [12]. Upon DMBA binding, like in the presence of 2,3,7,8-Tetrachlorodibenzo-p-dioxin (TCDD), AHR translocates to the nucleus where it heterodimerizes with the AHR nuclear translocator (ARNT) and binds to AHR DNA recognition sites, also named xenobiotic response elements (XRE) [13]. Most AHR ligands display anti-estrogenic properties. This could be explained at the molecular levels by several mechanisms including estrogen catabolism, ubiquitination and degradation of both estrogen receptors, negative interaction between responsive elements or co-activator squelching [14]. However, recent studies showed that pro-estrogenic properties could also be observed according to the status of the estrogen receptor (bound versus unbound to its ligand) [15]. Interestingly, a co-localisation of AHR and ERβ was documented in the Anterior Pituitary [16] and the brain [17,18].

Given the long-term dysregulation of the activity of HPG and HPA axes, two major neuroendocrine axes strongly positively and/ or negatively connected [19] and of the well documented effects of estrogens on the HPG and HPA axes, we hypothesized that DMBA can induce changes in specific area of the brain of the expression of genes encoding AHR, ERS1and ERS2 and induce the unbalanced functioning of the HPG and HPA axes and in the reduced melatonin secretion.

After DMBA administration, the expression of genes encoding AHR, ERS1 and ERS2 was registered in the Hypothalamus which is involved in the control of neuroendocrine functions, and in the Pineal Gland, which is involved in the control of Melatonin secretion.

The expression of genes encoding GNRH1, Corticotropin Releasing Hormone (CRH) and Hydroxy-Indo-O-Methyl-Transferase (ASMT), the rate limiting enzyme for the synthesis of Melatonin, were also recorded in the same extracts of Hypothalamus and Pineal Gland.

Last, the expression of all investigated genes was also recorded in the same extracts in the hippocampus, a structure of the brain which is not involved in the control of neuroendocrine functions, but in cognitive functions.

Materials and Methods

Animals

Ethics statement: The present study has been conducted according to the European rules and the CNRS instruction on Animal Welfare. The animal studies described in this manuscript were conducted in accordance with accepted standards of animal care. The study was approved by the ethical committee of Paris Descartes University. All surgery was performed under chloral anesthesia, and all efforts were made to minimize suffering.

SD female rats (Charles River) were purchased at 49 to 51 days of age. They were housed (5 animals per cage), under controlled temperature (21+1°C). The animal housing room diurnal cycle was 12 hours light/12 hours' darkness (light on: from 7 a.m. to 7 p.m.) The animals receive UAR food and water at libidum.

After 6-8 days of acclimatation, the rats received, at 55-57 days of age, either 75 mg/kg of DMBA dissolved in 1 ml of sesame oil or 1 ml vehicle alone, on the day of estrous of the estrous cycle. Rats were treated at 55-57 days of life, since the induction of the mammary cancer is maximal at this time of life [1]. Then, DMBA-treated and control-treated rats were ovariectomized 5 days after administration of the treatments, to avoid a possible effect of variations of gonadal hormones on DMBA action. The ovariectomy was not performed before the administration of DMBA since the induction of the mammary tumors requires the presence of the ovary; when the ovary was present, the first palpable mammary tumors appear by 60 days after the induction of the carcinogenic process [6]. Rats were then sacrificed by decapitation one month later, at a time when there was still no palpable mammary tumor.

Then the Pineal Gland, the Hippocampus and the Hypothalamus (Hypothalami were removed using the anterior border of the optic chiasma, the posterior border of mammillary bodies and lateral hypothalamic sulci to a depth of 2.5 mm as dissection limits), were removed and immediately frozen in liquid nitrogen and stored at -80°C until extraction.

Two series of experiments were performed, with 7 and 15 animals per DMBA-treated or Control-treated group, in the first and the second experiment, respectively.

RNA extraction and RT-PCR

Total RNA from the Pineal Gland, the Hippocampus and the Hypothalamus were obtained with the RNeasy mini kit for lipid tissues (Qiagen) according to the manufacturer's instructions. Sample quality was controlled with the 260/280 nm absorption ratio determination (Nano drop ND-1000, Thermo Scientific). For real-time PCR analysis, 1.25 μg of total RNA was reverse transcribed with the multiscribe™ reverse transcriptase of the high capacity cDNA archive kit (Applied Biosystems). cDNA were amplified on a thermal cycler (ABI-Prism 7900HT from Applied Biosystems) using specific oligonucleotides and the Sybr Green fluorescence method(SYBR Select Master MIX from Life Technologies). Specific sequences of forward and reverse primers were respectively as follows:

AHR: 5'-TTCCCTTATGAGTGCCTTG-3' and 5'-CCTGAGTGTGTCTGATTTCC-3';

ERS1: 5'-TGCTCCTAACTTGCTCTTG-3' and 5'-GATGTGGTCCTTCTCTTCC-3';

ERS2:5'-TGAGCACCTTGAGTCCAGAG-3' and 5'-CAGTCCCACCATTAGCACC-3';

CRH: 5'-CTGTCCCCCAACTCCAC-3' and 5'-GCTAACTGCTCTGCCCTG-3';

GNRH1: 5'-CTGGTCCTATGGGTTGC-3' and 5'-AGTTCTGGGGTTCTGCC-3';

ASMT: 5'-CTCCTGCTGTCACTCAAC-3' and 5'-CAAAACTTCCTGTCCCC-3';

For each couple of primers, PCR efficiency and specificity were tested with serial dilutions of samples and melting curve analysis, respectively. Data were normalized with the ribosomal 18S RNA level as a reference and quantification was carried out by comparison of the number of cycles required to reach reference and target threshold values (δ-δ Ct method).

Statistical analysis

The main purpose of this study was to compare the gene expression between control group and DMBA group within the Pineal Gland, the Hippocampus and the Hypothalamus. Results of two independent experiments were pooled before statistical analysis. Mean and standard deviation were presented with 95% confidence interval. The Mann-Whitney test was performed to compare gene expression between control and DMBA group. All analyses were performed in SAS 9.1 (Cary, NC). The significance level was at least 0.05.

Results

Results are shown in figures 1 to 3.

In the PINEAL GLAND (Figure 1), mRNA levels of the AHR, ERS1, ERS2, GNRH1 and ASMT were significantly different between DMBA and control groups. Transcript abundance in the DMBA group was lower than in controls for AHR, ERS1 and ERS1. However, transcripts from DMBA-treated animals were more abundant than in the control group for GNRH1 and ASMT. All other mRNA levels were not found significantly different between DMBA and control groups.

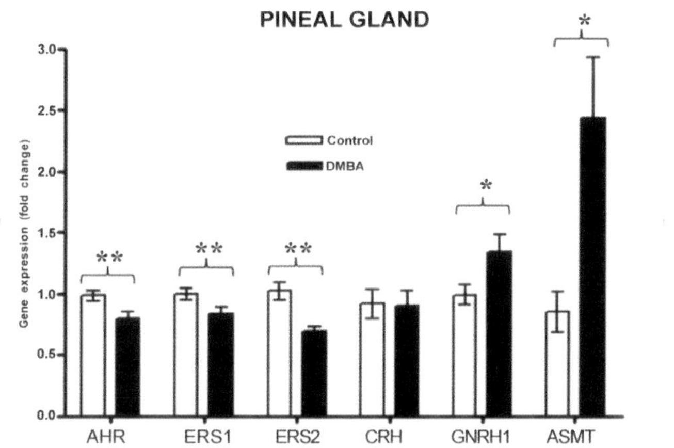

Figure 1: Relative gene expression levels within the Pineal Gland.

Expression levels were normalized to those of 18S. Empty bars indicate the normalized levels of gene expression for the control group. Asterisks represent statistically-significant differences between the DMBA group and the corresponding control group.

Mean ± SE of 18-20 determinations

*$p<0.05$; **$p<0.01$

In the HIPPOCAMPUS (Figure 2), the expression of all investigated genes was similar in DMBA and control groups.

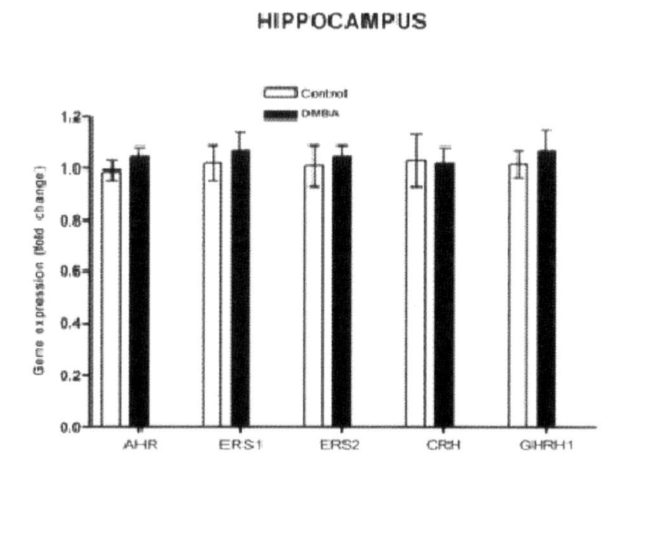

Figure 2: Relative gene expression levels within the Hippocampus.

Mean ± SE of 18-20 determinations

In the HYPOTHALAMUS (Figure 3), the expression of the genes encoding AHR, ERS1, ERS2, CRH, CRH and GNRH1 were significantly different between DMBA and control groups. In the DMBA-treated animals, the abundance of AHR, ERS1, ERS2 and CRH transcripts was significantly lower than in the control group. However, GNRH1 mRNA levels were significantly higher in the DMBA group than in controls.

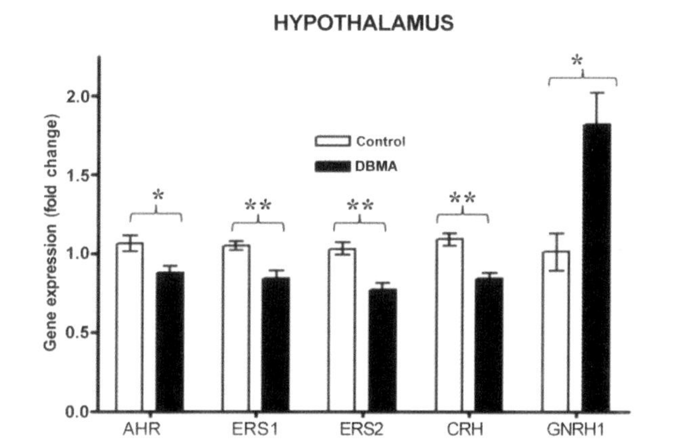

Figure 3: Relative gene expression levels within the Hypothalamus

Expression levels were normalized to those of 18S. Empty bars indicate the normalized levels of gene expression for the control group. Asterisks represent statistically-significant differences between the DMBA group and the corresponding control group.

Mean ± SE of 18-20 determinations

*$P< 0.05$; **$p<0.01$

Discussion

The present results clearly provide strong evidence that changes in brain gene expression were observed only in the Pineal Gland and the Hypothalamus one month after exposure to DMBA. An almost identical parallel decrease was recorded for the expression of AHR, ERS1 and ERS2 genes. The long-term decrease in the expression of the AHR gene and in the expression of both ERS1 and ERS2 genes is probably due to the interaction of DMBA with these three receptors. Indeed, DMBA is an AHR ligand that rapidly leads to nuclear translocation of the receptor and to transcriptional activation of target genes after its heterodimerization with ARNT. However, this process also causes the degradation of the AHR, which is sometimes described as a negative feedback. This mechanism might not be sufficient to explain the observed down-regulation because DMBA is not a persistent organic pollutant and this negative feedback might be then difficult to maintain after one month which is the period between DMBA treatment and the sacrifice of animals.

Most AHR ligands were also historically described as anti-estrogens [14]. For example, female Sprague-Dawley rats treated with TCDD, an AHR high affinity ligand, display delayed incidence of mammary tumors [20]. Only few studies were carried out on the nervous system of mammals with DMBA [21] but alternative ligands, including TCDD, were sometimes used. Experimental studies showed that TCDD-exposed animals display multiple symptoms including defects of motor coordination or spatial memory [22-24]. The associated mechanisms have not been discovered yet but the anti-estrogenic properties of AHR ligands might be important to consider; estrogens and ERs indeed regulate several developmental or homeostatic process related to the nervous system [25]. The interactions between the AHR and ERs have been characterized at the molecular level and might be considered to understand the effects of DMBA on ERs in our study. First, AHR ligands increase the expression of several cytochromes P450 including CYP1A1 and CYP1B1 which catabolize 17β-Estradiol and decrease its concentration [12,26,27]. Second, both AHR and ERs share common co-activators (CBP/p300); competition might occur if both signaling pathways are simultaneously activated [28]. Third, the dioxin receptor responsive element (XRE) was early on described in the promoter of 17β-Estradiol responsive genes [28]. The proximity of the XRE with the 17β-Estradiol response element very likely supports interactive action between AHR, ERS1 and ERS2 [16].

Finally, recent studies highlighted a new property of AHR, showing that the receptor also forms a nuclear complex with ERS1 and CUL4B (an E3 ubiquitin ligase) triggering the ubiquitination of ERS1 and subsequently its degradation [29]. Interestingly, this is only observed if ERS1 is bound to 17β- Estradiol; conversely, if ERS1 is unbound, AHR acts as a co-activator on estrogen-responsive promoters suggesting that the interaction between both receptors is more complex than previously described; this AHR might be alternatively described as a modulator of estrogenic pathways [15]. A co-localization of the AHR with ERS2 was already demonstrated at the brain level, thus suggesting that an interaction might occur between these receptors [30,31]. The decreased expression of ERS1 and ERS2 in our study might be due to an activated AHR pathway that stimulates the ubiquitination process. Alternatively, genetic or epigenetic mechanisms could also take place to explain the long-term effect of DMBA and needs to be explored because it could represent a novel type of crosstalks between AHR and ERs.

DMBA was previously shown to mimic most of the biological effects of 17β-Estradiol [32] and its effects on ERs were documented [33].

The DMBA effects on GNRH1, ASMT and CRH transcripts most likely result from the direct or indirect action of DMBA throughout changes in AHR and ERs gene expression.

At the hypothalamic level, the reverse relationship between the expression of GNRH1 and CRH genes is in agreement with the well-documented reverse relationship between the activity of HPG and HPA axes [19]. Interestingly, the expression of the ASMT gene, encoding the rate-limiting enzyme for the synthesis of melatonin, was markedly up-regulated by DMBA. However, DMBA reduces the secretion of melatonin from the Pineal Gland [11].

All together the most important findings of the present study are that DMBA induces identical long term decreases in the expression of AHR, ERS1 and ERS2 genes, in the Pineal Gland and the Hypothalamus,two neuroendocrine structures, whereas no effect is detected at the Hippocampus level, a non-neuroendocrine structure.

Whether or not the decreases seen for the expression of AHR, ERS1 and ERS2 genes in the Pineal Gland and the Hypothalamus play a role in the promotion of the carcinogenic process remains to be demonstrated.Follow up studies will involve protein expression of the investigated genes.

Acknowledgment

We thank Krystel El Hage for her help during the preparation of the manuscript.

References

1. Huggins C, Grand LC, Brillantes FP (1961) Mammary cancer induced by a single feeding of polymucular hydrocarbons, and its suppression. Nature 189: 204-207.
2. Daniel FB, Joyce NJ (1983) DNA adduct formation by 7,12-dimethylbenz[a]anthracene and its noncarcinogenic 2-fluoro analogue in female Sprague-Dawley rats. J Natl Cancer Inst 70: 111-118.
3. Russo J, Tait L, Russo IH (1983) Susceptibility of the mammary gland to carcinogenesis. III. The cell of origin of rat mammary carcinoma. Am J Pathol 113: 50-66.
4. Russo J, Tay LK, Russo IH (1982) Differentiation of the mammary gland and susceptibility to carcinogenesis. Breast Cancer Res Treat 2: 5-73.
5. Dao TL (1962) The role of ovarian hormones in initiating the induction of mammary cancer in rats by polynuclear hydrocarbons. Cancer Res 22: 973-981.
6. Kerdelhue B, El Abed A (1979) Inhibition of preovulatory gonadotropin secretion and stimulation of prolactin secretion by 7,12-dimethylbenz(a)anthracene in Sprague-Dawley rats. Cancer Res 39: 4700-4705.
7. el Abed A, Kerdelhue B, Castanier M, Scholler R (1987) Stimulation of estradiol-17 beta secretion by 7,12-dimethylbenz (a) anthracene during mammary tumor induction in Sprague-Dawley rats. J Steroid Biochem 26: 733-738.
8. Kerdelhue B, Peck EJ Jr (1981) In vitro LHRH release: correlation with the LH surge and alteration by a mammary carcinogen. Peptides 2: 219-222.
9. Jakubowski M, Lenoir V, Jimenez-Linan M, Duval P, Israel L, et al. (2002) Long-term effects of the mammary carcinogen 7,12-dimethylbenz(a) anthracene on hypothalamic gonadotropin-releasing hormone and its pituitary receptor gene expression, during the

promotion stage, in female Sprague-Dawley rats. Breast Cancer Res Treat 73: 23-29.

10. Yon de Jonage-Canonico MB, Lenoir V, Scholler R, Kerdelhué B (2005) Long-term dysregulation of circadian and 17-beta estradiol-induced LH, prolactin and corticosterone secretion after dimethylbenz (a) anthracene administration in the Sprague-Dawley female rat. Breast Cancer Res Treat 92: 47-50.

11. De Jonage-Canonico MB, Lenoir V, Martin A, Scholler R, Kerdelhué B (2003) Long term inhibition by estradiol or progesterone of melatonin secretion after administration of a mammary carcinogen, the dimethyl benz(a)anthracene, in Sprague-Dawley female rat; inhibitory effect of Melatonin on mammary carcinogenesis. Breast Cancer Res Treat 79: 365-377.

12. Huang P, Rannug A, Ahlbom E, Håkansson H, Ceccatelli S (2000) Effect of 2,3,7,8-tetrachlorodibenzo-p-dioxin on the expression of cytochrome P450 1A1, the aryl hydrocarbon receptor, and the aryl hydrocarbon receptor nuclear translocator in rat brain and pituitary. Toxicol Appl Pharmacol 169: 159-167.

13. Barouki R, Aggerbeck M, Aggerbeck L, Coumoul X (2012) The aryl hydrocarbon receptor system. Drug Metabol Drug Interact 27: 3-8.

14. Coumoul X (2007) [Dioxin and estradiol, a "complex" story]. Med Sci (Paris) 23: 701-702.

15. Ohtake F, Takeyama K, Matsumoto T, Kitagawa H, Yamamoto Y, et al. (2003) Modulation of oestrogen receptor signalling by association with the activated dioxin receptor. Nature 423: 545-550.

16. Ruegg J, Swedenborg E, Wahlstrom D, Escande A, Balaguer P, et al. (2008) The transcription factor aryl hydrocarbon receptor nuclear translocator functions as an estrogen receptor beta-selective coactivator, and its recruitment to alternative pathways mediates antiestrogenic effects of dioxin. MolEndocrinol 22: 304-316.

17. Frye CA, Bo E, Calamandrei G, Calzà L, Dessì-Fulgheri F, et al. (2012) Endocrine disrupters: a review of some sources, effects, and mechanisms of actions on behaviour and neuroendocrine systems. J Neuroendocrinol 24: 144-159.

18. Kajta M, WÃ³jtowicz AK, MaÄ‡kowiak M, LasoÅ„ W (2009) Aryl hydrocarbon receptor-mediated apoptosis of neuronal cells: a possible interaction with estrogen receptor signaling. Neuroscience 158: 811-822.

19. Kerdelhue B, Jones GS, Gordon K, Seltman H, Lenoir V, et al. (1995) Activation of the hypothalamo-anterior pituitary corticotropin-releasing hormone, adrenocorticotropin hormone and beta-endorphin systems during the estradiol 17 beta-induced plasma LH surge in the ovariectomized monkey. J Neurosci Res 42: 228-235.

20. Holcomb M, Safe S (1994) Inhibition of 7,12-dimethylbenzanthracene-induced rat mammary tumor growth by 2,3,7,8-tetrachlorodibenzo-p-dioxin. Cancer Lett 82: 43-47.

21. Granberg L, Ostergren A, Brandt I, Brittebo EB (2003) CYP1A1 and CYP1B1 in blood-brain interfaces: CYP1A1-dependent bioactivation of 7,12-dimethylbenz(a)anthracene in endothelial cells. Drug MetabDispos 31: 259-265.

22. Nishijo M, Kuriwaki J, Hori E, Tawara K, Nakagawa H, et al. (2007) Effects of maternal exposure to 2,3,7,8-tetrachlorodibenzo-p-dioxin on fetal brain growth and motor and behavioral development in offspring rats. ToxicolLett 173: 41-47.

23. Seo BW, Sparks AJ, Medora K, Amin S, Schantz SL (1999) Learning and memory in rats gestationally and lactationally exposed to 2,3,7,8-tetrachlorodibenzo-p-dioxin (TCDD). NeurotoxicolTeratol 21: 231-239.

24. Thiel R, Koch E, Ulbrich B, Chahoud I (1994) Peri- and postnatal exposure to 2,3,7,8-tetrachlorodibenzo-p-dioxin: effects on physiological development, reflexes, locomotor activity and learning behaviour in Wistar rats. Arch Toxicol 69: 79-86.

25. Carpenter KD, Korach KS (2006) Potential biological functions emerging from the different estrogen receptors. Ann N Y Acad Sci 1092: 361-373.

26. Coumoul X, Diry M, Robillot C, Barouki R (2001) Differential regulation of cytochrome P450 1A1 and 1B1 by a combination of dioxin and pesticides in the breast tumor cell line MCF-7. Cancer Res 61: 3942-3948.

27. Tsuchiya Y, Nakajima M, Yokoi T (2005) Cytochrome P450-mediated metabolism of estrogens and its regulation in human. Cancer Lett 227: 115-124.

28. Safe S, Wormke M, Samudio I (2000) Mechanisms of inhibitory aryl hydrocarbon receptor-estrogen receptor crosstalk in human breast cancer cells. J Mammary Gland Biol Neoplasia 5: 295-306.

29. Ohtake F, Baba A, Takada I, Okada M, Iwasaki K, et al. (2007) Dioxin receptor is a ligand-dependent E3 ubiquitin ligase. Nature 446: 562-566.

30. Baba T, Mimura J, Nakamura N, Harada N, Yamamoto M, et al. (2005) Intrinsic function of the aryl hydrocarbon (dioxin) receptor as a key factor in female reproduction. Mol Cell Biol 25: 10040-10051.

31. Cao J, Patisaul HB, Petersen SL (2011) Aryl hydrocarbon receptor activation in lactotropes and gonadotropes interferes with estradiol-dependent and -independent preprolactin, glycoprotein alpha and luteinizing hormone beta gene expression. Mol Cell Endocrinol 333: 151-159.

32. Pasqualini C, Sarrieau A, Dussaillant M, Corbani M, Bojda-Diolez F, et al. (1990) Estrogen-like effects of 7,12-dimethylbenz(a)anthracene on the female rat hypothalamo-pituitary axis. J Steroid Biochem 36: 485-491.

33. Garcia-Segura LM, Diolez-Bojda F, Lenoir V, Naftolin F, Kerdelhué B (1992) Estrogen-like effects of the mammary carcinogen 7,12-dimethylbenz(alpha)anthracene on hypothalamic neuronal membranes. Brain Res Bull 28: 625-628.

Cellular Metabolism of Estradiol in Models for Select Molecular Subtypes of Clinical Breast Cancer

Nitin Telang*

Palindrome Liaisons Consultants, Cancer Prevention Research Program, Montvale, New Jersey, USA

***Corresponding author:** Nitin Telang, Ph.D., Cancer Prevention Research Program, Palindrome Liaisons Consultants, 10 Rolling Ridge Road, Suite B, Montvale, NJ 07645-1559, USA, E-mail: entitytoo@gmail.com

Abstract

The mitogenic ovarian steroid hormone 17β-estradiol (E_2) is associated with progression of Estrogen Receptor Positive (ER^+) breast cancer, and ER represents a major therapeutic target for endocrine therapy. In addition to the ER dependent signal transduction, cellular oxidative metabolism of the ER ligand E_2 generates several metabolites with pleotropic growth modulatory effects on breast cancer cells, providing valuable leads for novel therapeutic approach. The molecular classification of clinical breast cancer has defined cancer subtypes based on differential expression of the genes for hormones and growth factor receptors, thereby facilitating subtype targeted therapeutic interventions. However, de novo or acquired resistance to conventional endocrine and targeted small molecule based treatment limits the therapeutic efficacy and promotes therapy resistant disease progression. These aspects emphasize the need for identification of new efficacious non-toxic lead compounds. The present review summarizes critical experiments conducted to i) develop and optimize human tissue derived cell culture models for select molecular subtypes of clinical breast cancer, ii) determine the status of homeostatic growth control, cellular metabolism of 17β-estradiol (E_2) and cancer risk in the developed models, and iii) evaluate the therapeutic efficacy and identify possible mechanisms of action of select herbal extracts/phyto-chemical. Additionally, this review discusses the evidence for the role of E_2 metabolism in breast carcinogenesis and therapy. The data generated from the cell culture experiments demonstrate that the models for select molecular sub-types exhibit aberrant hyper-proliferation, altered cellular metabolism of E_2 and enhanced cancer risk. Select mechanistically distinct herbal extracts and natural phyto-chemical at their respective maximum cytostatic concentrations modulate cellular metabolism of E_2 favoring generation of anti-proliferative metabolites and inhibit anchorage independent growth, thus reducing cancer risk. Collectively, these data validate the present mechanism based cell culture approach to identify and prioritize novel efficacious lead compounds for subtype targeted therapy of clinical breast cancer.

Keywords: Breast cancer models; Estradiol metabolism; Therapeutic target

Introduction

The ovarian steroid hormone 17β-estradiol (E_2) represents a major hormone involved in promotion of breast cancer. E_2 functions as a physiological ligand for Estrogen Receptor (ER), a well-established nuclear transcription factor that via a complex signaling cascade drives the expression of several E_2 responsive genes, promoting proliferation of normal and tumor derived breast epithelial cells. In addition to the ER dependent biological functions of E_2, cellular Cyp450 mediated oxidative metabolism of E_2 is involved in various biological functions including normal mammary cell proliferation and modulation of breast cancer growth [1,2].

Global gene expression profiling based on differential expression of hormone and growth factor receptor genes has classified the molecular subtypes of clinical breast cancer, and thereby, has provided important molecular insights in breast cancer pathogenesis and identified mechanism based, subtype targeted therapeutic interventions [3].

Conventional targeted therapy for hormone responsive breast cancer includes selective estrogen receptor modulators and aromatase inhibitors for the Luminal A subtype, and small molecule inhibitors of growth factor function together with the anti-estrogens for the Luminal B subtype. HER-2 targeted therapy represents the treatment of choice for the endocrine resistant HER-2 enriched subtype, while the triple negative subtype responds to anthracyline/taxol based chemotherapy and to PARP inhibitors [4-8]. However, long-term treatment with conventional chemo-endocrine therapeutics as well as with newer targeted therapeutics is frequently associated with de novo or acquired resistance that limits the efficacy of therapeutic intervention, in part due to progression of drug resistant cancer stem cells [4,7,9]. These aspects emphasize a need to identify and evaluate promising novel lead compounds for their efficacy on select molecular subtypes of clinical breast cancer.

The present review summarizes the experimental data on the development and characterization of reliable cell culture models for select molecular subtypes of clinical breast cancer, on validation of cellular metabolism of E_2 as an endocrine biomarker, and on evidence for efficacy of mechanistically distinct herbal extracts and a naturally occurring phyto-chemical on the developed models.

Experimental Models, Biomarkers and Test Agents

Models

The human mammary carcinoma derived MCF-7 cells express the receptors for Estrogen (ER) and Progesterone (PR) but lack the expression of Human Epidermal Growth Factor-2 (HER-2). The MCF-7 cells represented the model for the Luminal A molecular subtype of clinical breast cancer [10]. The human mammary epithelial cell line 184-B5/HER is stably transfected with HER-2 oncogene and unlike the parental 184-B5 cells, exhibits tumorigenic transformation [11]. This cell line represented a model for the HER-2 enriched molecular subtype of clinical breast cancer. The human mammary carcinoma derived MDA-MB-231 cell line lacks the expression of ER, PR and HER-2 [10,12]. This cell line represented the model for the triple negative molecular subtype of clinical breast cancer.

Biomarkers

Population doubling time and saturation density represented the quantitative endpoint biomarkers for the status of homeostatic growth control. Estrogen metabolite ratios represented the biomarkers for endocrine responsiveness. Anchorage independent (AI) growth in vitro and tumor development in vivo represented the quantitative endpoint biomarkers for the risk for cancer development.

The cellular metabolism of E_2 was evaluated by determining the formation of select metabolites including Estrone (E_1), 2-hydroxyestrone (2-OHE$_1$), 16α-hydroxyestrone (16α-OHE$_1$) and estriol (E_3), using stable isotope dilution and GC-MS analysis or tritium exchange assay [13]. Since E_1 functions as the common precursor for 2-OHE$_1$ and 16α-OHE$_1$, and since 16α-OHE$_1$ is converted to E_3 [2,13], the data on the cellular metabolism of E_2 is expressed as 2-OHE$_1$: 16α-OHE$_1$ and E_3: 16α-OHE$_1$ ratios.

Test Agents

Non-fractionated herbal extracts were prepared from the bark of Lycium barbarum (LBB) and the fruit of Lycium barbarum (LBF), from the fruit of Cornus officinalis (CO), and from the leaf and stem of Epimedium grandiflorum (EG) according to the published protocol [14,15]. The naturally occurring phyto-chemical Indole-3-Carbinol (I3C, Sigma Chemical Co., St. Louis, MO) was solubilized in Di-Methyl Sulfoxide (DMSO). Initial dose response experiments using the herbal extracts and I3C identified the respective maximum cytostatic concentrations for individual test agent. Each test agent at its respective maximum cytostatic concentration was used for the experiments on E_2 metabolism and AI growth.

Status of homeostatic growth control and risk for cancer development: The data presented in Table 1 compares the modulation in population doubling time, saturation density, E_2 metabolism, AI growth and tumor development in the models for select molecular sub types of clinical breast cancer. Relative to the non-tumorigenic 184-B5 cells the models for luminal A, HER-2 enriched and triple negative subtypes exhibited about a 55.6% decrease in population doubling times, and a 19.3 to 47.3% increase in saturation density. Overall, these data are consistent with the published data on aberrant hyper-proliferation, accelerated cell cycle progression, down-regulated cellular apoptosis and enhanced cancer risk in oncogene transfected mouse and human mammary epithelial cell culture models, as well as in human mammary carcinoma derived cell culture models [16].

The data on the E_2 metabolite ratio demonstrated that relative to the non-tumorigenic 184-B5 cells, the models for the three molecular subtypes exhibited an 85.7%, 88.1% and 90.5% decrease in the 2-OHE$_1$:16α-OHE$_1$ ratio. This down-regulation was predominantly due to increased formation of 16α-OHE$_1$. In this context it is noteworthy that similar alteration in E_2 metabolism has been documented in mammary epithelial cells that have been initiated for tumorigenic transformation using chemical carcinogens, retrovirus or oncogenes [17].

Biomarker End Point	Cell Culture Model			
	184-B5	MCF-7	184-B5/HER	MDA-MB-231
Population Doubling (hr.)[a]	34	15.2	15	15
Saturation Density ($x10^5$)[b]	22.3 ± 1.2	26.6 ± 1.7	32.8 ± 1.5	32.9 ± 2.3
2-OHE$_1$: 16α-OHE$_1$ Ratio[c]	4.2 ± 0.3	0.8 ± 0.2	0.5 ± 0.1	0.4 ± 0.2
AI Colony Formation[d]				
Incidence	0/18	18/18	18/18	18/18
Mean Colony Number	----	30.9 ± 2.4	23.0 ± 2.6	38.9 ± 1.6
Tumor Formation[e]				
Incidence	0/10	10-Oct	10-Oct	10-Oct
Latency	24 weeks	3-5 weeks	3-5 weeks	3-5 weeks

Table 1: Homeostatic Growth Control and Cancer Risk in Cell Culture Models for Molecular Subtypes of Clinical Breast Cancer. [a]Determined from the exponential growth phase. [b]Determined at day 7 post-seeding of $1.0x10^5$ cells. [c]Determined at day 3 post-seeding of $3.0x10^6$ cells. E_2 at a concentration of 20 nm was used as the substrate for the stable isotope dilution and GC-MS analysis. [d]Anchorage Independent (AI) colonies counted at day 21 post-seeding of 1,000 cells. [e]Palpable tumors after sub-cutaneous transplantation.

It is also noteworthy that the formation of 16a-OHE$_1$ is up-regulated in patients with breast and endometrial cancer [18-20], and that the human breast organoids of intact Terminal Duct Lobular Units (TDLU) obtained from the non-involved areas of breast cancer patients exhibit a higher extent of 16α-OHE$_1$ formation relative to the TDLU obtained from the patients undergoing reduction mammoplasty [21,22]. Collectively, these observations suggest that altered cellular metabolism of E_2 may represent a cause and/or consequence of tumorigenic transformation in E_2 responsive target cells, and more importantly, suggest a potential "field effect" for the relative risk for breast cancer progression.

Furthermore, unlike the 184-B5 cells the three models exhibited a 23.0 to 38.9 fold increase in the number of AI colonies in vitro, and retained their tumorigenic potential in vivo as evidenced by a 100% tumor incidence with a latency of 3-5 weeks, thus demonstrating that AI colony formation represents an in vitro surrogate end point biomarker for cancer risk. These data from the three models demonstrate cancer cell phenotype specific expression of the end point biomarkers, thereby suggesting that the models for the three molecular subtypes of clinical breast cancer have lost homeostatic growth control, have altered cellular metabolism of E_2, and have retained the risk of developing cancer.

Modulation of end point biomarkers by herbal extracts

The data presented in Table 2 compares the status of E_2 metabolite ratio and AI growth in response to treatment with herbal extracts in the model for Luminal A molecular subtype. The 2-OHE$_1$: 16α-OHE$_1$ ratio was increased by 3.7 fold, 12 fold and 16 fold respectively in response to treatment with EG, LBB and CO. In addition, the E_3: 16α-OHE$_1$ ratio was increased by about 25 fold in response to treatment with LBF and LBB. These data suggest that EG and CO function predominantly via favoring the formation of anti-proliferative 2-OHE$_1$ [14,23]. On the other hand, LBB and LBF function via increased formation of 2-OHE$_1$ as well as via accelerated conversion of the pro-mitogenic16α-OHE$_1$ to relatively inert E_3 [15].

Model: MCF-7		**End Point Biomarker**		
Treatment[a]	Concentration	2-OHE$_1$: 16α-OHE$_1$[b]	E_3: 16α-OHE$_1$[b]	AI Colonies[c]
E_2	20 nM	0.4 ± 0.1[d]	0.1 ± 0.1[h]	36.0 ± 1.5[k]
E_2+LBB	0.05%	5.2 ± 1.3[e]	2.3 ± 0.3[i]	2.5 ± 1.0[l]
E_2+LBF	1.0%	0.1 ± 0.09	2.6 ± 0.3[j]	4.8 ± 1.2[m]
E_2+CO	0.1%	6.8 ± 1.7[f]	0.4 ± 0.1	4.0 ± 1.2[n]
E_2+EG	1.0%	1.9 ± 0.5[g]	0.6 ± 0.2	4.9 ± 1.5[o]

Table 2: Modulation of End Point Biomarkers in Model for Luminal A Molecular Subtype of Breast Cancer. [a]E_2 at 20 nM and herbal extracts at their respective maximum cytostatic concentrations. [b]Concentrations of individual E_2 metabolites determined by stable isotope dilution and GC-MS analysis after a 48 hr treatment. Mean±SD, N=3 per treatment group. [c]Anchorage independent (AI) colonies counts at day 21 post-seeding of 1,000 cells per well of six-well plates. Mean±SD, N=18 per treatment group. $^{d<e,\ d<f,\ d<g}$ Data analyzed by 1-way ANOVA and Dunnett's multiple comparison test ($\alpha<0.05$). $^{h<I,\ h<j}$Data analyzed by 1-way ANOVA and Dunnett's multiple comparison test ($\alpha<0.05$). $^{k>l,\ k>m,\ k>n,\ k>o}$ Data analyzed by 1-way ANOVA and Dunnett's multiple comparison test ($\alpha < 0.05$).

E_2 is a well-established physiological ligand for ER, a ligand activated nuclear transcription factor that dictates E_2 mediated cellular activities and represents a therapeutic target for selective estrogen receptor modulators [4]. In addition to ER dependent functions, cellular metabolism of E_2 impacts on cell proliferation [2]. Thus, experimental modulation of E_2 metabolic profile may provide novel mechanistic leads to identify potential therapeutic targets. In this context it is noteworthy that E_2 metabolites exhibit pleotropic growth modulatory effects. Thus, 2-OHE$_2$, 2-OHE$_1$ and E_3 inhibit cellular proliferation, while 4-OHE$_1$ and 16α-OHE$_1$ are pro-mitogenic and induce DNA adduct formation and/or DNA damage/repair in mammary epithelial cells, as well as in tumor derived epithelial cells [2,24-27].

Treatment with the herbal extracts resulted in an 87% to a 93% reduction in the number of AI colonies. The observed reduction in the number of AI colonies in response to treatment with herbal extracts provides evidence for the efficacy of these extracts towards reduction of breast cancer risk [14,15,23].

Since long-term treatment with estrogen receptor modulators or aromatase inhibitors frequently gives rise to therapy resistant tumors [4,5], the present data provide potential clinically translatable leads that the herbal extracts from LBB, LBF, CO and EG may be efficacious for endocrine therapy resistant clinical breast cancer. Furthermore, the present experimental approach may also facilitate identification and prioritization of additional new herbal extracts with potential efficacy for endocrine therapy resistant clinical breast cancer.

Modulation of end point biomarkers by Indole-3-Carbinol (I3C)

The data presented in Table 3 examines the effect of I3C on the model for HER-2 enriched clinical breast cancer. I3C at its maximum cytostatic concentration induced an 18.4 fold increase in the 2-OHE$_1$; 16α-OHE$_1$ ratio, and a 55.1% decrease in the number of AI colonies.

Model: 184-B5/HER		**End Point Biomarker**	
Treatment[a]	Concentration	2-OHE$_1$: 16α-OHE$_1$[b]	AI Colonies[c]
DMSO	0.1%	0.5 ± 0.2[d]	20.5 ± 1.4[f]
I3C	50 μM	9.7 ± 2.1[e]	9.2 ± 3.3[g]

Table 3: Modulation of End Point Biomarkers in Model for HER-2 Enriched Molecular Sub type of Breast cancer. [a]I3C at its maximum cytostatic concentration. [b]Concentration of individual E_2 metabolites determined by the tritium exchange assay after a 48 hr treatment. Mean ± SD, N=3 per treatment group. Data analyzed by the 2-sample t-test comparing with the data from the DMSO group (Control). [c]Anchorage independent (AI) colony counts at day 21 post seeding of 1,000 cell per well of Six well plates. Mean±SD, N=18 per treatment group. Data analyzed by the 2-sample t test comparing the data from the DMSO group (Control). $^{d\text{-}e}P=0.004$, $^{f\text{-}g}P=0.01$

The data presented in Table 4 examines the effects of I3C in the model for triple negative clinical breast cancer. In response to the treatment with I3C at its maximum cytostatic concentrations, the MDA-MB-231 cells exhibited a 5 fold increase in the 2-OHE_1: 16α-OHE_1 ratio. In addition, I3C treatment induced a 62.2% decrease in the number of AI colonies. These data on the models for HER-2 enriched and the triple negative breast cancer essentially confirm and extend the previously published data [28] that demonstrate the anti-proliferative effects of I3C via cell cycle regulation and induction of cellular apoptosis. In this context it is noteworthy that I3C has been demonstrated to cooperate with the selective estrogen receptor modulator tamoxifen to induce cell cycle arrest in MCF-7 cells [29] and operates via inhibition of CDK-6 inducing G_1 arrest in human breast cancer cells independent of ER signaling [30].

Model: MDA-MB-231		**End Point Biomarker**	
Treatment[a]	Concentration	2-OHE_1: 16α-OHE_1[b]	AI Colonies[c]
DMSO	0.1%	0.4 ± 0.1[d]	23.8 ± 2.2[f]
I3C	50 μM	2.4 ± 0.3[e]	9.0 ± 1.2[g]

Table 4: Modulation of End Point Biomarkers in Model for Triple Negative Breast Cancer. [a]I3C at its maximum cytostatic concentration. [b]Concentration of individual E_2 metabolites determined by the tritium exchange assay after a 48 hr treatment. Mean± SD, N=3 per treatment group. Data analyzed by the 2-sample t test comparing the data from the DMSO group (Control). [c]Anchorage independent (AI) colony counts at day 21 post-seeding of 1,000 cell per well of six well plates. Mean±SD, N=18 per treatment group. Data analyzed by the 2-sample t test comparing the data from the DMSO group (Control). [d-e]P= 0.001. [f-g]P=0.01.

Effective up-regulation of the E_2 metabolite ratio and inhibition of AI colony number by I3C in the models for HER-2 enriched and triple negative breast cancer taken together provide evidence for the efficacy of the natural phyto-chemical I3C independent of the status of ER, PR and/or HER-2 expression. Since long-term treatment with HER-2 targeted small molecule inhibitors or cytotoxic chemotherapeutic agents is associated with progression of therapy resistant tumors [4-8], the present data provides potential leads for the efficacy of I3C in HER-2 enriched and triple negative molecular subtypes of clinical breast cancer.

Conclusions

The data summarized in the present review permits the following conclusions.

- The cell culture models for select molecular subtypes of clinical breast cancer exhibit loss of homeostatic growth control, altered cellular metabolism of E_2 and enhanced cancer risk.
- E_2 metabolite ratio may represent a novel quantifiable surrogate end point biomarker for endocrine responsiveness of the cancer cell phenotype.
- Non-toxic herbal extracts and mechanistically distinct natural phyto-chemicals may represent promising alternatives for the treatment of chemo-endocrine therapy resistant clinical breast cancer.

Acknowledgements

The author is a past recipient of research funding through US National Cancer Institute grants/contracts CA-44741, CA-29502, and CN-75029-63, US Department of Defense IDEA Award DAMD-17-94-J-4208, and the Irving Weinstein Foundation. Active collaboration with former colleagues Drs. Meena Katdare, Dan Sepkovic, Leon Bradlow, George Wong and Michael Osborne is gratefully acknowledged.

References

1. Hankinson SE, Colditz GA, Willett WC (2004) Towards an integrated model for breast cancer etiology: the lifelong interplay of genes, lifestyle, and hormones. Breast Cancer Res 6: 213-218.
2. Yager JD, Davidson NE (2006) Estrogen carcinogenesis in breast cancer. N Engl J Med 354: 270-282.
3. Sørlie T, Perou CM, Tibshirani R, Aas T, Geisler S, et al. (2001) Gene expression patterns of breast carcinomas distinguish tumor subclasses with clinical implications. Proc Natl Acad Sci U S A 98: 10869-10874.
4. Musgrove EA, Sutherland RL (2009) Biological determinants of endocrine resistance in breast cancer. Nat Rev Cancer 9: 631-643.
5. Johnston SR, Dowsett M (2003) Aromatase inhibitors for breast cancer: lessons from the laboratory. Nat Rev Cancer 3: 821-831.
6. Baselga J, Swain SM (2009) Novel anticancer targets: revisiting ERBB2 and discovering ERBB3. Nat Rev Cancer 9: 463-475.
7. Hynes NE, Lane HA (2005) ERBB receptors and cancer: the complexity of targeted inhibitors. Nat Rev Cancer 5: 341-354.
8. Anders CK, Winer EP, Ford JM, Dent R, Silver DP, et al. (2010) Poly(ADP-Ribose) polymerase inhibition: "targeted" therapy for triple-negative breast cancer. Clin Cancer Res 16: 4702-4710.
9. Smalley M, Ashworth A (2003) Stem cells and breast cancer: A field in transit. Nat Rev Cancer 3: 832-844.
10. Neve RM, Chin K, Fridlyand J, Yeh J, Baehner FL, et al. (2006) A collection of breast cancer cell lines for the study of functionally distinct cancer subtypes. Cancer Cell 10: 515-527.
11. Zhai Y-F, Beitenmiller H, Wang B, Gould MN, Oakley C, Esselmann WJ, Welsh CW (1993) Increased expression of specific protein tyrosine phosphatases in human breast epithelial cells neoplastically transformed by the neu oncogene. Cancer Res. 53: 2272-2278.
12. Subik K, Lee JF, Baxter L, Strzepek T, Costello D, et al. (2010) The Expression Patterns of ER, PR, HER2, CK5/6, EGFR, Ki-67 and AR by Immunohistochemical Analysis in Breast Cancer Cell Lines. Breast Cancer (Auckl) 4: 35-41.
13. Sepkovic DW, Bradlow HL, Michnovicz J, Murtezuni S, Levy I, et al (1994) Catechol estrogen production in rat microsomes after treatment with Indole-3 carbinol, ascorbigen or ß-napthaflavone: A comparison of stable isotope dilution, gas chromatography-mass spectrophotometry and radiometric methods. Steroids 39: 318-323.
14. Telang NT, Li G, Sepkovic DW, Bradlow HL, Wong GY (2012) Anti-proliferative effects of Chinese herb Cornus officinalis in a cell culture model for estrogen receptor-positive clinical breast cancer. Mol Med Rep 5: 22-28.
15. Telang N, Li G, Sepkovic D, Bradlow HL, Wong GY (2014) Comparative efficacy of extracts from Lycium barbarum bark and fruit on estrogen receptor positive human mammary carcinoma MCF-7 cells. Nutr Cancer 66: 278-284.
16. Telang N, Katdare M (2012) Epithelial cell culture models for the prevention and therapy of clinical breast cancer (Review). Oncol Lett 3: 744-750.
17. Telang NT (1996) Oncogenes, estradiol biotransformation, and mammary carcinogenesis. Ann N Y Acad Sci 784: 277-287.
18. Schneider J, Kinne D, Fracchia A, Pierce V, Anderson KE, et al. (1982) Abnormal oxidative metabolism of estradiol in women with breast cancer. Proc Natl Acad Sci U S A 79: 3047-3051.

19. Fishman J, Schneider J, Hershcope RJ, Bradlow HL (1984) Increased estrogen-16 alpha-hydroxylase activity in women with breast and endometrial cancer. J Steroid Biochem 20: 1077-1081.
20. Fishman J, Osborne MP, Telang NT (1995) The role of estrogen in mammary carcinogenesis. Ann N Y Acad Sci 768: 91-100.
21. Telang NT, Axelrod DM, Wong GY, Bradlow HL, Osborne MP (1991) Biotransformation of estradiol by explant culture of human mammary tissue. Steroids 56: 37-43.
22. Osborne MP, Bradlow HL, Wong GY, Telang NT (1993) Upregulation of estradiol C16 alpha-hydroxylation in human breast tissue: a potential biomarker of breast cancer risk. J Natl Cancer Inst 85: 1917-1920.
23. Telang N, Li G, Katdare M, Sepkovic DW, Bradlow HL, Wong GYC (2013) Preventive efficacy of the Chinese nutritional herb Epimedium grandiflorum in a preclinical cell culture model for Luminal A molecular subtype of breast cancer. Proc. San Antonio Breast Cancer Symposium.
24. Schneider J, Huh MM, Bradlow HL, Fishman J (1984) Antiestrogen action of 2-hydroxyestrone on MCF-7 human breast cancer cells. J Biol Chem 259: 4840-4845.
25. Lottering ML, Haag M, Seegers JC (1992) Effects of 17 beta-estradiol metabolites on cell cycle events in MCF-7 cells. Cancer Res 52: 5926-5932.
26. Telang NT, Suto A, Wong GY, Osborne MP, Bradlow HL (1992) Induction by estrogen metabolite 16 alpha-hydroxyestrone of genotoxic damage and aberrant proliferation in mouse mammary epithelial cells. J Natl Cancer Inst 84: 634-638.
27. Suto A, Telang NT, Tanino H, Takeshita T, Ohmiya H, et al. (1999) In Vitro and In Vivo Modulation of Growth Regulation in the Human Breast Cancer Cell Line MCF-7 by Estradiol Metabolites. Breast Cancer 6: 87-92.
28. Telang NT, Katdare M, Bradlow HL, Osborne MP, Fishman J (1997) Inhibition of proliferation and modulation of estradiol metabolism: novel mechanisms for breast cancer prevention by the phytochemical indole-3-carbinol. Proc Soc Exp Biol Med 216: 246-252.
29. Cover CM, Hsieh SJ, Cram EJ, Hong C, Riby JE, et al. (1999) Indole-3-carbinol and tamoxifen cooperate to arrest the cell cycle of MCF-7 human breast cancer cells. Cancer Res 59: 1244-1251.
30. Cover CM, Hsieh SJ, Tran SH, Hallden G, Kim GS, et al. (1998) Indole-3-carbinol inhibits the expression of cyclin-dependent kinase-6 and induces a G1 cell cycle arrest of human breast cancer cells independent of estrogen receptor signaling. J Biol Chem 273: 3838-3847.

15

Evaluation of Carbohydrate and Lipid Metabolism and Risk of Obesity in Children after Brain Tumors Treatment

Maja Okońska[1*], Elżbieta Adamkiewicz-Drożyńska[2], Maria Korpal-Szczyrska[1], Dorota Birkholz-Walerzak[1] and Małgorzata Myśliwiec[1]

[1]*Department of Pediatric Diabetology, Clinic of Pediatrics, Diabetology and Endocrinology, Medical University of Gdańsk, ul. Dębinki 7, 80-952 Gdańsk, Poland*

[2]*Clinic of Pediatrics, Hematology and Oncology, Medical University of Gdańsk, ul. Dębinki 7, 80-952 Gdańsk, Poland*

[*]**Corresponding author:** Maja Okońska, Department of Pediatric Diabetology, Clinic of Pediatrics, Diabetology and Endocrinology, Medical University of Gdańsk, ul. Dębinki 7, 80-952 Gdańsk, Poland, E-mail: majkul@wp.pl

Abstract

The aim of the study was to assess the carbohydrate and lipid metabolism disturbances as well as weight in children after brain tumors treatment.

The study included 33 boys (53.2%) and 29 girls (46.8%) aged 11.6 ± 3.9. 22 patients underwent treatment for tumors of hypothalamic-pituitary(h-p) area: IA–surgery(19/22); IB–surgery and radiotherapy(3/22). 40 patients were treated for tumors outside the h-p area: IIA– with surgery, chemo-and radiotherapy(22/40); IIB–only with surgery(15/40); IIC–patients treated for optic nerve glioma with chemotherapy(3/40).

BMI was assessed before and after the treatment. OGTT, HbA1c, lipid profile and WHtR after treatment were assessed. Indices of insulin resistance: HOMA-IR, Quickie, Matsuda and de Fronzo were calculated.

63% overweight/obese patients of IA-group and 27% of IIA-group were observed. Hyperinsulinemia was noted in 44% of IA-group, 20% of IIA-group, and insulin resistance in 38% of IA and 15% of IIA. DM2 was diagnosed in 1 patient of IA-group, IFG in 1 patient of IIB, IGT in 1 patient of IA and 1 patient of IIC. Dyslipidemia was noted in 47% of IA-group, elevated level of LDL-cholesterol in 30% of IIA-group.

The excessive weight gain, hyperinsulinemia and dyslipidemia were observed primarily in children treated for hypothalamic-pituitary tumors.

Keywords: Brain tumor; Hyperinsulinemia; Obesity; Dyslipidemia

Abbreviations

Acth: Adrenocorticotropic Hormone; All: Acute Lymphoblastic Leukemia; BMI: Body Mass Index; BMI-SDS: Body Mass Index Standard Deviation Score; CNS - Central Nervous System; DM: Diabetes Mellitus; DM2: Diabetes Mellitus Type 2; FT4: Free Thyroxine; GH: Growth Hormone; GHD: Growth Hormone Deficiency; H-P: Hypothalamic-Pituitary; HBA1C: Hemoglobin A1c; HDL: High-Density Lipoprotein; Homa-IR: Homeostasis Model Assessment: Insulin Resistance Index; IFG: Impaired Fasting Glucose; IGT: Impaired Glucose Tolerance; LDL: Low-Density Lipoprotein; MB: Medulloblastoma; OGTT: Oral Glucose Tolerance Test; PNET: Primitive Neuroectodermal Tumor; RGH: Recombinant Growth Hormone; TC: Total Cholesterol; TG: Triglycerides; TSH: Thyroid-Stimulating Hormone; WHTR - Waist-To-Height Ratio

Introduction

Central Nervous System (CNS) neoplasms are the most common type of solid tumors in children and the second type of all children neoplasms after leukemias. A significant improvement in the treatment of this condition was possible due to development of neurosurgery, radiotherapy and chemotherapy. Majority of brain tumor survivors present chronic complications due to neoplastic process and oncology management [1,2]. An assessment of abnormalities of carbohydrate metabolism and its etiology in patients after brain tumors treatment is still an unacknowledged area of interest.

The aim of the study was to assess the type and the frequency of carbohydrate and lipid metabolism disturbances as well as weight in children after brain tumors treatment.

Materials and Methods

Patients characteristics

The study included 62 children: 33 boys (53.2%) and 29 girls (46.8%), who have finished brain tumors treatment. At the time of laboratory investigations the age of patients ranged from 3 years and 10 months to 17 years and 11 months. Mean age at the diagnosis was 7 years and 10 months. The average time from the end of oncology treatment to laboratory investigations was 2.9 years.

CNS neoplasms diagnosed by cytology included: gliomas in 23 patients (low grade gliomas - 22 patients, high grade gliomas - 1 patient); MB/PNET (11 patients), craniopharyngioma (18 patients), ependymoma in 3 patients and other types of tumor in 7 patients. 59 children had surgical treatment (a specimen for histopathological diagnosis was obtained during surgery) and 3 were treated with chemotherapy exclusively (diagnosis based on imaging study). Radiotherapy was performed in 25 patients, including 6 patients treated with both: surgery and radiotherapy and 19 treated with surgery, chemotherapy and radiotherapy.

Group division

Patients were divided into 5 groups due to tumor localization and the type of treatment: IA: 19 patients surgically treated for tumors of hypothalamic-pituitary area (h-p); IB: 3 patients treated by surgery and radiotherapy for tumors of h-p area; IIA: 22 patients who received complex treatment (surgery, chemotherapy, radiotherapy) due to tumors of other localization than h-p area; IIB: 15 patients surgically treated for tumors of other localization than h-p area; IIC: 3 patients with optic nerve gliomas treated with chemotherapy. Three most numerous groups (IA, IIA, IIB) were included in statistical analysis.

Medical history data

History data of diabetes occurrence in patients' family members: parents, grandparents, their siblings and patients' siblings were taken.

Pubertal stage

Pubertal development of the patients was assessed according to Tanner scale.

Body mass index and waist-to-hight ratio (WHtR)

Body mass index (BMI) (weight / height [kg/m^2]) was established before the diagnosis based on available medical history data of patients aged 4.7 ± 2.6. To evaluate the influence of oncological treatment on body mass disturbances BMI was calculated at diagnosis, after 6 months of treatment, at the end of the treatment and one year after the treatment. These data were compared to BMI at the time of laboratory assessment and one year after the study, as previously planned in the research protocol.

Being overweight was defined with BMI between 90 and 97 percentile and obesity was diagnosed in patients with BMI above 97 percentile according to polish population BMI-for-age-and-sex percentile charts [3]. BMI was presented by standard deviation score (BMI-SDS).

A single waist circumference measurement was assessed by measure tape (accuracy of measurement 0.5 cm) at the time of laboratory investigation. Waist-to-height ratio (WHtR) was calculated (waist circumference/ height [cm/cm]). Values below 0.5 were accepted as regular regardless of age or sex [4].

Laboratory investigation

Laboratory tests were made 2.9 ± 2.5 years after oncology treatment.

Pituitary growth hormone (GH) reserve was assessed by two different stimulation tests: Clonidine (0.15 mg / m^2 per oral) and Insulin (0.1 j/kg intravenously) or Glucagon (0.03 mg/kg intramuscularly). GH night profile was also assessed (5 evaluations every 30 minute during sleep). Pituitary insufficiency was diagnosed when maximal GH serum concentration in all tests was below 10 ng/ml. Thyroid hormones (fasting TSH and fT4) and adrenal function (Cortisol and ACTH at 8 am and 11 pm) were assessed as well. Methods of immunochemiluminescency were used to perform all biochemical tests.

In all patients Oral Glucose Tolerance Test (OGTT) was performed. Serum glucose concentrations were assessed by spectrophotometry and insulin concentrations by immunochemiluminescency. Impaired fasting glucose (IFG), impaired glucose tolerance (IGT) and diabetes mellitus (DM) were defined using World Health Organization criteria [5]. Patients were diagnosed with hyperinsulinemia when insulin level was higher than 15 μU/ml in a fasting state, more than 150 μU/ml in OGTT or more than 75 μU/ml in the 2nd hour of OGTT [6].

Serum HbA1c level was measured by high quality fluid chromatography.

Lipid profile was assessed by immunoenzymatic method (total cholesterol - TC, triglycerides - TG, high density lipids: HDL). Low density lipids (LDL) were calculated by Friedewald formula (TC-[TG/5+HDL]).

Insulin Resistance Indices

Based on the glucose and insulin levels established in OGTT insulin resistance indices were calculated: HOMA-IR (fasting insulin [mU/ml] × fasting glucose [mmol/l] / 22.5), normal level ≤ 3.16 [6,7]; Matsuda and de Fronzo (10000 / √(fasting insulin [mU/ml] × fasting glucose [mg/dl] × mean glucose concentration in OGTT [mg/dl] × mean insulin concentration in OGTT [mU/ml]), normal level ≥5 [6,8-10]; Quickie (1 / (log fasting insulin [uU/ml] + log fasting glucose [mmol/l]), normal level >0.34 [6,11].

Statistical analysis

The statistical analysis included a describing analysis and a decision analysis. The describing analysis consisted of graphic presentations and numeric results. The statistical decision analysis comprised Mann-Whitney U test and Wilcoxon signed-rank test for dependent variables. An investigation of the dependence between attributes was based on Fisher test and χ^2 test. In a statistical testing, the accepted p-value was $p = 0.05$. If the statistical significance level was lower than 0.05, the decision about relevance or frequency was made. Calculations were performed by Statistica 8.0 and statistical calculations R 2.8.0.

Results and Discussion

Patient's hormonal status during laboratory investigation

A growth hormone deficiency was diagnosed in majority of patients from groups: IA (18/19), IB (3/3), IIA (17/22) and only in 2 patients from IIB-group. Nobody in IIC-group was GH-deficient. The therapy with the recombinant GH (rGH) was introduced in the majority of patients from IA-group (13/18) and in 3 of IIA-group. The rest of GH-deficient patients in IIA-group remained under observation because of greater risk of tumor recurrence.

Primary hypothyroidism was diagnosed in 4 IIA-patients and in 1 patient from group IIB. All patients from groups IA and IB and 3 patients from IIA-group revealed secondary hypothyroidism.

Pituitary-adrenal axis insufficiency was observed in all patients from group I. Diabetes insipidus was shown in 89.5% of patients of IA group and all patients of IB group. Every deficient patient received an appropriate substitute treatment.

Pubertal stage during laboratory investigation

The most of IA-group (15 patients), all patients from IB-group, 5 patients from IIA and 7 patients from IIB-group were pre-pubertal (Tanner I). 11 patients from IIA-group, all patients from IIC-group, 4 patients in IA-group and 4 patients in IIB-group were pubertal (Tanner II-III). Maturity stage (Tanner IV-V) was observed in 6 patients from IIA-group and 4 patients from group IIB.

Weight assessment

Most of patients with h-p tumors (IA: 12/19) revealed an excessive weight gain after treatment, more frequently than patients from other groups: IIA: 6/22, IIB: 3/15 (IA vs. IIA: $p < 0.023$; IA vs. IIB: $p < 0.041$). 26.3% (5/19) of IA-patients were overweight, whereas patients from other groups were twice less frequent overweight (IIA - 3/22 and IIB: 2/15). Obesity was diagnosed in 31.6% (6/19) of IA-patients and in 13.6% (3/22) of patients treated complex for tumors outside the h-p area (IIA). The location of a tumor in the hypothalamic-pituitary area and the age below 10 years at diagnosis significantly influenced the excessive weight gain ($p<0.012$; $p<0.029$ respectively) and the obesity ($p<0.041$). An excessive weight gain was more frequently observed in patients in a pre-pubertal stage at the moment of the laboratory investigation ($p<0.032$). It was established that neither intracranial hypertension with consciousness disorders nor steroid treatment had influence on weight gain and obesity after completed therapy.

Analysis of BMI variations

The most significant increase of BMI-SDS after the completed therapy was observed in patients with hypothalamic-pituitary tumors treated exclusively with surgery (IA). The highest BMI was noted 12 months after the end of the treatment. The rGH treatment had significant influence on BMI-SDS reduction for patients qualified for this therapy.

BMI-SDS values in patients with tumors outside the hypothalamic-pituitary location showed dependence on different types of treatment. Patients receiving complex treatment (IIA) had lower BMI-SDS after completed therapy than before it ($p<0.006$). Lesser BMI-SDS before treatment (-0.6 ± 1.09) was observed in patients treated exclusively with surgery (IIB) (Figure 1).

WHtR

IA-patients presented significantly higher WHtR values (0.5 ± 0.1), than other patients (IA vs. IIA: $p<0.027$; IA vs. IIB: $p<0.008$).

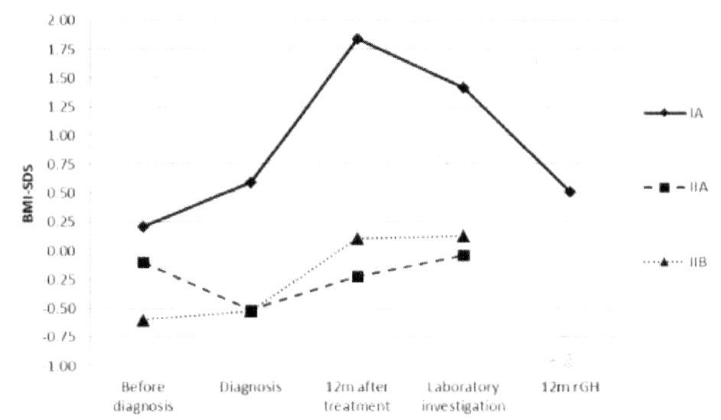

Figure 1: BMI-SDS changes in 3 main groups. IA – group of patients treated surgically for tumors of hypothalamic-pituitary area; IIA – group of patients treated for tumors outside the h-p area with surgery, chemo- and radiotherapy; IIB – group of patients treated surgically for tumors outside the h-p area. Before diagnosis- historical data; Diagnosis – at the moment of diagnosis; 12 m after treatment – 12 months after oncology treatment; Laboratory investigation – laboratory tests after oncology treatment; 12 m rGH- after 12 months of treatment with recombinant growth hormone.

Glucose [mg/dl]	Serum glucose concentrations					Statistical differences		
	IA	IB	IIA	IIB	IIC	p(IA/IIA)	p(IA/IIB)	p(IIA/IIB)
	n=16	n=2	n=20	n=15	n=3			
In a fasting state	79.05 ± 5.33	77.33 ± 7.23	81.90 ± 5.17	81.27 ± 7.27	90.67 ± 1.16	p>0.05	p>0.05	p>0.05
In 2nd hour of OGTT	113.69 ± 3.90	104.50 ± 16.26	93.35 ± 17.94	92.87 ± 15.27	124.00 ± 21.93	p<0.019*	p<0.010*	p>0.05
Mean concentration in OGTT	107.30 ± 24.22	93.40 ± 12.16	103.22 ± 17.98	100.40 ± 11.90	109.44 ± 6.15	p>0.05	p>0.05	p>0.05

Table 1: Serum glucose concentrations in OGTT (mean values and standard deviations) in particular groups. IA- group of patients treated surgically for tumors of hypothalamic-pituitary area; IB - group of patients treated with surgery and radiotherapy for tumors of hypothalamic-pituitary area; IIA –group of patients treated with surgery, chemo- and radiotherapy for tumors outside the h-p area; IIB – group of patients treated surgically for tumors outside the h-p area; IIC- patients with optic nerve glioma treated with chemotherapy. Analysis was made by Fisher test. Values marked by "*" were calculated by U Mann-Whitney test. Statistically important differences were marked as bold.

Carbohydrate metabolism assessment: family history

A diabetes occurrence in family members was more common in patients with tumors outside the h-p area receiving complex treatment (IIA) than in other groups, however the difference was not significant.

Glucose concentration in OGTT

Impaired fasting glucose (IFG) was noted only in one patient treated for an optic nerve glioma (IIC). A mean glucose level at 2nd hour of OGTT was significantly higher in patients surgically treated for h-p tumors (IA) in comparison to patients with other localization of tumor (IA vs. IIA: $p<0.019$; IA vs. IIB: $p<0.010$). Impaired glucose tolerance (IGT) was diagnosed in one patient from IA-group and one from IIC-group. The type 2 diabetes was diagnosed in one patient from IA-group [Table 1].

The post-operative steroid treatment did not influence fasting glucose, glucose tolerance or diabetes occurrence in the patients.

Assessement of HbA1c

For all patients HbA1c values were within normal ranges. The highest HbA1c values were noted for patients with h-p tumors (IB: 5.53 ± 0.15%; IA: 5.38 ± 0.37%) and the lowest for patients receiving complex treatment for tumors outside the h-p area (IIA: 5.18 ± 0.33%). The difference between groups was not significant.

Insulin concentration in OGTT

Fasting insulin concentration above 15 μU/l was observed significantly more frequent in subjects who underwent surgical treatment for h-p tumors (IA) than in other groups (IA vs. IIA: p<0.016; IA vs. IIB: p<0.049). In those patients mean fasting insulin concentration was higher than in others (IA vs. IIA: p<0.03) [Table 2].

The highest average concentration of insulin in 1st hour of OGTT was observed in patients treated for tumors outside the h-p area (IIA: 60.07 ± 57.26 μU/ml), whereas in 2nd hour of OGTT it was supreme in IA-group. For those patients concentrations above 75μU/ml were more frequently seen in comparison to the others, but the difference was not significant.

The highest maximum concentration of insulin in OGTT was noted in patients of IA-group (130.09 ± 143.05 μU/ml). Five of them revealed insulin concentration above 150μU/ml [Table 2].

Elevated insulin concentrations were related to being overweight and obese (p<0.008).

	Serum insulin concentrations in OGTT and insulin resistance indices					Statistical differences		
	IA	IB	IIA	IIB	IIC	p(IA/IIA)	p(IA/IIB)	p(IIA/IIB)
	n=16	n=2	n=20	n=15	n=3			
Fasting insulin [μU/ml]	12.11 ± 8.51	7.80 ± 0.00	5.88 ± 3.41	12.11 ± 21.71	12.37 ± 4.37	p<0.03*	p>0.05	p>0.05
Fasting insulin > 15 μU/ml	6/16 (37.5%)	0/2 (0%)	1/20 (5%)	1/15 (6,7%)	1/3 (33.3%)	p<0.016	p<0.049	p>0.05
Insulin in 2nd hour of OGTT [μU/ml]	69.13 ± 112.74	25.30 ± 0.00	37.71 ± 38.87	31.26 ± 24.44	60.57 ± 29.70	p>0.05	p>0.05	p>0.05
Insulin in 2nd hour of OGTT >75 μU/ml	3/16 (18.8%)	0/2 (0%)	2/20 (9.5%)	1/15 (6.7%)	1/3 (33%)	p>0.05	p>0.05	p>0.05
Max insulin in OGTT > 150 μU/ml	5/16 (31.3%)	0/2 (0%)	2/20 (9.5%)	0/15 (0%)	0/3 (0%)	p<0.003	p<0.001	p>0.05
HOMA-IR (>3,16)	6/16 (37.5%)	0/2 (0%)	0/20 (0%)	1/15 (6.7%)	1/3 (33.3%)	p<0.012	p>0.05	p>0.05
Quickie (<0,34)	11/16 (68.8%)	2/2 (100%)	11/20 (55%)	8/15 (53.3%)	3/3 (100%)	p>0.05	p>0.05	p>0.05
Matsuda and de Fronzo (<5)	6/16 (37.5%)	0/2 (0%)	2/20 (10%)	2/15 (13.3%)	1/3 (33.3%)	p>0.05	p>0.05	p>0.05

Table 2: Serum insulin concentrations in OGTT and insulin resistance indices in particular groups. IA- group of patients treated surgically for tumors of hypothalamic-pituitary area; IB - group of patients treated with surgery and radiotherapy for tumors of hypothalamic-pituitary area; IIA –group of patients treated with surgery, chemo- and radiotherapy for tumors outside the h-p area; IIB – group of patients treated surgically for tumors outside the h-p area; IIC- patients with optic nerve glioma treated with chemotherapy. Analysis was made by Fisher test. Values marked by "*" were calculated by U Mann-Whitney test. Statistically important differences were marked as bold.

Insulin resistance indices

Patients treated for h-p tumors (IA) revealed HOMA-IR values above 3.16 more frequently than other subjects (IA vs. IIA p<0.012). Quickie index values below 0.34 were observed in most of the patients; however differences between groups were not significant. Matsuda and de Fronzo index lower than 5 revealed mostly patients treated for h-p tumors (IA) [Table 2].

Hyperinsulinemia and abnormal insulin resistance indices: HOMA-IR (p<0.001), Matsuda (p<0.001) and Quickie (p<0.024) were related.

Obesity was diagnosed more frequently in patients with abnormal HOMA-IR and Matsuda indices values (p<0.049 and p<0.047 respectively). An excessive weight gain was dependent on abnormal values of these indices as well (p<0.009 and p<0.01 respectively).

Lipids profile

Elevated total cholesterol was noted in a half of IA-group and almost a half of IIA-group, but the second one revealed the highest average concentration of total cholesterol and LDL-cholesterol. The average concentration of HDL-cholesterol in patients treated surgically for h-p tumors was lower than in other groups (IA vs. IIA p < 0.029). Reduced HDL-cholesterol was noted more frequently in IA-group (IA vs.IIA p < 0.043).

The highest concentration of triglycerides was observed in patients with tumors of hypothalamic-pituitary area (IA), significantly higher than in other groups (IA vs. IIB: p<0.002; IA vs. IIA: p < 0.025). Elevated triglycerides were more frequently observed in IA-group (10/19) than in others (IA vs. IIA: p < 0.009; IA vs. IIB: p < 0.037) [Table 3].

	Serum concentrations of Total cholesterol, LDL, HDL, Triglycerides					Statistical differences		
	IA n=18	IB n=2	IIA n=20	IIB n=15	IIC n=3	p (IA/IIA)	p (IA/IIB)	p (IIA/IIB)
Total cholesterol [mg/dl]	192.84 ± 56.40	199.67 ± 52.00	204.43 ± 64.83	167.87 ± 31.16	148.67 ± 13.80	p>0.05	p>0.05	p<0.028*
Elevated total cholesterol	9/18(50.0%)	1/2 (50.0%)	8/20 (40%)	4/15(26.7%)	0/3 (0.0%)	p>0.05	p>0.05	p>0.05
LDL cholesterol [mg/dl]	117.50 ± 49.16	121.00 ± 25.46	137.10 ± 61.78	104.73 ± 22.89	78.33 ± 18.04	p>0.05	p>0.05	p<0.033*
Elevated LDL cholesterol	5/18 (27.8%)	1/2 (50.0%)	6/20 (30.0%)	2/15 (13.3%)	0/3 (0.0%)	p>0.05	p>0.05	p>0.05
HDL cholesterol [mg/dl]	41.11 ± 10.63	52.50 ± 10.61	48.30 ± 8.97	48.4 ± 14.29	53.67 ± 11.37	p<0.029	p>0.05	p>0.05
Reduced HDL cholesterol	7/18 (38.9%)	0/2 (0.0%)	2/20 (10.0%)	4/15 (26.7%)	0/3 (0.0%)	p<0.043	p>0.05	p>0.05
Triglicerides [mg/dl]	162.26 ± 100.77	151.33 ± 130.78	96.43 ± 41.32	78.33 ± 34.33	84.00 ± 9.54	p<0.025*	p<0.002*	p>0.05
Elevated trigliceriides	10/18 (55.6%)	1/2 (50.0%)	1/20 (5.0%)	1/15 (6.7%)	0/3 (0.0%)	p<0.009	p<0.037	p>0.05

Table 3: Serum lipids concentrations in particular groups. IA- group of patients treated surgically for tumors of hypothalamic-pituitary area; IB - group of patients treated with surgery and radiotherapy for tumors of hypothalamic-pituitary area; IIA –group of patients treated with surgery, chemo- and radiotherapy for tumors outside the h-p area; IIB – group of patients treated surgically for tumors outside the h-p area; IIC- patients with optic nerve glioma treated with chemotherapy. Analysis was made by Fisher test. Values marked by "*" were calculated by U Mann-Whitney test. Statistically important differences were marked as bold.

Discussion

Patients with brain tumors who participated in the study were diverse. The subjects differed by histology of the tumor and its localization in the brain. The selection of patients was limited because the study included only those patients who already finished treatment in one clinical centre.

Current studies in patients who completed oncological therapy describe various abnormalities of carbohydrate metabolism. An excessive weight gain is the most frequent observed complication [7,8,9-15]. Many authors emphasize that the main cause of obesity during or after oncology management is the neoplastic process itself (tumors of h-p area), steroid treatment in brain edema prophylaxis, pituitary insufficiency - particularly growth hormone deficiency, other endocrinopathies, lifestyle changes and accompanying neurological symptoms [18,19].

Childhood Cancer Survivor Study [9] evaluated adults treated for brain tumors in childhood. It reveal that the risk of obesity comparing to healthy adults is similar. On the other hand, Pietilä et al. [8] describe significant frequency of obesity and carbohydrate metabolism abnormalities in patients after brain tumors management. Patients in this study underwent treatment for brain tumors of various locations. In few patients tumors were situated in hypothalamus and sella turcica area. The majority of patients were treated exclusively with surgery. Obesity was diagnosed in 35% of patients (21% with the central one). Adiposity was observed more frequently in patients receiving radiotherapy for the whole brain, after damage of hypothalamic-pituitary area by neoplastic process, in patients with growth hormone deficiency and with decreased physical activity [8].

In our study the group with the highest risk of developing obesity were patients treated for tumors located in hypothalamic-pituitary area (60% of all patients with excessive weight gain).

No dependence between weight gain and chemotherapy or radiotherapy was noted.

Numerous authors inform that excessive weight gain frequently correlates with increased appetite. It relates mostly to patients treated for hypothalamic-pituitary tumors [8,14,20-22]. As far as some authors are concerned, hypothalamic obesity may develop even some years after hypothalamic tumors management [22], though there are observations that first symptoms may be present shortly after surgery [23].

Excessive weight gain related to an increased appetite is most common for patients after surgical treatment or radiotherapy of craniopharyngioma [10,12,13,15-17,21]. Meuric et al. [24] evaluated patients with craniopharyngioma after extensive treatment and primary damage of hypothalamus and observed correlation between weight gain and increased insulin secretion. Hyperinsulinemia can develop either before the surgical treatment or after completed therapy [21-25]. The cause of increased insulin concentration in the serum indirectly explained animal studies. The damage of ventromedial nucleus in hypothalamus of rats was the cause of hyperphagia and increased serum insulin concentration, which led to obesity [26]. In this study the correlation between hyperinsulinemia and increased activity of parasympathetic system was shown. Other studies also confirm the hypothesis that increased insulin secretion may cause the hypothalamic obesity. It is considered that positive influence of Octreotide treatment in this type of obesity is by insulin secretion inhibition [14,27].

Pinto et al. [23] observed that carbohydrate metabolism abnormalities intensified during and after oncology treatment. There is a hypothesis, that the craniopharyngioma itself and the surgery in addition modified the insulin secretion. The correlation between hyperinsulinemia and the weight gain is described for healthy population as well [28].

In our study, in half of the patients who underwent surgical treatment for h-p tumors, elevated insulin concentrations after treatment were observed. The location of the tumor in this area had a significant influence on weight gain and hyperinsulinemia. There was dependence between hyperinsulinemia and an excessive weight gain. For the patients receiving complex treatment for tumors outside the h-p area increased fasting insulin concentrations were noted only in 5% of patients and elevated insulin concentrations in OGTT were seen in 15% of patients. In this group only 27% were overweight or obese. 20% of patients surgically treated for tumors outside the h-p area revealed weight gain. Elevated insulin concentrations in OGTT were noted for 13% of them. The imbalance between patients with tumors of different areas testifies that the tumor location in the h-p area has the greatest influence on weight gain and insulin resistance after treatment.

Carbohydrate metabolism disorders as diabetes mellitus and impaired glucose tolerance were described after treatment for brain tumors in hypothalamic-pituitary area [29,30]. Crowley et al. diagnosed diabetes mellitus in 11.5% of patients after surgical treatment of craniopharyngioma [29]. Furthermore, in Deepak et al. study diabetes mellitus was diagnosed in 9% of those patients [30]. In the other survey [31] diabetes mellitus incidence was 3.7%. In our present study type 2 diabetes mellitus was diagnosed only in one patient (1.6%) treated with surgery for craniopharyngioma. Impaired glucose tolerance was noted in one patient treated for h-p tumor and another treated exclusively with chemotherapy for optic nerve glioma. The highest average HbA1c value was observed in patients treated for h-p tumors [32].

For patients with abnormal glucose or insulin concentrations, the insulin resistance assessment is required. It can be evaluated by indirect calculation of insulin resistance indices. A more adequate method is the glucose clamp technique [33,34], but because of the complexity of the method, it is not routinely used in the clinical practice. Yeni-Komshian et al. [35] compared different insulin resistance indices with the glucose clamp technique and observed that fasting insulin concentration was the most sensitive insulin resistance index. A fasting glucose to insulin ratio and HOMA-IR index also showed high sensitivity, however they were less sensitive than fasting insulin.

In our study elevated fasting insulin concentrations, HOMA-IR and Matsuda abnormal values were noted more frequently in patients treated surgically for h-p tumors. Some patients treated with surgery followed by radio- and chemotherapy for tumors outside the h-p area also revealed insulin resistance. This was mostly accompanied by overweight and obesity. In the literature only few authors assessed insulin resistance indices for patients after complex treatment of brain tumors. Usually patients with h-p tumors and craniopharyngioma were described [15,36]. There are also studies concerning patients after treatment of acute lymphoblastic leukemia [37]. In those groups increased percentage of abnormal values of assessed indices has been observed comparing to control groups [15,36,37].

Steroid treatment in cancer therapy is an important factor influencing carbohydrate metabolism abnormalities [38,39]. The steroid use in therapeutic protocols of acute lymphoblastic leukemia (ALL) increases frequency of obesity and carbohydrate metabolism abnormalities [40-42]. On the other hand, in the studies assessing large population of ALL survivors, prophylactic radiotherapy was essential factor influencing obesity rate. Exclusive chemotherapy did not influence the obesity rate [43]. In our study correlation between chemotherapy and radiotherapy with the excessive weight gain was not observed. In brain tumor therapeutic schedules in children steroid treatment is used commonly in pre-operative period in order to decrease intracranial pressure, and less frequently in later treatment stages. Our results did not confirm correlation between carbohydrate metabolism disorders and the type of treatment.

An important constituent of the abdominal obesity assessment is a measurement of waist and hip circumferences and calculation of indices. In our study WHtR (waist-to-height ratio) index was used. It is widely accepted as a very good index assessing abdominal obesity and it is an excellent prognostic factor for abdominal obesity complications, especially in children [4,44,45]. In our study 26% of patients treated for h-p tumors revealed abnormal values of this index. Lower prevalence of abdominal obesity was noted in patients with tumors of other than h-p location.

While analyzing the causes of obesity, mainly abdominal type, hypopituitarism and decreased growth hormone secretion has to be taken into consideration. Many authors mentioned growth hormone deficiency (GHD) as one of the main factors increasing the risk of obesity and dyslipidemia in patients after treatment of brain tumors [46-48] and other neoplasms, mainly ALL [49,50]. In the present study patients with damaged hypothalamic-pituitary area by neoplastic process with accompanying GHD, more frequently revealed excessive weight gain and dyslipidemia. After the year of treatment with recombinant growth hormone significant reduction of SDS BMI was observed.

In our previous study influence of treatment with recombinant growth hormone (rGH) on metabolic functions in patients after craniopharyngioma with pituitary insufficiency was assessed [48]. Growth hormone therapy caused significant BMI, LDL-cholesterol and HbA1c reduction one year after treatment.

Conclusions

In summary our study showed that patients after treatment of brain tumors localized in hypothalamic-pituitary area have the highest risk of abnormalities in carbohydrate metabolism, hyperinsulinemia in particular.

Moreover, age below 10 years at diagnosis and tumor localization in hypothalamic-pituitary area is related with more frequent excessive weight gain.

This single study is not sufficient to assess a reversibility of found abnormalities and there is a need of further observation.

References

1. Krawczuk-Rybak M (2008) [Improvement of the quality of life in children and adolescents after anticancer treatment - a challenge for doctors in XXI century]. Med Wieku Rozwoj 12: 987-994.
2. Han JW, Kwon SY, Won SC, Shin YJ, Ko JH, et al. (2009) Comprehensive clinical follow-up of late effects in childhood cancer survivors shows the need for early and well-timed intervention. Ann Oncol 20: 1170-1177.
3. Palczewska I, Niedzwiecka Z, Wskazniki rozwoju (2001) somatycznego dzieci i mlodziezy warszawskiej. Med Wieku Rozwoj 5: suppl. 1-2.
4. Mokha JS, Srinivasan SR, Dasmahapatra P, Fernandez C, Chen W, et al. (2010) Utility of waist-to-height ratio in assessing the status of central obesity and related cardiometabolic risk profile among normal weight and overweight/obese children: the Bogalusa Heart Study. BMC Pediatr 10: 73.
5. WHO (2006) Definition and diagnosis of diabetes mellitus and intermediate hyperglycemia: report of a WHO/IDF consultation. WHO Document Production Services, Geneva, Switzerland.
6. Ten S, Maclaren N (2004) Insulin resistance syndrome in children. J Clin Endocrinol Metab 89: 2526-2539.
7. Szurkowska M, Szafraniec K, Gilis-Januszewska A, Szybinski Z, Huszno B (2005) Insulin resistance indices in population-based study and their predictive value in defining metabolic syndrome. Przegl Epidemiol 59: 743-751.
8. Pietilä S, Mäkipernaa A, Sievänen H, Koivisto AM, Wigren T, et al. (2009) Obesity and metabolic changes are common in young childhood brain tumor survivors. Pediatr Blood Cancer 52: 853-859.
9. Gurney JG, Ness KK, Stovall M, Wolden S, Punyko JA, et al. (2003) Final height and body mass index among adult survivors of childhood brain cancer: childhood cancer survivor study. J Clin Endocrinol Metab 88: 4731-4739.
10. Lustig RH, Post SR, Srivannaboon K, Rose SR, Danish RK, et al. (2003) Risk factors for the development of obesity in children surviving brain tumors. J Clin Endocrinol Metab 88: 611-616.
11. Brauner R, Trivin C, Zerah M, Souberbielle JC, Doz F, et al. (2006) Diencephalic syndrome due to hypothalamic tumor: a model of the relationship between weight and puberty onset. J Clin Endocrinol Metab 91: 2467-2473.
12. Lek N, Prentice P, Williams RM, Ong KK, Burke GA, et al. (2010) Risk factors for obesity in childhood survivors of suprasellar brain tumours: a retrospective study. Acta Paediatr 99: 1522-1526.
13. Roth C, Wilken B, Hanefeld F, Schröter W, Leonhardt U (1998) Hyperphagia in children with craniopharyngioma is associated with hyperleptinaemia and a failure in the downregulation of appetite. Eur J Endocrinol 138: 89-91.
14. Lustig RH, Rose SR, Burghen GA, Velasquez-Mieyer P, Broome DC, et al. (1999) Hypothalamic obesity caused by cranial insult in children: altered glucose and insulin dynamics and reversal by a somatostatin agonist. J Pediatr 135: 162-168.
15. Trivin Ch, Busiah K, Mahlaoui N, Recasens C, Souberbielle JC, et al. (2009) Childhood craniopharyngioma: greater hypothalamic involvement before surgery is associated with higher homeostasis model insulin resistance index. BMC Pediatr, 9: 24.
16. Müller HL, Bueb K, Bartels U, Roth C, Harz K, et al. (2001) Obesity after childhood craniopharyngioma--German multicenter study on pre-operative risk factors and quality of life. Klin Padiatr 213: 244-249.
17. Müller HL, Emser A, Faldum A, Bruhnken G, Etavard-Gorris N, et al. (2004) Longitudinal study on growth and body mass index before and after diagnosis of childhood craniopharyngioma. J Clin Endocrinol Metab 89: 3298-3305.
18. de Haas EC, Oosting SF, Lefrandt JD, Wolffenbuttel BH, Sleijfer DT, et al. (2010) The metabolic syndrome in cancer survivors. Lancet Oncol 11: 193-203.
19. Brook Ch, Spoudeas HA (2001) Clinical Pediatric Endocrinology. Blackwell Science, Oxford.
20. Oberfield SE, Garvin JH Jr (2000) Thalamic and hypothalamic tumors of childhood: endocrine late effects. Pediatr Neurosurg 32: 264-271.
21. Srinivasan S, Ogle GD, Garnett SP, Briody JN, Lee JW, et al. (2004) Features of the metabolic syndrome after childhood craniopharyngioma. J Clin Endocrinol Metab 89: 81-86.
22. Pinkney J, Wilding J, Williams G, MacFarlane I (2002) Hypothalamic obesity in humans: what do we know and what can be done? Obes Rev 3: 27-34.
23. Pinto G, Bussières L, Recasens C, Souberbielle JC, Zerah M, et al. (2000) Hormonal factors influencing weight and growth pattern in craniopharyngioma. Horm Res 53: 163-169.
24. Meuric S, Brauner R, Trivin C, Souberbielle JC, Zerah M, et al. (2005) Influence of tumor location on the presentation and evolution of craniopharyngiomas. J Neurosurg 103: 421-426.
25. Daousi C, Dunn AJ, Foy PM, MacFarlane IA, Pinkney JH (2005) Endocrine and neuroanatomic features associated with weight gain and obesity in adult patients with hypothalamic damage. Am J Med 118: 45-50.
26. Inoue S, Bray GA (1977) The effects of subdiaphragmatic vagotomy in rats with ventromedial hypothalamic obesity. Endocrinology 100: 108-114.
27. Lustig RH, Hinds PS, Ringwald-Smith K, Christensen RK, Kaste SC, et al. (2003) Octreotide therapy in pediatric hypothalamic obesity: a double-blind, placebo-controlled trial. J Clin Endocrinol Metab, 88: 2586-2592.
28. Chiarelli F, Marcovecchio ML (2008) Insulin resistance and obesity in childhood. Eur J Endocrinol 159 Suppl 1: S67-74.
29. Crowley RK, Hamnvik OP, O'Sullivan EP, Behan LA, Smith D, et al. (2010) Morbidity and mortality in patients with craniopharyngioma after surgery. Clin Endocrinol (Oxf) 73: 516-521.
30. Deepak D, Furlong NJ, Wilding JP, MacFarlane IA (2007) Cardiovascular disease, hypertension, dyslipidaemia and obesity in patients with hypothalamic-pituitary disease. Postgrad Med J 83: 277-280.
31. Verhelst J, Kendall-Taylor P, Erfurth EM, Price DA, Geffner M, et al. (2005) Baseline Characteristics and Response to 2 Years of Growth Hormone (GH) Replacement of Hypopituitary Patients with GH Deficiency due to Adult-Onset Craniopharyngioma in Comparison with Patients with Nonfunctioning Pituitary Adenoma: Data from KIMS (Pfizer International Metabolic Database). J Clin Endocrinol Metab 90: 4636-4643.
32. Adams LA, Feldstein A, Lindor KD, Angulo P (2004) Nonalcoholic fatty liver disease among patients with hypothalamic and pituitary dysfunction. Hepatology 39: 909-914.
33. DeFronzo RA, Tobin JD, Andres R (1979) Glucose clamp technique: a method for quantifying insulin secretion and resistance. Am J Physiol 237: E214-223.
34. Szulinska M, Pupek-Musialik D, Bogdanski P, Miczke A, Bryl W (2006) Evaluation of insulin resistance with euglicemic clamp in obese patients. Endokrynologia, Otylosc, Zaburzenia Przemiany Materii 2: 5-11.
35. Yeni-Komshian H, Carantoni M, Abbasi F, Reaven GM (2000) Relationship Between Several Surrogate Estimates of Insulin Resistance and Quantification of Insulin-Mediated Glucose Disposal in 490 Healthy Nondiabetic Volunteers. Diabetes Care 23: 171–175.
36. Roth CL, Gebhardt U, Müller HL (2011) Appetite-regulating hormone changes in patients with craniopharyngioma. Obesity (Silver Spring) 19: 36-42.
37. Lowas S1, Malempati S, Marks D (2009) Body mass index predicts insulin resistance in survivors of pediatric acute lymphoblastic leukemia. Pediatr Blood Cancer 53: 58-63.
38. Brouwer CA, Gietema JA, Kamps WA, de Vries EG, Postma A (2007) Changes in body composition after childhood cancer treatment: impact on future health status--a review. Crit Rev Oncol Hematol 63: 32-46.
39. Gardner D, Shoback D (2011) Greenspan's basic & clinical endocrinology. (9 edn.) McGraw-Hill Medical Companies, China.

40. Oeffinger KC (2008) Are survivors of acute lymphoblastic leukemia (ALL) at increased risk of cardiovascular disease? Pediatr Blood Cancer 50: 462-467.

41. Surapolchai P, Hongeng S, Mahachoklertwattana P, Pakakasama S, Winaichatsak A, et al. (2010) Impaired Glucose Tolerance and Insulin Resistance in Survivors of Childhood Acute Lymphoblastic Leukemia: Prevalence and Risk Factors. J Pediatr Hematol Oncol 32: 383-389.

42. Oeffinger KC, Buchanan GR, Eshelman DA, Denke MA, Andrews TC, et al. (2001) Cardiovascular risk factors in young adult survivors of childhood acute lymphoblastic leukemia. J Pediatr Hematol Oncol 23: 424-430.

43. Oeffinger KC, Mertens AC, Sklar CA, Yasui Y, Fears T, et al. (2003) Obesity in adult survivors of childhood acute lymphoblastic leukemia: a report from the Childhood Cancer Survivor Study. J Clin Oncol 21: 1359-1365.

44. Hara M, Saitou E, Iwata F, Okada T, Harada K (2002) Waist-to-height ratio is the best predictor of cardiovascular disease risk factors in Japanese schoolchildren. J Atheroscler Thromb 9: 127-132.

45. Kahn HS, Imperatore G, Cheng YJ (2005) A population-based comparison of BMI percentiles and waist-to-height ratio for identifying cardiovascular risk in youth. J Pediatr 146: 482-488.

46. Heikens J, Ubbink MC, van der Pal HP, Bakker PJ, Fliers E, et al. (2000) Long term survivors of childhood brain cancer have an increased risk for cardiovascular disease. Cancer 88: 2116-2121.

47. Geffner M, Lundberg M, Koltowska-Häggström M, Abs R, Verhelst J, et al. (2004) Changes in Height, Weight, and Body Mass Index in Children with Craniopharyngioma after Three Years of Growth Hormone Therapy: Analysis of KIGS (Pfizer International Growth Database). J Clin Endocrinol Metab 89: 5435-5440.

48. Okonska M, Birkholz D, Korpal-Szczyrska M, Adamkiewicz-Drozynska E, Alska A, et al. (2010) The evaluation of the influence of growth hormone therapy on growing process and metabolic functions in patients after treatment of craniopharyngioma. Pediatric Endocrinology, Diabetes and Metabolism 16: 19-24.

49. Link K, Moëll C, Garwicz S, Cavallin-Ståhl E, Björk J, et al. (2004) Growth hormone deficiency predicts cardiovascular risk in young adults treated for acute lymphoblastic leukemia in childhood. J Clin Endocrinol Metab 89: 5003-5012.

50. Gurney JG, Ness KK, Sibley SD, O'Leary M, Dengel DR, et al. (2006) Metabolic syndrome and growth hormone deficiency in adult survivors of childhood acute lymphoblastic leukemia. Cancer 107: 1303-1312.

16

Central Functions of Glucagon-like Peptide-1: Roles in Energy Regulation and Neuroprotection

Rachel T McGrath[1,2*], Sarah J Glastras[1,2], Samantha L Hocking[1,2], Iona Tjoeng[3], Martin Krause[2,3] and Gregory R Fulcher[1,2]

[1]Department of Diabetes, Endocrinology and Metabolism, Royal North Shore Hospital, St Leonards, NSW 2065, Australia

[2]University of Sydney, Northern Clinical School, St Leonards, NSW 2065, Australia

[3]Department of Neurology, Royal North Shore Hospital, St Leonards, NSW 2065, Australia

[*]**Corresponding author:** Rachel McGrath, Department of Diabetes, Endocrinology & Metabolism, Level 3, Acute Services Building, Royal North Shore Hospital, St Leonards, Sydney, NSW 2065, Australia, Email: Rachel.McGrath@health.nsw.gov.au

Abstract

The identification of the glucagon-like peptide-1 receptor in the central nervous system has led to an array of studies exploring the functions of central GLP-1 signalling. Originally identified as a gastrointestinal incretin hormone responsible for the potentiation of insulin secretion following ingestion of nutrients, the role of GLP-1 has been expanded to include specific neural activities. Two distinct actions of GLP-1 receptor activation in the brain have been identified, namely the regulation of appetite via promotion of satiety, as well as anti-inflammatory and anti-apoptotic activity to promote neuronal cell survival. Both of these features are now being exploited clinically, with GLP-1 receptor agonists, initially designed and marketed for the treatment of hyperglycaemia in type 2 diabetes, now being directed towards use in obesity and as potential neuroprotective agents. This review gives a summary of the functional role of GLP-1 in the central nervous system, in terms of promoting satiety, modulating food intake and aiding in the regulation of peripheral glycaemia. In addition, the molecular mechanisms underpinning the beneficial effects of central GLP-1 receptor agonist therapy in protecting against neuronal cell inflammation and death, including neurodegenerative processes, are described.

Keywords: Glucagon-like peptide-1; Central nervous system; Glucose metabolism; Satiety; Neuroprotection

Introduction

Glucagon-like Peptide-1

Glucagon-like peptide-1 (GLP-1) is a peptide hormone secreted from specific populations of cells in both the distal gut and central nervous system (CNS). In response to nutrient intake, GLP-1 exerts its insulinotropic activity via direct stimulation of pancreatic β-cells to potentiate insulin secretion in a glucose-dependent manner [1]. Thus, the principal metabolic function of GLP-1 is that of an incretin hormone. GLP-1 further lowers blood glucose levels by slowing gastric emptying, thereby reducing postprandial hyperglycaemia. In addition, GLP-1 participates in the gut-to-brain axis by transmitting nutritional signals to the CNS, resulting in increased satiety [2].

The GLP-1 peptide is produced through posttranslational processing of proglucagon in the intestinal L-cells and preproglucagon neurons in the hindbrain [3]. Native GLP-1 is 37 amino acids in length and is proteolysed by prohormone convertase 1/3 to give rise to the major active circulating peptide; GLP-1(7-36)-amide [4]. This peptide engages and activates the GLP-1R on the surface of pancreatic β-cells when plasma glucose levels ≥5 mMol/L, resulting in a rise in intracellular Ca2+ and consequent secretion of insulin. GLP-1 mediated signalling also reduces the expression of pro-inflammatory and pro-apoptotic mediators, leading to enhanced pancreatic β-cell viability [5,6].

Regulation of endogenous GLP-1 activity occurs through rapid proteolytic inactivation in the circulation by dipeptidyl peptidase-4 (DPP-4), such that GLP-1 has a half-life of approximately 3 minutes. While the short half-life of GLP-1 limits the therapeutic utility of the native protein as a diabetes treatment, the development of degradation resistant forms of GLP-1 and inhibitors of DPP-4 (DPP-4i) has proved an important therapeutic advance in the management of type 2 diabetes [7]. Furthermore, due to the glucose-dependent nature of incretin-mediated insulin release, GLP-1 receptor agonists and DPP-4i are associated with a minimal risk of inducing hypoglycaemia [8].

The GLP-1 receptor (GLP-1R) has been localised in tissues outside the pancreas, including the heart, kidney and brain [9]. It is widely distributed throughout the central nervous system (CNS), with expression in the thalamus, hypothalamus, hippocampal region, cerebellum, cortex and brain stem [10]. Interestingly, GLP-1 has also been identified as a neuropeptide, and is produced by preproglucagon neurons of the nucleus of the solitary tract (NTS) located in the caudal brainstem [11,12]. Furthermore, GLP-1 positive cells have been identified in the hippocampus and cortex in rodents and GLP-1 is secreted from microglial cells via a cyclic AMP (cAMP) dependent pathway [13]. It has also been observed that the GLP-1 peptide can cross the blood brain barrier [14].

The pleiotropic actions of GLP-1 to preserve β-cell function and reduce inflammation have led to the hypothesis that GLP-1 receptor activation could also have beneficial effects in the CNS. In addition to the regulation of satiety following a meal, experimental data also suggest an important role of GLP-1 in neuroprotection. An overview of these data is provided below, with a focus on the effect of GLP-1 receptor activation in the modulation of food intake and glucose homeostasis, as well as the neuroprotective and anti-inflammatory properties of GLP-1 in ischaemic stroke and neurodegenerative disorders.

Central Activity of Glucagon-Like Peptide-1

Regulation of food intake

Ingestion of food leads to GLP-1 secretion from entero endocrine L-cells in the distal gut. As a consequence, insulin release from the pancreas is stimulated in a glucose-dependent fashion and satiety is increased through both central and peripheral effects [15]. There are several possible mechanisms through which GLP-1 modulates food intake. Firstly, GLP-1 transmits nutritional signals to the brain via activation of the enteric nervous system and/or vagus nerve in the gastrointestinal tract [16,17]. It has also been suggested that a small proportion of GLP-1 may escape degradation by DPP-4 and enter the systemic circulation to cross the blood brain barrier, where it may directly activate its receptor and increase satiety [18]. Moreover, food intake may lead to the release of GLP-1 from neurons in the nucleus of the solitary tract (NTS), and the activation the GLP-1R in the CNS [19]. GLP-1 additionally adds to the regulation of energy intake by decreasing gastrointestinal motility, thereby contributing to feelings of fullness [20].

In the absence of nutrient ingestion, central administration of GLP-1 limits food intake [18]. Intracerebro ventricular (ICV) injection of GLP-1 in rodents slowed gastric emptying, through non-adrenergic and non-cholinergic pathways [21]. The mechanisms through which this centrally mediated reduction in gastric motility occurs have not been completely elucidated, however a role for vagal afferent nerves has been proposed. Nutrient stimulated secretion of GLP-1 from the distal gut led to activation of hepatic vagal nerves [22], and the suppression of food intake mediated by peripherally administered GLP-1 was abolished in vagotomised individuals [23]. Targeted administration of GLP-1 receptor agonists in the hypothalamus and hindbrain diminished food intake, suggesting that both of these cerebral areas are important for GLP-1 mediated anorexia [24,25]. Furthermore, GLP-1 reactive nerve fibres extend from the NTS to the hypothalamus, a major centre in the brain for regulation of eating behaviour, and activation of hypothalamic GLP-1R inhibits feeding and promotes satiety [19,26]. In addition, ICV administration of the GLP-1 receptor agonist, exendin-4, gave rise to activation of neuropeptide Y, neurotensin, ghrelin and proopiomelanocortin neurons in the hypothalamus, leading to upregulated expression of appetite-regulating neuropeptides [27]. More recently, it was found that nestin-Cre mediated site-specific knockdown of the GLP-1 receptor in the hypothalamus and brain stem rendered high-fat fed rodents resistant to reductions in body weight and food intake induced by the long-acting GLP-1 analogue, liraglutide [28].

Several of the cellular pathways through which GLP-1R activation in the CNS modulates appetite have been identified. GLP-1 stimulates signalling cascades downstream of cAMP and protein kinase A (PKA) in the NTS, resulting in inhibition of food intake [29]. In particular, hindbrain GLP-1R activation suppresses energy intake via a PKA-mediated reduction in adenosine monophosphate protein kinase (AMPK) activity and concurrent upregulation of mitogen-activated protein kinase (MEK)/extracellular signal-related kinase-1/2 (ERK-1/2) pathways [24]. This has been proposed to ultimately lead to Ca2+-dependent depolarisation of GLP-1R expressing neurons, and long-term cAMP response element-binding protein (CREB)-mediated transcriptional changes in genes responsible for regulation of food intake [30]. Surprisingly, a role for the central cytokines interleukin-1β (IL-1β) and IL-6 was found in GLP-1 mediated suppression of food intake [31]. Ablation of IL-1β or IL-6 activity through either receptor blockade or knock-out gave rise to a reduction in GLP-1 mediated anorexia and loss of body weight in mice.

In clinical studies, infusion of GLP-1 led to increased satiety and reduced energy intake in obese individuals and also in patients with type 2 diabetes [32,33]. Similarly, GLP-1 dose-dependently reduced nutrient intake in lean and overweight individuals [34]. Interestingly, functional magnetic resonance imaging (fMRI) of the brain has shown that infusion of GLP-1 attenuates blood-oxygen level dependent signal changes in fasted individuals who were presented with images of food [35]. Likewise, continuous administration of exenatide, a GLP-1 analogue, reduced food intake in obese men which correlated with enhanced hypothalamic activity, as measured by fMRI [36]. The favourable effects of GLP-1 on reducing appetite and food intake have been exploited in a recent clinical trial, where liraglutide therapy for 56 weeks resulted in clinically significant weight loss in non-diabetic obese individuals [37] With additional human studies underway [38,39], it is highly likely that a new therapeutic indication for GLP-1 will be established in the coming years, to aid in the reduction of excess body weight in obese individuals through augmentation of central GLP-1R mediated appetite suppression.

Glycaemic Control and Peripheral Glucose Homeostasis

While the chief physiological function of GLP-1 is in the glucose-dependent stimulation of insulin secretion to regulate systemic glycaemia, a glucose lowering effect of GLP-1 has also been recognised in the brain. In healthy male subjects administered glucose via IV infusion, GLP-1 leads to decreased glucose concentrations in all cerebral areas with an increase in glucose metabolism through enhanced hexokinase activity during hyperglycaemia [40]. Similarly, glucose transport across the blood brain barrier (BBB) is down-regulated by GLP-1 in healthy individuals with normal blood glucose levels [41]. In the presence of hypoglycaemia, GLP-1 does not affect brain-glucose concentrations, nor does it influence glucose metabolism or transfer across the BBB [42].

A further role of central GLP-1 is to regulate peripheral glucose homeostasis (Figure 1). As evidenced in animal studies, stimulation of the GLP-1R in the CNS leads to increased insulin secretion and greater hepatic glycogen storage, during hyperglycaemia [43]. Interestingly, GLP-1 signalling in the CNS facilitates glucose-uptake into skeletal muscle in an insulin-dependent and non-insulin dependent manner, as seen in MIRKO mice, a muscle insulin receptor knock-out model. In another study, ICV administration of GLP-1 in rodents augmented glucose-dependent insulin release, and decreased glucose production in the liver [44]. Moreover, it was demonstrated that antagonism of arcuate GLP-1 receptors in the rat brain increased the magnitude of glycaemic excursion during a glucose tolerance test. GLP-1 regulates peripheral glucose levels via activation of the afferent nervous system, through slowed gastric emptying and a concomitant reduction in absorption of glucose into the bloodstream [45]. Furthermore, GLP-1 can promote enhanced energy expenditure, through CNS signalling pathways; ICV administration of GLP-1 gave rise to increased thermogenesis in brown adipose tissue of C57BL/6 mice, which the authors suggest contributes to the mechanisms by which GLP-1 regulates energy balance [46].

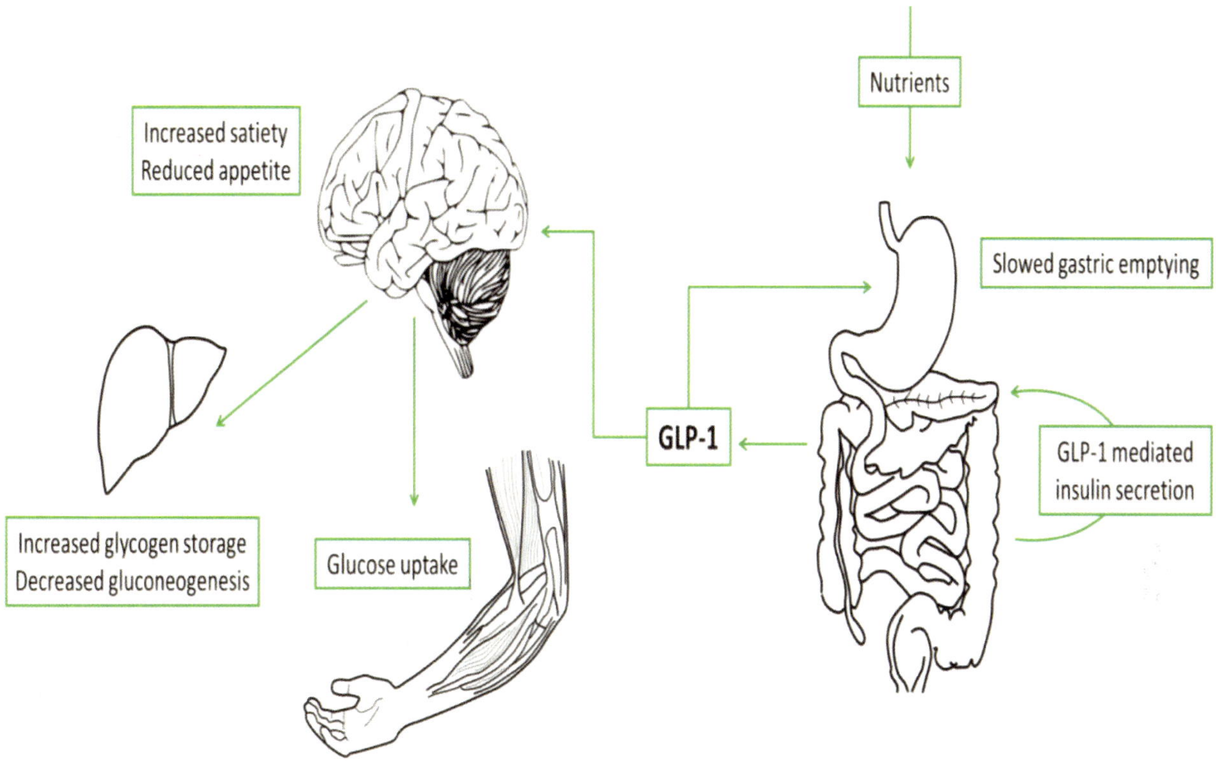

Figure 1: Functions of GLP-1 in the regulation of glycaemia. Upon ingestion of food, GLP-1 is secreted from the L cells in the lower gut and potentiates (glucose-dependent) insulin secretion from pancreatic β-cells, whilst also stimulating centrally mediated signals that give rise to a reduction in appetite, and peripheral uptake of glucose in both liver and muscle.

Sisley et al. recently observed that CNS expression of the GLP-1R is not necessary for peripheral glucose regulation, as administration of liraglutide reduced glucose excursions in the absence of neuronal GLP-1R [28]. This implies that pancreatic GLP-R activation is sufficient for the glucose lowering activity of GLP-1; however previous evidence suggests a direct role of central GLP-1R activation in the modulation of systemic glucose homeostasis [43,44]. Finally, administration of the GLP-1 receptor agonist liraglutide to patients with type 2 diabetes gave rise to a decrease in fasting endogenous glucose release due to a reduction in hepatic glycogenolysis, although the role of central GLP-1R signalling in this process is unclear [47].

Glucagon-like Peptide-1 and Neuroprotection

Anti-inflammatory properties of GLP-1 in the brain

The cytoprotective and anti-inflammatory effects of GLP-1 have been demonstrated in several cell types, including pancreatic islets and endothelial cells [48-50]. In addition, a recent study has shown that stimulation of the GLP-1 receptor reduces the inflammatory response in the kidneys of diabetic rodents, independent of GLP-1 blood-glucose lowering activity [51]. In each of these studies, improvements in cell viability and a concomitant reduction in the expression of pro-inflammatory adhesion molecules and cytokines was observed.

In vitro experiments initially revealed that GLP-1 exerts neuroprotective activity in neuronal cell culture, [52] promotes cell survival and proliferation, and prevents apoptosis and oxidative-stress-associated cell death in mammalian glial and hippocampal cells (Figure 2). The pathways involved in GLP-1 mediated neuronal cell proliferation are downstream of protein kinase A and phosphoinositide 3-kinase activity, and enhanced cell survival arises through modulation of apoptotic signal expression (decreased bax and caspase-3, and increased bcl-2; Figure 3) [53-56]. GLP-1 further regulates inflammatory cytokine expression in the brain; lipopolysaccharide (LPS) challenge in activated microglia and astrocytes gave rise to a significant increase in IL-1β, and this increase was attenuated in the presence of GLP-1 [57]. This finding is in contrast to that observed by Shirazi and colleagues, who showed that GLP-1 promotes IL-1β expression in the brain, to reduce food intake and appetite. Thus, GLP-1 may differentially influence the expression of central cytokines, dependent on the initial stimulus or upon which signalling pathway is activated. More recently, it was found that the GLP-1 receptor agonist liraglutide enhanced cell viability and prevented cytotoxicity and apoptosis in human neuroblastoma cells exposed to methylglyoxal stress [58]. The mechanisms through which this increase in cell viability occurs include activation of the transcription factor p90RSK, which modulates the expression of genes associated with the cellular response to stress.

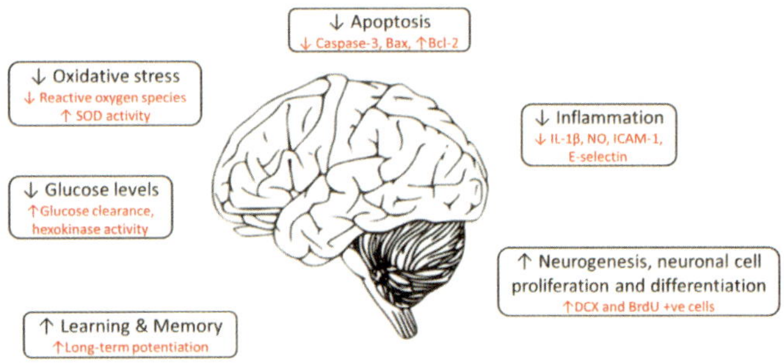

Figure 2: Glucagon-like peptide-1 activity in the brain gives rise to neuroprotection, through various molecular mechanisms. The mechanisms through which GLP-1 elicits a neuroprotective effect in the brain are outlined. General mechanisms are indicated in black, with specific molecular pathways in red. GLP-1 enhances neurogenesis, neuronal cell proliferation and differentiation, as evidenced by increases in the cell proliferation markers DCX and BrdU. Stimulation of the GLP-1 receptor prevents apoptosis, with a decrease in pro-apoptotic signalling molecules caspase-3 and bax, as well as greater levels of anti-apoptotic bcl-2 observed. Favourable effects on learning and memory are also seen, as reflected by enhancements in long-term potentiation, a marker of synaptic plasticity and a major mechanism underlying the processes of memory and learning in the brain. Oxidative stress is ameliorated through a reduction in reactive oxygen species. Finally, GLP-1 lowers blood glucose levels in the brain, preventing hyperglycaemia associated inflammation and cell death during ischaemia [40].

The role of GLP-1 in attenuating neuroinflammation has been also demonstrated using animal models. Both liraglutide and its metabolite GLP-1 (9-36) decreased the expression of pro-inflammatory markers such as ICAM-1 and E-selectin after intracerebral haemorrhage in mice [59]. Indeed, it was also found that liraglutide reduced the number of neutrophils in the perihaematoma region, further downregulating neuroinflammation. In addition, chronic irradiation-induced inflammation in rodent brains was ameliorated by treatment with GLP-1, with lower levels of markers such as interleukin-6 and nitrite observed [60,61]. GLP-1 receptor stimulation through treatment with the GLP-1 analogue exendin-4 minimised mild traumatic brain injury induced deficits in mice, again through reduction of oxidative stress associated inflammation [62]. This study demonstrated that administration of GLP-1 gave rise to increased levels of neuronal cell survival in response to challenge with the oxidative stress mediator hydrogen peroxide, and also protected cells against glutamate-induced toxicity.

Due to the modulatory effects of GLP-1 on neuroinflammation, a key process in the pathogenesis of neurodegenerative disorders and cerebral injury, it has been proposed that GLP-1 may be a viable treatment option for targeting inflammation in the brain, and as such, further clinical studies in this area are warranted

GLP-1 and Ischaemic Stroke

Diabetes is an established risk factor for the development of ischaemic events, such as stroke. Persistently high blood glucose after stroke correlates with larger infarct volume, and hyperglycaemia is an independent predictor for increased functional impairment, disability and mortality [63-66]. The mechanisms through which hyperglycaemia may exert a deleterious effect in ischaemic stroke include heightened lactic acidosis, enhanced production of free radicals, oxidative stress and augmentation of inflammation. As previously described, GLP-1 effectively lowers hyperglycaemia in the brain and furthermore, ameliorates oxidative stress and inflammation in preclinical models of brain injury and inflammatory challenge [40]. In addition, GLP-1 therapy resulted in favourable effects in a rodent model of ischaemic stroke and concomitant type 2 diabetes, with a dose-dependent reduction in hyperglycaemia, inflammation and neuronal tissue damage [67]. Treatment of mice with the DPP-4 inhibitor linagliptin significantly enhanced circulating levels of GLP-1, and lowered both fasting and fed blood glucose levels. Treated mice also showed a marked decrease in ischaemic brain damage [68].

In a recent clinical study, patients with acute ischaemic stroke were given subcutaneous exenatide for glycaemic control. It was observed that blood glucose levels were effectively regulated, with minimal incidence of hyperglycaemia and no symptomatic hypoglycaemia [69]. These promising preliminary results suggest that GLP-1 therapy may be a viable treatment option for individuals with hyperglycaemia in ischaemic stroke, with negligible glycaemic variability, and low risk of hypoglycaemia. This may lead to improved outcomes for patients with acute stroke, as hypoglycaemia has been associated with poorer outcomes and an increased risk of morbidity and mortality [70].

The mechanisms through which GLP-1 exerts its beneficial effects in stroke, in addition to glycaemic control, have been determined in a variety of preclinical models. Administration of exendin-4 was shown to reduce brain damage and improve functional outcome in a transient middle cerebral artery occlusion stroke model, independent of its blood glucose lowering activity [71,72]. Likewise, treatment of rats with exendin-4 confers significant neurological protection following cerebral ischemia as a consequence of middle cerebral artery occlusion with a reduction in infarct size, oxidative stress levels and neurological deficit [73]. In particular, exendin-4 was found to increase the levels of superoxide dismutase (SOD), an antioxidative enzyme that reduces the concentration of harmful superoxide within cells. More recently, GLP-1 treated rats showed an improvement in behavioural score and smaller infarct volumes after stroke [74]. A reduction in reactive oxygen metabolites and an increase in the levels of vascular endothelial growth factor (VEGF) were seen, reinforcing the premise that GLP-1 down-regulates oxidative stress and promotes oxygenation. It has also been observed that administration of exendin-4 to rodents protects against ischaemia-induced activation of microglial cells, thereby preventing premature microglial cell death [75].

Interestingly, GLP-1 exerts cardioprotective activity in patients with myocardial infarction (MI) and ischaemic heart disease. In a small cohort of non-diabetic patients, treatment with GLP-1 led to an improvement in left ventricular function (LVF) and a reduction in ischaemic dysfunction after coronary balloon occlusion during percutaneous coronary intervention [76]. Infusion of GLP-1 to patients after acute MI enhanced LVF and increased recovery in the peri-infarct area, and exenatide was shown to improve myocardial salvage after ST-segment elevation MI [77,78]. Epidemiological data has further found that individuals taking exenatide had a lower incidence of cardiovascular disease, including stroke [79]. These results, taken together with the above animal data, suggest that GLP-1 therapy may lead to favourable outcomes after ischaemic injury, both in the heart and CNS. Indeed, GLP-1 may exert a dual protective effect in the ischaemic brain, in terms of preventing hyperglycaemia associated neurological damage, and directly ameliorating neuro inflammation and oxidative stress associated cell death.

Protective Role of GLP-1 in Neurodegenerative Disorders

The risk of developing neurodegenerative disorders such as dementia and Parkinson's disease is significantly increased in individuals with diabetes [80,81]. The pathogenesis of neurological impairment and injury in these disorders includes premature neuronal cell death, oxidative stress and neuro inflammation, processes that may be attenuated by GLP-1 signalling in the brain. Interestingly, GLP-1 receptor knockout mice demonstrated impaired learning, memory and cognitive ability, as well as a reduction in recovery after neurological insult, suggesting an intrinsic role for endogenous GLP-1 in maintaining normal brain activity [82,83].

Pre-clinical models of neuro degeneration have been used to show that GLP-1 therapy is beneficial in preserving neurological function. In a mouse model of Alzheimer's disease, both short- and long-term administration of the GLP-1 receptor agonist, liraglutide, resulted in increased neuronal cell survival and proliferation, and enhanced neurogenesis [84]. Furthermore, several studies have demonstrated that GLP-1 preserves synaptic plasticity and further reduces the accumulation of the pathogenic β-amyloid protein in the brain of preclinical models of Alzheimer's disease [61,85]. Administration of GLP-1 dose-dependently conserved spatial memory in rats exposed to β-amyloid, by protecting hippocampal long-term potentiation between neurons. Similarly, GLP-1 was found to be protective against neuro degeneration in a Parkinson's disease model; administration of exendin-4 reduced functional impairment and also increased the number of neuronal precursor cells, showing protection against loss of neurons [86,87]. Treatment with exendin-4 increased levels of L-DOPA and tyrosine hydroxylase after challenge with 6-OHDA (a selective inducer of Parkinsonism), suggesting that GLP-1 can rescue dopaminergic neurons after damage has occurred. Finally, GLP-1 improves motor performance and extends survival in a murine model of Huntington's disease [88].

GLP-1 is currently being explored as a potential neuroprotective agent in patients with dementia and Parkinson's disease [89]. A recent pilot study investigated the effect of exenatide treatment in addition to regular therapy on neurological function in non-diabetic individuals with Parkinson's disease. Exenatide was well tolerated and patients in the treated group showed a significant reduction in disease progression and improvements in motor and cognitive skills [90]. Phase 1 studies have also been completed for a novel GLP-1 delivery system, where CellBeads® containing mesenchymal stem cells that overexpress GLP-1 are inserted directly at the site of injury in patients with haemorrhagic stroke, with the aim of eliciting GLP-1 mediated protection against neuronal cell damage [91]. Two further clinical trials have been described, where the effect of liraglutide on glucose metabolism and functional outcome in Alzheimer's disease, and in reducing reperfusion injury after acute stroke will be studied [92,93]. Moreover, GLP-1 has also been suggested as a prospective treatment option for the cognitive impairments observed in individuals with mood disorders [94].

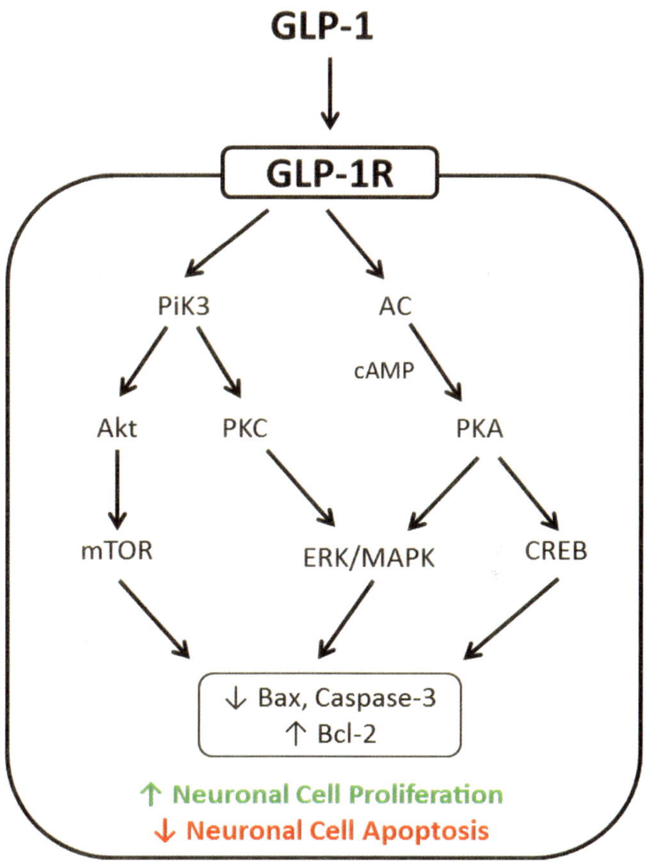

Figure 3: Summary of the principal signalling pathways through which glucagon-like peptide-1 receptor activation promotes neuronal cell survival. Stimulation of the GLP-1R on the surface of neuronal calls activates protective signalling pathways, downstream of phosphoinoside kinase 3 (PiK3) and adenylate cyclase (AC) [63]. Activation of protein kinase A (PKA) leads to modulation of pro-survival gene expression via the extracellular signal-related kinase/mitogen-activated protein kinase (ERK/MAPK) and cAMP response element-binding protein (CREB) pathways [52,56]. Similarly, protein kinase C (PKC) and Akt signal through ERK/MAPK and mTOR (mammalian target of rapamycin), respectively, to promote neuronal cell proliferation and modulate levels of apoptotic gene expression (decreased Bax and Caspase-3; increased Bcl-2).

Conclusions

Characterisation of GLP-1R activation in the CNS, in both in-vitro and pre-clinical models has enabled an understanding of the dual regulatory activities of central GLP-1 signalling. First, GLP-1R activation leads to increased satiety and a reduction in food intake [95]. Second, GLP-1 signalling in the brain regulates peripheral glucose metabolism, through modulation of glucose uptake. Thus, GLP-1 has an important role in energy homeostasis; initially to regulate food intake limiting nutrient ingestion and further to influence how nutrient-derived energy is metabolised peripherally.

Another consequence of central GLP-1R activation is in the protection of neuronal cells against damage and premature cell death. This neuroprotective activity of GLP-1 is achieved through ameliorating inflammation and oxidative stress, processes that occur in the brain after an ischaemic event and also during neurodegeneration. In addition, GLP-1 may additionally protect against the neurological consequences of hyperglycaemia. In turn, this could potentially lead to improved outcomes in acute stroke and neurodegeneration with several studies showing a correlation between stress hyperglycaemia and functional outcome, morbidity and mortality [96]. Furthermore, it has recently been hypothesised that GLP-1 agonists could lower blood glucose levels without the risk of hypoglycaemia in critically ill patients, thereby minimising the occurrence of treatment-related morbidity [97].

By further elucidating the molecular mechanisms responsible for the beneficial effects of GLP-1R activation in the brain, it may be possible to harness the neuroprotective properties of GLP-1 for the targeted treatment of ischaemic stroke and neurodegenerative disease. Moreover, clinical trials are currently underway where GLP-1 analogues are being utilised as anti-obesity therapies, due to their potent effects on satiety and food intake [98-101]. As such, GLP-1 could soon be added to our armamentarium as a therapeutic target above and beyond its usefulness as a glucose-regulating agent in type 2 diabetes.

References

1. Drucker DJ (2006) The biology of incretin hormones. Cell Metab 3: 153-165.
2. Burcelin R, Serino M, Cabou C (2009) A role for the gut-to-brain GLP-1-dependent axis in the control of metabolism. Curr Opin Pharmacol 9: 744-752.
3. Baggio LL, Drucker DJ (2007) Biology of incretins: GLP-1 and GIP. Gastroenterology; 132: 2131-2157.
4. Dhanvantari S, Seidah NG, Brubaker PL (1996) Role of prohormone convertases in the tissue-specific processing of proglucagon. Mol Endocrinol 10: 342-355.
5. Brubaker PL, Drucker DJ (2004) Minireview: Glucagon-like peptides regulate cell proliferation and apoptosis in the pancreas, gut, and central nervous system. Endocrinology 145: 2653-2659.
6. Yusta B, Baggio LL, Estall JL, Koehler JA, Holland DP, et al. (2006) GLP-1 receptor activation improves beta cell function and survival following induction of endoplasmic reticulum stress. Cell Metab 4: 391-406.
7. Drucker DJ, Nauck MA (2006) The incretin system: glucagon-like peptide-1 receptor agonists and dipeptidyl peptidase-4 inhibitors in type 2 diabetes. Lancet 368: 1696-1705.
8. Meloni AR, DeYoung MB, Lowe C, Parkes DG (2013) GLP-1 receptor activated insulin secretion from pancreatic Î^{2}-cells: mechanism and glucose dependence. Diabetes Obes Metab 15: 15-27.
9. Holst JJ (2007) The physiology of glucagon-like peptide 1. Physiol Rev 87: 1409-1439.
10. Alvarez E, Martínez MD, Roncero I, Chowen JA, García-Cuartero B, et al. (2005) The expression of GLP-1 receptor mRNA and protein allows the effect of GLP-1 on glucose metabolism in the human hypothalamus and brainstem. J Neurochem 92: 798-806.
11. Larsen PJ, Holst JJ (2005) Glucagon-related peptide 1 (GLP-1): hormone and neurotransmitter. Regul Pept 128: 97-107.
12. Trapp S, Richards JE (2013) The gut hormone glucagon-like peptide-1 produced in brain: is this physiologically relevant? Curr Opin Pharmacol 13: 964-969.
13. Kappe C, Tracy LM, Patrone C, Iverfeldt K, Sjöholm Å (2012) GLP-1 secretion by microglial cells and decreased CNS expression in obesity. J Neuroinflammation 9: 276.
14. Kastin AJ, Akerstrom V, Pan W (2002) Interactions of glucagon-like peptide-1 (GLP-1) with the blood-brain barrier. J Mol Neurosci 18: 7-14.
15. Rodriquez de Fonseca F, Navarro M, Alvarez E, Roncero I, Chowen JA, et al. (2000) Peripheral versus central effects of glucagon-like peptide-1 receptor agonists on satiety and body weight loss in Zucker obese rats. Metabolism 49: 709-717.
16. Burcelin R, Cani PD, Knauf C (2007) Glucagon-like peptide-1 and energy homeostasis. J Nutr 137: 2534S-2538S.
17. Näslund E, Hellström PM (2007) Appetite signaling: from gut peptides and enteric nerves to brain. Physiol Behav 92: 256-262.
18. Dailey MJ, Moran TH (2013) Glucagon-like peptide 1 and appetite. Trends Endocrinol Metab 24: 85-91.
19. Vrang N, Hansen M, Larsen PJ, Tang-Christensen M (2007) Characterization of brainstem preproglucagon projections to the paraventricular and dorsomedial hypothalamic nuclei. Brain research 1149: 118-126.
20. Näslund E, Gutniak M, Skogar S, Rössner S, Hellström PM (1998) Glucagon-like peptide 1 increases the period of postprandial satiety and slows gastric emptying in obese men. Am J Clin Nutr 68: 525-530.
21. ImeryÃ¼z N, YeÄŸen BC, Bozkurt A, CoÅŸkun T, Villanueva-PeÃ ±acarrillo ML, et al. (1997) Glucagon-like peptide-1 inhibits gastric emptying via vagal afferent-mediated central mechanisms. Am J Physiol 273: G920-927.
22. Nakabayashi H, Nishizawa M, Nakagawa A, Takeda R, Niijima A (1996) Vagal hepatopancreatic reflex effect evoked by intraportal appearance of tGLP-1. Am J Physiol 271: E808-813.
23. Plamboeck A, Veedfald S, Deacon CF, Hartmann B, Wettergren A, et al. (2013) The effect of exogenous GLP-1 on food intake is lost in male truncally vagotomized subjects with pyloroplasty. Am J Physiol Gastrointest Liver Physiol 304: G1117-1127.
24. Hayes MR, Leichner TM, Zhao S, Lee GS, Chowansky A, et al. (2011) Intracellular signals mediating the food intake-suppressive effects of hindbrain glucagon-like peptide-1 receptor activation. Cell Metab 13: 320-330.
25. Schick RR, Zimmermann JP, vorm Walde T, Schusdziarra V (2003) Peptides that regulate food intake: glucagon-like peptide 1-(7-36) amide acts at lateral and medial hypothalamic sites to suppress feeding in rats. American journal of physiology Regulatory, integrative and comparative physiology; 284: R1 427-435.
26. Turton MD, O'Shea D, Gunn I, Beak SA, Edwards CM, et al. (1996) A role for glucagon-like peptide-1 in the central regulation of feeding. Nature 379: 69-72.
27. Dalvi PS, Nazarians-Armavil A, Purser MJ, Belsham DD (2012) Glucagon-like peptide-1 receptor agonist, exendin-4, regulates feeding-associated neuropeptides in hypothalamic neurons in vivo and in vitro. Endocrinology; 153: 2208-22.
28. Sisley S, Gutierrez-Aguilar R, Scott M, Alessio DA, Sandoval DA, et al. (2014) Neuronal GLP1R mediates liraglutide's anorectic but not glucose-lowering effect. J Clin Invest 124: 2456-2463.
29. Hayes MR, De Jonghe BC, Kanoski SE (2010) Role of the glucagon-like-peptide-1 receptor in the control of energy balance. Physiology & behavior; 100: 503-510.
30. Hayes MR (2012) Neuronal and intracellular signaling pathways mediating GLP-1 energy balance and glycemic effects. Physiol Behav 106: 413-416.
31. Shirazi R , Palsdottir V, Collander J, Anesten F, Vogel H, et al. (2013) Glucagon-like peptide 1 receptor induced suppression of food intake, and body weight is mediated by central IL-1 and IL-6. Proc Natl Acad Sci U S A 110: 16199-16204.
32. Naslund E, Barkeling B, King N (1999) Energy intake and appetite are suppressed by glucagon-like peptide-1 (GLP-1) in obese men.

International journal of obesity and related metabolic disorders: journal of the International Association for the Study of Obesity 23: 304-311.

33. Gutzwiller JP, Drewe J, Göke B, Schmidt H, Rohrer B, et al. (1999) Glucagon-like peptide-1 promotes satiety and reduces food intake in patients with diabetes mellitus type 2. Am J Physiol 276: R1541-1544.
34. Verdich C, Flint A, Gutzwiller JP, Näslund E, Beglinger C, et al. (2001) A meta-analysis of the effect of glucagon-like peptide-1 (7-36) amide on ad libitum energy intake in humans. J Clin Endocrinol Metab 86: 4382-4389.
35. De Silva A, Salem V, Long CJ, Makwana A, Newbould RD, et al. (2011) The gut hormones PYY 3-36 and GLP-1 7-36 amide reduce food intake and modulate brain activity in appetite centers in humans. Cell Metab 14: 700-706.
36. Schlogl H, Kabisch S, Horstmann A (2013) Exenatide-induced reduction in energy intake is associated with increase in hypothalamic connectivity. Diabetes care; 36: 1933-1940.
37. Wadden TA, Hollander P, Klein S, Niswender K, Woo V, et al. (2013) Weight maintenance and additional weight loss with liraglutide after low-calorie-diet-induced weight loss: the SCALE Maintenance randomized study. Int J Obes (Lond) 37: 1443-1451.
38. Kelly AS, Rudser KD, Nathan BM, Fox CK, Metzig AM, et al. (2013) The effect of glucagon-like peptide-1 receptor agonist therapy on body mass index in adolescents with severe obesity: a randomized, placebo-controlled, clinical trial. JAMA Pediatr 167: 355-360.
39. (2013) Treatment of Antipsychotic-associated Obesity With a GLP-1 Analogue (TAO).
40. Gejl M, Egefjord L, Lerche S (2012) Glucagon-like peptide-1 decreases intracerebral glucose content by activating hexokinase and changing glucose clearance during hyperglycemia. Journal of cerebral blood flow and metabolism: official journal of the International Society of Cerebral Blood Flow and Metabolism 32: 2146-2152.
41. Lerche S, Brock B, Rungby J, Bøtker HE, Møller N, et al. (2008) Glucagon-like peptide-1 inhibits blood-brain glucose transfer in humans. Diabetes 57: 325-331.
42. Gejl M, Lerche S, Egefjord L, Brock B, Møller N, et al. (2013) Glucagon-like peptide-1 (GLP-1) raises blood-brain glucose transfer capacity and hexokinase activity in human brain. Front Neuroenergetics 5: 2.
43. Knauf C, Cani PD, Perrin C (2005) Brain glucagon-like peptide-1 increases insulin secretion and muscle insulin resistance to favor hepatic glycogen storage. The Journal of clinical investigation 115: 3554-3563.
44. Sandoval DA, Bagnol D, Woods SC, D'Alessio DA, Seeley RJ (2008) Arcuate glucagon-like peptide 1 receptors regulate glucose homeostasis but not food intake. Diabetes 57: 2046-2054.
45. Sandoval D (2008) CNS GLP-1 regulation of peripheral glucose homeostasis. Physiol Behav 94: 670-674.
46. Lockie SH, Heppner KM, Chaudhary N, Chabenne JR, Morgan DA, et al. (2012) Direct control of brown adipose tissue thermogenesis by central nervous system glucagon-like peptide-1 receptor signaling. Diabetes 61: 2753-2762.
47. Degn KB, Juhl CB, Sturis J (2004) One week's treatment with the long-acting glucagon-like peptide 1 derivative liraglutide (NN2211) markedly improves 24-h glycemia and alpha- and beta-cell function and reduces endogenous glucose release in patients with type 2 diabetes. Diabetes; 53: 1187-1194.
48. Cechin SR, Pérez-Álvarez I, Fenjves E, Molano RD, Pileggi A, et al. (2012) Anti-inflammatory properties of exenatide in human pancreatic islets. Cell Transplant 21: 633-648.
49. Krasner NM, Ido Y, Ruderman NB, Cacicedo JM (2014) Glucagon-like peptide-1 (GLP-1) analog liraglutide inhibits endothelial cell inflammation through a calcium and AMPK dependent mechanism. PLoS One 9: e97554.
50. Ceriello A, Novials A, Ortega E, Canivell S, La Sala L, et al. (2013) Glucagon-like peptide 1 reduces endothelial dysfunction, inflammation, and oxidative stress induced by both hyperglycemia and hypoglycemia in type 1 diabetes. Diabetes Care 36: 2346-2350.
51. Kodera R, Shikata K, Kataoka HU (2011). Glucagon-like peptide-1 receptor agonist ameliorates renal injury through its anti-inflammatory action without lowering blood glucose level in a rat model of type 1 diabetes. Diabetologia; 54: 965-978.
52. Velmurugan K, Bouchard R, Mahaffey G, Pugazhenthi S (2012) Neuroprotective actions of glucagon-like peptide-1 in differentiated human neuroprogenitor cells. J Neurochem 123: 919-931.
53. Perry T, Haughey NJ, Mattson MP, Egan JM, Greig NH (2002) Protection and reversal of excitotoxic neuronal damage by glucagon-like peptide-1 and exendin-4. J Pharmacol Exp Ther 302: 881-888.
54. Holst JJ, Burcelin R, Nathanson E (2011) Neuroprotective properties of GLP-1: theoretical and practical applications. Curr Med Res Opin 27: 547-558.
55. Liu WJ, Jin HY, Lee KA, Xie SH, Baek HS, et al. (2011) Neuroprotective effect of the glucagon-like peptide-1 receptor agonist, synthetic exendin-4, in streptozotocin-induced diabetic rats. Br J Pharmacol 164: 1410-1420.
56. Li Y, Tweedie D, Mattson MP, Holloway HW, Greig NH (2010) Enhancing the GLP-1 receptor signaling pathway leads to proliferation and neuroprotection in human neuroblastoma cells. J Neurochem 113: 1621-1631.
57. Iwai T, Ito S, Tanimitsu K, Udagawa S, Oka J (2006) Glucagon-like peptide-1 inhibits LPS-induced IL-1beta production in cultured rat astrocytes. Neurosci Res 55: 352-360.
58. Sharma MK, Jalewa J, Hölscher C (2014) Neuroprotective and anti-apoptotic effects of liraglutide on SH-SY5Y cells exposed to methylglyoxal stress. J Neurochem 128: 459-471.
59. Hou J, Manaenko A, Hakon J, Hansen-Schwartz J, Tang J, et al. (2012) Liraglutide, a long-acting GLP-1 mimetic, and its metabolite attenuate inflammation after intracerebral hemorrhage. Journal of cerebral blood flow and metabolism: official journal of the International Society of Cerebral Blood Flow and Metabolism 32: 2201-2210.
60. Parthsarathy V, Hölscher C (2013) The type 2 diabetes drug liraglutide reduces chronic inflammation induced by irradiation in the mouse brain. Eur J Pharmacol 700: 42-50.
61. McClean PL, Parthsarathy V, Faivre E, Hölscher C (2011) The diabetes drug liraglutide prevents degenerative processes in a mouse model of Alzheimer's disease. J Neurosci 31: 6587-6594.
62. Rachmany L, Tweedie D, Li Y, Rubovitch V, Holloway HW, et al. (2013) Exendin-4 induced glucagon-like peptide-1 receptor activation reverses behavioral impairments of mild traumatic brain injury in mice. Age (Dordr) 35: 1621-1636.
63. Hölscher C (2014) Central effects of GLP-1: new opportunities for treatments of neurodegenerative diseases. J Endocrinol 221: T31-41.
64. Plummer MP, Meier JJ, Deane AM (2013) The gut-brain axis in the critically ill: is glucagon-like peptide-1 protective in neurocritical care? Crit Care 17: 163.
65. Lindsberg PJ, Roine RO (2004) Hyperglycemia in acute stroke. Stroke 35: 363-364.
66. Baird TA, Parsons MW, Phanh T (2003) Persistent poststroke hyperglycemia is independently associated with infarct expansion and worse clinical outcome. Stroke; a journal of cerebral circulation; 34: 2208-2214.
67. Darsalia V, Mansouri S, Ortsäter H, Olverling A, Nozadze N, et al. (2012) Glucagon-like peptide-1 receptor activation reduces ischaemic brain damage following stroke in Type 2 diabetic rats. Clin Sci (Lond) 122: 473-483.
68. Darsalia V, Ortsäter H, Olverling A, Darlöf E, Wolbert P, et al. (2013) The DPP-4 inhibitor linagliptin counteracts stroke in the normal and diabetic mouse brain: a comparison with glimepiride. Diabetes 62: 1289-1296.
69. Daly SC, Chemmanam T, Loh PS, Gilligan A, Dear AE, et al. (2013) Exenatide in acute ischemic stroke. Int J Stroke 8: E44.
70. Hsu PF, Sung SH, Cheng HM, Yeh JS, Liu WL, et al. (2013) Association of clinical symptomatic hypoglycemia with cardiovascular events and

total mortality in type 2 diabetes: a nationwide population-based study. Diabetes Care 36: 894-900.

71. Li Y, Perry T, Kindy MS (2009). GLP-1 receptor stimulation preserves primary cortical and dopaminergic neurons in cellular and rodent models of stroke and Parkinsonism. Proceedings of the National Academy of Sciences of the United States of America; 106: 1285-1290.
72. Teramoto S, Miyamoto N, Yatomi K (2011). Exendin-4, a glucagon-like peptide-1 receptor agonist, provides neuroprotection in mice transient focal cerebral ischemia. Journal of cerebral blood flow and metabolism: official journal of the International Society of Cerebral Blood Flow and Metabolism; 31: 1696-1705.
73. Briyal S, Gulati K, Gulati A (2012) Repeated administration of exendin-4 reduces focal cerebral ischemia-induced infarction in rats. Brain Res 1427: 23-34.
74. Sato K, Kameda M, Yasuhara T, Agari T, Baba T, et al. (2013) Neuroprotective effects of liraglutide for stroke model of rats. Int J Mol Sci 14: 21513-21524.
75. Lee CH, Yan B, Yoo KY (2011). Ischemia-induced changes in glucagon-like peptide-1 receptor and neuroprotective effect of its agonist, exendin-4, in experimental transient cerebral ischemia. Journal of neuroscience research; 89: 1103-1113.
76. Read PA, Hoole SP, White PA (2011). A pilot study to assess whether glucagon-like peptide-1 protects the heart from ischemic dysfunction and attenuates stunning after coronary balloon occlusion in humans. Circulation Cardiovascular interventions; 4: 266-272.
77. Nikolaidis LA, Mankad S, Sokos GG, Miske G, Shah A, et al. (2004) Effects of glucagon-like peptide-1 in patients with acute myocardial infarction and left ventricular dysfunction after successful reperfusion. Circulation 109: 962-965.
78. Lønborg J, Vejlstrup N, Kelbæk H, Bøtker HE, Kim WY, et al. (2012) Exenatide reduces reperfusion injury in patients with ST-segment elevation myocardial infarction. Eur Heart J 33: 1491-1499.
79. Best JH, Lavillotti K, DeYoung MB, Garrison LP (2012). The effects of exenatide bid on metabolic control, medication use and hospitalization in patients with type 2 diabetes mellitus in clinical practice: a systematic review. Diabetes, obesity & metabolism; 14: 387-398.
80. Ott A, Stolk RP, van Harskamp F, Pols HA, Hofman A, et al. (1999) Diabetes mellitus and the risk of dementia: The Rotterdam Study. Neurology 53: 1937-1942.
81. Biessels GJ, Staekenborg S, Brunner E, Brayne C, Scheltens P (2006) Risk of dementia in diabetes mellitus: a systematic review. Lancet Neurol 5: 64-74.
82. Abbas T, Faivre E, Hölscher C (2009) Impairment of synaptic plasticity and memory formation in GLP-1 receptor KO mice: Interaction between type 2 diabetes and Alzheimer's disease. Behav Brain Res 205: 265-271.
83. During MJ, Cao L, Zuzga DS, Francis JS, Fitzsimons HL, et al. (2003) Glucagon-like peptide-1 receptor is involved in learning and neuroprotection. Nat Med 9: 1173-1179.
84. Parthsarathy V, Hölscher C (2013) Chronic treatment with the GLP1 analogue liraglutide increases cell proliferation and differentiation into neurons in an AD mouse model. PLoS One 8: e58784.
85. Han WN, Hölscher C, Yuan L, Yang W, Wang XH, et al. (2013) Liraglutide protects against amyloid-Î² protein-induced impairment of spatial learning and memory in rats. Neurobiol Aging 34: 576-588.
86. Harkavyi A, Abuirmeileh A, Lever R, Kingsbury AE, Biggs CS, Whitton PS (2008). Glucagon-like peptide 1 receptor stimulation reverses key deficits in distinct rodent models of Parkinson's disease. Journal of neuroinflammation; 5: 19.
87. Bertilsson G, Patrone C, Zachrisson O (2008). Peptide hormone exendin-4 stimulates subventricular zone neurogenesis in the adult rodent brain and induces recovery in an animal model of Parkinson's disease. Journal of neuroscience research; 86: 326-338.
88. Martin B, Golden E, Carlson OD, Pistell P, Zhou J, et al. (2009) Exendin-4 improves glycemic control, ameliorates brain and pancreatic pathologies, and extends survival in a mouse model of Huntington's disease. Diabetes 58: 318-328.
89. Hölscher C (2012) Potential role of glucagon-like peptide-1 (GLP-1) in neuroprotection. CNS Drugs 26: 871-882.
90. Olmos IA, Dickson J, Kefalopoulou Z, Djamshidian A, Ell P, et al. (2013) Exenatide and the treatment of patients with Parkinson's disease. J Clin Invest 123: 2730-2736.
91. (2013) GLP-1 for the Treatment of Stroke Patients With Space-occupying Intracerebral Hemorrhage.
92. Evaluating Liraglutide in Alzheimer's Disease (ELAD)
93. McIntyre RS, Powell AM, Beilin OK, et al.(2013) The role of GLP-1 analogues in reducing reperfusion injury after acute stroke in patients with impaired swallowing. The neuroprotective effects of GLP-1: possible treatments for cognitive deficits in individuals with mood disorders. Behavioural brain research; 237: 164-171.
94. Lockie SH (2013) Glucagon-like peptide-1 receptor in the brain: role in neuroendocrine control of energy metabolism and treatment target for obesity. J Neuroendocrinol 25: 597-604.
95. Capes SE, Hunt D, Malmberg K, Pathak P, Gerstein HC (2001) Stress hyperglycemia and prognosis of stroke in nondiabetic and diabetic patients: a systematic overview. Stroke 32: 2426-2432.
96. Schwartz S, DeFronzo RA (2013) Is incretin-based therapy ready for the care of hospitalized patients with type 2 diabetes?: The time has come for GLP-1 receptor agonists! Diabetes Care 36: 2107-2111.
97. Effect of Liraglutide on Body Weight in Non-diabetic Obese Subjects or Overweight Subjects With Co-morbidities: Obesity and Pre-diabetes.
98. The Effects of Exenatide (Byetta) on Energy Expenditure and Weight Loss in Nondiabetic Obese Subjects.
99. Isacson R, Nielsen E, Dannaeus K, Bertilsson G, Patrone C, et al. (2011) The glucagon-like peptide 1 receptor agonist exendin-4 improves reference memory performance and decreases immobility in the forced swim test. Eur J Pharmacol 650: 249-255.
100. Ma T, Du X, Pick JE, Sui G, Brownlee M, et al. (2012) Glucagon-like peptide-1 cleavage product GLP-1 (9-36) amide rescues synaptic plasticity and memory deficits in Alzheimer's disease model mice. J Neurosci 32: 13701-13708.
101. Kimura R, Okouchi M, Fujioka H, Ichiyanagi A, Ryuge F, et al. (2009) Glucagon-like peptide-1 (GLP-1) protects against methylglyoxal-induced PC12 cell apoptosis through the PI3K/Akt/mTOR/GCLc/redox signaling pathway. Neuroscience 162: 1212-1219.

Peroxisome Proliferator-Activated Receptor γ as a Therapeutic Target in Human Breast Cancer

Julie M. Hall* **and Matthew L. Robinson**

Department of Pharmaceutical Sciences, Campbell University, College of Pharmacy & Health Sciences, Buies Creek, NC, USA

***Corresponding author:** Julie M. Hall, Campbell University, College of Pharmacy & Health Sciences, Box 1090, Buies Creek, NC 27506, USA,
E-mail: halljm@campbell.edu

Abstract

Objective: Peroxisome proliferator-activated receptor γ (PPARγ) is aberrantly expressed in most breast tumors, suggesting the potential of agents that target this receptor in treatment and chemoprevention of breast cancer. However, whether PPARγ leads to the promotion or reduction of tumor formation has remained controversial and is further complicated by the ability of its available thiazolidinedione (TZD) ligands to activate another PPAR subtype, PPARδ.

Method: To examine the role of each receptor in breast cancer biology, we performed a systematic evaluation of PPARγ and PPARδ agonists on the growth of human estrogen receptor (ER)-positive and -negative breast cancer cells.

Results: In this manner we found that TZD-activated PPARγ was highly effective in suppressing the proliferation of estrogen-dependent cancer cells. Activated PPARδ, however, displayed growth-enhancing effects independent of estradiol and regardless of the ER status of the cells. Strikingly, in ER-negative cancer cells expressing a favorable PPARδ/γ ratio, TZDs promoted growth in a PPAR γ-independent manner by direct activation of PPARδ. A screen for ligands with increased receptor selectivity compared to TZDs revealed that GW7845 functioned as a full agonist of PPARγ, yet this agent lacked the ability to activate PPARδ and elicit its associated mitogenic effects.

Conclusion: These studies indicate that selective PPAR γ modulators (SPPARγMs) that lack agonist activity on PPARδ may be clinically useful in future cancer treatment and chemoprevention.

Keywords: PPAR γ; Thiazolidinedione (TZD); Breast cancer; Estrogen; ER; Subtype-selective; Proliferation

Introduction

Breast cancer is currently the most prevalent malignancy among women in industrialized countries, and one in eight women living in the United States will develop the disease at some point in her lifetime. It is estimated that over 230,000 women will be newly diagnosed with breast cancer in the United States this year, accounting for 30% of cancers found in women [1]. Despite the increase in diagnostic technologies, incidence rates of distant-stage disease have remained stable over the past several decades [2]. A series of mechanistically distinct therapeutics are currently in clinical use, including those targeting estrogen and growth factor signaling pathways [3-5]. Unfortunately, difficulties in mode of delivery, adverse cardiovascular effects, associated bone loss and development of resistance over time have provided limitations for sustained use of the many of these agents [5-9]. To date there still exists an unmet need for novel breast cancer therapeutics with improved tolerance, specificity and safety. Thus, further molecular characterization of the disease should aid in guiding both the most appropriate use of existing therapies and subsequent identification of new drug targets [3,10].

The PPARs (α, δ, γ), are nuclear hormone receptors that regulate lipid metabolism and homeostasis by regulating cell growth, differentiation and survival [11]. In addition to normal physiology, each receptor is associated with pathways linked to carcinogenesis, and thus, emerging evidence indicates a role for PPARs in the etiology of cancer [12]. While the link between each subtype and carcinogenesis is unclear, there is notable aberrant expression of PPARγ and its coactivator PGC-1α in both ER-positive and ER–negative human breast tumors, where low levels of these factors are associated with poor clinical outcomes [13].

Given these observations, it is not surprising that PPAR γ has recently become a prospective target for prevention and treatment of breast cancers [14]. While the available PPARγ ligands were developed for their ability to normalize blood glucose levels in patients with type II diabetes, analogous to the selective estrogen receptor modulator (SERM) concept, it has been proposed that selective PPARγ modulators (SPPARγ Ms) may be clinically useful in future cancer chemoprevention [14]. However, the development of such agents has been hindered by the uncertainty as to whether PPARγ activation or inhibition is the desired effect. In vitro and in vivo studies have revealed that PPARγ physiological ligands (prostaglandins; lipids) and pharmacological ligands (thiazolidinediones (TZDs)) effectively inhibit growth and induce apoptosis in human breast cancer cells and tumors, yet not in normal breast epithelial cells [15-19]. Yet other studies using several cancer cell lines, animal models, and a variety of PPARγ agonists have shown discordant results, perhaps due to differences in tumor type, grade, species and pharmacological dose

[20,21]. Thus, despite early concurrence as to the protective effects of the receptor, whether PPARγ leads to the promotion or reduction of tumor formation currently remains somewhat controversial.

The apparent confounding effects of available PPARγ ligands on PPARδ have the potential to further complicate the development of SPPARγMs as breast cancer therapeutics. A biological impact of 'receptor crossover' was demonstrated in human macrophages. Specifically, TZDs, which possess established anti-inflammatory actions through activation of PPARy, were shown to display unanticipated pro-inflammatory activities in a PPARγ-independent manner through direct activation of PPARδ [22]. Whether similar, nonspecific activities of PPARγ ligands could occur in breast cancers is not clear, nor is it know whether this phenomenon might explain the one clinical trial to date evaluating TZDs in metastatic breast cancer patients, which failed to demonstrate efficacy of troglitazone as a breast cancer therapeutic [23]. Regardless, the potential for 'receptor crossover' suggests that the ratio of PPARγ to PPARδ expression could alter both tumor biology and drug pharmacology. This is particular alarming given that the two receptors are co-expressed in most breast cancers and PPARδ has been implicated in promoting development and expansion of tumors from several tissue origins [24-27]. Clearly, an understanding of the role of each receptor in regulating growth of cancer cells should allow for future development of safer, yet effective PPAR modulators with potential therapeutic use for cancer. We undertook these studies therefore with the intent to determine the impact of PPARγ and PPARδ expression in breast cancer and to evaluate the contribution of each receptor to breast cancer biology.

Materials and Methods

Biochemicals

PCR reagents were obtained from BIO-RAD (Hercules, CA). 17β-estradiol and GW9662 were purchased from Sigma (St. Louis, MO). Rosiglitazone, pioglitazone, troglitazone, ciglitazone, and carbaprostacyclin were purchased from Cayman Chemical (Ann Arbor, MI). GSK660 was a gift from Drs. Andrew Billin and Barry Shearer (GlaxoSmithKline). The FluoReporter Blue Fluorometric dsDNA Quantitation Kit, transfection reagents, and PCR oligos were purchased from Life Technologies (Grand Island, NY).

Mammalian cell culture and ligand treatments

All cell lines were obtained from American Type Culture Collection (Manassas, VA). MCF-7, ZR-75 and T47D (human ER-positive breast cancer) cells and MDA MB-231 (human ER-negative breast cancer) cells were maintained in DMEM F12 medium supplemented with 10% fetal calf serum (FCS), 2 mM glutamine, 0.1 mM nonessential amino acids, and 1 mM sodium pyruvate (Life Technologies). HeLa (human cervical cancer) cells were maintained in MEM supplemented with 10% FCS. Cell were grown in a 37°C incubator with 5% CO_2. For RNA analysis, cells were plated at 60% confluency in 6-well culture dishes in 2 ml phenol red-free DMEM F12 containing 8% charcoal-stripped FCS (HyClone Laboratories, Inc., Logan, UT) for 24 h prior to treatment. Media was then replaced and supplemented with ethanol (vehicle), 17β-estradiol, rosiglitazone, carbaprostacyclin, pioglitazone, troglitazone, ciglitazone, GSK660 or GW7845. Note figure legends for details on concentrations of agents used in specific experiments. For some studies GW9662 (PPARγ antagonist) or GSK660 (PPARδ antagonist) was co-administered with vehicle or treatments. For cell proliferation assays, cells were induced with vehicle, 17β-estradiol or other agents.

RNA isolation and quantitative PCR

RNA was isolated from cultured BG-1 cells using the RNeasy kit (Qiagen, Valencia, CA). One μg of RNA was reverse transcribed using the BioRad iScript cDNA synthesis kit. The ABI PRISM® 7900HT Real Time PCR System was used to amplify and quantitate levels of target gene cDNA. Quantitative PCR (qPCR) reactions were performed using 0.1 μl of cDNA, 10 μM gene-specific primers, and 2x SYBR Green Mastermix (Applied Biosystems). Data are the mean +/-STDEV of three biological replicates performed in triplicate. All experiments were repeated a minimum of three times. The following primers were used: CXCL12,

5'-GTGGTCGTGCTGGTCCTC-3' (for) and 5'-GATGCTTGACGTTGGCTCTG-3' (rev), Cyclin D1, 5'-GCTGCGAAGTGGAAACCATC-3' (for) and 5'-CCTCCTTCTGCACACATTTGAA-3' (rev), p21, 5'-TGTCCGTCAGAACCCATGC-3'(for) and 5'-AAAGTCGAAGTTCCATCGCTC-3' (rev), pS2, 5'-CGGGGAGTGAGAAACCCTC-3' (for) and 5'-CACTGGAGTCGAAACAGCATC-3' (rev), PR 5'-ACCCGCCCTATCTCAACTACC-3' (for) and 5'-AGGACACCATAATGACAGCCT-3' (rev), ID3, 5'-GAGAGGCACTCAGCTTAGCC-3' (for) and 5'-TCCTTTTGTCGTTGGAGATGAC-3' (rev), and 36B4 5'-GGACATGTTGCTGGCCAATAA-3' (for) and 5'-GGGCCCGAGACCAGTGTT-3' (rev).

Cell proliferation assays

For standard assays, cells were seeded and adhered in 96-well plates at 2.5 x 10^4 cells/well. Cells were incubated in the absence or presence of ligands for 96 h in phenol red-free DMEM F12 containing 8% charcoal-stripped FCS (100 μl/well). After 96 h, cell proliferation was measured using the FluoReporter® Blue Fluorometric dsDNA Quantitation Kit according to the manufacturers' protocols (Life Technologies). All values were corrected for fluorescence values read from blank controls containing media with no cells. Sextuplicate biological replicates were used for each treatment condition in each experiment, and data are the mean +/-STDEV of the 6 replicates. All experiments were repeated a minimum of three independent times.

Mammalian cell transfections

HeLa cells were used for transactivation and mammalian-two-hybrid assays. For transient transfections, cells were plated in 24-well plates 24 h before transfection. Lipofectin-mediated transfection has been described in detail previously [22]. Briefly, prior to transfection, the media was replaced with phenol-free MEM containing 8% charcoal-stripped serum (Hyclone), 0.1 mM non-essential amino acids and 1 mM sodium pyruvate (Life Technologies). A DNA-Lipofectin mixture containing a total of 3 μg of plasmid for each triplicate sample was added to the cells. For transactivation assays, each triplicate contained 2 μg DR1-Luc, 0.1 μg pCMV-βgal, 0.1 μg pcDNA3-PPAR(γ or δ), and 0.8 μg PBSII filler vector. For mammalian two-hybrid assays, each triplicate contained 1.5 μg 5x-Gal4-TATA-Luc, 0.1 μg pCMV-βgal, 0.7 μg pVP16-PPAR (γ or δ) and 0.7 μg pM-ASC-2. Receptor ligands were added to cells 4 h following transfection. Cells were assayed 40 h following transfection. Luminescence was measured on a Fusion luminometer (Perkin Elmer) and β-galactosidase activity on a Multiskan MS plate reader (Thermo Labsystems). Results are expressed as normalized luciferase activity (normalized with β-Gal for transfection efficiency) per triplicate sample of cells in a representative experiment; error bars indicate the S.E.M. of triplicate determinations. Each experiment was repeated at least three independent times with very similar results.

Results

It has been well established that gene expression patterns have the ability to define clinically relevant risk factors in disease prognosis [28-30]. The aberrant over-representation of PPARs in breast cancers, together with their suspect roles in tumor biology, prompted us to investigate the relationship between PPARγ and δ expression, receptor activity, and associated impact on cancer biology. Thus, in the following series of studies, human breast cancer cell lines, containing endogenous expression of both PPAR subtypes, were used as a simplified system to study the respective roles of the two receptors.

PPARγ agonists attenuate estradiol-dependent growth of human breast cancer cells

The majority of human breast tumors over-express ERα and grow in response to estrogens, making this signaling system a primary target for therapeutic intervention [31]. Given that ER+ breast cancer cells also express PPARγ, the impact of TZDs on the growth of ER-positive breast cancer cells was examined. However, no effects of pharmacological doses of rosiglitazone or other TZDs were observed when administered in the absence of estrogen stimulation despite the detection of biologically active PPARγ in all cell lines examined (Figure 1A and not shown).

Given that the growth of ER+ cancer cells is estrogen-dependent, agents that when co-administered display anti-estrogenic (anti-proliferative) activity are of keen therapeutic interest. Thus, the effect of rosiglitazone on estrogen-stimulated growth of three ERα/PPARγ-positive breast cancer cell lines was next examined (Figure 1A). Each of the MCF-7, ZR-75, and T47D cell lines displayed a mitogenic response to estradiol that was partially (T47D-50% inhibition) to completely (MCF-7) attenuated with co-administration of rosiglitazone. Interestingly, the degree of inhibition positively correlated with the expression levels of PPARγ in each of the three cell lines. Co-administration of the PPARγ-selective antagonist GW9662 rendered cells resistant to the antiproliferative effects of rosiglitazone, demonstrating the observed growth inhibitory effects were receptor-dependent (Figure 1B). Annexin V staining confirmed that the observations made in these experiments reflected changes in proliferation rather than in apoptosis. Together these data indicate that agonist-activated PPARγ can effectively attenuate the growth of estradiol-dependent breast cancer cells.

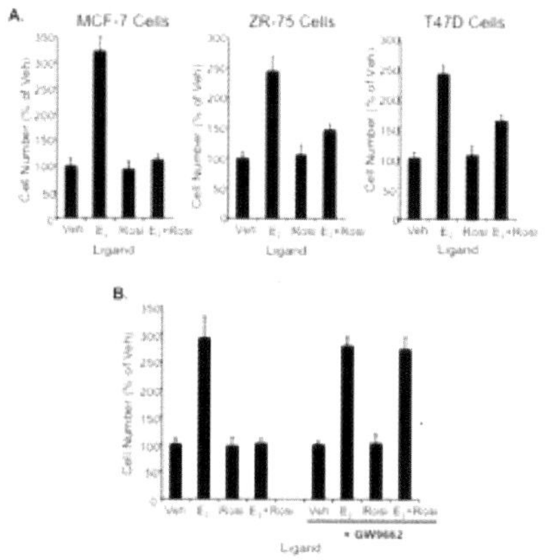

Figure 1: PPARγ agonists attenuate estradiol-dependent growth of human breast cancer cells. A, Estradiol stimulation of breast cancer cell proliferation is attenuated by PPARγ. MCF-7, ZR-75 and T47D cells were seeded in 96-well plates and treated with vehicle (Veh) (ethanol), 17β-estradiol (E2) (10 nM), rosiglitazone (Rosi) (1 μM), or E2+Rosi for 92 h and then assayed for cell growth. Graphical data are represented as % increase in cell number over vehicle (set at 100%). Data points represent the average of quadruplicate samples for each condition in a representative experiment. Proliferation assays were optimized for each cell type as described previously. B, MDA MB-231 cells were seeded in 96-well plates and treated as above in the absence or presence of GW9662 (1 μM) for 92 h. Cell proliferation (quadruplicate samples per treatment) was assayed as described above.

PPARγ agonists oppose estradiol in modulating expression of key regulators of growth

In most target tissues PPARγ expression is associated with cell differentiation and ERα with proliferation [32,33], and these activities are reflected in the gene expression profiles of each receptor [34,35]. Given that both receptors are expressed in breast cancer cells [13,31] and were found to display opposing effects on cell growth (Figure 1), it seemed possible that the signaling pathways of the activated receptors might converge at the genomic level.

To address this possibility, the gene expression patterns of MCF-7 cells administered estradiol, rosiglitazone or both agents were evaluated by microarray analysis. Quantitative real-time PCR (qPCR) was used to verify the effects of each receptor on the expression of several genes that exhibited differential expression profiles in the microarrays. Figure 2 shows the qPCR results from MCF-7 cells administered estrogen in the presence or absence of PPARγ agonist. Strikingly, rosiglitazone completely suppressed estrogen-stimulated induction of two known regulators of breast cancer growth, C-X-C motif chemokine 12 (CXCL12) and Cyclin D1. Furthermore, rosiglitazone displayed inverse agonist activity, decreasing CXCL12 and Cyclin D1 mRNA expression below that observed in vehicle treated cells. This effect was not specific for rosiglitazone as all other PPARγ ligands tested, both TZDs and others, displayed similar activity on CXCL12 expression in this assay. Rosiglitazone and estradiol also displayed opposing effects on the cell cycle inhibitor p21, although in this instance the estradiol-mediated response was dominant when the two agents were co-administered.

Although ER and PPAR signaling may converge in some aspects of cell growth, the receptors likely have independent gene targets associated with other cellular activities. This in fact was reflected in our gene validation analysis, as the expression of the estrogen responsive progesterone receptor (PR), pS2 and ID3 mRNAs remained unchanged with the addition of PPARγ agonists (Figure 2B). These data indicate that PPARγ agonists can oppose estradiol in modulating expression of key regulators of growth in human breast cancer cells, an activity consistent with the suppressive effects of these agents on estrogen-dependent proliferation.

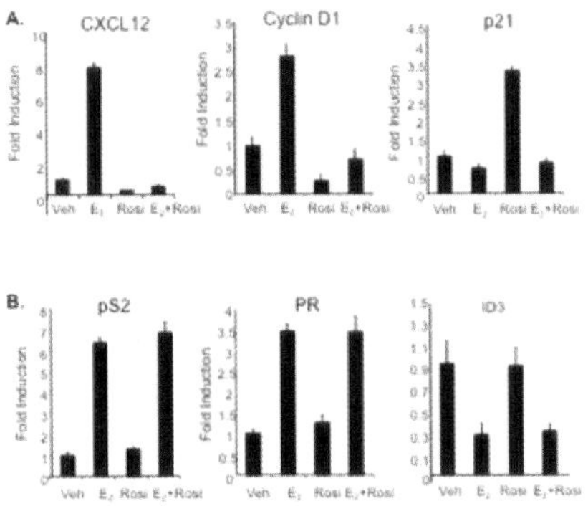

Figure 2: PPARγ agonists oppose estradiol in modulating expression of key regulators of growth in breast cancer cells. A, Real-time PCR analysis of endogenous CXCL12, Cyclin D1 and p21 expression or B, endogenous pS2, PR and ID3 expression in MCF-7 cells. MCF-7 cells were grown for 48 h in phenol-red free DMEM + 10% stripped FCS and then treated with vehicle (Veh) (ethanol), 17β-estradiol (E2) (10 nM), rosiglitazone (Rosi) (1 μM), or E2+Rosi. After 24 h, cells were harvested for total RNA, which was used for real-time PCR. Graphical data are represented as fold induction over vehicle (set at 1). Data points represent the average of triplicate amplification reactions for each condition in a representative experiment.

PPARγ promotes growth of human breast cancer cells

The effect of activated PPARδ on breast cancer cell growth was next examined. Notably, the PPARδ agonist carbaprostacyclin (Carb) enhanced proliferation of MCF-7 and T47D cells in a manner comparable to that of estrogen (Figure 3A). Co-administration of Carb did not enhance the effects of estradiol, however, additive effects of the two agents were seen when assayed at lower, sub-efficacy doses (not shown). The specific PPARδ antagonist GSK660 [36] completely attenuated Carb-induced growth, demonstrating that the growth-stimulatory effects were receptor-mediated (Figure 3A). Interestingly, the inverse agonist effects of GSK660 suggest that PPARδ might have constitutive growth-promoting effects. This possibility is supported by previous findings that the receptor displays significant basal activity in the absence of an added ligand [22,37]. As a control, HeLa cells, which lack detectable activity of both ER and PPARs, exhibited no effects of any of the agents tested; this further ensured that the observed growth inhibitory activity of GSK660 were not due to a general effect on cell survival (Figure 3B). Thus, PPARδ stimulates the growth of human breast cancer cells, and this activity appears to be manifest in both a ligand-independent and -dependent manner.

Rosiglitazone can stimulate breast cancer cell growth by activating PPARδ.

The results thus far have suggested contrasting roles of the two PPAR subtypes in breast cancer, whereas PPARγ may be protective, yet PPARδ activity might be unfavorable.

In this context, previous observations that saturating doses TZDs can activate PPARδ are concerning given that as agonists of PPARγ one would expect TZDs to be protective in cancer [22]. Since whether PPARγ-independent activities of these ligands could occur in breast cancers is not clear, to test this possibility, the impact of different pharmacological doses of TZDs on growth of breast cancer cells was next examined. While Rosi administered at a subsaturating quantity (100 nM) had no significant impact in the assay, at a micromolar dose Rosi displayed growth-stimulatory effects in a manner comparable to that of the PPARδ agonist Carb (Figure 3C). Co-administration of the PPARδ agonist GSK660 completely attenuated these effects, suggesting that the mitogenic activity of Rosi was in fact occurring by activation of PPARδ. This was further supported by the inability of the PPARγ specific antagonist GW9662 to block Rosi-stimulated proliferation. Thus, at saturating concentrations Rosi can function as a PPARδ agonist and elicit the growth-promoting activity of the receptor in human breast cancer cells.

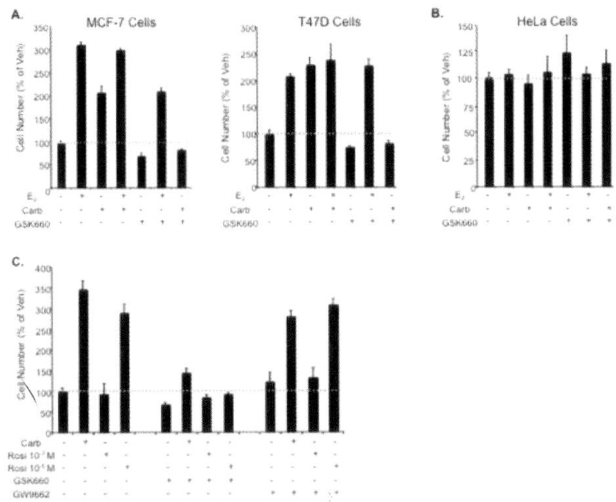

Figure 3: PPARδ promotes growth of human breast cancer cells. (A) MCF-7, ZR-75 and T47D cells or (B) HeLa cells were seeded in 96-well plates and treated with vehicle (Veh) (ethanol), 17β-estradiol (E2) (10 nM), carbaprostacyclin (Carb) (1 μM), GSK660 (1 μM) or a combination of agents for 96 h. Cells were harvested for proliferation assays. Graphical data are represented as % increase in cell number over vehicle (set at 100%). Data points represent the average of quadruplicate samples for each condition in a representative experiment. (C) MDA MB-231 cells were seeded in 96-well plates and treated as indicated for 48 h. Cell proliferation (quadruplicate samples per treatment) was assayed and analyzed as above.

GW7845 is a PPARδ-Sparing PPARγ agonist

One of the key goals of this study was to assess whether drugs that target PPARγ might have promise as future breast cancer therapeutics. While it appears that activation of PPARγ would be the desired effect of such agents, unfortunately, available receptor agonists have undesirable feature of cross-reactivity with PPARδ.

We therefore undertook a screen for ligands with increased receptor selectivity compared to TZDs. The ability of a series of 30 known PPARγ agonists and SSPARγMs to activate PPARγ, PPARα and PPARδ was evaluated in mammalian cells.

Specifically, PPAR negative HeLa cells were used for these assays, enabling us to measure the transcriptional responses of each receptor in isolation. HeLa cells were transfected with expression plasmids for either PPARγ PPARα or PPARδ in combination with a DR1-luc reporter. All results shown reflect receptor activity at maximal efficacy for a particular agent (Figure 4A). None of the test compounds were capable of activating PPARα (not shown); this was not entirely surprising given the indications that this receptor is somewhat more discriminatory in ligand preferences [38-40]. However, in evaluation of PPARγ and PPARδ in the assay, one compound, GW7845, functioned as a subtype-selective, full agonist of PPARγ (Figure 4A). Specifically, while all 4 TZDs as shown previously were effective activators of PPARδ, GW7845 displayed modest inverse agonist activity on the receptor. Others, however, have also demonstrated that GW7845 does indeed bind PPARδ and modulate its structure [41,42].

Classical nuclear receptor agonists function by binding to the receptor and inducing an activating conformational change that facilitates recruitment of transcriptional coactivators. The observation that GW7845 was a PPAR subtype-selective agonist suggested that the agent might differ in its ability to promote cofactor recruitment to PPARγ and PPARδ. Mammalian two-hybrid assays were next used to compare the ability of GW7845 and TZDs to facilitate an interaction between the AF-2 domain of PPARγ/δ and the nuclear receptor interacting domain (NR-box) of the coactivator Activating Signal Cointegrator 2 (ASC-2) (Figure 4B). HeLa cells were transfected with pM-ASC-2 (NR-Box), containing the yeast Gal4 transcription factor DNA-binding domain fused to the ASC-2 NR-Box, and VP16-PPARγ or VP16-PPARδ which are chimeras of the strong Herpes Simplex virus VP16 activation domain fused to N-terminus of each PPAR. Transcriptional readout, a measurement of protein-protein interactions in the assay, was obtained by cotransfection of a luciferase reporter vector containing five tandem Gal4 binding sites (5xGal4-Luc). Notably, a substantial amount of ASC-2 interaction with both PPARγ and δ was observed in the absence of ligand (Figure 4C). This likely reflects the fact that in the absence of an added activating ligand PPARs reside in an active conformation, as shown previously [22,37]. Despite the high basal level of ASC-2 binding, GW7845 enhanced the interaction with PPARγ in a manner comparable to that of all four TZDs (Figure 4C). Likewise, Carb and TZDs enhanced cofactor binding to PPAR δ; these interactions were completely antagonized by GSK660, indicating that all compounds were binding in the known ligand-binding pocket of the receptor. GW7845, conversely, demonstrated inverse agonist activity in the ability to partially disrupt the basal interaction of PPAR δ with ASC-2. Thus, GW785 is mechanistically and functionally distinct from other known PPAR modulators, as the agonist activity of this agent is PPARγ-selective.

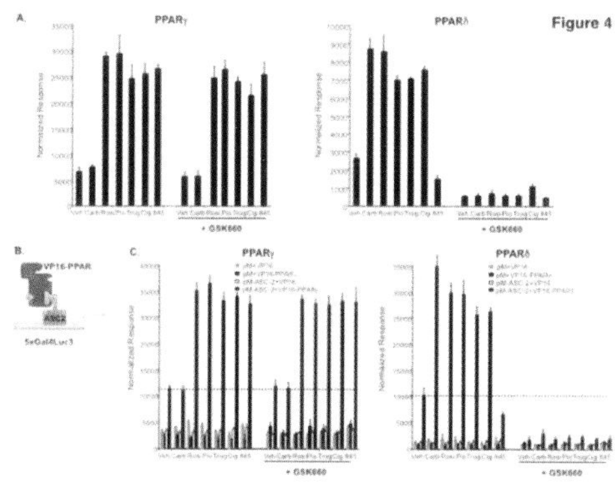

Figure 4: GW7845 is a selective PPARγ agonist. (A), PPAR transcriptional activity was measured by mammalian cell transfection assays. HeLa cells were transfected with a PPARγ or PPARδ expression vector in combination with a DR1-Luc reporter plasmid and a β-galactosidase normalization vector. After transfection, cells were treated with vehicle (Veh) or 1 μM carbaprostacyclin (Carb), or 1 μM TZDs: rosiglitazone (Rosi), pioglitazone (Pio), troglitazone (Trog) or ciglitazone (Cig), or 100 nM GW7845 in the absence or presence of 1 μM PPARδ antagonist GSK660 for 40 h. Cells were harvested and assayed for luciferase activity; all luciferase assay values were normalized to β-gal controls. Data points are the average of triplicate determinations in a representative experiment, and the average coefficient of variance for each value is <10%. (B) Schematic of mammalian two-hybrid assay. (C) HeLa cells were transfected with VP16 and pM control vectors, pM-ASC-2 (NR-box), and VP16-PPARγ (VP16-PPARδ or VP16-PPARγ expression vectors in combination with a 5x-Gal4-TATA-Luc reporter plasmid and a β-galactosidase normalization vector. After transfection, cells were treated, assayed and analyzed as in A.

GW7845 manifests the anti-proliferative effects of PPARγ without inducing the proliferative effects of activated PPARδ.

Given that TZD-activated PPARγ is effective at suppressing growth in estrogen-dependent breast cancer cells (Figure 1), it would be predicted that GW7845 as a full receptor agonist should behave similarly. Thus, the effect of GW7845 on estrogen-stimulated growth of two ERα/PPARγ-positive breast cancer cell lines was next examined (Figure 5A). Both the MCF-7 and ZR-75 cells displayed a mitogenic response to estradiol that was completely attenuated with co-administration of GW7845. Furthermore, GW7845 displayed a modest anti-proliferative activity when administered alone, further suggesting that this compound might possess inverse agonist activity on PPARδ as seen beforehand (Figures 4A, 4B and 5A).

Despite the apparent protective effects of TZDs, their ability to activate the proliferative effects of PPARδ at high doses is concerning (Figure 3B). If as our studies have suggested GW7845 is indeed superior to the TZDs in receptor selectivity, at saturating doses this agent should not display agonist activity through PPARδ. In investigating this possibility, as seen before (Figure 3B), Rosi when present at a micromolar concentration enhanced proliferation in a

PPARδ-dependent in a manner that was comparable to that of full agonist Carb (Figure 5B). Given the potency of GW7845 is 1-2 log values superior to that of TZDs [18], 10-fold lower doses than those used for Rosi were administered. Regardless, GW7845 failed to evoke a proliferative response in the assay (Figure 5B). Thus the PPAR subtype-selective activities of GW7845 are reflected in both its receptor pharmacology (Figure 4) and biology in breast cancer cells (Figure 5).

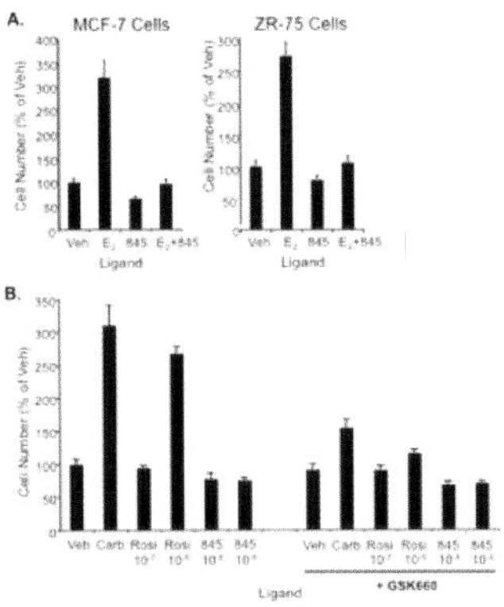

Figure 5: GW7845 manifests the anti-proliferative effects of PPARγ without inducing the proliferative effects of PPARγ. (A) MCF-7 and ZR-75 cells were seeded in 96-well plates and treated with vehicle (Veh), 17β-estradiol (E2) (10 nM), GW7845 (100 nM), or E2+GW7845 for 96 h. Cells were harvested for proliferation assays. Graphical data are represented as % increase in cell number over vehicle (set at 100%). Data points represent the average of quadruplicate samples for each condition in a representative experiment. (B) MDA MB-231 cells were seeded in 96-well plates and treated with vehicle (Veh), carbaprostacyclin (Carb) (1 μM), rosiglitazone (Rosi) (100 nM or 10 μM), GW7845 (10 nM or 1 μM) in the absence or presence of GSK660 (1 μM) for 96 h. Cell proliferation (quadruplicate samples per treatment) was assayed and analyzed as above.

Discussion

PPARγ-selective agonists as promising therapeutics for breast cancer

Together, the observations made in this study suggest a potential therapeutic value of subtype-selective PPARγ agonists in treatment of breast cancer. This was evidenced by the efficacy with which GW7845 suppressed the growth of estrogen-dependent cancer cells. Clearly this agent has an advantage over available PPARγ ligands such as TZDs, which we show can manifest agonist activity through PPARδ and elicit mitogenic actions of the receptor in breast cancer cells. In fact it appears that PPARγ-selectivity need only be in regards to the agonist activity of a compound, as GW7845, while acting as a PPARγ-selective agonist could also display antagonist activity through PPARδ. This was supported by observations that GW7845 promoted binding of transcriptional coactivators to PPARγ and corepressors to PPARδ [42]. Importantly, both the agonist and antagonist activities of GW7845 contribute to its anti-proliferative role in breast cancer cells. Thus, PPAR 'pan-compounds,' with dual PPARγ agonist/PPARδ antagonist activities, could be highly effective as breast cancer therapeutics as they would capitalize on the protective actions of PPARγ whilst blocking both the constitutive and ligand-activated proliferative effects of PPARδ. As a potent and highly selective PPARδ antagonist has been characterized [36], it may be possible to use structural information from this molecule to create a GW7845-like chemical with enhanced antagonist activity on PPARδ. Additionally, as the available PPARγ ligands were developed for their ability to normalize blood glucose levels in patients with type II diabetes, it is likely that anti-proliferative effects can be optimized further.

An important implication of our study was the potential to develop PPARγ modulators in treatment of ER-positive breast cancer. Given the high percentage (approximately 70%) of breast tumors that express both ERα and PPARγ the effectiveness with which activated PPARγ could interfere with ER signaling was striking. It was of further note that with the complexity of the gene expression profiles induced by ER in breast cancer cells [34] PPARγ influenced expression of only a small handful of estrogen-regulated genes. Thus, the activated receptor could completely attenuate estrogen-dependent cell proliferation without interfering with other ER functions. This high degree of process-specificity is something lacking in many of the currently available breast cancer therapeutics that target ER signaling yet often relay adverse side-effects. For example, the aromatase inhibitors (AIs), anastrozole and letrozole (Arimidex, Femara), which block estrogen biosynthesis in all tissues, are known to cause bone loss, hot flashes, arthralgia and myalgia, and significantly increase the risk of cardiovascular disease and osteoporosis [43-45]. While fewer side-effects are generally associated with the selective estrogen receptor modulator (SERM) tamoxifen (Nolvadex), this agent does markedly increase the incidence of endometrial cancer, endometriosis, thrombosis and stroke; furthermore, drug-resistance is a currently a serious problem associated with both tamoxifen and the AIs [44-46]. Thus, while tremendous efforts have been made by the pharmaceutical industry to create better AIs and SERMs, PPARγ agonists, in their ability to function as process-targeted ER-modulators, may in fact fulfill both the need for effective and safer therapeutics for ER-positive breast cancers.

Unlike the available ER-targeted therapeutics for breast cancer, PPARγ modulators may also have utility in prevention and treatment of ER-negative tumors. Notably, GW7845 was shown to decrease the incidence, number, and weight of tumors in a nitrosomethylurea-experimental rat model of ER-negative mammary carcinogenesis [18]. In the current study, a modest yet significant effect of GW7845 on growth of ER-negative cancer cells was observed. However, unlike the studies with ER+ cells, which included stimulation with estrogen, the ER-negative cancer cells studies excluded the use of growth activators and rather examined effects of PPAR ligands only on basal proliferation. This is may be an important oversight, as there is emerging evidence that PPARγ may interfere with several signal transduction pathways associated with growth activators that are over-represented in ER-negative tumors. For example, HER-2/neu and epidermal growth factor receptor (EGFR) are over-expressed in 20-30% breast carcinomas, the majority of which are ER-negative. PPARγ agonists were shown to both cause dose-dependent decreases in levels of HER-2/neu and EGFR in human breast epithelial cells and to display inhibitory cross-talk with these receptors [47-49]. Increased Wnt signaling is also implicated in the development of mammary carcinomas, and notably, PPARγ can function to suppress tumorigenesis and/or Wnt signaling by targeting phosphorylated ßcatenin to the proteasome [50]. As a follow up to the current study, therefore, we intend to test the effects of PPARγ modulators on the EGFR, HER2 and Wnt pathways of cell growth with anticipation that in a scenario of "activated-proliferation" receptor agonists will demonstrate much more dramatic inhibitory effects.

PPARs as predictive biomarkers in breast cancer

Previous studies noted that low levels of PPARγ are correlated with decreased survival in breast cancer patients whereas PPARγ expression is correlated with increased survival rate. Specifically, ligand-activated PPARγ upregulates the tumor suppressor 'phosphatase and tensin homolog' (PTEN), an event thought to help mediate the antiproliferative effect of the receptor in breast and other cancer types [51,52]. Furthermore, it seems that the mere presence of the receptor is protective even in the absence of pharmacological intervention. Whether the ligand constitutive activity of the receptor is adequate to confer protection is not known, although it is also anticipated that sufficient quantities of endogenous ligands for receptor activation might be present in breast tissues.

Recently, clinical data has also revealed that PPARδ expression in breast tumors is associated with poor prognosis (our unpublished data). Likewise, there exists strong evidence linking the receptor to related pathologies in other tissues. Analysis of PPARδ in matched normal and tumor samples revealed a remarkable upregulation of the receptor in colon carcinomas [53]. Others suggested a supporting role of the receptor in events controlling initiation and progression of cancers in the colon. Specifically, marked increases in PPARδ expression are evident from normal intestinal mucosa to pre-cancerous polyps to colorectal cancer cells, to cancer cells with malignant morphology [54]. In contrast, PPARγ was demonstrated to be protective in colon carcinoma cells, as the increases in receptor expression induced by the tumor suppressor Zac, were associated with anti-proliferative effects [55]. Together, these observations indicate that association of PPAR and PPARδ with differing outcomes in cancer may be more broadly applicable, and likewise, the two receptors may be useful predictive biomarkers for other types of cancers. Our observations also suggest factors that increased expression of PPARγ or PPARδ has the potential to influence breast cancer biology and patient survival rates.

The concept that PPARγ may function as a protective agent in some cancers may explain some of the correlations that have been made between diet and breast cancer. Interestingly, trans fatty acid intake at levels of human consumption can decrease PPARγ levels in women by 40% in reproductive tissues. In fact, decreases in receptor levels in the ovary due to high intake of trans fatty acids were recently associated with a increased incidence of infertility. Apparently the changes in PPARγ levels were sufficient to interfere with fertility, as when the women began a treatment regimen of PPARγ agonists there was a consistent and significant increase in ovulatory function [56]. In addition to potential effects of dietary fats, α and γ tocopherol (Vitamin E) can upregulate the expression of the receptor in colon cancer cells, where PPARγ is considered an important molecular target for chemoprevention [57]. There are reports that levels of HDL cholesterol positively correlate with PPARγ expression; while a direct association is not clear, it is known that cardiovascular health is often associated with decrease risk of breast and other cancers [58]. Regardless, it will be interesting to determine whether dietary-related changes in PPAR expression can significantly impact the incidence, progression and reoccurrence of cancers.

In summary, in this study we report that at therapeutically relevant levels TZDs can activate PPARδ and elicit its mitogenic effects, whereas in the same contexts PPARγ-specific agonists can effectively inhibit the growth of human breast cancer cells and tumors. These discoveries provide an explanation for several puzzling observations made previously, such as the ability of TZDs to manifest PPARγ-independent effects and the controversy surrounding whether PPARγ enhances or reduces cancer risk. Given the observed growth-promoting activity of the human PPARδ, we suggest that PPARγ modulators with increased specificity show promise as safer, more effective therapeutics for breast tumors and perhaps other cancers.

Acknowledgements

The authors would like to thank Drs. Andrew Billin and Barry Shearer (GlaxoSmithKline) for their generous gift of the PPARδ antagonist GSK660. An American Association of College of Pharmacy (AACP) New Investigator Award and an Internal Research Grant from Campbell University (to J.M.H.) supported this work.

References

1. American Cancer Society (2015) What are the Key Statistics for Breast Cancer. http://www.cancer.org/cancer/breastcancer/detailedguide/breast-cancer-key-statistics. Accessed May 3, 2015.
2. Komen SG (2015) Breast cancer statistics.
3. Doyle DM, Miller KD (2008) Development of new targeted therapies for breast cancer. Cancer Treat Res 141: 119-134.
4. Lin NU, Winer EP (2008) Optimizing Endocrine Therapy for Estrogen Receptor-Positive Breast Cancer: Treating the Right Patients for the Right Length of Time. J Clin Oncol 26: 1919-1921.
5. Lin NU, Winer EP (2008) Advances in adjuvant endocrine therapy for postmenopausal women. J Clin Oncol 26: 798-805.
6. Hadji P, Bundred N (2007) Reducing the risk of cancer treatment-associated bone loss in patients with breast cancer. Semin Oncol 34: S4-10.
7. Iorns E, Turner NC, Elliott R, Syed N, Garrone O, et al. (2008) Identification of CDK10 as an important determinant of resistance to endocrine therapy for breast cancer. Cancer Cell 13: 91-104.
8. Perez EA (2007) Safety profiles of tamoxifen and the aromatase inhibitors in adjuvant therapy of hormone-responsive early breast cancer. Ann Oncol 18 Suppl 8: 26-35.
9. Urruticoechea A (2007) The oestrogen-dependent biology of breast cancer. Sensitivity and resistance to aromatase inhibitors revisited: a molecular perspective. Clin Transl Oncol 9: 752-759.
10. Muscat GE, Eriksson NA, Byth K, Loi S, Graham D, et al. (2013) Research resource: nuclear receptors as transcriptome: discriminant and prognostic value in breast cancer. Mol Endocrinol 27: 350-365.
11. Moore KJ, Rosen ED, Fitzgerald ML, Randow F, Andersson LP, et al. (2001) The role of PPAR-gamma in macrophage differentiation and cholesterol uptake. Nat Med 7: 41-47.
12. Michalik L, Desvergne B, Wahli W (2004) Peroxisome-proliferator-activated receptors and cancers: complex stories. Nat Rev Cancer 4: 61-70.
13. Jiang WG, Douglas-Jones A, Mansel RE (2003) Expression of peroxisome-proliferator activated receptor-gamma (PPARgamma) and the PPARgamma co-activator, PGC-1, in human breast cancer correlates with clinical outcomes. Int J Cancer 106: 752-757.
14. Sporn MB, Suh N, Mangelsdorf DJ (2001) Prospects for prevention and treatment of cancer with selective PPARgamma modulators (SPARMs). Trends Mol Med 7: 395-400.
15. Zaytseva YY, Wallis NK, Southard RC, Kilgore MW (2011) The PPARgamma antagonist T0070907 suppresses breast cancer cell

proliferation and motility via both PPARgamma-dependent and -independent mechanisms. Anticancer Res 31: 813-23.

16. Lea MA, Sura M, Desbordes C (2004) Inhibition of cell proliferation by potential peroxisome proliferator-activated receptor (PPAR) gamma agonists and antagonists. Anticancer Res 24: 2765-2771.
17. Nunez NP, Liu H, Meadows GG (2005) PPAR-gamma ligands and amino acid deprivation promote apoptosis of melanoma, prostate, and breast cancer cells. Cancer Lett 236: 133-141.
18. Suh N, Wang Y, Williams CR, Risingsong R, Gilmer T, et al. (1999) A new ligand for the peroxisome proliferator-activated receptor-gamma (PPAR-gamma), GW7845, inhibits rat mammary carcinogenesis. Cancer Res 59: 5671-5673.
19. Wang PS, Chou FS, Porchia L, Saji M, Pinzone JJ (2008) Troglitazone inhibits cell migration, adhesion, and spreading by modulating cytoskeletal rearrangement in human breast cancer cells. Mol Carcinog 47: 905-915.
20. Mueller E, Sarraf P, Tontonoz P, Evans RM, Martin KJ, et al. (1998) Terminal differentiation of human breast cancer through PPAR gamma. Mol Cell 1: 465-470.
21. Saez E, Rosenfeld J, Livolsi A, Olson P, Lombardo E, et al. (2004) PPAR gamma signaling exacerbates mammary gland tumor development. Genes Dev 18: 528-540.
22. Hall JM, McDonnell DP (2007) The molecular mechanisms underlying the proinflammatory actions of thiazolidinediones in human macrophages. Mol Endocrinol 21: 1756-1768.
23. Burstein HJ, Demetri GD, Mueller E, Sarraf P, Spiegelman BM, Winer EP (2003) Use of the peroxisome proliferator-activated receptor (PPAR) gamma ligand troglitazone as treatment for refractory breast cancer: a phase II study. Breast Cancer Res Treat 79: 391-397.
24. Peters JM, Foreman JE, Gonzalez FJ (2011) Dissecting the role of peroxisome proliferator-activate receptor- β/δ (PPAR β/δ) in colon, breast, and lung carcinogenesis. Cancer Metastasis Rev 30: 619-640.
25. Daikoku T, Tranguch S, Chakrabarty A, Wang D, Khabele D, et al. (2007) Extracellular signal-regulated kinase is a target of cyclooxygenase-1-peroxisome proliferator-activated receptor-delta signaling in epithelial ovarian cancer. Cancer Res 67: 5285-5292.
26. Jarvis MC, Gray TJ, Palmer CN (2005) Both PPARgamma and PPARdelta influence sulindac sulfide-mediated p21WAF1/CIP1 upregulation in a human prostate epithelial cell line. Oncogene 24: 8211-8215.
27. Yin Y, Russell RG, Dettin LE, Bai R, Wei ZL, et al. (2005) Peroxisome proliferator-activated receptor delta and gamma agonists differentially alter tumor differentiation and progression during mammary carcinogenesis. Cancer Res 65: 3950-3957.
28. Garcia-Escudero R, Paramio JM (2008) Gene expression profiling as a tool for basic analysis and clinical application of human cancer. Mol Carcinog 47: 593-579.
29. van 't Veer LJ, Dai H, van de Vijver MJ, He YD, Hart AA, et al. (2002) Gene expression profiling predicts clinical outcome of breast cancer. Nature 415: 530-536.
30. Wei JS, Greer BT, Westermann F, Steinberg SM, Son CG, et al. (2004) Prediction of clinical outcome using gene expression profiling and artificial neural networks for patients with neuroblastoma. Cancer Res 64: 6883-6891.
31. McDonnell DP, Chang CY, Norris JD (2001) Capitalizing on the complexities of estrogen receptor pharmacology in the quest for the perfect SERM. Ann N Y Acad Sci 949: 16-35.
32. Hall JM, Couse JF, Korach KS (2001) The multifaceted mechanisms of estradiol and estrogen receptor signaling. J Biol Chem 276: 36869-36872.
33. Rosen ED, Spiegelman BM (2001) PPARgamma : a nuclear regulator of metabolism, differentiation, and cell growth. J Biol Chem 276: 37731-37734.
34. Frasor J, Danes JM, Komm B, Chang KC, Lyttle CR, Katzenellenbogen BS (2003) Profiling of estrogen up- and down-regulated gene expression in human breast cancer cells: insights into gene networks and pathways underlying estrogenic control of proliferation and cell phenotype. Endocrinology 144: 4562-4574.
35. Gupta RA, Brockman JA, Sarraf P, Willson TM, DuBois RN (2001) Target genes of peroxisome proliferator-activated receptor gamma in colorectal cancer cells. J Biol Chem 276: 29681-29687.
36. Shearer BG, Steger DJ, Way JM, Stanley TB, Lobe DC, et al. (2008) Identification and characterization of a selective peroxisome proliferator-activated receptor beta/delta (NR1C2) antagonist. Mol Endocrinol 22: 523-529.
37. Mettu NB, Stanley TB, Dwyer MA, Jansen MS, Allen JE, et al. (2007) The nuclear receptor-coactivator interaction surface as a target for peptide antagonists of the peroxisome proliferator-activated receptors. Mol Endocrinol 21: 2361-2377.
38. Cronet P, Petersen JF, Folmer R, Blomberg N, Sjoblom K, et al. (2001) Structure of the PPARalpha and -gamma ligand binding domain in complex with AZ 242; ligand selectivity and agonist activation in the PPAR family. Structure 9: 699-706.
39. Forman BM, Chen J, Evans RM (1997) Hypolipidemic drugs, polyunsaturated fatty acids, and eicosanoids are ligands for peroxisome proliferator-activated receptors alpha and delta. Proc Natl Acad Sci USA 94: 4312-4317.
40. Kliewer SA, Sundseth SS, Jones SA, Brown PJ, Wisely GB, et al. (1997) Fatty acids and eicosanoids regulate gene expression through direct interactions with peroxisome proliferator-activated receptors alpha and gamma. Proc Natl Acad Sci USA 94: 4318-4323.
41. Liu KG, Lambert MH, Ayscue AH, Henke BR, Leesnitzer LM, et al. (2001) Synthesis and biological activity of L-tyrosine-based PPARgamma agonists with reduced molecular weight. Bioorg Med Chem Lett 11: 3111-3113.
42. Stanley TB, Leesnitzer LM, Montana VG, Galardi CM, Lambert MH, et al. (2003) Subtype specific effects of peroxisome proliferator-activated receptor ligands on corepressor affinity. Biochemistry 42: 9278-9287.
43. Panday K, Gona A, Humphrey MB (2014) Medication-induced osteoporosis: screening and treatment strategies. Ther Adv Musculoskelet Dis 6: 185-202.
44. Bird BR, Swain SM (2008) Cardiac toxicity in breast cancer survivors: review of potential cardiac problems. Clin Cancer Res 14: 14-24.
45. Conte P, Frassoldati A (2007) Aromatase inhibitors in the adjuvant treatment of postmenopausal women with early breast cancer: Putting safety issues into perspective. Breast J 13: 28-35.
46. Patel RR, Sharma CG, Jordan VC (2007) Optimizing the antihormonal treatment and prevention of breast cancer. Breast Cancer 14: 113-122.
47. Dannenberg AJ, Subbaramaiah K (2001) Treating cancers associated with overexpression of class I family of receptor tyrosine kinases. In: USP Office 6,291,496: 1-16.
48. Konopleva M, Zhang W, Shi YX, McQueen T, Tsao T, et al. (2006) Synthetic triterpenoid 2-cyano-3,12-dioxooleana-1,9-dien-28-oic acid induces growth arrest in HER2-overexpressing breast cancer cells. Mol Cancer Ther 5: 317-328.
49. Chen A, Xu J Activation of PPAR{gamma} by curcumin inhibits Moser cell growth and mediates suppression of gene expression of cyclin D1 and EGFR (2005) Am J Physiol Gastrointest Liver Physiol 288: G447-456.
50. Liu J, Wang H, Zuo Y, Farmer SR (2006) Functional interaction between peroxisome proliferator-activated receptor gamma and beta-catenin. Mol Cell Biol 26: 5827-5837.
51. Rovito D, Giordano C, Vizza D, Plastina P, Barone I, et al. (2013) Omega-3 PUFA ethanolamides DHEA and EPEA induce autophagy through PPARγ activation in MCF-7 breast cancer cells. J Cell Physiol 228: 1314-1322.
52. Teresi RE, Waite KA (2008) PPAR, PTEN, and the Fight against Cancer. PPAR Res 2008: doi: 10.1155/2008/932632.
53. Gupta RA, Tan J, Krause WF, Geraci MW, Willson TM, et al. (2000) Prostacyclin-mediated activation of peroxisome proliferator-activated receptor delta in colorectal cancer. Proc Natl Acad Sci U S A 97: 13275-13280.

54. Takayama O, Yamamoto H, Damdinsuren B, Sugita Y, Ngan CY, et al. (2006) Expression of PPARdelta in multistage carcinogenesis of the colorectum: implications of malignant cancer morphology. Br J Cancer 95: 889-895.

55. Barz T, Hoffmann A, Panhuysen M, Spengler D (2006) Peroxisome proliferator-activated receptor gamma is a Zac target gene mediating Zac antiproliferation. Cancer Res 66: 11975-11982.

56. Chavarro JE, Rich-Edwards JW, Rosner BA, Willett WC (2007) Dietary fatty acid intakes and the risk of ovulatory infertility. Am J Clin Nutr 85: 231-237.

57. Friedrich MJ (2004) To "E" or not to "E," vitamin E's role in health and disease is the question. Jama 292: 671-673.

58. Han J, Hajjar DP, Zhou X, Gotto AM Jr, Nicholson AC (2002) Regulation of peroxisome proliferator-activated receptor-gamma-mediated gene expression. A new mechanism of action for high density lipoprotein. J Biol Chem 277: 23582-23586.

18

Testosterone and Cardiovascular Disease in Men

Emmanuela Quental Callou de Sa[2*], **Francisco Carleial Feijó de Sá**[1], **Augusto Saboia Neto**[1] **and Juliana Viana Pinheiro**[1]

[1]*Department of Internal Medicine, Universidade Federal do Cariri, Barbalha, Ceará, Brazil*

[2]*Coordinator, Department of Endocrinology, Universidade Federal do Cariri, Barbalha, Ceará, Brazil*

[*]**Corresponding author:** Emmanuela Quental Callou de Sá, Universidade Federal do Cariri, Barbalha, Ceará, Brazil, E-mail: eqcallou@gmail.com

Abstract

In this Century Cardiovascular Disease (CVD) is the most common isolated cause of death in developed countries. Many studies have suggested that men with low testosterone levels present higher incidence of components of metabolic syndrome and are at a greater risk of developing CVD.

Testosterone can affect the development of atherosclerosis in the coronary arteries. While this androgen seems to have a cardioprotective effect by benefiting endothelial function, inducing vasodilation, and reducing fat mass, insulin resistance and chronic inflammation, it also appears to increase endothelin, thromboxane A2 and reactive oxygen species and renal smooth muscle cells.

The relation between testosterone and coronary disease in men has been the focus of study of many authors. Most studies point to a neutral and/or protective effect of endogenous testosterone in male cardiovascular health. Unfortunately, many intervention studies have not been able to confirm this effect with testosterone therapy.

More studies are needed to elucidate the pathogenic mechanisms of testosterone in cardiovascular health and to evaluate androgen receptor polymorphisms and their physiological responses to testosterone.

Key words

Testosterone; Cardiovascular Disease; Coronary; Hormonal Therapy; Review Aging

Introduction

In the beginning of the 20th Century Cardiovascular Disease (CVD) was responsible for less than 10% of all deaths worldwide. In this century CVD has become the isolated leading cause of death in industrialized nations [1]. The male gender has traditionally been associated with a higher risk of CVD [2]. One explanation for this was elevated serum levels of testosterone known to be atherogenic.

Except for some indirect evidence, many studies have suggested that men with low levels of testosterone have higher incidence of the components of metabolic syndrome as well as a higher risk of developing CVD in their lifetime [2,3].

It is estimated ten percent of Myocardial Infarction (MI) patients do not have classic cardiovascular risk factors [4] and as a result new investigations for non-classic risk factors have emerged. Thus there has been a sharp increase in studies on the role of testosterone in the pathogenesis of ischemic cardiovascular disease.

This review summarizes the current evidence on the association between endogenous testosterone and CVD in men.

Testosterone and Aging

In men the most important serum androgen is testosterone, which is almost exclusively secreted by the testes. There it is produced more specifically by Leydig cells in response to the stimulus of a gonadotropin called Luteinizing Hormone (LH) [6].

In plasma, approximately 2% of testosterone travels freely, 44% are bound to Sex Hormone Binding Globulin (SHBG) and the remaining 54% are bound to albumin and other proteins. The portions that are free or bound to albumin are readily available to tissues and are called Bioavailable Testosterone (BT).

In men testosterone levels are highest after 30 years of age and start declining thereafter at about 1-2% every year [6]. There are different aspects to the changes in testosterone levels in age men: there are reduced testicular response to the gonadotropic stimuli associated with an unsatisfactory compensation by the hypothalamus-pituitary axis [7] and there is an aged-associated increase of SHBG levels by about 1.2% per year, so that the decrease Free Testosterone (FT) and BT serum levels is larger than that of Total Testosterone (TT) [8,9].

As men age, this fall in the serum levels of testosterone intensifies: about one in every five men over the age of 60 and half of men over 80 have levels of testosterone below the lowest levels considered physiological in young men [8]. This relative deficiency is most commonly manifested with an increase in body fat and a reduction in both bone mass and muscle strength [8] contributing to the fat redistribution and to reduce in lean body mass [11,12]. Such loss in muscle mass at this age could explain the higher risk of falling, balance problems, obstructive sleep apnea, obesity, Diabetes Mellitus 2 (DM2), depression, chronic obstructive pulmonary disease, kidney and liver diseases and other functional limitations [13-15].

Testosterone and Endothelial Dysfunction

Endothelial dysfunction refers to an imbalance in the endothelial production of mediators that regulate vascular tonus, platelet aggregation, coagulation and fibrinolysis. It is frequently referred to as a worsening of the endothelium dependent relaxation caused by the bioavailability of nitric oxide (NO) and other vasodilating substances. Thus it can be found in many metabolic and/or cardiovascular diseases.

Testosterone is a vasoactive hormone with a predominantly vasodilating role in many vascular beds [16]. This androgen can exert its effects over the cardiovascular system through genomic models, by activating the androgen receptor (AR), and through non-genomic models, by activating the steroid receptors in the plasma membrane, which can also lead to blockage of the calcium L channels and opening of the calcium activated potassium channels [17]. The acute and chronic administration of testosterone has shown beneficial effects in ischemic myocardium induced by exercise in men with coronary arterial disease (CAD) [18,19].

The immunosuppressant effect of androgens has been well understood and greater levels of auto-immune diseases in women and hypogonadic men are thought to be due to a down regulation of pro-inflammatory cytokines caused by testosterone [20]. Testosterone is capable of stimulating the production of an anti-inflammatory cytokine called interleukin 10 (IL-10) [21] and reducing other pro-inflammatory cytokines such as tumor necrosis factor α (TNFα), interleukin 1(IL-1) and interleukin 6β [22,23] commonly elevated in elderly patients in subclinical inflammatory states [25].

A recent study of orchidectomized mice by Freeman et al. observed that androgenic supplementation was associated with a decline in inflammatory markers; while sub physiological testosterone levels were associated with an elevation of these markers, suggesting that the modulation of these hormonally responsive pathways could contribute to the development of the vascular pathogenesis [34].

In the last few years chronic inflammation has emerged as an important independent predictor of CAD. C-reactive Protein (CRP) is the most well studied inflammatory biomarker and today it is the most important among all the available ones, functioning as an independent risk factor for MI, stroke, peripheral vascular disease and sudden death [26]. Kupelian et al. [27], in a population based observational study of a sectional cohort with 1559 men with urologic symptoms, found an inverse association between testosterone and CRP, providing evidence to support testosterone's role in the inflammatory process. Finally, Wickramatilake et al. [28] demonstrated, in a case-control study of 206 men with CAD submitted to coronary angiography, that CVD patients had lower levels of testosterone and higher levels of CRP compared to the control group's. While CRP did show a positive association with the degree of atherosclerosis, testosterone did not. Inversely, in a similar study of 400 healthy men by Nakhai-Pour et al. [29], levels of TT and BT were not statistically associated to CRP in spite adjusting for age.

Testosterone also affects endothelial function by modulating the release of NO. This promotes vasodilation, inhibits platelet aggregation and adhesion of leukocytes to the endothelium, migration and growth of smooth muscle cells and oxidation of LDL-cholesterol (LDL-c). In a study using endothelial cell culture, Campelo et al. [30] demonstrated that testosterone increases the production of NO via AR.

Finally, testosterone also has vasoconstrictor effects. The administration of 200mg of testosterone cypionate to healthy men in a double-blind, randomised, placebo-controlled trial revealed increased platelet aggregation by modulating the expression of thromboxane A2 receptors [31]. In another study, testosterone was implicated for impairing coronary vasodilation in response to adenosine in isolated mice heart models [32]. Such effect was attributed to and acutely mediated by the release of thromboxane, which is a potent vasoconstrictor and platelet aggregate.

Endothelins are potent endogenous vasoconstricting peptides. The relation between testosterone and endothelin 1 (ET-1) is complex with some studies suggesting that testosterone increases levels of ET-, mediating vasoconstriction, while others suggest that the levels of these peptides are higher in hypogonadism situations [33].

Recently Chignalia et al. [34] proposed that testosterone induces the generation of Reactive Oxygen Species (ROS) in renal smooth muscle cells. Since ROS in the kidneys reduce the bioavailability of NO and increases vasoconstriction [35], it is possible that this androgen can contribute to the loss in renal function and vascular dysfunction via ROS production.

As discussed so far, testosterone modulates the mechanisms associated with endothelial dysfunction that occurs during old age. Although testosterone levels are associated with endothelial dysfunction and increased CVD, this relation of cause and effect still remains controversial. Some authors advocate that reduced levels of testosterone could function as a old age marker, and such reduction corresponding only to an epiphenomenon [36]. In reality, elevated levels of this androgen in the elderly reflect good health and a reduced risk for cardiovascular events [37].

Testosterone and Cardiovascular Risk Factors

Low levels of endogenous testosterone have been associated with the presence of many components of metabolic syndrome, including dyslipidemia, visceral obesity, Systemic Arterial Hypertension (SAH), DM2, hepatic steatosis, and others [18,38-40].

Important meta-analysis and prospective studies have demonstrated a negative association between testosterone and the incidence of Diabetes Mellitus in men [41-43]. However the temporal nature of this association is still controversial, with some arguments in each direction. Some have suggested that diabetes mellitus in mice cause a reduction in the number of Leydig cells [44] resulting in lower levels of testosterone, while other authors have put forth that elevated levels of this androgen increase lean mass and reduce the levels of TNF-α and insulin resistance [41-43].

Morbidly obese patients with peripheral insulin resistance frequently have low levels of TT, which increase with weight loss. The mechanisms responsible for the reduction in the levels of testosterone in obese men are not fully understood. The reduction in FT in severe obesity is not associated to an increase in LH suggesting a form of hypogonadotropic hypogonadism. One postulated hypothesis would be a dysfunction in the testicular hypothalamic-pituitary axis characterized by the reduction of peaks of LH [45]. Another suggested mechanism would be an increase in the peripheral conversion of androgens into estrogens by the enzyme aromatase, which is present in elevated concentrations in adipose tissue [45]. Furthermore, obesity is one of many conditions that can result in low levels of SHBG, with insulin being an important inhibitor of the production of this globulin in the liver [45]. This way, individuals with insulin resistance tend to present with lower values of TT.

Through the activation of β-adrenergic AR expressed in adipose cells, androgens stimulate hormone sensitive lipase and inhibit the activity of lipoproteic lipase, the main enzyme that regulates the intake of glucose in adipose tissues [46]. As a result testosterone is able to reduce the fat reserves in adipose tissue by stimulating lipolysis. This explains the increase in body fat mass associated with low levels of testosterone observed in hypogonadism patients.

Some interventionist prospective studies have revealed beneficiary effects of testosterone therapy in the parameters for metabolic syndrome. Kalinchenko et al. [47], in a study with 184 men with metabolic syndrome and low levels of testosterone, demonstrated that treatment for 30 weeks with Intramuscular (IM) testosterone undecanoate reduced Body Mass Index (BMI), Waist Circumference (WC), insulin levels, CRP, IL-1β and TNF-α in comparison with placebo but there was no significant change in levels of glucose, IL-6 and IL-10 and in lipid profile. In another prospective, longitudinal study by Yassin et al. [48] of 261 men, treatment with IM testosterone undecanoate during five years reduced WC, BMI, cholesterol, LDL-c, triglycerides, fasting glucose, glycated hemoglobin and arterial pressure (AP) but did not produce an increase in HDL-cholesterol (HDL-c) .

Haddad et al. [49] in a meta-analysis of 30 randomised placebo-controlled studies, with 1642 men, 808 of which treated with testosterone in the commercially available forms (IM, transdermical, oral and buccal) showed negligible effects of testosterone on the levels of lipids, AP, glicemic control and cardiovascular events.

Finally, Kelly et al. [50] in a study with orchidectomized mice, with androgen receptor deficiency and with a cholesterol rich diet, observed the effect of testosterone therapy over regulatory enzymes in the synthesis of fatty acids. In the testosterone supplementation group there were smaller fat deposits in hepatocytes when compared to placebo. Such result suggests a different mechanism of action of testosterone, independent of AR, over the regulation of the main lipogenic enzymes and protection against hepatic steatosis.

Testosterone and Cardiovascular Disease

Atherosclerosis is a complex pathology characterized by endothelial dysfunction, vascular inflammation and lipid buildup in the intima layer of blood vessels. The development of atherosclerosis is promoted not only by systemic factors, but also metabolic, vascular and inflammatory dysfunctions of the vessels' walls.

Testosterone can affect the development of atherosclerosis in coronary arteries. While it seems to have cardioprotective effects by benefiting endothelial function, inducing vasodilation and reducing insulin resistance and chronic inflammation [40,51,52], it also appears to increase endothelin, thromboxane A2 and ROS in renal smooth muscle cells [31,32,34,35].

The relationship between testosterone and CAD in men has been the focus of study of many authors. Most of the studies point to a neutral and/or protective effect of endogenous testosterone in cardiovascular health.

In this line of research, Callou de Sá *et al.*[53], in a case-control study of 144 patients who underwent elective coronary angiography found a neutral effect of TT, BT, FT and free androgen index in the prevalence of CAD. Similarly, Vikan et al. [52] in a study with 1318 men followed for 9.1 years, did not find an association between TT and FT and the incidence of MI. Araujo et al. [55] in a meta-analysis with 11831 participants did not find a statistically significant correlation between reduced levels of testosterone and cardiovascular mortality either.

On the other hand, Hyde *et al.*[56]in a population based prospective study of 3637 elderly men followed by 5.1 years, found that reduced FT levels were associated with higher mortality by CVD. Furthermore, Li Li *et al.*[56], in a study of 803 patients who underwent elective coronary angiography, demonstrated reduced levels of TT to be associated with CAD and with it's severity determined by the Gensini score.

Despite the beneficial effects of endogenous testosterone in men's cardiovascular health well described in the literature, a number of studies were not able to replicate these beneficial effects with testosterone therapy. In fact, when observed studies involving interventions with testosterone therapy and CVD, results vary greatly between authors.

In the TOM study [57], elderly participants with limited mobility and low levels of testosterone were randomly assigned to either a placebo group or a therapy group receiving transdermic gel with 100 mg of testosterone during six months. It had to be discontinued prematurely due to a higher incidence of cardiovascular events in the testosterone group. Similarly, Xu *et al.*[58] in a meta-analysis of 27 randomised placebo-controlled trials, with 2994 participants, 1733 of which used testosterone, found RR 1.54 for cardiovascular events (95% CI,1.09 to 2.18) for the testosterone group. In accordance with these results Vigen et al. [59] in a retrospective cohort study of 8709 men with low levels of testosterone who underwent coronary angiography, of which 1223 received testosterone therapy, showed increased mortality, MI and stroke rates in the testosterone group.

Haddad *et al.*[49] in a previously cited meta-analysis showed only negligible effects of testosterone in cardiovascular events OR 1.86 (95% CI, 0.78 to 4.23). Similarly Fernandez-Balsells et al. [60], in a meta-analysis of 51 studies with 2716 men who used testosterone did not find a significant difference in mortality by all causes, arrhythmias, coronary bypass surgery or MI between the testosterone group and the control group.

On the other hand, Toma *et al.*[61], in a meta-analysis of randomised controlled trials of 198 men with heart failure, found testosterone therapy was associated with a significant improvement in exercise capacity compared with placebo (New York Heart Association functional class improved by ≥1 grade, increase in the 6-minute walk test and the peak oxygen consumption in exercise).

Finally, many authors agree that low testosterone levels could be interpreted as a factor, which when associated with old age contributes to an increase in comorbidities [51], or could help reveal previously existing hidden pathologies [16,39,51] functioning as a biomarker for old age [16,51]. High levels of this androgen in the elderly reflect good health and a reduced risk of cardiovascular events [16,51].

Conclusion

Endogenous testosterone exerts a neutral and/or beneficial effect in the male cardiovascular system. This androgen favors vasodilation, has a pro and anti-aggregate role, and reduces the fat mass, inflammatory biomarkers, insulin resistance and the incidence of diabetes mellitus. Lending support to this line of thought, some observational studies point to a larger prevalence of cardiovascular disease and cardiovascular mortality in populations with reduced serum levels of this hormone. On the other hand, interventional studies in which testosterone replacement was used do not reach a uniform consensus with regards to the cardiovascular endpoints, with some suggesting higher risk, some neutral and others describing lower risk. It is important to keep in mind that this study describes the cardiovascular effects of testosterone replacement therapy and does not investigate improvements in the quality of life of the patients. Testosterone replacement therapy in men with hypogonadism by pituitary or testicular diseases deserves special consideration. More studies are needed to try to describe the pathogenic mechanisms of testosterone in cardiovascular health and to investigate polymorphisms of the androgen receptor in the physiological response to it.

References

1. WHO - World Health Organization (1998) Life in the 21st century: A vision for all. The world health report.
2. Arnlöv J, Pencina MJ, Amin S, Nam BH, Benjamin EJ, et al. (2006) Endogenous sex hormones and cardiovascular disease incidence in men. Ann Intern Med 145: 176-184.
3. Turhan S, Tulunay C, Güleç S, Ozdöl C, Kilickap M, et al. (2007) The association between androgen levels and premature coronary artery disease in men. Coron Artery Dis 18: 159-162.
4. Yusuf S, Hawken S, Ounpuu S, Dans T, Avezum A, et al. (2004) Effect of potentially modifiable risk factors associated with myocardial infarction in 52 countries (the INTERHEART study): case-control study. Lancet 364: 937-952.
5. Gebara OC, Vieira NW, Meyer JW, Calich AL, Tai EJ, et al. (2002) [Cardiovascular effects of testosterone]. Arq Bras Cardiol 79: 644-649.
6. Feldman HA, Longcope C, Derby CA, Johannes CB, Araujo AB, et al. (2002) Age trends in the level of serum testosterone and other hormones in middle-aged men: longitudinal results from the Massachusetts male aging study. J Clin Endocrinol Metab 87: 589-598.
7. Kaufman JM, Vermeulen A (2005) The decline of androgen levels in elderly men and its clinical and therapeutic implications. Endocr Rev 26: 833-876.
8. Muller M, den Tonkelaar I, Thijssen JH, Grobbee DE, van der Schouw YT (2003) Endogenous sex hormones in men aged 40-80 years. Eur J Endocrinol 149: 583-589.
9. Feldman HA, Longcope C, Derby CA, Johannes CB, Araujo AB, et al. (2002) Age trends in the level of serum testosterone and other hormones in middle-aged men: longitudinal results from the Massachusetts male aging study. J Clin Endocrinol Metab 87: 589-598.
10. Harman SM, Metter EJ, Tobin JD, Pearson J, Blackman MR (2001) Longi- tudinal effects of aging on serum total and free testosterone levels in healthy men. Baltimore Longitudinal Study of Aging. J Clin Endocrinol Metab 86:724-731.
11. Dunajska K, Milewicz A, Szymczak J, Jêdrzejuk D, Kuliczkowski W, et al. (2004) Evaluation of sex hormone levels and some metabolic factors in men with coronary atherosclerosis. Aging Male 7: 197-204.
12. Iannuzzi-Sucich M, Prestwood KM, Kenny AM (2002) Prevalence of sarcopenia and predictors of skeletal muscle mass in healthy, older men and women. J Gerontol A Biol Sci Med Sci 57: 772-777.
13. Simon D, Charles MA, Nahoul K, Orssaud G, Kremski J, et al. (1997) Association between plasma total testosterone and cardiovascular risk factors in healthy adult men: The Telecom Study. J Clin Endocrinol Metab 82: 682-685.
14. Khaw KT, Dowsett M, Folkerd E, Bingham S, Wareham N, et al. (2007) Endogenous testosterone and mortality due to all causes, cardiovascular disease, and cancer in men: European prospective investigation into cancer in Norfolk (EPIC-Norfolk) Prospective Population Study. Circulation 116: 2694-2701.
15. Shores MM, Matsumoto AM, Sloan KL, Kivlahan DR (2006) Low serum testosterone and mortality in male veterans. Arch Intern Med 166: 1660-1665.
16. Kelly DM, Jones TH (2013) Testosterone: a vascular hormone in health and disease. J Endocrinol 217: R47-71.
17. Webb CM, McNeill JG, Hayward CS, de Zeigler D, Collins P (1999) Effects of testosterone on coronary vasomotor regulation in men with coronary heart disease. Circulation 100: 1690-1696.
18. Wu J, Hadoke PW2, Mair I2, Lim WG2, Miller E2, et al. (2014) Modulation of neointimal lesion formation by endogenous androgens is independent of vascular androgen receptor. Cardiovasc Res 103: 281-290.
19. English KM, Steeds RP, Jones TH,Diver MJ, Channer KS (2000) Low-dose transdermal testosterone therapy improves angina threshold in men with chronic stable angina: A randomized, double-blind, placebo-controlled study. Circulation 102:1906-1911
20. Bain J (2007) The many faces of testosterone. Clin Interv Aging 2: 567-576.
21. Liva SM, Voskuhl RR (2001) Testosterone acts directly on CD4+ T lymphocytes to increase IL-10 production. J Immunol 167: 2060-2067.
22. Malkin CJ, Pugh PJ, Jones RD, Kapoor D, Channer KS, et al. (2004) The effect of testosterone replacement on endogenous inflammatory cytokines and lipid profiles in hypogonadal men. J Clin Endocrinol Metab 89: 3313-3318.
23. Saad F, Aversa A, Isidori AM, Zafalon L, Zitzmann M, et al. (2011) Onset of effects of testosterone treatment and time span until maximum effects are achieved. Eur J Endocrinol 165: 675-685.
24. Singh T, Newman AB (2011) Inflammatory markers in population studies of aging. Ageing Res Rev 10: 319-329.
25. Freeman BM, Mountain DJ, Brock TC, Chapman JR, Kirkpatrick SS, et al. (2014) Low testosterone elevates interleukin family cytokines in a rodent model: a possible mechanism for the potentiation of vascular disease in androgen-deficient males. J Surg Res 190:319-27.
26. Silva D, Pais de Lacerda A (2012) [High-sensitivity C-reactive protein as a biomarker of risk in coronary artery disease]. Rev Port Cardiol 31: 733-745.
27. Kupelian V, Chiu GR, Araujo AB, Williams RE, Clark RV, et al. (2010) Association of sex hormones and C-reactive protein levels in men. Clin Endocrinol (Oxf) 72: 527-533.
28. Wickramatilake CM, Mohideen MR, Withanawasam BP, Pathirana C (2014) Testosterone and high-sensitive C-reactive protein in coronary artery disease patients awaiting coronary artery bypass graft. Andrologia .
29. Nakhai Pour HR, Grobbee DE, Muller M, van der Schouw YT (2007) Association of endogenous sex hormone with C-reactive protein levels in middle-aged and elderly men. Clin Endocrinol (Oxf) 66: 394-398.
30. Campelo AE, Cutini PH, Massheimer VL (2012) Testosterone modulates platelet aggregation and endothelial cell growth through nitric oxide pathway. J Endocrinol 213: 77-87.
31. Ajayi AA, Mathur R, Halushka PV (1995) Testosterone increases human platelet thromboxane A2 receptor density and aggregation responses. Circulation 91: 2742-2747.
32. Ceballos G, Figueroa L, Rubio I, Gallo G, Garcia A, et al. (1999) Acute and nongenomic effects of testosterone on isolated and perfused rat heart. J Cardiovasc Pharmacol 33: 691-697.
33. Tostes RC, Fortes ZB, Callera GE, Montezano AC, Touyz RM, et al. (2008) Endothelin, sex and hypertension. Clin Sci (Lond) 114: 85-97.
34. Chignalia AZ, Schuldt EZ, Camargo LL, Montezano AC, Callera GE, et al. (2012) Testosterone induces vascular smooth muscle cell migration by

NADPH oxidase and c-Src-dependent pathways. Hypertension 59: 1263-1271.

35. Lopes RA, Neves KB, Carneiro FS, Tostes RC (2012) Testosterone and vascular function in aging. Front Physiol 3: 89.

36. Horstman AM, Dillon EL, Urban RJ, Sheffield-Moore M (2012) The role of androgens and estrogens on healthy aging and longevity. J Gerontol A Biol Sci Med Sci 67: 1140-1152.

37. Sá EQ, Sá FC, Guedes AD, Verreschi IT (2009) [Serum testosterone and cardiovascular disease in men]. Arq Bras Endocrinol Metabol 53: 915-922.

38. Oskui PM, French WJ, Herring MJ, Mayeda GS, Burstein S, et al. (2013) Testosterone and the cardiovascular system: a comprehensive review of the clinical literature. J Am Heart Assoc 2: e000272.

39. Hackett G, Kirby M2, Sinclair AJ3 (2014) Testosterone deficiency, cardiac health, and older men. Int J Endocrinol 2014: 143763.

40. Corona G, Monami M, Rastrelli G, Aversa A, Sforza A, et al. (2011) Type 2 diabetes mellitus and testosterone: a meta-analysis study. Int J Androl 34: 528-540.

41. Ding EL, Song Y, Malik VS, Liu S (2006) Sex differences of endogenous sex hormones and risk of type 2 diabetes: a systematic review and meta-analysis. JAMA 295: 1288-1299.

42. Colangelo LA, Ouyang P, Liu K, Kopp P, Golden SH, et al. (2009) Association of endogenous sex hormones with diabetes and impaired fasting glucose in men: multi-ethnic study of atherosclerosis. Diabetes Care 32: 1049-1051.

43. Pitteloud N, Hardin M, Dwyer AA, Valassi E, Yialamas M, et al. (2005) Increasing insulin resistance is associated with a decrease in Leydig cell testosterone secretion in men. J Clin Endocrinol Metab 90: 2636-2641.

44. Vermeulen A (1996) Decreased androgen levels and obesity in men. Ann Med 28: 13-15.

45. Mårin P, Odén B, Björntorp P (1995) Assimilation and mobilization of triglycerides in subcutaneous abdominal and femoral adipose tissue in vivo in men: effects of androgens. J Clin Endocrinol Metab 80: 239-243.

46. Kalinchenko SY, Tishova YA, Mskhalaya GJ, Gooren LJ, Giltay EJ, et al. (2010) Effects of testosterone supplementation on markers of the metabolic syndrome and inflammation in hypogonadal men with the metabolic syndrome: the double-blinded placebo-controlled Moscow study. Clin Endocrinol (Oxf) 73: 602-612.

47. Yassin DJ, Doros G, Hammerer PG, Yassin AA (2014) Long-term testosterone treatment in elderly men with hypogonadism and erectile dysfunction reduces obesity parameters and improves metabolic syndrome and health-related quality of life. J Sex Med 11:1567-1576.

48. Haddad RM, Kennedy CC, Caples SM, Tracz MJ, Boloña ER, et al. (2007) Testosterone and cardiovascular risk in men: a systematic review and meta-analysis of randomized placebo-controlled trials. Mayo Clin Proc 82:29-39.

49. Kelly DM, Nettleship JE2, Akhtar S2, Muraleedharan V3, Sellers DJ4, et al. (2014) Testosterone suppresses the expression of regulatory enzymes of fatty acid synthesis and protects against hepatic steatosis in cholesterol-fed androgen deficient mice. Life Sci 109: 95-103.

50. Yeap BB (2014) Sex steroids and cardiovascular disease. Asian J Androl 16: 239-247.

51. Li L, Guo CY, Jia EZ, Zhu TB, Wang LS, et al. (2012) Testosterone is negatively associated with the severity of coronary atherosclerosis in men. Asian J Androl 14: 875-878.

52. Callou de Sá EQ, Feijó de Sá FC, e Silva Rde S, de Oliveira KC, Guedes AD, et al. (2011) Endogenous oestradiol but not testosterone is related to coronary artery disease in men. Clin Endocrinol (Oxf) 75: 177-183.

53. Vikan T, Schirmer H, Njølstad I, Svartberg J (2009) Endogenous sex hormones and the prospective association with cardiovascular disease and mortality in men: the Tromsø Study. Eur J Endocrinol 161: 435-442.

54. Araujo AB, Dixon JM, Suarez EA, Murad MH, Guey LT, et al. (2011) Clinical review: Endogenous testosterone and mortality in men: a systematic review and meta-analysis. J Clin Endocrinol Metab 96: 3007-3019.

55. Hyde Z, Norman PE, Flicker L, Hankey GJ, Almeida OP, et al. (2012) Low free testosterone predicts mortality from cardiovascular disease but not other causes: the Health in Men Study. J Clin Endocrinol Metab 97: 179-189.

56. Basaria S, Coviello AD, Travison TG, Storer TW, Farwell WR, et al. (2010) Adverse events associated with testosterone administration. N Engl J Med 363: 109-122.

57. Xu L, Freeman G, Cowling BJ, Schooling CM (2013) Testosterone therapy and cardiovascular events among men: a systematic review and meta-analysis of placebo-controlled randomized trials. BMC Medicine 11:108-116.

58. Vigen R, O'Donnell CI, Barón AE, Grunwald GK, Maddox TM, et al. (2013) Association of testosterone therapy with mortality, myocardial infarction, and stroke in men with low testosterone levels. JAMA 310: 1829-1836.

59. Fernández-Balsells MM, Murad MH, Lane M, Lampropulos JF, Albuquerque F, et al. (2010) Clinical review 1: Adverse effects of testosterone therapy in adult men: a systematic review and meta-analysis. J Clin Endocrinol Metab 95: 2560-2575.

60. Toma M, McAlister FA, Coglianese EE, Vidi V, Vasaiwala S, et al. (2012) Testosterone supplementation in heart failure: a meta-analysis. Circ Heart Fail 5: 315-321.

Post-Saline Infusion Plasma Aldosterone Concentrations are Well Correlated with the Lateralized Ratio of Adrenal Venous Sampling in Patients of Primary Aldosteronism

Yuko Tsushima[1,2], **Ken Terui**[1,2*], **Koshi Makita**[1,2], **Yuko Asari**[1,2], **Noriko Ishigame**[1,2], **Yuki Nakada**[1,2], **Aya Sugiyama**[1,2], **Shingo Murasawa**[1,2], **Satoshi Yamagata**[1,2], **Yutaka Watanuki**[1,2], **Shinobu Takayasu**[1,2], **Takeshi Nigawara**[1,2], **Kazunori Kageyama**[1,2] **and Makoto Daimon**[1,2]

[1]*Department of Endocrinology and Metabolism, Hirosaki University Graduate School of Medicine, Hirosaki, Japan*

[2]*Department of Endocrinology, Diabetes and Metabolism, Hirosaki University School of Medicine and Hospital, Hirosaki, Japan*

[*]**Corresponding author**: Ken Terui, Department of Endocrinology and Metabolism, Hirosaki University Graduate School of Medicine, 5 Zaifu-cho, Hirosaki, Japan, E-mail: terui@hirosaki-u.ac.jp

Abstract

Objective: Adrenal venous sampling (AVS) is the most reliable test to distinguish between unilateral and bilateral primary aldosteronism (PA). However, AVS is invasive, risky, and expensive, and alternative diagnostic methods are desirable. This study aimed to investigate the diagnostic power of saline infusion test (SIT) to distinguish between unilateral and bilateral PA.

Design: Retrospective database analysis.

Subjects and Methods: We selected 111 patients with PA diagnosed by confirmatory tests who underwent both SIT and successful AVS. Thirty-two patients had lateralized ratio (LR) over 4.0 and 79 patients had LR less than 4.0. Multiple regression analysis and receiver operating characteristic (ROC) analysis were used to examine whether the SIT had good diagnostic power to distinguish between patients with high LR and those with low LR.

Results: The patients with high LR had significantly lower serum potassium levels ($P<0.0001$, Mann-Whitney's U Test) and higher plasma aldosterone concentrations after SIT (Post-PAC) ($P<0.0001$). It was revealed that Post-PAC levels were independently associated with the LR by multiple regression analysis ($P=0.0112$). ROC analysis revealed that the diagnostic accuracy of SIT was very high for distinguishing between patients with high LR and those with low LR. The optimal cut-off value of Post-PAC for the diagnosis of patients with low LR was less than 9.3 ng/dl.

Conclusions: SIT is useful for distinguishing between patients with high LR and low LR. It might be possible to omit AVS in patients with a Post-PAC value less than 9.3 ng/dl.Combining the results of serum potassium levels and imaging examinations with SIT might be a potential strategy for PA subtypes.

Keywords: Primary aldosteronism; Saline infusion test; Aldosterone-renin ratio; Adrenal venous sampling; Lateralized ratio

Introduction

Primary aldosteronism (PA) is currently considered to be the most frequent cause of secondary hypertension [1,2]. To screen for PA, the plasma aldosterone to renin ratio (ARR) is assessed in hypertensive patients [3]. If the ARR is higher than normal limits, confirmatory tests are requested, such as captopril challenge test (CCT), saline infusion test (SIT), fludrocortisone suppression test, and oral sodium loading test.

The Endocrine Society advocates the use of the four confirmatory tests in their clinical practice guidelines for PA. A conclusive diagnosis of PA is reached based on at least one positive test result [3,4]. The Japan Endocrine Society proposes the use of three confirmatory tests, that is, CCT, SIT, and furosemide plus upright test (FUT) [5]. Based on these guidelines, two positive test results are needed for diagnosis. There is no consensus whether any confirmatory test is a gold standard for diagnosis.

After PA is diagnosed, the subtype should be identified in order to select the appropriate treatment for PA: surgical or medical treatment. In aldosterone-producing adenoma (APA) patients, hypersecretion of aldosterone is usually one-sided, that is, from one of the adrenal glands [6]. In patients with idiopathic hyperaldosteronism (IHA), hypersecretion is usually from both adrenal glands. Currently, adrenal venous sampling (AVS) is the most reliable test to distinguish between unilateral and bilateral PA [7,8]. To identify patients with PA, AVS is a reliable but invasive, risky, and costly procedure.7 Therefore, alternative diagnostic methods are needed. A new guideline of the Endocrine Society recommends medical treatment without AVS if a patient is unable or unwilling to undergo surgery [4].

Küpers et al. proposed a clinical prediction score to diagnose unilateral PA. Their results suggest that AVS can be omitted in patients with a typical APA of at least 8 mm on computed tomography (CT), hypokalemia, and/or a high estimated glomerular filtration rate (eGFR) [9].

Arteaga et al. reported that SIT was useful for the differentiation of patients with APA from those with IHA [10]. Nanba et al. proposed that the shortened SIT be used to predict unilateral PA in Japanese patients [11]. Nevertheless, both these studies involved small patient populations.

The present study was performed to test whether the standard SIT has good diagnostic power for distinguishing between patients with unilateral and bilateral PA. To examine this hypothesis, we determined the best cut-off value to evaluate the diagnostic efficiency of SIT.

Patients and Methods

Patients

We retrospectively analyzed hypertensive patients with elevated ARR [>20; PAC in ng/dl and plasma renin activity (PRA) in ng/ml/h] (n=323) who were admitted to the Department of Endocrinology, Diabetes and Metabolism of Hirosaki University School of Medicine and Hospital from 2008 to 2016.

Before determination of ARR, mineralocorticoid receptor blockers, diuretics, beta-adrenergic blockers, angiotensin converting enzyme inhibitors and angiotensin receptor blockers were withdrawn for at least 2 weeks. These drugs should be changed to other drugs such as calcium channel blockers and alpha-adrenergic blockers. According to the Japanese guidelines, all of the patients had at least two of the three confirmatory tests for diagnosis of PA (CCT, SIT, or FUT). In this study, we re-evaluated the diagnosis of PA by CCA or FUT only. Overall, 295 patients had at least one positive test result of CCA or FUT, while 28 had negative results for all two tests. Of the 295 patients with positive test results, 278 underwent AVS, while the remaining 17 patients did not undergo AVS because they opted against surgery. AVS was successfully performed in 209 patients. This study involved 111 patients who underwent both SIT and successful AVS (Figure 1).

Hypokalemic patients were given adequate oral potassium supplements before SIT to maintain serum potassium levels higher than 3.0 mmol/L. SIT was not performed in patients with severe uncontrolled hypertension, cardiac arrhythmia, and cardiac or renal insufficiency. The study was approved and registered as an institutional case-notes review at the Institutional Review Board of Hirosaki University School of Medicine and Hospital (Registration No. 2015-252).

Saline infusion test

Patients were administered an intravenous drip infusion of 2 L of 0.9 NaCl over 4 h. After infusion, the PAC (Post-PAC) was measured [5,12].

Adrenal venous sampling

AVS was performed by expert radiologists to diagnose whether a unilateral or bilateral aldosterone-producing lesion was present. AVS was performed with cosyntropin infusion, as previously reported [13]. The lateralized ratio (LR) was calculated as (adrenal venous blood aldosterone/cortisol ratio on the high-value side)/(adrenal venous blood aldosterone/cortisol ratio on the low-value side). The contralateral ratio (CLR) was also calculated as (adrenal venous blood aldosterone/cortisol ratio on the low-value side)/(venous blood aldosterone/cortisol ratio in the inferior vena cava).

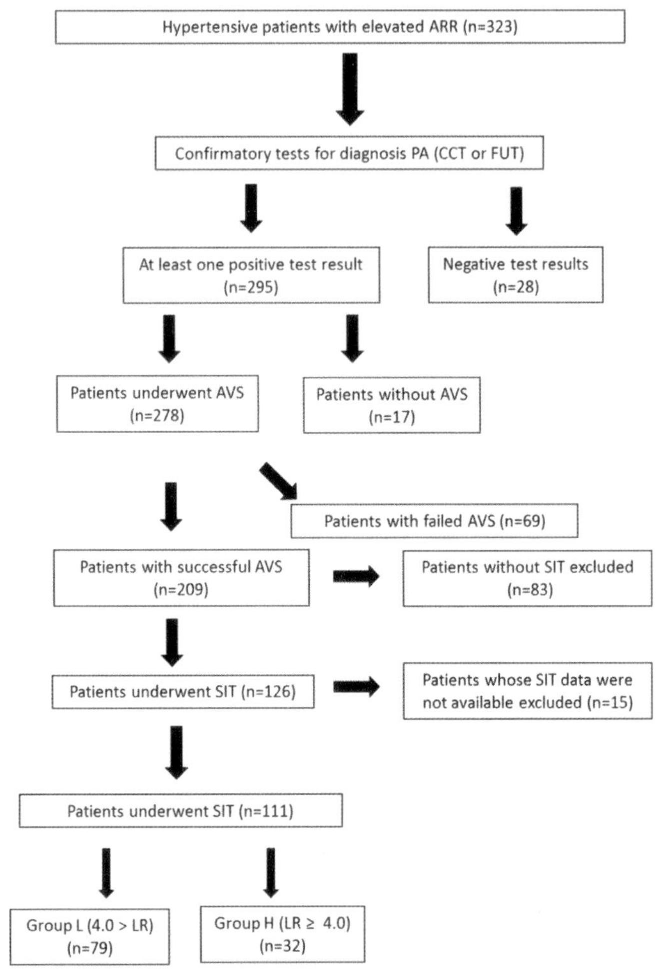

Figure 1: Flowchart of the study population. ARR: Plasma Aldosterone to Renin Ratio; PA: Primary Aldosteronism; AVS: Adrenal Venous Sampling; CCT: Captopril Challenge Test; FUT: Furosemide Plus Upright Test; SIT: Saline Infusion Test.

Statistical analysis

All the data are presented as medians with interquartile ranges. We used Mann-Whitney's U Test to compare medians between unilateral and bilateral groups. $P<0.05$ was considered to indicate statistical significance.

Spearman's rank-order correlation analysis was used to examine the relationship between the clinical parameters and LR.

A multiple regression analysis was performed for correlation between LR as a dependent variable and clinical parameters including Post-PAC as independent variables. Because the data had a non-normal distribution, logarithmic conversion was carried out. Factors with P values less than 0.05 on univariate analyses were considered for inclusion in the model, and forward selection and backward elimination methods were used to choose the explanatory variables.

The diagnostic accuracy of the SIT for differential diagnoses between bilateral and unilateral PA groups was assessed using the receiver operating characteristic (ROC) curve and the area under the ROC curve (AUC_{ROC}).

Results

Characteristics of the study population

We classified all the patients with PA in one group had LR over 4.0 (group H) or the other group (group L). The clinical characteristics of the two groups are summarized in Table 1. The number of patients of group L was higher than that of patients of group H. Age, height, body weight, and body mass index showed no significant differences between the two groups. Serum potassium levels were significantly lower in patients of group H than in those of group L. Basal PAC levels and ARR in patients of group H were higher than those in patients of group L. Post-PAC values were significantly higher in patients of group H than in those of group L.

Variables	Total	Group L (4.0> LR)	Group H (LR ≥ 4.0)	P value
N (M/F)	111 (44/67)	79 (27/52)	32 (17/15)	0.0645
Age (year) [median (IQR)]	53.0 [46.0-61.0]	53.0 [48.0-61.0]	58.0 [46.0-65.0]	0.1527
Height (cm) [median (IQR)]	159.6 [153.0-168.0]	158.8 [152.5-166.7]	164.8 [158.1-168.9]	0.0881
Body weight (kg) [median (IQR)]	65.9 [55.5-75.9]	63.5 [55.1-75.7]	67.6 [55.9-78.5]	0.4983
BMI (kg/m^2) [median (IQR)]	25.6 [22.1-28.2]	25.6 [22.3-28.6]	24.6 [22.0-28.1]	0.9046
Serum potassium (mmol/l) [median (IQR)]	3.7 [3.3-3.9]	3.8 [3.6-4.0]	3.1 [2.5-3.4]	<0.0001
eGFR (ml/min/1.73 m^2) [median (IQR)]	84.1 [71.0-96.2]	84.9 [73-95.3]	85.2[68.5-101.7]	0.792
Basal PAC (ng/dl) [median (IQR)]	145.5 [11.4-23.0]	13.4 [10.4-17.8]	26.1 [18.9-39.8]	<0.0001
Basal PRA (ng/ml/hr) [median (IQR)]	0.3 [0.2-0.4]	0.3 [0.2-0.4]	0.2 [0.1-0.4]	0.1215
ARR [median (IQR)]	59 [36-117]	49 [33-86]	133 [71-230]	<0.0001
Post-PAC (ng/dl) [median (IQR)]	8.9 [6.5-14.5]	7.9 [5.9-9.2]	26.2 [18.9-39.8]	<0.0001
Post-PRA (ng/ml/hr) [median (IQR)]	0.2 [0.1-0.3]	0.2 [0.1-0.3]	0.2 [0.1-0.3]	0.3919
Contra-lateralized ratio [median (IQR)]	1.4 [0.7-2.1]	1.8 [1.3-2.2]	0.4 [0.3-0.6]	<0.0001
Lateralized ratio [median (IQR)]	1.8 [1.3-5.2]	1.5 [1.2-2.0]	10.4 [7.0-17.4]	

Table 1: Characteristics of the study population.

Univariate and multiple regression analyses of continuous variables for LR

Univariate correlation analysis between each continuous variable and LR was performed (Table 2). Serum potassium, basal PAC, basal ARR, and Post-PAC (Figure 2) were positively correlated with LR, whereas eGFR was not.

Variables	Correlation coefficient	P value
Age	-0.0438	0.6478
Height	0.1809	0.0575
Body weight	0.029	0.7628
BMI	-0.0747	0.436
eGFR	-0.0875	0.3611
Serum potassium	-0.5032	<0.001
Basal PAC	0.5714	<0.001
Basal PRA	-0.1694	0.0755
Basal ARR	0.4936	<0.001
Post-PAC	0.6414	<0.001
Post-PRA	0.6414	0.8677
Contra-lateralized ratio	-0.757	<0.001

Table 2: Univariate analysis of continuous variables for lateralized ratio.

To further examine whether these parameters were associated with LR, stepwise multiple linear regression analysis was performed. Post-PAC and serum potassium levels were independently associated with LR among the factors analyzed (Table 3).

Diagnostic accuracy of SIT

The Post-PAC values were significantly lower in group L than in group H (Figure 3).

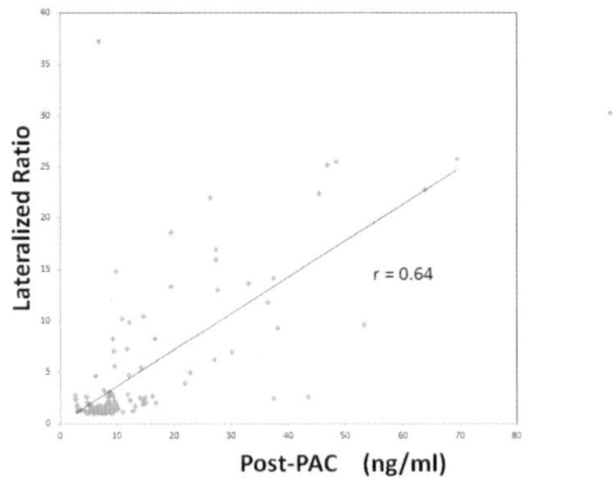

Figure 2: Relationship between plasma aldosterone concentration after saline infusion tests (Post-PAC) and the lateralized ratio (LR) of adrenal venous sampling.

Variables	PRC	SPRC	P value
Serum potassium	-1.629	-0.2988	<0.001
Basal PAC	0.2173	0.1168	0.414
Basal ARR	0.1158	0.0966	0.2896
Post-PAC	0.4947	0.36	0.0112
PRC: partial regression coefficient; SPRC: standardized partial regression coefficient			

Table 3: Multiple linear regression analysis for lateralized ratio.

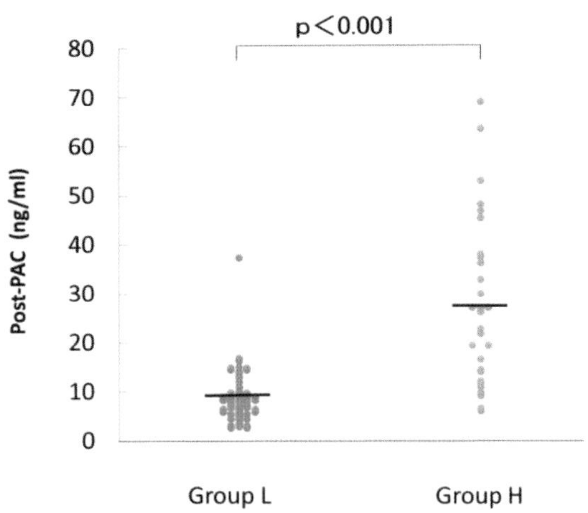

Figure 3: Scattergram of plasma aldosterone concentrations after saline infusion tests (Post-PAC) in group L and group H.

We analyzed the diagnostic accuracy of the SIT for differential diagnosis between patients with group L and group H. AUC_{ROC} was approximately 0.9, and the optimal cut-off value of Post-PAC was <9.3 ng/dl. These results showed a sensitivity of 76% and specificity of 94%, respectively (Figure 4). The Youden index identified the same optimal cut-off value.

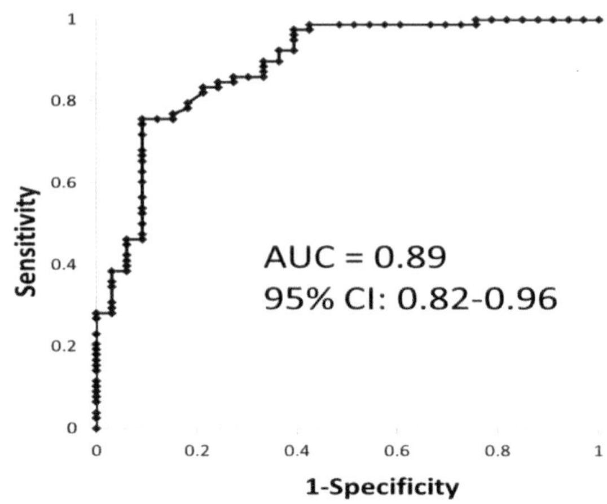

Figure 4: Receiver operating characteristic curves for plasma aldosterone concentrations after saline infusion tests (Post-PAC) for differential diagnosis between group L and group H.

Discussion

After a diagnosis of PA, the subtype should be identified. While AVS is the most reliable test to distinguish between unilateral and bilateral PA and is used to make management decisions [7,12], AVS is an invasive, risky, and costly procedure [7,9]. The need for an alternative diagnostic method has posed a challenging problem in this field.

Küpers et al. proposed a clinical prediction score to diagnose unilateral PA [9]. Their results suggest that AVS could be omitted in patients with a typical APA measuring at least 8 mm, with serum potassium levels <3.5 mmol/L and/or eGFR of at least 100 ml/min/1.73 m^2. In our findings, serum potassium levels were also positively correlated with LR by univariate correlation analysis. In contrast, eGFR was not correlated with LR. Riester et al. reported that the prediction score proposed by Küpers et al. has high accuracy only in young patients but cannot substitute for AVS in elderly patients [14]. Furthermore, in the present study, stepwise multiple linear regression analysis revealed that Post-PAC of SIT and serum potassium levels were independently associated with LR among the analyzed parameters.

Some papers have reported that confirmatory tests for PA are useful for distinguishing between unilateral and bilateral PA. Jiang et al. reported that the ACTH stimulation test with 1 mg dexamethasone was useful for differentiating patients with unilateral PA from patients with bilateral PA [15]. We reported that ACTH stimulation test suggest that there is a high likelihood of laterlizing on AVS [16]. Arteaga et al. reported that SIT and CT scan were useful in the differentiation of patients with APA from those with IHA [10]. They evaluated 20 patients with PA, 14 patients with APA who were surgically treated, and 6 patients with IHA. In the SIT method used in their study, the patients were administered 1.25 L of 0.9% saline solution over 2 h. They reported that after infusion, a PAC/cortisol ratio of <2.2 was diagnostic of IHA. On the other hand, Magill et al. reported that CT imaging was unreliable for the differentiation of PA and that AVS was essential to identify the PA subtype [17].

Nanba et al. [11] reported the shortened SIT method, wherein patients were administered 2 L of 0.9% saline solution over 4 h as usual; they proposed that PAC at 2 h would be more useful for predicting unilateral PA. They evaluated 39 patients with PA, including 18 patients with unilateral PA and 21 patients with bilateral PA. In their paper, the optimal cut-off value of PAC at 2 h was greater than 119 pg/ml and the AUC_{ROC} was about 0.89, with a sensitivity of 89% and specificity of 81%. Recently, the importance of SIT as a confirmatory test for PA has become controversial. Weigel et al. reported that SIT was the most widely used confirmatory test for PA in Germany, due to practicability, costs, and compliance [18]. On the other hand, Nanba et al. investigated the diagnostic significance of confirmatory tests in Japanese hypertensive patients [12] and reported that the positive rate on SIT was low, being <65%. Li et al. reported that PAC after SIT remained higher than 5 ng/dl in a great majority of Chinese patients with essential hypertension as well as in healthy subjects [19]. Thus, it seems that SIT lacks adequate efficacy as a confirmatory test for PA but has diagnostic power for differentiation of PA subtypes in Asian patients.

In the present study, we found that standard SIT was useful for differentiating between patients with low LR and high LR in a larger population of patients than those assessed in the two above-mentioned papers concerning SIT [10,11]. The optimal cut-off value of Post-PAC was <9.3 ng/dl, with a very high accuracy for the diagnosis of low LR patients. Our findings suggest that AVS can be omitted in patients with Post-PAC <9.3 ng/dl in standard SIT. For these patients, medical treatment may be selected directly without further invasive tests. Patients with Post-PAC of 9.3 ng/dl and above in standard SIT are likely to have unilateral PA; therefore, AVS is needed for these patients. Omitting AVS for approximately half of the patients with PA based on SIT results may enable a reduction in the risks and costs of the time-consuming AVS procedure.

Some limitations of our study should be mentioned. This study was a retrospective analysis, and recall bias cannot be excluded. In order to diagnose PA in our patients, we used the diagnostic criteria of Japanese guidelines for Japanese patients. Additional studies are needed for clarifying the usefulness of the standard SIT in other populations. Recently, a French group reported that SIT had a good predictive value for unilateral PA; however, 30% of patients with Post-PAC <5 ng/dl in SIT had unilateral secretion of aldosterone by AVS results [20]. These results disagree with our findings, that is, the PAC after SIT was over 9.3 ng/dl in almost all patients (94%) with high LR in our study. The reason underlying this difference may be the use of different AVS methods in the two studies and the presence or absence of ACTH stimulation [21]. While we used the cut-off value of the LR that was at least 4.0, more permissive cut-off value of LR was used in many previous studies. Because Umakoshi et al. reported that such permissive cut-off values could be seen even in non-PA patiets [22], we used a cut-off value of LR with a high specificity for unilateral PA patients.

Considering our findings alone, approximately 6% of patients with high LR would not undergo AVS and subsequent surgical treatment. Recently, Dekkers et al. reported that treatment of PA based on CT scan or AVS findings did not show significant differences in the intensity of medical treatment or clinical benefits [23]. Combining the results of serum potassium levels and imaging examinations such as CT with SIT might be a potential strategy for differentiating between patients with unilateral and bilateral PA.

In conclusion, standard SIT was useful for distinguishing between patients with low LR and high LR. Post-PAC of SIT and serum potassium levels were closely related to LR than other parameters, including eGFR. For the diagnosis of patients with low LR, the optimal cut-off value of Post-PAC was less than 9.3 ng/dl. Accordingly, combining the results of serum potassium levels and imaging examinations with SIT might be a potential strategy for PA subtypes.

References

1. Williams JS, Williams GH, Raji A, Jeunemaitre X, Brown NJ, et al. (2006) Prevalence of primary hyperaldosteronism in mild to moderate hypertension without hypokalaemia. J Hum Hypertens 20: 129-136.
2. Rossi GP, Bernini G, Caliumi C, Desideri G, Fabris B, et al. (2006) A prospective study of the prevalence of primary aldosteronism in 1,125 hypertensive patients. J Am Coll Cardiol 48: 2293-2300.
3. Funder JW, Carey RM, Fardella C, Gomez-Sanchez CE, Mantero F, et al. (2008) Case detection, diagnosis, and treatment of patients with primary aldosteronism: An endocrine society clinical practice guideline. J Clin Endocrinol Metab 93: 3266-3281.
4. Funder JW, Carey RM, Mantero F, Murad MH, Reincke M, et al. (2016) The management of primary aldosteronism: Case detection, diagnosis, and treatment: An endocrine society clinical practice guideline. J Clin Endocrinol Metab 101: 1889-1916.
5. Nishikawa T, Omura M, Satoh F, Shibata H, Takahashi K, et al. (2011) Guidelines for the diagnosis and treatment of primary aldosteronism. The Japan Endocrine Society 2009. Endocr J 58: 711-721.
6. Biglieri EG, Irony I, Kater CE (1989) Identification and implications of new types of mineralocorticoid hypertension. J Steroid Biochem 32: 199-204.
7. Sonoyama T, Sone M, Miyashita K, Tamura N, Yamahara K, et al. (2011) Significance of adrenocorticotropin stimulation test in the diagnosis of an aldosterone-producing adenoma. J Clin Endocrinol Metab 96: 2771-2778.
8. Young WF, Stanson AW, Thompson GB, Grant CS, Farley D, et al. (2004) Role for adrenal venous sampling in primary aldosteronism. Surgery 136: 1227-1235.
9. Küpers EM, Amar L, Raynaud A, Plouin PF, Steichen O (2012) A clinical prediction score to diagnose unilateral primary aldosteronism. J Clin Endocrinol Metab 97: 3530-3537.
10. Artega E, Klein R, Biglieri EG (1985) Use of the saline infusion test to diagnose the cause of primary aldosteronism. Am J Med 79: 722-728.
11. Nanba K, Tsuiki M, Umakoshi H, Nanba A, Hirokawa, et al. (2015) Shortened saline infusion test for subtype prediction in primary aldosteronism. Endocrine 50: 802-806.
12. Nanba K, Tamanaha T, Nakao K, Kawashima ST, Usui T, et al. (2012) Confirmatory testing in primary aldosteronism. J Clin Endocrinol Metab 97: 1688-1694.
13. Rossi GP, Auchus RJ, Brown M, Lenders JW, Naruse M, et al. (2014) An expert consensus statement on use of adrenal vein sampling for the subtyping of primary aldosteronism. Hypertension 63: 151-160.
14. Riester A, Fischer E, Degenhart C, Reiser MF, Bidlingmaier M, et al. (2014) Age below 40 or a recently proposed clinical prediction score cannot bypass adrenal venous sampling in primary aldosteronism. J Clin Endocrinol Metab 99: E1035- E1039.
15. Jiang Y, Zhang C, Wang W, Su T, Zhou W, et al. (2015) Diagnostic value of ACTH stimulation test in determining the subtype of primary aldosteronism. J Clin Endocrinol Metab 100: 1837-1844.
16. Terui K, Nigawara T, Kageyama K, Moriyama T, Sakihara S, et al. (2016) Evaluation of the (1-24) adrenocorticotropin stimulation test for the diagnosis of primary aldosteronism. J Renin Angiotensin Aldosterone Syst 17: 1-6.

17. Magill SB, Raff H, Shaker JL, Brickner RC, Knechtges TE, et al. (2001) Comparison of adrenal vein sampling and computed tomography in the differentiation of primary aldosteronism. J Clin Endocrinol Metab 86: 1066-1071.

18. Weigel M, Riester A, Hanslik G, Lang K, Willenberg HS, et al. (2015) Post-saline infusion test aldosterone levels indicate severity and outcome in primary aldosteronism. Eur J Endocrinol 172: 443-450.

19. Li Y, Liu Y, Li J, Wang X, Yu Y (2016) Sodium infusion test for diagnosis of primary aldosteronism in Chinese population. J Clin Endocrinol Metab 101: 89-95.

20. Cornu E, Steichen O, Nogueira-Silva L, Küpers E, Pagny JY, et al. (2016) Suppression of aldosterone secretion after recumbent saline infusion does not exclude lateralized primaryaldosteronism. Hypertension 68: 989-994.

21. Satoh F, Abe T, Tanemoto M, Nakamura M, Abe M, et al. (2007) Localization of aldosterone-producing adrenocortical adenomas: Significance of adrenal venous sampling. Hypertens Res 30: 1083-1095.

22. Umakoshi H, Naruse M, Wada N, Ichijo T, Kamemura K, et al. (2016) Adrenal venous sampling in patients with positive screening but negative confirmatory testing for primary aldosteronism. Hypertension 67: 1014-1019.

23. Dekkers T, Prejbisz A, Schultze Kool LJ, Groenewoud HJ, Velema M, et al. (2016) Adrenal vein sampling versus CT scan to determine treatment in primary aldosteronism: An outcome-based randomized diagnostic trial. Lancet Diabetes Endocrinol 4: 739-746.

Stage-Specific Expression Profiles of Anti-Müllerian Hormone and its Type II Receptor in Germ Cells during Spermatogenic Cycle of Rats

Kenji Ohyama[1*], **Masanori Ohta**[1], **Yoshinao Z Hosaka**[2], **Tetsuji Ohyama**[3] **and Yoshiaki Yamano**[4]

[1]*Interdisciplinary Graduate School of Medicine and Engineering, University of Yamanashi, Yamanashi, Japan*

[2]*Laboratory of Veterinary Anatomy, Faculty of Agriculture, Tottori University, Tottori, Japan*

[3]*Biostatistics Center, Kurume University, Fukuoka, Japan*

[4]*Laboratory of Veterinary Biochemistry, Faculty of Agriculture, Tottori University, Tottori, Japan*

[*]**Corresponding Author**: Kenji Ohyama, Interdisciplinary Graduate School of Medicine and Engineering, University of Yamanashi, 1110 Shimokato, Chuo-city, Yamanashi 409-3898, Japan, E-mail: ohyakenj@yahoo.co.jp

Abstract

Although anti-Müllerian hormone (AMH) is present in seminiferous tubules, its physiological roles in testis remain unclear. We defined expression patterns of AMH and its type II receptor (AMHR2) in germ cells during spermatogenic cycles. To this end, we performed *in situ* hybridization of *Amh* and *Amhr2*, and immunohistochemical staining using antibodies against AMH and AMHR2 in testes from rats aged 10, 15, 21, 35, and 49 days (d). In addition, quantitative RT-PCR analyses were performed to determine relative expression levels of *Amh, Amhr2, synaptonemal complex protein 1 (Scp1)* and *round spermatid basic protein 1 (Rsbn1),* and *Smads 1, 5, and 8* in germ cells isolated from 49d testes. In 49d testes, synthesis of AMH and AMHR2 corresponded with spermatocyte expression of *Amh* and *Amhr2*. Spermatocytes of stages VII-XIV synthesized AMH, and AMH staining was decreased in round spermatids and was not detectable in elongated spermatids. Spermatocytes of stages VII-XIV synthesized AMHR2, and round and elongated spermatids continued expressing AMHR2. The strongest staining of AMH was observed in spermatocytes at stage VIII, and that of AMHR2 was observed in round spermatids at the same stage. When isolated germ cells were cultured with anti-AMH antibody, expression levels of *Amh* and *Amhr2* were significantly increased, those of *Smads 1, 5 and Scp1* increased simultaneously, and that of *Rsbn1* decreased. We speculate that the AMH-SMADs axis is associated with morphological change from round to elongated spermatids at stage VIII.

Keywords: Anti-Müllerian hormone; Testis; Spermatogenesis; Germ cell; SMAD protein

Introduction

Anti-Müllerian hormone (AMH) is also known as Müllerian inhibiting substance (MIS), and is a member of the TGF-β superfamily [1]. AMH plays an essential role in the regression of Müllerian ducts and descent of the testes during sexual differentiation of male fetuses [2,3]. Fetal Sertoli cells secrete AMH until birth, even after Müllerian ducts regression [4,5]. Moreover, male transgenic mice overexpressing *Amh* manifest feminized genitalia [6], in accordance with decreased Leydig cell numbers and testosterone secretion [7]. Conversely, *Amh* knockout mice manifested Leydig cell hyperplasia and infertility [8,9]. It is therefore likely that AMH plays an important role in fetal Leydig cell function [10,11].

Postnatally, expression of *Amh* and *Amhr2* has been observed in rat testes and ovaries [12,13]. During postnatal maturation of the testis, Sertoli cells change morphologically and functionally from immature type to mature type cells, although slightly immature Sertoli cells persist even in mature testes [14].

However, there were few reports that examine AMH-producing cells of postnatal mature testes in detail. Recently, we were the first to show expression of AMH and AMH type II receptor (AMHR2) in spermatocytes from rats aged 21 days (21d) using immunohistochemical (IHC) staining and *in situ* hybridization (ISH). In agreement, germ cells from 21d rat testes expressed *Amh* and *Amhr2* [15].

During the development of spermatogenesis in maturing rat testis, germ cells of neonatal testes are only spermatogonia, and spermatocytes appear during weaning prior to formation of round and elongated spermatids [16]. Spermatogonia and spermatocytes are present in 21d rat testis, whereas round and elongated spermatids are not. Moreover, in postnatal maturing rat testis, Sertoli cells and spermatocytes express and synthesize AMH and AMHR2 [15].

AMH signals are initiated by binding to an AMHR2, and can activate other signaling pathways such as those of β-catenin or NFkB [17]. In previous reports of AMH-AMHR2 signal transduction, AMH was shown to bind AMHR2 and activate the SMAD 1, 5, and 8 signaling pathway through one or several type 1 receptors [18].

SMAD proteins are intracellular mediators of TGF signaling and in postnatal mouse testes; SMAD1 was detected in spermatocytes and round spermatids [19], whereas SMAD5 was detected mainly in spermatogonia [20]. AMH activates the SMAD1, 5, and 8 signaling pathway through AMHR2 and inhibits SMAD6 [20]. We also reported that 21d testes and isolated germ cells expressed *Smad1, 5,* and *8* [15].

These data indicated that AMH is involved in spermatogenesis. However, although AMH is present in seminiferous tubules, its physiological roles in mature testis are not entirely clear. Thus, in this study we characterized expression patterns of AMH and AMHR2 in germ cells from mature rat testis during the spermatogenic cycle.

Materials and Methods

Animals

All experiments were approved by the Animal Care and Use Committee of the University of Yamanashi, Japan.

Normal Sprague-Dawley (SD) rats aged 5, 10, 16, 30, and 44 days (d) were purchased from Japan SLC and were housed for 5 days in an air-conditioned animal room at an ambient temperature of 22°C and a relative humidity of 55% ± 10% under a 12 h light/12 h dark cycle. Male rats were bred with maternal rats until postnatal day 20 (20d). The day of birth was designated as 0d and testes were collected from 10, 15, 21, 35 and 49d rats for use in assays.

In situ hybridization (ISH)

To determine the localization of *Amh* and *Amhr2* in 49d rat testis, ISH was performed using antisense probes comprising 55-mer oligonucleotides, which were labeled at the 5′-end using digoxigenin (DIG). Two non-overlapping probes were designed based on the *Amh* and *Amhr2* sequences and were commercially synthesized (BEX, Tokyo, Japan). *Amh* and *Amhr2* antisense probe sequences were previously reported [15]. Paraffin-embedded rat testis sections of 8 μm in thickness, were prepared and mounted on glass slides, which were pre-coated with 3-aminopropyltriethoxysilane (Shin-Etsu Chemical Co., Tokyo, Japan). All hybridization steps, including washing and visualization, were performed using a commercial kit (IsHyb *In situ* Hybridization Kit; Biochain Institute, Newark, CA) according to the manufacturer's instructions. Probe signals were detected with an alkaline phosphatase-conjugated anti-DIG antibody and nitroblue tetrazolium/5-bromo-4-chloro-3-indolyl-phosphate (NBT/BCIP) solution. ISH was performed by mixing two individual mRNA probes (AS1 and AS2), and specificity of hybridization was confirmed using sense oligonucleotide probes located at the same position as the antisense probes, which were used as a negative controls.

AMH and AMHR2 antibodies

AMH and AMHR2 polyclonal antibodies [15] were raised by Operon Biotechnologies K.K. custom synthesis service (Tokyo, Japan). Briefly, the AMH peptides, C+KFQEPPPGGASRWE (143-156) and CAWPQSDRNPRYGNH (485-499) were synthesized, and mixed, and rabbits were immunized four times with the mixture and with the carrier protein KLH every week. In identical procedures, the antigen peptides, CDPVPRAHPSPSSTL (92-106) and CSATDPRGLRELLED (470-484) were used to raise the AMHR2 antibody in rabbits. Polyclonal antisera were purified using affinity column chromatography with synthesized antigens.

Immunohistochemical (IHC) staining

Testes from 10d-49d rats were fixed in buffered neutral formalin, were embedded in paraffin, and were sectioned (5-μm, thickness) for IHC staining, following the procedure prescribed by Morpho Technology (Sapporo, Japan). IHC procedures were performed as previously reported [15]. Briefly, fixed tissues were deparaffinized, rehydrated, and washed with tris-buffered solution (TBS). Antigen retrieval was then performed using a high temperature antigen unmasking technique, in which sections were incubated with EDTA buffer solution (pH 9.0) at 95°C for 20 min. Sections were then rinsed with TBS, and endogenous peroxidase activity was inactivated with 0.1% H_2O_2 at room temperature for 10 min. Tissue sections were then immunostained using an automated staining system (Autostainer Plus, Dako). Sections were incubated with anti-AMH antibody (1:100 dilution) or anti-AMHR2 antibody (1:100 dilution) at room temperature for 60 min and were then washed with TBS. Sections were then incubated with Histofine® Simple Stain MAX-PO(R) (Nichirei, Tokyo) at room temperature for 30 min, and were visualized with DAB solution at room temperature for 5 min. Sections were counterstained with hematoxylin for 1.5 min and negative controls were processed simultaneously by omitting the primary antibodies.

Germ-cell isolation

Germ cells were isolated from 49d testes to examine the effects of the AMH antibody on AMH expression. Testicular cells were isolated as described previously by Galardo et al. [21] with minor modifications [15]. Germ cells were isolated from 4 testes of 49d rats in each experiment. Testes were decapsulated and treated with 0.1% collagenase type 2 (Worthington Biochemical Corp., Lakewood, NJ) and 10 U/ml DNase I (D7291, Sigma-Aldrich, St Louis, MO) in 20 ml of Hanks' balanced salt solution (HBSS) for 10 min at 35°C in a Bio Shaker (BR-30L, Taitec, Tokyo) at 100 oscillations per min. Collagenase solution was diluted with 20 ml of HBSS and seminiferous tubules were allowed to sediment for 2 min. Supernatants were then discarded and the tubular pellets were digested with 20 ml of 0.1% trypsin (Gibco) in HBSS for 20 min at 35°C in a Bio Shaker at 100 oscillations per min. Trypsin-digested solutions were supplemented with 10 ml of 10% fetal calf serum (FCS) in HBSS and were filtered with a Steriflip 100 μm nylon net filter (Millipore) and then centrifuged at 400 × g for 5 min. Cell pellets were re-suspended in a 1:1 mixture of DMEM-Ham's F-12 medium supplemented with 10% FCS, 15-mM $NaHCO_3$, 100 IU/ml penicillin, 2.5 mg/ml amphotericin B, and 20-mM HEPES (pH 7.4; DMEM-F12). Isolated cells from seminiferous tubules were seeded in 10 culture plates (10 cm^2/plate) and were cultured at 35°C in a 5% CO_2 incubator for 6 h. During this period, Sertoli cells were attached to the surface of the plate. Attached cells (Sertoli cells) were washed twice with HBSS, and cultured again with DMEM-F12 for 12 h. These cells were then washed twice with HBSS, scraped, centrifuged, and frozen for total RNA isolation. Floating germ cells were collected by carefully removing the medium and centrifuging at 400 × g for 5 min. Germ cell pellets were re-suspended in HBSS and were loaded on a discontinuous four-layer (20%, 25%, 32%, and 37%) Percoll density gradient (Percoll PLUS, GE Healthcare Bio-Sciences) for gradient centrifugation at 800 × g for 30 min at 4°C. The fraction between the 25%-32% Percoll interface was collected. To remove Percoll, 4 volumes of HBSS were added to the recovery solution, and were centrifuged at 400 × g for 5 min at 4°C. Germ cell pellets were re-suspended in DMEM-F12, and were then cultured in 10 cm^2 plates at 35°C in a CO_2 incubator for 12 h. Few Sertoli cells remained in the germ cell population, and these were attached to the dish surface. Floating germ cells were obtained by carefully removing the medium and were precipitated from the medium by centrifugation at 400 × g for 5 min. Germ cell pellets were re-suspended in 60 ml of DMEM-F12 (without FCS), and cell suspensions were then divided into 6 plates (10 ml/plate). Subsequently, 50 μl of anti-AMH antibody was added to 3 of 6 plates (final dilution 200 X). Re-suspended germ cells in these 6 plates were cultured at 35°C in a CO_2 incubator for 2 h, and were then centrifuged.

Germ cell pellets collected from 6 plates were frozen for total RNA isolation and subsequent quantitative real-time polymerase chain reaction (qRT-PCR). Experiments were performed in triplicate.

Quantitative real-time polymerase chain reaction

Total RNA was extracted from germ cells and Sertoli cells that were isolated from 49d rat testes, using RNeasy Mini Kit (QIAGEN, Tokyo). Subsequently, cDNA was synthesized from 1 μg of total RNA template using a High Capacity cDNA Reverse Transcription Kit (Applied Biosystems, Foster City, CA). For qRT-PCR, triplicated samples containing 9 μl of cDNA with 10 μl of Taqman Universal PCR Master Mix (Applied Biosystems) and 1 μl of 20 X Assays-on-demand Gene Expression Product (Applied Biosystems) were pre-incubated at 50°C for 2 min and then at 95°C for 10 min. Amplification was performed by 40 cycles of reaction at 95°C for 15 s and 60°C for 1 min. Fluorescence intensity was quantitatively analyzed using an ABI Prism 7500 Sequence Detection System (Applied Biosystems). Genes that were analyzed using PCR included *Amh, Amhr2, Scp1, Rsbn1, Ngfr, Rhox5, and Smads 1, 5,* and *8* (Table 1). Testicular expression of individual genes in whole testis from 49 d rats was set at 1.0. Relative expression levels of genes in isolated germ cells were normalized to that of β-*actin*.

Gene	Assay ID
Amh	Rn00563731_g1
Amhr2	Rn00513843_m1
SCP1	Rn00513843_m1
Rsbn1	Rn00554492_m1
Ngfr	Rn00561634_m1
Rhox5	Rn02132641_s1
Smad1	Rn00565555_m1
Smad5	Rn00572484_m1
Smad8	Rn00594023_m1
Beta actin	Rn00667869_m1

Table 1: List of candidate genes.

Statistical analysis

Relative expression levels of *Amh, Amhr2, Scp1, Rsbn1, and Smads 1, 5, and 8* in isolated germ cells were log-transformed, and the effects of anti-AMH antibody were analyzed separately using linear regression models that were adjusted for the order of experiments. P-values of less than 0.05 were considered indicative of statistical significance.

Results

ISH of *Amh* and *Amhr2*

Figure 1 demonstrates signals of *Amh* and *Amhr2* in stages I-IV, VIII and IX-XI in ISH analyses of 49d seminiferous tubules. Although signal intensities of *Amh* and *Amhr2* varied from weak to strong, *Amh* and *Amhr2* signals in spermatocytes were detected at all stages of the spermatogenic cycle and especially during stage VIII (Figures 1b and 1e). Signals of *Amh* and *Amhr2* in round and elongated spermatids were negative at all stages, but were unclear in spermatogonia, and were faint in Sertoli cells.

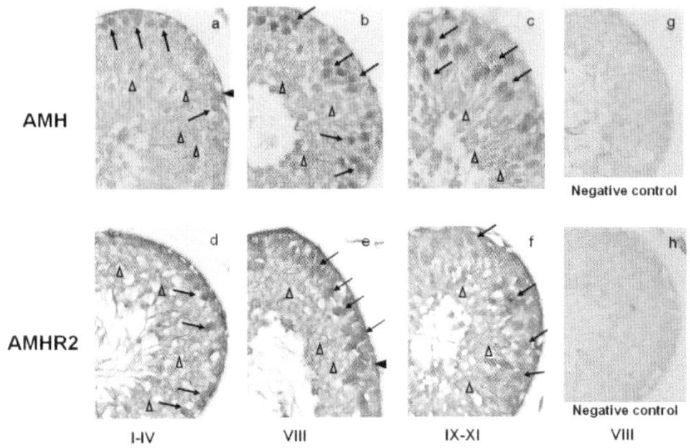

Figure 1: *In situ* hybridization of *Amh* and *Amhr2* in seminiferous tubules from 49 day old (49d) rat testis. I-IV, VIII, and IX-XI indicate stages of spermatogenic cycle. Solid arrows indicate positive spermatocytes. Solid arrowheads indicate Sertoli cells. Open arrowheads indicate negative round (a, b, d, e) and elongated (c, f) spermatids. *Amh* and *Amhr2* expression levels varied from weak staining (a, d), through mild (c, f), to strong (b, e).

IHC staining of AMH and AMHR2

Figure 2 demonstrates age-related changes in AMH and AMHR2 IHC staining. Only spermatogonia and Sertoli cells were present in the seminiferous tubules of 10d testis, whereas few spermatocytes appeared in those of 15d testes. In 10d testes, AMH and AMHR2 stainings were strong in Sertoli cells, but were not present in spermatogonia (Figures 2a and 2e). When spermatocytes appeared in the seminiferous tubules of 15d testes, AMH and AMHR2 staining's observed in Sertoli cells and were weakly present in spermatocytes, but were absent in spermatogonia (Figures 2b and 2f). In 21d testis, many spermatogonia had differentiated into spermatocytes, but no spermatids were observed. Strong AMH and AMHR2 staining's observed in spermatocytes, but were absent in Sertoli cells and spermatogonia (Figures 2c and 2g). Spermatocytes had differentiated into spermatids in 35d seminiferous tubules, and AMH staining was strong in spermatocytes, weak in Sertoli cells, and not present in elongated spermatids and spermatogonia (Figure 2d). In contrast, AMHR2 staining was strong in spermatocytes and elongated spermatids, but was unclear in Sertoli cells (Figure 2h).

Figures 3 and 4 shows the spermatogenic stage-specific IHC staining of AMH and AMHR2 in 49d seminiferous tubules. In spermatocytes, AMH staining was negative or weak at stage I-IV (Figure 3a), but was strong at stages VII-XIV. The strongest AMH staining was observed at stage VIII (Figure 3c and Figure 4a). In contrast, AMH staining was clearly observed in round spermatids at stages I-IV (Figure 3a), but was decreased at stage VII, and was diminished in elongated spermatids at stages VIII-XIV (Figures 3c, 3d and 3e. Figure 4a). AMHR2 staining was negative or weak in spermatocytes at stages I-IV (Figure 3f), but was strong at stages VII-XIV. Unlike the staining of AMH in spermatids, AMHR2 staining was present in round and elongated spermatids at all stages, and was especially strong in cell membranes of round spermatids at stage VII-VIII (Figures 4b and 4c). Moreover, AMHR2 staining was observed in residual bodies (Figure 4c). AMH and AMHR2 staining's were absent in spermatogonia at all stages, and were clear in Sertoli cells at stages I-IV.

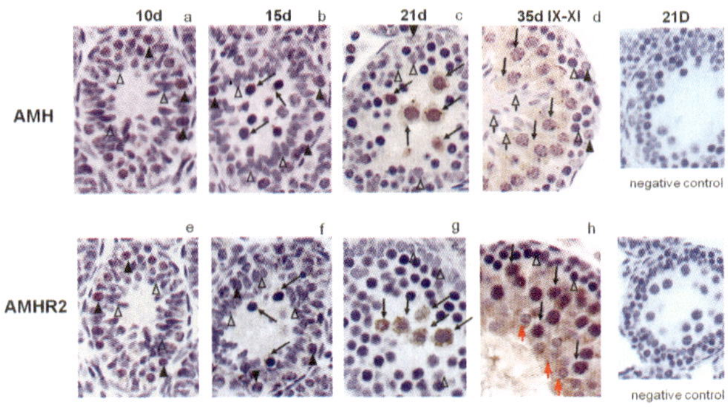

Figure 2: Immunohistochemical (IHC) staining of AMH and AMHR2 in seminiferous tubules of 10d, 15d, 21d, and 35d testes (IX-XI indicates stage of spermatogenic cycle). Solid arrowheads indicate positive Sertoli cells (a, b, c, d, e, and f). Open arrowheads indicate negative spermatogonia (a-h). Solid arrows indicate positive spermatocytes (b, c, d, g, and h). Open arrows indicate negative elongated spermatids (d). Red solid arrows indicate positive elongated spermatids (h).

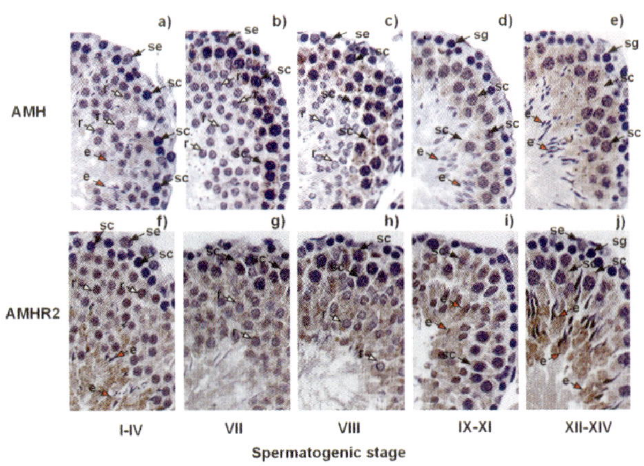

Figure 3: IHC staining of AMH and AMHR2 at spermatogenic stages in semuniferous tubules of a 49D testis. Sg: spermatogonia; sc: spermatocyte; r: round spermatid; e: elongated spermatid; se: Sertoli cell. IHC stainings of AMH and AMHR2 in spermatocytes were negative or weak at stages I-IV (a, f), but were strong at stages VII-XIV (b-e, g-j). AMH staining of round spermatids was strong at stages I-IV (a), and was faint at stage VII (b). AMH staining of elongated spermatids was negative at all stages (a, d, e). AMHR2 stainings of round and elongated spermatids were strong at all stages from I-XIV. AMH and AMHR2 staining of Sertoli cells was weakly positive at stages I-IV and VII.

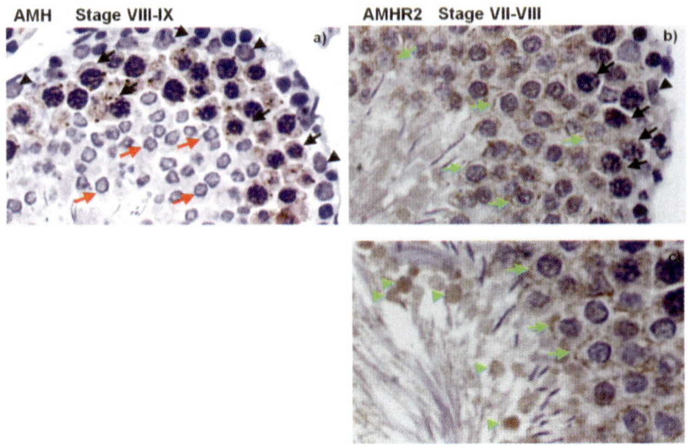

Figure 4: IHC staining of AMH and AMHR2 at spermatigenic stage VIII. AMH staining (a) was strong in spermatocytes (solid arrow), was faint in Sertoli cells (solid arrow head), and negative in round spermatids (red arrow). AMHR2 staining (b,c) was strong in spermatocytes (solid arrow), was faint in Sertoli cells (solid arrow head) and was strong in cell membranes of round spermatids (green arrow). AMHR2 staining (c) was positive in residual bodies (green arrow head).

Expression levels of *Amh, Amhr2, Scp1, Rsbn1, Ngfr, Rhox5,* and *Smads1, 5,* and *8* in germ cells and Sertoli cells isolated from 49d testes

Figure 5 shows expression levels of *Amh, Amhr2, Ngfr,* and *Rhox5* in isolated germ cells and Sertoli cells. Expression of *Ngfr* (immature Sertoli cell specific gene) and *Rhox5* (mature Sertoli cell specific gene) was not observed in isolated germ cells. Isolated Sertoli cells expressed *Amh, Ngfr,* and *Rhox5,* but not *Amhr2.*

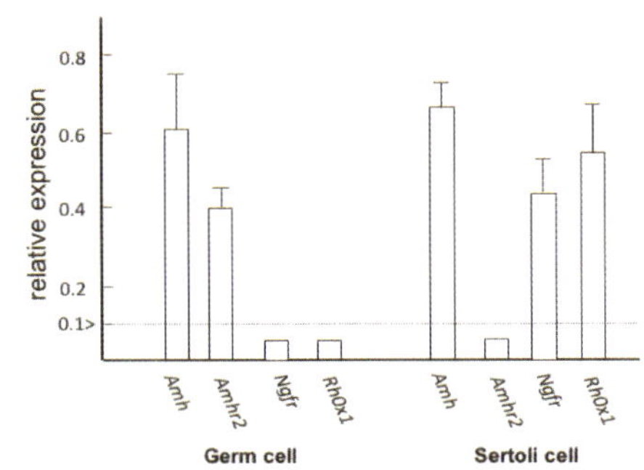

Figure 5: Relative expression of *Amh, Amhr2, Ngfr* and *Rhox1* in isolated germ cells and Sertoli cells of 49d testes. Testicular expression at 49d was set at 1.0; Data are presented as means and standard deviations.

As shown in Figure 6, germ cells from 49d testes expressed *Amh, Amhr2, Scp1 and Rsbn1,* and *Smads 1, 5,* and *8.* After incubation of isolated germ cells with anti-AMH antibody, expression levels of *Amh, Amhr2, Scp1, Smad1 and Smad5* were significantly increased, whereas that of *Rsbn1* was significantly decreased.

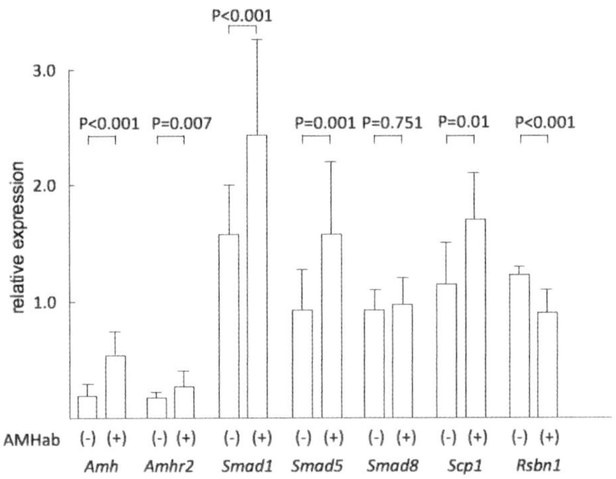

Figure 6: Effect of AMH antibody on expression levels of *Amh, Amhr2, Smads* (*1, 5, 8*), *Scp1* and *Rsbn1* in isolated germ cells of 49d testes. Testicular expression at 49d was set at 1.0; Data are presented as means and standard deviations.

Discussion

Josso et al. were the first to report evidence that Sertoli cells in fetal testes produce AMH [22]. Based on studies of fetal testes, it was thought that AMH was produced only by Sertoli cells in males. During postnatal spermatogenesis, Sertoli cells and spermatogonia are present in 10d rat testes, and whereas spermatocytes appear after 15d testis, round spermatids do not appear in testes until 21d. Recently, we showed that spermatocytes of rat testes synthesize AMH and AMHR2 at 21d [15]. Similarly, several recently reports show AMH expression in oocytes and primordial follicles [23,24], although other studies show that AMH is absent in oocytes of all follicular categories [25,26]. Hence, although the present experiments indicate that germ cells of matured gonads express AMH, the physiological role of AMH in gonads remains unclear.

In this study, we first clarified that spermatocytes expressed and synthesized AMH and AMHR2 during spermatogenic cycle in 49 d rat testes. The stage-specific expression profiles of AMH and AMHR2 in spermatocytes, spermatids and Sertoli cells are showed in Table 2.

Spermatocytes expressed *Amh* and *Amhr2,* and synthesized AMH and AMHR2. IHC staining of AMH in spermatocytes was negative or weak during stage I-IV of the spermatogenic cycle, but became strong during stages VII-XIV. Moreover, the intensity of AMH staining in spermatocytes during the spermatogenic cycle corresponded with that of *Amh* expression in spermatocytes. In contrast, *Amh* expression was not detected in spermatids, despite positive staining of AMH protein, suggesting that during differentiation of spermatocytes to round spermatids, AMH is transferred from spermtocytes to round spermatids. Accordingly, staining of the transferred AMH in round spermatids decreased with the progression of the spermatogenic cycle, was diminished at stage VIII, and was not observed in elongated spermatids. AMH staining was also weak in Sertoli cells at stage I to IV. Taken together, these data indicate that AMH is predominantly produced by spermatocytes rather than Sertoli cells in matured testes.

Variables	Stage	I-IV	VII	VIII	XII-XIV
Spermatocyte	AMH	(-)	++	++	+
	AMHR2	(-)	++	++	+
Round spermatid	AMH	+	±		
	AMHR2	+	+		
Elongated spermatid	AMH	(-)		(-)	(-)
	AMHR2	+		++	+
Sertoli cell	AMH	+	(-)	(-)	(-)
	AMHR2	+	(-)	(-)	(-)

Table 2: Stage-specific expression of AMH and AMHR2 during spermatogenic cycle.

In this study, we first clarified that spermatocytes expressed and synthesized AMH and AMHR2 during spermatogenic cycle in 49 d rat testes. The stage-specific expression profiles of AMH and AMHR2 in spermatocytes, spermatids and Sertoli cells are showed in Table 2.

Spermatocytes expressed *Amh* and *Amhr2,* and synthesized AMH and AMHR2. IHC staining of AMH in spermatocytes was negative or weak during stage I-IV of the spermatogenic cycle, but became strong during stages VII-XIV. Moreover, the intensity of AMH staining in spermatocytes during the spermatogenic cycle corresponded with that of *Amh* expression in spermatocytes. In contrast, *Amh* expression was not detected in spermatids, despite positive staining of AMH protein, suggesting that during differentiation of spermatocytes to round spermatids, AMH is transferred from spermtocytes to round spermatids. Accordingly, staining of the transferred AMH in round spermatids decreased with the progression of the spermatogenic cycle, was diminished at stage VIII, and was not observed in elongated spermatids. AMH staining was also weak in Sertoli cells at stage I to IV. Taken together, these data indicate that AMH is predominantly produced by spermatocytes rather than Sertoli cells in matured testes.

Moreover, expression patterns of *Amhr2* and AMHR2 in spermatocytes closely resembled those of *Amh* and AMH, with high expression during stages VII-XIV. *Amhr2* expression was not detected in spermtids, despite positive staining of AMHR2, suggesting that AMHR2 was transferred from spermatocytes to round spermatids. However, unlike the expression pattern of AMH, AMHR2 was observed in round spermatids and elongated spermatids. AMHR2 staining was clearly observed at cell membranes of round spermatids, especially during stages VII-VIII. Moreover, AMHR2 was present in residual bodies at stage VIII. Because spermatocytes synthesize both AMH and AMHR2, these data indicate that 1) AMH acts on spermatocytes in an autocrine fashion during stages VII-XIV, 2) AMH is mainly produced by spermatocytes and acts on round and elongated spermatids through AMHR2 in a paracrine fashion from stages VIII to XIV, especially at stage VIII, and 3) AMH from Sertoli cells acts on elongated spermatids during the early stages I-IV. These observations suggest that AMH contributes to morphological changes from round to elongated spermatid forms at stages VIII-IX, and to morphological changes in elongated spermatids.

In our experiments with isolated testicular cells, expression of Sertoli cell specific genes (*Ngfr* and *Rhox5*) was not observed in isolated germ cells. The result indicates that cultured germ cells did not have the contamination of Sertoli cells. In cultured germ cells isolated from 49d testes, expression levels of *Amh, Amhr2, Smad1, and Smad5* were significantly increased by the addition of AMH antibody. In a previous study, AMH through AMHR2 activated the SMAD1/5/8 signaling pathway and inhibited SMAD6 [20]. SMAD1 was also detected in spermatocytes and round spermatids [19], and SMAD5 was detected mainly in spermatogonia [20]. In the present study, although spermatogonia did not express *Amhr2* and AMHR2, expression levels of *Smads1* and *5* were increased in isolated germ cells, indicating that SMADs1 and 5 are present in spermatocytes and spermatids. Moreover, treatment with anti-AMH antibody led to increased *Scp1* expression and decreased *Rsbn* expression in isolated germ cells. *Scp1* is pachytene spermatocyte specific gene and *Rsbn1* is round spermatids specific gene. These results may suggest that AMH mainly secreted by spermatocytes controls differentiation from spermatocytes to round spermatids and morphological changes from round spermatids to elongated form.

In AMHR2 expressing ovarian granulose cell tumor cells, exogenous AMH activated SMADs 1 and 5, and augmented caspase-3 activity, a marker of apoptosis induction [27]. Caspase-3 is present in spermatocytes and residual bodies and may be associated with germ cell apoptosis [28]. During terminal morphological spermatogenic changes, spermatid cytoplasm's are eliminated and finally collected in residual bodies that display several apoptotic features. Male mice with a targeted deletion of the septin4 gene (*Sept4*) are sterile due to abnormal spermatozoa with attached residual cytoplasm. In accordance, caspase inhibitor XIAP was induced following mutation of *Sept4* [29]. These reports suggest that AMH activates caspase-3 through AMHR2-SMAD signaling in germ cells, and that caspase-3 contributes to cytoplasmic apoptosis in elongated spermatids.

In conclusion, the present data show that the spermatocytes stage-specifically express and synthesize AMH and AMHR2 during the spermatogenic cycle, and that AMH and AMHR2 are transferred to spermatids. AMH was expressed in spermatocytes at stages VII-XIV, and AMHR2 was most strongly expressed in round spermatids at stage VIII, and then in elongated spermatids and residual bodies. Finally, *Smad 1* and *5* expressions were increased in response to AMH in cultured isolated germ cells, indicating that the AMH-SMAD pathway may be associated with morphological changes from round to elongated spermatids at stage VIII. However, the inferred cytoplasmic apoptosis of spermatids remains to be fully established. Future studies are required to define further details of the physiological role of AMH during spermatogenic cycles.

Acknowledgment

The authors wish to thank Takashi Okamoto (Laboratory of Veterinary Biochemistry, Faculty of Agriculture, Tottori University) and Yoshiko Tanabe (Interdisciplinary Graduate School of Medicine and Engineering, University of Yamanashi) for their excellent technical assistance.

This work was supported by Grant-in-aid for Scientific Research (C 24591504) of Japan Society for the Promotion of Science.

Disclosure

None of the authors have any potential conflicts of interest associated with this research.

References

1. Cate RL, Mattaliano RJ, Hession C, Tizard R, Farber NM, et al. (1986) Isolation of the bovine and human genes for Müllerian inhibiting substance and expression of the human gene in animal cells. Cell 45: 685-698.
2. Vigier B, Watrin F, Magre S, Tra D, Josso N (1987) Purified bovine AMH induces a characteristic freemartin effect in fetal rat prospective ovaries exposed to it in vitro. Development 100: 43-55.
3. Hutson JM, Donahoe PK (1986) The hormonal control of testicular descent. Endocr Rev 7: 270-283.
4. Koopman P, Munsterberg A, Capel B, Vivian N, Lovell-Badge R (1990) Expression of a candidate sex-determining gene during mouse testis differentiation. Nature 348: 450-452.
5. Munsterberg A, Lovell-Badge R (1991) Expression of the mouse anti-Müllerian hormone gene suggests a role in both male and female sex differentiation. Development 113: 613-624.
6. Behringer RR, Cate RL, Froelick GJ, Palmiter RD, Brinster RL (1990) Abnormal sexual development in transgenic mice chronically expressing Müllerian inhibiting substance. Nature 345: 167-170.
7. Racine C, Rey R, Forest MG, Louis F, Ferre A, et al. (1998) Receptors for anti-müllerian hormone on Leydig cells are responsible for its effects on steroidogenesis and cell differentiation. Proc Natl Acad Sci 95: 594-599.
8. Mishima Y, Rey R, Finegold MJ, Matzuk MM, Josso N, et al. (1996) Genetic analysis of the Müllerian-inhibiting substance signal transduction pathway in mammalian sexual differentiation. Genes Dev 10: 2577-2587.
9. Behringer RR, Finegold MJ, Cate RL (1994) Müllerian inhibiting substance function during mammalian sexual development. Cell 79: 415-425.
10. Rouiller-Fabre V, Carmona S, Merhi RA, Cate R, Habert R, et al. (1998) Effect of anti-Müllerian hormone on Sertoli and Leydig cell function in fetal and immature rats. Endocrinology 139: 1213-1220.
11. Wu X, Arumugan R, Baker SP, Lee MM (2005) Pubertal and adult Leydig cell function in Müllerian inhibiting substance-deficient mice. Endocrinology 146: 589-595.
12. Baarends WM, Hoogerbrugge JW, Post M, Visser JA, De Rooij DG, et al. (1995) Anti-müllerian hormone and anti-müllerian hormone receptor

type II receptor messenger ribonucleic acid expression during postnatal testis development in the adult testis of the rat. Endocrinology 136: 5614–5622.

13. Baarends WM, Uilenbroek JT, Kramer P, Hoogerbrugge JW, van Leeuwen EC, et al. (1995) Anti-müllerian hormone and anti-müllerian hormone type II receptor messenger ribonucleic acid expression in rat ovaries during postnatal development, the estrous cycle, and gonadotropin-induced follicle growth. Endocrinology 136: 4951-4962.
14. Nistal M, Abaurrea MA, Paniagua R (1982) Morphological and histometric study on the human Sertoli cell from birth to the onset of puberty. J Anat 134: 351-363.
15. Ohyama K, Ohta M, Hosaka YZ, Tanabe Y, Ohyama T, et al. (2015) Expression of anti-Müllerian hormone and its type II receptor in germ cells of maturing rat testis. Endocrine J 62: 997-1006.
16. Malkov M, Fisher Y, Don J (1998) Developmental schedule of the rat testis determined by flow cytometry. Biol Reprod 59: 84-92.
17. Josso N, di Clemente N (2003) Transduction pathway of anti-Müllerian hormone, a sex-specific member of the TGF-beta family. Trends Endocrinol Metab 14: 91-97.
18. Di Clemente N, Josso N, Gouedard L, Belville C (2003) Components of the anti-Müllerian hormone signaling pathway in gonads. Mol Cell Endocrinol 211: 9-14.
19. Zhao GQ, Hogan BL (1997) Evidence that mothers-against-dpp-related 1 (Madr1) plays a role in the initiation and maintenance of spermatogenesis in the mouse. Mech Dev 61: 63-73.
20. Pellegrini M, Grimaldi P, Rossi P, Geremia R, Dolci S (2003) Developmental expression of BMP4/ALK3/SMAD5 signaling pathway in the mouse testis: A potential role of BMP4 in spermatogonia differentiation. J Cell Sci 116: 3363-3372.
21. Galardo MN, Regueira M, Riera MF, Pellizzari EH, Cigorraga SB, et al. (2014) Lactate regulates rat male germ cell function through reactive oxygen species. PLos One 9: e88024.
22. Josso N (1973) In vitro synthesis of müllerian-inhibiting hormone by seminiferous tubules isolated from the calf fetal testis. Endocrinology 93: 829-834.
23. Amorim CA, Jacobs S, Devireddy RV, Van Langendonckt A, Vanacker J, et al. (2013) Successful virtification and autografting of baboon (papio anubis) ovarian tissue. Hum Reprod 28: 2146-2156.
24. Weenen C, Laven JS, Von Bergh AR, Cranfield M, Groome NP, et al. (2004) Anti-Müllerian hormone expression pattern in the human ovary: Potential implications for initial and cyclic follicle recruitment. Mol Hum Reprod 10: 77-83.
25. Durlinger AL, Gruijters MJ, Kramer P, Kares B, Ingraham HA, et al. (2002) Anti-Müllerian hormone inhibits initiation of primordial follicle growth in the mouse ovary. Endocrinol 143: 1076-1084.
26. Rocha RMP, Lima LF, Carvalho AA, Chaves RN, Bernuci MP, et al. (2016) Immunolocalization of the Anti-Müllerian hormone (AMH) in caprine follicles and the effects of AMH on in vitro culture pre-antral follicles enclosed in ovarian tissue. Reprod Dom Anim 51: 212-219.
27. Anttonen M, Farkkila A, Tauriala H, Kauppinen M, Maclaughlin DT, et al. (2011) Anti-Müllerian hormone inhibits growth of AMH type II receptor-positive human ovarian granulose cell tumor cells by activating apoptosis. Laboratory Invest 91: 1605-1614.
28. Kim JM, Ghosh SR, Weil ACC, Zirkin BR (2001) Caspase-3 and caspase-activated deoxyribonuclease are associated with testicular germ cell apoptosis resulting from reduced intratesticular testosterone. Endocrinol 142: 3809-3816.
29. Kissel H, Georgescu MM, Larisch S, Manova K, Hunnicutt GR, et al. (2005) The sept4 septin locus is required for sperm terminal differentiation in mice. Developmental Cell 8: 353-364.

Synthetic Epoxy-Pregnan Steroids: Effects on Anxiety Behavior in Rats

Rey M[1], Ghini AA[2] and Coirini H[1,3,*]

1Laboratorio de Neurobiología, Instituto de Biología y Medicina Experimental (IBYME-CONICET), Vuelta de Obligado 2490, (C1428ADN), Ciudad Autónoma de Buenos Aires, Argentina.

2Departamento de Química Orgánica, Unidad de Microanálisis y Métodos Físicos aplicados a Química Orgánica (UMYMFOR-CONICET) Facultad de Ciencias Exactas y Naturales, Universidad de Buenos Aires (FCEN-UBA), Pabellón 2, Ciudad Universitaria, Intendente Güiraldes 2160, (C1428EHA) Ciudad Autónoma de Buenos Aires, Argentina

3Departamento de Bioquímica Humana, Facultad de Medicina, Universidad de Buenos Aires, Paraguay 2155, 5to Piso, (C1121ABG) Ciudad Autónoma de Buenos Aires, Argentina.

[*]**Corresponding author:** Prof. Dr. Héctor Coirini, Laboratorio de Neurobiología, Instituto de Biología y Medicina Experimental (IBYME-CONICET), Vuelta de Obligado 2490, (C1428ADN), Ciudad Autónoma de Buenos Aires, Argentina, E-mail: hcoirini@ibyme.conicet.gov.ar

Abstract

Neurosteroids like 3α-OH-5α-pregnan-20-one (allopregnanolone) and 3α-OH-5β-pregnan-20-one (pregnanolone) modulate the γ-aminobutyric acid-A ($GABA_A$) receptor function and produce several effects that can be considered for therapeutical pruposes like antidepressant and anxiolyticts, in a similar way to benzodiazepines. However, their rapid metabolism is a great disadvantage for medicinal treatments consideration. Synthetic steroid analogues with more bioavailability and stability arise like a solution to overcome these limitations. In previous studies, we evaluated the performance of a synthetic steroid group (*Epoxies*, similar to allopregnanolone and pregnanolone) throughout different assays in rat cerebral cortex and hippocampus, including neuroprotection and $GABA_A$ receptor modulation obtaining promising results. Taking into account the anxiolytic effect of allopregnanolone and pregnanolone, in this work we evaluated the effect of an intracranial administration (in dorsal hippocampus) of two synthetic steroids, *Epoxy 1* and *Epoxy 2*, in an anxiety animal model to provide knowledge about the possible *in vivo* effects of these steroids. Allopregnanolone and pregnanolone produced increases in vertical and horizontal exploration behaviors, interpreted as anxiolytic-like effects. However, the two *Epoxies* capable to modulate $GABA_A$ receptor binding have no effect on anxiety at the dose evaluated. These features make them suitable for other therapeutical purposes where the anxiogenic behaviors are not involved.

Keywords: Neurosteroids; Synthetic analogues; Allopregnanolone; Pregnanolone; Open field

Introduction

Inside the central nervous system, the *in situ* synthesized steroids (neurosteroids, NS) are capable of modify the brain excitability [1,2]. Due to their chemical structure, the steroids may produce positive or negative modulations over receptors, like the γ-aminobutyric acid-A ($GABA_A$) receptor [3,4]. Among the positive modulators of this receptor are two progesterone's metabolites: the 5α-pregnane-3α-ol-20-one (allopregnanolone, **A**) and its isomer 5α-pregnane-3β-ol-20-one (pregnanolone, **P**) [5]. In the last decades, the relevance of NS, like **A** and **P**, also has been increasing due to their multiple roles in normal and pathological behavior, ageing processes, damaged tissue regeneration and neuroprotection [6-9].

The interest on these steroids arises specifically from their potential activity as anticonvulsants, anesthetics, anxiolytic or sedative-hypnotic agents [10] useful for the treatment of several neurological and psychiatric disorders [5]. But, the main limitation for the therapeutical administration of these NS is their rapid *in vivo* biotransformation to other metabolites. Therefore, synthetic steroids (SS) analogues with better bioavailability and efficacy have an important therapeutic potential in brain disorders, becoming an alternative approach for different pathologies [11,12].

In the last decades, a significant increase around NS physiology and synthetic analogues development has been observed. The medicinal chemistry of neuroactive steroids (NAS) has been focused in the development of SS analogues preserving the absolute configuration of naturally occurring steroids. Structure/activity studies of the progesterone metabolites, indicate that the 3α-hydroxyl configuration is required for binding and activity maintenance [13], while modifications in some carbon atoms do not affect their functions [14-16]. In previous works we evaluated the performance of a SS group *Epoxies* (similar to **A** and **P**) through different assays as well as neuroprotection and inhibition/stimulation binding of specific ligands of the $GABA_A$ receptor in rat cerebral cortex and hippocampus [17,18]. The main feature of these *Epoxies* is the presence of an oxygen bridge that holds the A/B angle of steroidal nucleus in a controlled way, conferring conformational restricted analogues [19]. In those studies, we demonstrated that, of all the *Epoxies* tested, the *Epoxy 1* (3α-hydroxy-2β,19-epoxy-5α-pregnan-20-one; **A** analogue) and the *Epoxy 2* (3α-hydroxy-6,19-epoxypregn-4-ene-20-one; **P** analogue) produced the most similar effects to **A** and **P** [17,18].

On the other hand, severe psychiatric conditions like anxiety and stress-related disorders affect daily performance in tasks and represent a high cost to public health. Thus, the search of new and improve therapeutical alternatives remains currently. Also, the fact that neurosteroidogenic agents lack benzodiazepine-like side effects shows promise in the treatment of anxiety and depression [11]. Administration of **A** or **P** produces anxiolytic, ataxic, hypnotic-anesthetic and anticonvulsant effects as well as locomotor stimulation [5,20-30], being able to mimic the actions of benzodiazepines. Taking into account their effects as modulators of the $GABA_A$ receptor-ion-channel complex [5] mentioned before, the mechanism underlying their anxiolytic properties appears to be due to a potentiation of neural inhibition via this receptor [31-34]. Previous studies suggest that **A** increases the channel conductance of $GABA_A$ receptor-gated Cl^- in hippocampal neurons, promoting anxiolytic-like effects [35-37]. This supports the hypothesis about the role that the dorsal (CA1) hippocampus area plays in emotional processes and NS modulation of anxiety and exploration. It has also been postulated that the dorsal region of this brain structure is involved in memory-related functions, whereas the ventral region mediates fear and anxiety responses[38]. In contrast to these anatomical and functional considerations, the recent results of Mòdol *et al.* [39] demonstrate that the dorsal (CA1) area of the hippocampus is also implicated in the modulation of anxiety-related behaviors. Their studies indicate that the hippocampal administration of **A** produces an anxiolytic-like profile and also increases exploratory behavior, observed trough the enhancement of the number of entries into the open arms in the elevated plus-maze device. This suggests that CA1 region together with other brain structures (such as the amygdala or the medial septum) could be an important target for explaining the NS effects on exploration, anxiety, learning and memory [39]. **P** administration in the dorsal hippocampus or in the lateral septum also produces dose-dependent anxiolytic-like effects in several animal models [36]. Moreover, both steroids have shown a comparable potency eliciting anxiolytic effects [24,27,31]. In addition, the ability of these and other NS to decrease anxiety-induced behavior has been demonstrated in several tests such as light/dark transition, rearing events and open-field [22,34,40]. In fact, there is evidence that the anxiolytic action of progesterone is mediated by its reduced metabolites, **A** and **P** [41,42]. Based in the previous results obtained with the *Epoxies* in the $GABA_A$ receptor modulation and the neuroprotective actions [17,18], and the anxiolytic-like effects mediated by **A** and **P**, the aim of this work was to evaluate the effects of two of these SS (*Epoxy 1* and *Epoxy 2*) administration over the animal behavior. These analysis were performed in an anxiety model (open-field test), assessing horizontal and vertical exploration and the anxiolytic-like effects; comparing results between synthetic and natural steroids.

Materials and Methods

Steroids

Two natural steroids (**A** and **P**) and two synthetic analogues, 3α-hydroxy-1β,11α-epoxy-5α-pregnan-20-one (*Epoxy 1*, **A** analogue) [43] and 3α-hydroxy-6,19-epoxypregn-4-ene-20-one (*Epoxy 2*, **P** analogue) [44] were used. Steroid concentration used for microinfusion (6.7 μg/μl) was selected according to our previous results [17,18]. The solutions were prepared using cyclodextrin 30% in artificial cerebrospinal fluid (aCSF) as vehicle one hour before the administration.

Experimental animals

Ninety day old adult male Sprague Dawley rats (400 g; n=48) were housed under standard laboratory conditions with a 12-h light-dark cycle, with food and water *ad libitum* on a temperature (21°C) and humidity (40-70%) controlled vivarium. The animal surgical procedures and treatments were evaluated by the Ethics Committee of the Instituto de Biología y Medicina Experimental (IBYME), CABA, Argentine, and approved according to the described on the protocol CE 040-Jun/2014, in accordance with guidelines defined by the European Community Council Directive (86/609/EEC) and the National Institutes of Health Guide for the Care and Use of Laboratory Animals.

Male rats were anesthetized with ketamine-xylazine (40:4 mg/Kg i.p.; Holliday, Richmond, Argentina) and placed in a stereotaxic apparatus (David Kopf Instruments, Tujunga CA, USA). Handmade 23-gauge stainless steel cannulae with 30-gauge removable inserts (dummy cannulae) were unilaterally implanted on the dorsal hippocampus using flat skull coordinates (anteroposterior, -2.3 mm; mediolateral, ± 1.6 mm; dorsoventral, 2.8 mm; from Bregma) according to the atlas Paxinos and Watson [45]. Three stainless steel screws and dental cement were used to fix the cannulae to the skull surface. After the surgery, animals were subcutaneously injected with a nonsteroidal anti-inflammatory (Meloxican 2 mg/Kg body weight, Boehringer Ingelheim, Argentina). A painkiller (Tramadol chlorhydrate 0.15 g/L; Finadiet SACIFI, Argentina) and an antibiotic (Enrofloxaxine 5 mg/L; Afford SA, Argentina) were administered in the drinking water for the next 3 days.

Bilateral implants in some brain areas have been widely used to explore the anxiolytic and/or antidepressant like-effects [46-48]. Although, the choice of unilateral cannulation (with left/right alternations) performed in this work, was based in previous reports that described anxiolytic and antidepressant effects with unilateral microinjections of **A** [49] or progesterone [50], without behavioral differences between brain sides.

Microinfusion procedure

Animals were allowed to recover for 10 days before performing the behavioral trials. Vehicle (cyclodextrin 30% in aCSF) or steroids (**A**, **P**, *Epoxy 1* and *Epoxy 2*; 2 μg) were administered in 0.3 μl using a 30-gauge injection needle connected by PC-40 tubing (Rivero SA, Argentina) to a 10 μl glass syringe (Hamilton, Reno NV, USA; 0.1 μl/min). After the 3 minutes of microinfusion, the injection needle was kept in place for 1 additional minute to allow diffusion away from the cannula tip before the dummy cannula reposition. According to the condition, 5 groups of animals (n=8) were established: Vehicle (cyclodextrin 30% in aCSF treatment), **A** (**A** treatment), **P** (**P** treatment), *Epoxy 1* (*Epoxy 1* treatment) and *Epoxy 2* (*Epoxy 2* treatment). Animals were hand restrained during all microinfusion procedure.

Behavioral testing

The open-field task [51,52] was used in accordance with the methods described by McCarthy *et al.* [53]. Behavioral testing occurred between 10:00 and 15:00h. The open-field device (housed in a dimly lit room with controlled temperature 21°C and humidity 40-70%) consisted of 75 cm side squared box divided in 25 quadrants, with 30 cm height walls and an open roof. All animals were allowed to explore the device for 15 minutes (precondition test) one day before steroids microinfusion. At the next day, one minute after the dummy cannula relocation, animals were placed in the center of the device and were allowed to explore it for 300 seconds. The animal activity was videotaped with a digital camera suspended above the test apparatus. The behavioral parameters evaluated were: *Freezing* (duration of the animal in a completely stationary state), *Active time* (determined as total time test minus *Freezing* time), *Line Crossing* (number of grid lines crossed with all four paws), the frequency and duration of *Grooming* (when the animal licks and/or scratches itself while it stays still) and *Rearing* (when the animal stands up on its hind legs). After each trial, the apparatus was thoroughly cleaned with damp and dry towels to prevent olfactory cues. Behavioral videos were scored by two observers who were blind to the rat's treatment condition.

Histology

At the end of the behavioral testing period, animals were rendered unconscious by CO_2 and killed by decapitation. The brains were removed, frozen and stored at -80ºC. Coronal sections (40 µm thick) obtained with a cryostat were mounted on subbed slides and stained with cresyl violet [54] for microscopic visualization of cannulae placements. The results from animals with accurately placed cannulae were used for the statistical analyses.

Statistical analysis

Statistical analyses were performed with commercial softwares GraphPad Prism (Graphpad Software Inc., v.4) and Statview (SAS Institute Inc. v5.0.1). The effects of intracranial microinfusions on the behavioral parameters were analyzed by a one-way ANOVA and comparisons between each steroid and vehicle were made by Newman-Keuls post hoc test. Differences were considered significant when $p<0.05$.

Results

Histological analysis

Cannulae tip localizations in the brain from those animals used for statistical analyses are schematically represented in Figure 1a. They were mainly placed on the dorsal (CA1) area of the hippocampus throughout the rostral-caudal extent. Cresyl violet staining was used for the visualization (Figure 1b). Cannulae distribution was more frequently positioned in -2.40 mm anteroposterior; 1.3 and 2.4 mm mediolateral (left or right sides) and 2.6 mm dorsoventral from Bregma (Figure 1c; Paxinos and Watson [45]). Animals with bad placed cannulae (n=8) were discarded for statistical analyses.

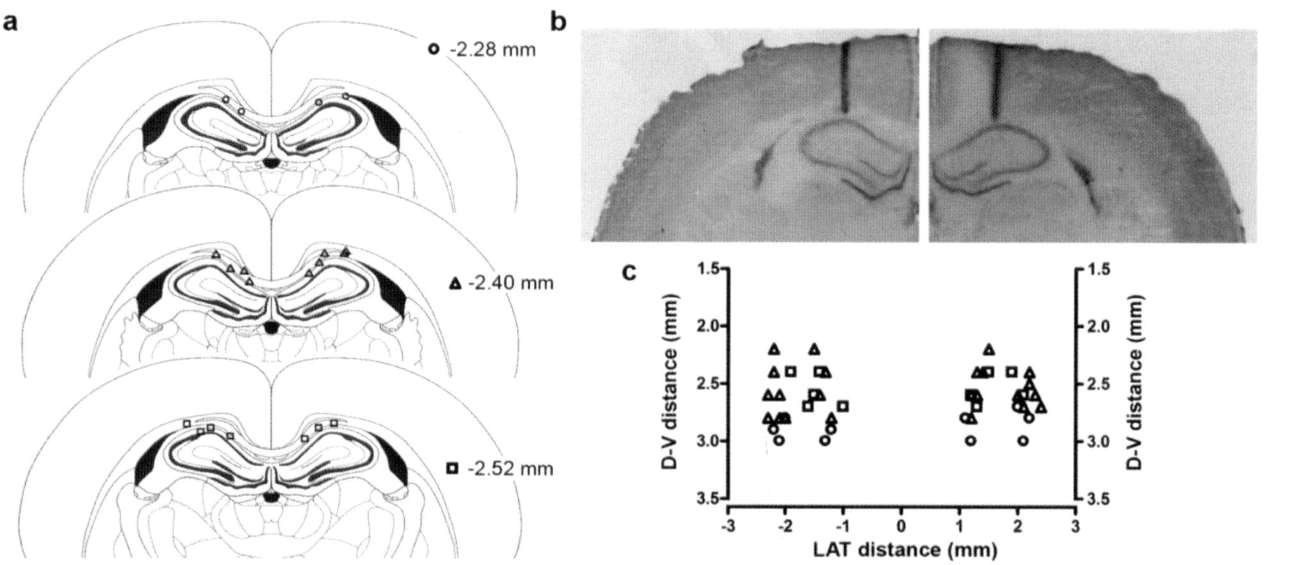

Figure 1: a Schematic representation of the well placed point of injection illustrating cannulae tip localizations throughout the rostral-caudal extent of the CA1 area of the hippocampus (anteroposterior, -2.3 mm; mediolateral, ± 1.6 mm; dorsoventral, 2.8 mm; from Bregma). Each symbol refers to different anteroposterior distance from Bregma according to Paxinos and Watson Atlas (1998; ○:n=11; Δ:n=19; □:n=10). **b** Representative photomicrographs of half coronal section, cresyl violet-stained, showing unilateral cannulae tip placements (left or right; magnification x2). **c** Cannulae distributions according to dorsoventral (D-V) and mediolateral (LAT) distance in mm.

Active time

The amount of time in which animals were in activity was determined as the total time of the test (300 sec) minus the *Freezing* time (when the animals remain completely immobile). A significant increase on *Active time* was observed with **A** and **P** treatments compared to control (143% and 147% respectively; $p<0.05$). These increases can be translated as an augmentation in total locomotor activity and horizontal and vertical explorations (Figure 2a). Although, no effects were observed with *Epoxy 1* and *Epoxy 2* treatments.

Line crossing

Ambulation was quantified as the number of grid lines crossed with all four paws within the 300 sec of testing. **A** and **P** administrations produced significant increases of this parameter compared to vehicle (114% and 136% respectively; $p<0.05$; Figure 2b). That can be interpreted as an increase in horizontal exploration activity, although no effects were observed with *Epoxy 1* and *Epoxy 2* administrations.

Grooming and grooming ratio

The frequency and duration of each occurrence (when the animal licks and scratches itself) was measured throughout the 300 sec of testing. A significant increase in *Grooming* duration was observed only with **P** microinfusion (428% compared to control; $p<0.05$; Figure 2c). However, no significant effects were observed on the duration of each *Grooming* event indicated by the *"Grooming ratio"* (defined like *Grooming* duration/*Grooming* frequency; Figure 2d). No effects were observed with the other three steroids in any of both variables.

Rearing and rearing ratio

The frequency and duration of each occurrence (when the animal stands up on its hind legs) was measured in the 300 sec of testing. Significant increases in total *Rearing* duration were observed with **A** and **P** treatments compared to vehicle (265% and 271% respectively; $p<0.05$; Figure 2e). The increase of this parameter can be interpreted as an augmentation of vertical exploration activity, although no effects were observed on the duration of each *Rearing* event indicated by the *"Rearing ratio"* (defined like Rearing duration/*Rearing* frequency; Figure 2f). No effects were observed with *Epoxy 1* and *Epoxy 2* administrations in any of both parameters.

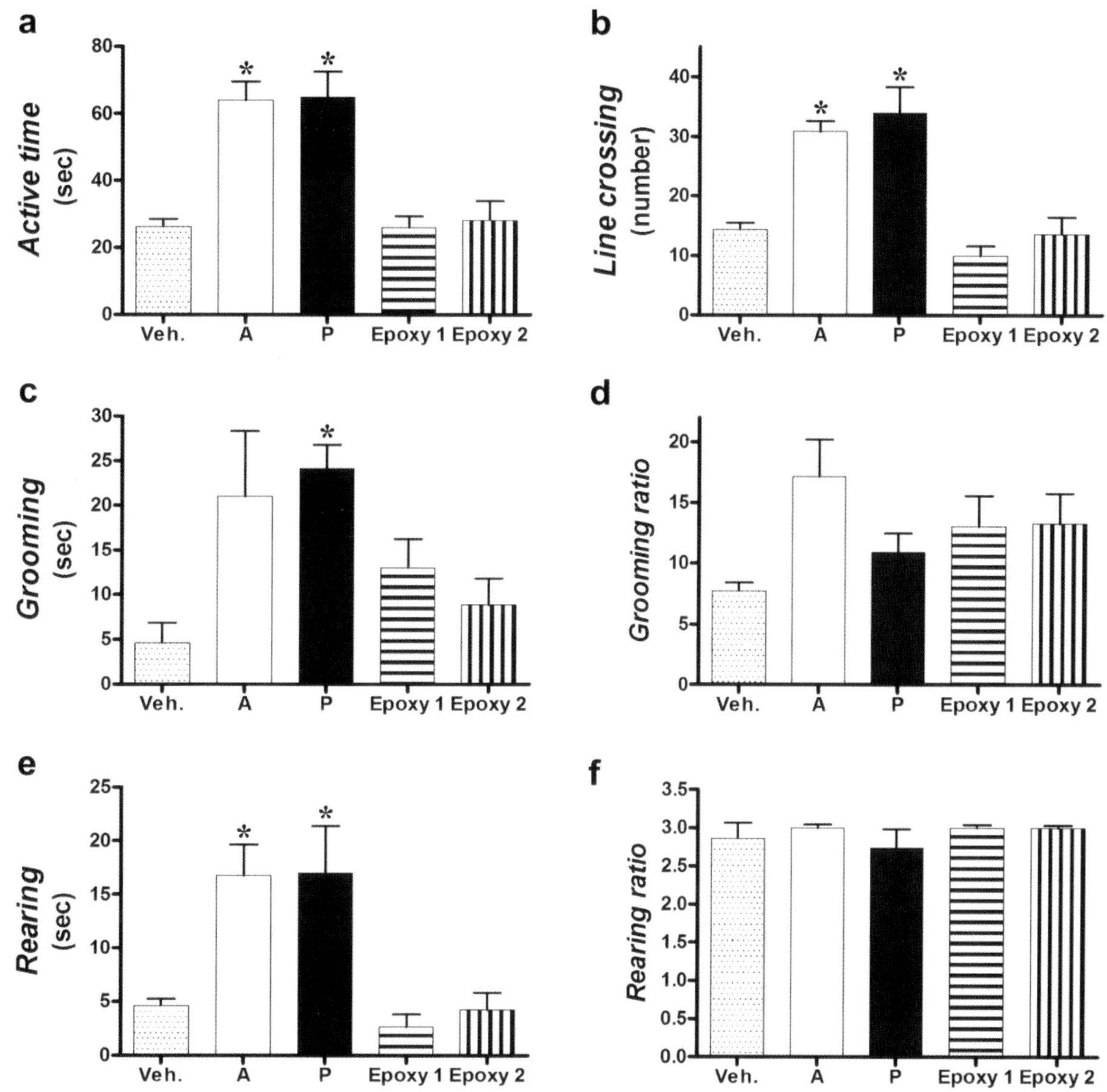

Figure 2: Unilateral microinfusion (0.3 µl) on dorsal hippocampus of vehicle (Veh., cylcodextrin 30% in aCSF) or steroid (**A**, **P**, *Epoxy 1* and *Epoxy 2*; 2 µg) and changes in open-field behavioral parameters: **a** *Active time* (difference between total time test and freezing in sec) **b** *Line crossing* (number of grid lines crossed with all four paws), **c** *Grooming* (when the animal licks or scratches itself while stays still in sec) and **d** ratio (duration/frequency) and **e** *Rearing* (when the animal stands up on its hind legs in sec), and f ratio (duration/frequency). Significant effect was determined by one-way ANOVA: $F_{Active\ time}(4,35)=15.3$; $p<0.001$, $F_{Line\ crossing}(4,35)=18.2$; $p<0.001$, $F_{Grooming}(4,35)=2.8$; $p<0.05$, $F_{Grooming\ ratio}(4,24)=1.1$; $p=0.12$, $F_{Rearing}(4,35)=13.3$; $p<0.001$ and $F_{Rearing\ ratio}(4,28)=0.5$; $p=0.75$, sub index in each F indicates the variable analysed. *p<0.05 Newman-Keuls post hoc test.

Correlation between Active time and Line crossing

Analysis of *Line crossing* variable based on *Active time*, showed a positive correlation factor of 0.74, when all the treatments were considered toghether (Figure 3 **C**). When this correlation was performed for each treatment, significant effects of **P** and its analogue, *Epoxy 2* (r2=0.77 and r2=0.69 respectively; Figure 3 **P** and Figure 3 *Epoxy 2*) were observed, but with lower *Active time* for the *Epoxy 2* than **P**. On the other hand, the *Epoxy 1* showed similar pattern than its natural analogue **A** and vehicle, with no significant ANOVA p values (Figure 3).

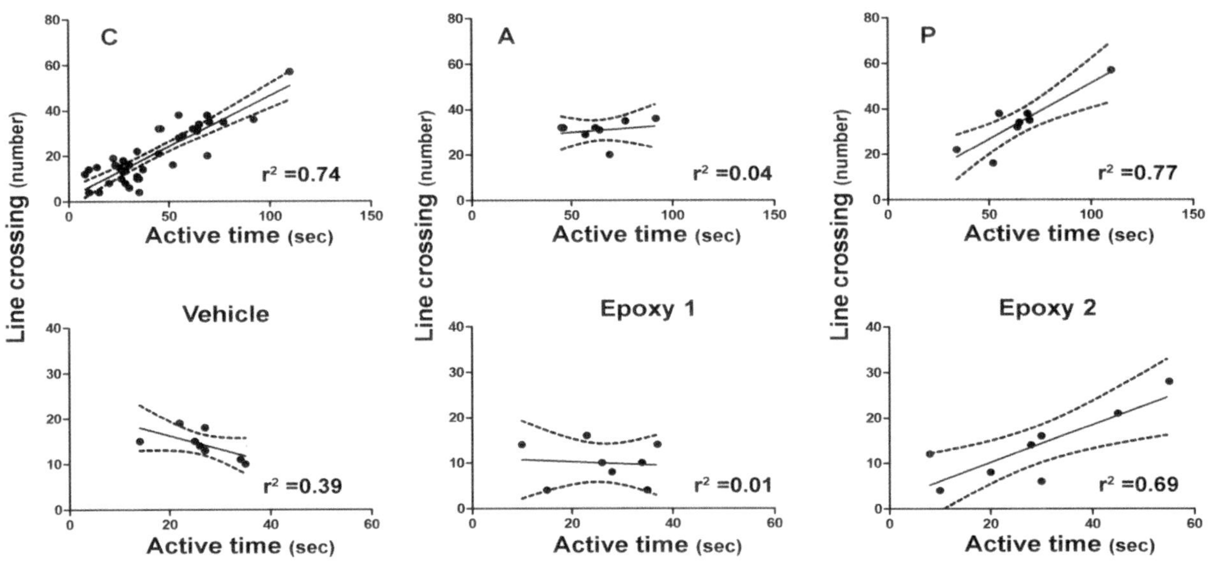

Figure 3: Correlation between *Line crossing* and *Active time* behavioral parameters, under all conditions together (**C**) or for each microinfusion treatment (Vehicle, **A**: allopregnanolone, **P**: pregnanolone, *Epoxy 1* and *Epoxy 2*). Each point represents a value corresponding to an individual animal test. Correlation coefficients are showed in each panel. Significant effects were determined by one-way ANOVA: $F_C(1,40)=108.2$; $p<0.0001$, $F_{Vehicle}(1,6)=3.9$; p=0.09, $F_A(1,6)=0.3$; p=0.62, $F_P(1,6)=20.5$; p=0.004, $F_{Epoxy\ 1}(1,6)=0.1$; p=0.82 and $F_{Epoxy\ 2}(1,6)=19.6$; p=0.01, sub index in each F indicates the treatment analyzed. Dotted lines indicate the 95% confidence intervals.

Discussion

Anxiety is an unpleasant nervous state of inner restlessness. Although benzodiazepines and barbiturates are among the treatments of choice for this kind of pathologies, they may induce various side effects [55]. Their actions may be mediated by the $GABA_A$ receptor located within the hippocampal formation, which mediates postsynaptic inhibition [56].

Progesterone and its reduced metabolites, **A** and **P**, were found to produce anxiolytic-like effects similar to benzodiazepines [36,57,58]. In the brain, *in situ* synthetized NS are capable of modulating neuronal excitability by rapid non-genomic actions [59] acting as potent modulators of $GABA_A$ receptor-mediated neurotransmission [5]. They can locally influence neuronal activity through their effects as paracrine messengers [60]. Thus, NS may have important effects on the regulation of the behavior in humans and in different murine models.

On the other hand, the hippocampal formation is important for the acquisition of short-term memory [61] and it has been also related to anxiety behaviors. Recently, reports described an association between dorsal hippocampus and the modulation of anxiety behavior [39]. Moreover, other studies have shown a significant correlation between low-anxiety or increased exploratory behaviors and **A** concentration in the hippocampus [52]. Several studies developed in rodents show that **A** and **P** reduce stress and anxiety-like behavior [1,36,62-67]. In fact, the blockade of progesterone's conversion to its metabolites impairs social behavior and induces anxiety-related behavior in rats [68].

The SS arise as a promising solution to the poor bioavailability and rapid metabolism of natural NS administration [12], but it is necessary to compare their biological effects in similar targets and doses of the NS.

In this work, an anxiety model developed to identify the pharmacological mechanisms and potential clinical effects of synthetic and natural steroids was used. Usually, this kind of model based on conflict situations can generate opposite motivational states induced by approach-avoidance situations, however it does not attempt to replicate all features and symptoms of a specific anxiety disorder. Rather, it tries to generate a state of anxiety that could be related to these disorders. Another important methodological consideration that needs to be taken into account is our choice to cannulate animals in a unilateral way (with left/right alternations). Although bilateral cannulae have been widely used to explore the anxiolytic and antidepressant-like effects [46-48], we relied in reports that have not found behavioral differences describing these effects between the brain sides with unilateral progesterone or **A** microinfusions [49,50]. In agreement with this information, we do not observe lateral influence on the horizontal and vertical exploratory activities either.

Here, we evaluated the anxiolytic properties of an equal dose of **A**, **P** or two synthetic steroid analogues (*Epoxy 1* and *Epoxy 2*) by microinfusions in dorsal hippocampus on the open-field test, quantifying horizontal and vertical exploration. The changes observed on the behavioral parameters by **A** and **P** can be interpreted as anxiolytic-like effects. Both natural NS enhanced the exploratory activity observed trough the *Line crossing*, *Grooming* and *Rearing* increases and *Freezing* decrease. However, in some cases **P** treatment produced the most potent anxiolytic-like effects. Although anxiolytic effects of **A** are widely described in literature [69-72], only few reports have shown that **P** administration is able to produce similar effects [28,36,57] with an improved efficacy in some cases [27].

Therefore, the results described in this work support these last findings and add more evidence to this topic. Moreover, none of the treatment affected the duration of *Grooming* and *Rearing* events observed through the absence of significant differences in their ratios.

Although **A** and **P** treatments produce a significant increase in the *Active time* and *Line crossing*, correlations analyses of *Line crossing* based *Active time* were not equal. Only a positive correlation of these parameters was observed with microinfusions of **P** or its analogue *Epoxy 2*. These differences may probably due to the molecular features of each steroid. These analyses allow to describe similar behavioral effects for steroids with similar A/B rings conformations and suggest that the SS and probably **A** doses should be administered in higher concentrations to probably produce anxiolytic-like effects. Although, these SS had a limited solubility in aqueous medium.

Previously, we described similar responses to **A** and **P** with these SS administrations in a variety of assays, including binding modulation of specific ligands to the $GABA_A$ receptor, the 3β-hydroxysteroid dehydrogenase activity alteration and neuroprotection in cerebral cortex and hippocampus cultures against a hypoxic event [17,18]. However, no effects were observed in these behavioral assays, we do not discard these SS for further *in vivo* evaluations that include another doses and more behavioral assays.

Summarizing, in this work we evaluated, in an open-field test, the *in vivo* anxiolytic-like effects of two synthetic analogues of **A** and **P** with a decreased molecular flexibility (that confers a favorable spatial arrangement for the steroid binding site). Only an increase in animal exploratory activities interpreted as anxiolytic-like effects were observed with **A** and **P** microinfusions. The lack of anxiolytic-like effect at the dose evaluated, and the previously reported modulation on the $GABA_A$ receptor [17,18] may these SS suitable for therapeutical treatments in other mood disorders where the GABAergic function is involved like early chronic psychosocial stress or depression. Nevertheless the action of these *Epoxies* should be further evaluated for these conditions.

Acknowledgment

This work was supported by grants from ANPCYT PICT-2006-727; CONICET PIP-860, PIP-243 and partially supported by UBACYT. M R was supported by a fellowship from CONICET.

References

1. Lambert JJ, Belelli D, Peden DR, Vardy AW, Peters JA (2003) Neurosteroid modulation of GABAA receptors. Prog Neurobiol 71: 67-80.
2. Akk G, Covey DF, Evers AS, Steinbach JH, Zorumski CF, et al. (2009) The influence of the membrane on neurosteroid actions at GABA(A) receptors. Psychoneuroendocrinology 34 Suppl 1: S59-66.
3. Majewska MD (1992) Neurosteroids: endogenous bimodal modulators of the GABAA receptor. Mechanism of action and physiological significance. Prog Neurobiol 38: 379-395.
4. Reddy DS (2003) Is there a physiological role for the neurosteroid THDOC in stress-sensitive conditions? Trends Pharmacol Sci 24: 103-106.
5. Gasior M, Carter RB, Witkin JM (1999) Neuroactive steroids: potential therapeutic use in neurological and psychiatric disorders. Trends Pharmacol Sci 20: 107-112.
6. Rupprecht R, di Michele F, Hermann B, Ströhle A, Lancel M, et al. (2001) Neuroactive steroids: molecular mechanisms of action and implications for neuropsychopharmacology. Brain Res Brain Res Rev 37: 59-67.
7. Mellon SH (2004) Synthesis, enzyme localization, and regulation of neurosteroids. In: Smith SS Editor. Neurosteroid effects in the central nervous system: the role of the GABAA receptor. Boca Raton: CRC Press 1-46.
8. Dubrovsky BO (2005) Steroids, neuroactive steroids and neurosteroids in psychopathology. Prog Neuropsychopharmacol Biol Psychiatry 29: 169-192.
9. Hirst JJ, Kelleher MA, Walker DW, Palliser HK (2014) Neuroactive steroids in pregnancy: key regulatory and protective roles in the foetal brain. J Steroid Biochem Mol Biol 139: 144-153.
10. Akk G, Covey DF, Evers AS, Steinbach JH, Zorumski CF, et al. (2007) Mechanisms of neurosteroid interactions with GABA(A) receptors. Pharmacol Ther 116: 35-57.
11. Reddy DS (2010) Neurosteroids: endogenous role in the human brain and therapeutic potentials. Prog Brain Res 186: 113-137.
12. Rey M, Coirini H (2015) Synthetic neurosteroids on brain protection. Neural Regen Res 10: 17-21.
13. Purdy RH, Morrow AL, Blinn JR, Paul SM (1990) Synthesis, metabolism, and pharmacological activity of 3a-hydroxy steroids which potentiate GABA-receptor-mediated chloride ion uptake in rat cerebral cortical synaptoneurosomes. J Med Chem 33: 1572-1581.
14. Souli C, Avlonitis N, Calogeropoulou T, Tsotinis A, Maksay G, et al. (2005) Novel 17beta-substituted conformationally constrained neurosteroids that modulate GABA A receptors. J Med Chem 48: 5203-5214.
15. Scaglione JB, Manion BD, Benz A, Taylor A, DeKoster GT, et al. (2006) Neurosteroid analogues. 11. Alternative ring system scaffolds: gamma-aminobutyric acid receptor modulation and anesthetic actions of benz[f]indenes. J Med Chem 49: 4595-4605.
16. Suñol C, García DA, Bujons J, Kristofíková Z, Matyás L, et al. (2006) Activity of B-nor analogues of neurosteroids on the GABA(A) receptor in primary neuronal cultures. J Med Chem 49: 3225-3234.
17. Rey M, Kruse MS, Alvarez LD, Ghini AA, Veleiro AS, et al. (2013) Neuroprotective action of synthetic steroids with oxygen bridge. Activity on GABAA receptor. Exp Neurol 249: 49-58.
18. Rey M, Veleiro AS, Ghini AA, Kruse MS, Burton G, et al. (2015) Effect of synthetic steroids on GABAA receptor binding in rat brain. Neuroscience 290: 138-146.
19. Veleiro AS, Burton G (2009) Structure-activity relationships of neuroactive steroids acting on the GABAA receptor. Curr Med Chem 16: 455-472.
20. Norberg L, Wahlström G, Bäckström T (1987) The anaesthetic potency of 3 alpha-hydroxy-5 alpha-pregnan-20-one and 3 alpha-hydroxy-5 beta-pregnan-20-one determined with an intravenous EEG-threshold method in male rats. Pharmacol Toxicol 61: 42-47.
21. Belelli D, Lan NC, Gee KW (1990) Anticonvulsant steroids and the GABA/benzodiazepine receptor-chloride ionophore complex. Neurosci Biobehav Rev 14: 315-322.

22. Wieland S, Lan NC, Mirasedeghi S, Gee KW (1991) Anxiolytic activity of the progesterone metabolite 5 alpha-pregnan-3 alpha-o1-20-one. Brain Res 565: 263-268.

23. Devaud LL, Purdy RH, Morrow AL (1995) The neurosteroid, 3 alpha-hydroxy-5 alpha-pregnan-20-one, protects against bicuculline-induced seizures during ethanol withdrawal in rats. Alcohol Clin Exp Res 19: 350-355.

24. Picazo O, Fernández-Guasti A (1995) Anti-anxiety effects of progesterone and some of its reduced metabolites: an evaluation using the burying behavior test. Brain Res 680: 135-141.

25. Wang MD, Wahlström G, Gee KW, Bäckström T (1995) Potency of lipid and protein formulation of 5 alpha-pregnanolone at induction of anaesthesia and the corresponding regional brain distribution. Br J Anaesth 74: 553-557.

26. Weiland NG, Orchinik M (1995) Specific subunit mRNAs of the GABAA receptor are regulated by progesterone in subfields of the hippocampus. Brain Res Mol Brain Res 32: 271-278.

27. Wieland S, Belluzzi JD, Stein L, Lan NC (1995) Comparative behavioral characterization of the neuroactive steroids 3 alpha-OH,5 alpha-pregnan-20-one and 3 alpha-OH,5 beta-pregnan-20-one in rodents. Psychopharmacology (Berl) 118: 65-71.

28. Carboni E, Wieland S, Lan NC, Gee KW (1996) Anxiolytic properties of endogenously occurring pregnanediols in two rodent models of anxiety. Psychopharmacology (Berl) 126: 173-178.

29. Finn DA, Roberts AJ, Lotrich F, Gallaher EJ (1997) Genetic differences in behavioral sensitivity to a neuroactive steroid. J Pharmacol Exp Ther 280: 820-828.

30. Palmer AA, Miller MN, McKinnon CS, Phillips TJ (2002) Sensitivity to the locomotor stimulant effects of ethanol and allopregnanolone is influenced by common genes. Behav Neurosci 116: 126-137.

31. Bitran D, Hilvers RJ, Kellogg CK (1991) Anxiolytic effects of 3 alpha-hydroxy-5 alpha[beta]-pregnan-20-one: endogenous metabolites of progesterone that are active at the GABAA receptor. Brain Res 561: 157-161.

32. Bitran D, Purdy RH, Kellogg CK (1993) Anxiolytic effect of progesterone is associated with increases in cortical allopregnanolone and GABAA receptor function. Pharmacol Biochem Behav 45: 423-428.

33. Fernández-Guasti A, Picazo O (1995) Flumazenil blocks the anxiolytic action of allopregnanolone. Eur J Pharmacol 281: 113-115.

34. Brot MD, Akwa Y, Purdy RH, Koob GF, Britton KT (1997) The anxiolytic-like effects of the neurosteroid allopregnanolone: interactions with GABA(A) receptors. Eur J Pharmacol 325: 1-7.

35. Reddy DS, Kulkarni SK (1997) Differential anxiolytic effects of neurosteroids in the mirrored chamber behavior test in mice. Brain Res 752: 61-71.

36. Bitran D, Dugan M, Renda P, Ellis R, Foley M (1999) Anxiolytic effects of the neuroactive steroid pregnanolone (3 alpha-OH-5 beta-pregnan-20-one) after microinjection in the dorsal hippocampus and lateral septum. Brain Res 850: 217-224.

37. Rupprecht R (2003) Neuroactive steroids: mechanisms of action and neuropsychopharmacological properties. Psychoneuroendocrinology 28: 139-168.

38. Bannerman DM, Rawlins JN, McHugh SB, Deacon RM, Yee BK, et al. (2004) Regional dissociations within the hippocampus--memory and anxiety. Neurosci Biobehav Rev 28: 273-283.

39. Mòdol L, Darbra S, Pallarès M (2011) Neurosteroids infusion into the CA1 hippocampal region on exploration, anxiety-like behaviour and aversive learning. Behav Brain Res 222: 223-229.

40. Pick CG, Peter Y, Terkel J, Gavish M, Weizman R (1996) Effect of the neuroactive steroid alpha-THDOC on staircase test behavior in mice. Psychopharmacology (Berl) 128: 61-66.

41. Mok WM, Krieger NR (1990) Evidence that 5 alpha-pregnan-3 alpha-ol-20-one is the metabolite responsible for progesterone anesthesia. Brain Res 533: 42-45.

42. Bitran D, Mc Leod M, Schiekh M (1995) Blockade of the bioconversion of progesterone to allopregnanolone prevents the anxiolytic effects and potentiation of cortical GABAA receptor function observed in progesterone treated ovariectomized rats. Soc Neurosci Abstr 19: 373-379

43. Eduardo SL, Ghini AA, Burton G (2003) Oxido-bridged neurosteroid analogues Synthesis of 2,19-oxido-allopregnanolone. ARKIVOC X: 468-476.

44. Veleiro AS, Rosenstein RE, Jaliffa CO, Grilli ML, Speroni F, et al. (2003) Synthesis and GABA(A) receptor activity of a 6,19-oxido analogue of pregnanolone. Bioorg Med Chem Lett 13: 343-346.

45. Paxinos G, Watson C (1998) The rat brain in stereotaxic coordinates (4thedn) Academic Press, San Diego California.

46. Engin E, Treit D (2007) The anxiolytic-like effects of allopregnanolone vary as a function of intracerebral microinfusion site: the amygdala, medial prefrontal cortex, or hippocampus. Behav Pharmacol 18: 461-470.

47. Frye CA, Paris JJ, Rhodes ME (2008) Estrogen is necessary for 5alpha-pregnan-3alpha-ol-20-one (3alpha,5alpha-THP) infusion to the ventral tegmental area to facilitate social and sexual, but neither exploratory nor affective behavior of ovariectomized rats. Pharmacol Biochem Behav 91: 261-270.

48. Nin MS, Salles FB, Azeredo LA, Frazon AP, Gomez R, et al. (2008) Antidepressant effect and changes of GABAA receptor gamma2 subunit mRNA after hippocampal administration of allopregnanolone in rats. J Psychopharmacol 22: 477-485.

49. Rodríguez-Landa JF, Contreras CM, Bautista-Martínez FE, Saavedra M, Bernal-Morales B, et al. (2005) Antidepressant-like effect of a microinjection of allopregnanolone in the dorsal hippocampus and lateral septal nucleus in the rat; involvement of GABAA receptor. Behav Pharmacol 16: S45.

50. Estrada-Camarena E, Contreras CM, Saavedra M, Luna-Baltazar I, López-Rubalcava C (2002) Participation of the lateral septal nuclei (LSN) in the antidepressant-like actions of progesterone in the forced swimming test (FST). Behav Brain Res 134: 175-183.

51. Blizard DA, Lippman HR, Chen JJ (1975) Sex differences in open-field behavior in the rat: the inductive and activational role of gonadal hormones. Physiol Behav 14: 601-608.

52. Frye CA, Petralia SM, Rhodes ME (2000) Estrous cycle and sex differences in performance on anxiety tasks coincide with increases in hippocampal progesterone and 3alpha,5alpha-THP. Pharmacol Biochem Behav 67: 587-596.

53. McCarthy MM, Felzenberg E, Robbins A, Pfaff DW, Schwartz-Giblin S (1995) Infusions of diazepam and allopregnanolone into the midbrain central gray facilitate open-field behavior and sexual receptivity in female rats. Horm Behav 29: 279-295.

54. Schumacher M, Coirini H, Pfaff DW, McEwen BS (1990) Behavioral effects of progesterone associated with rapid modulation of oxytocin receptors. Science 250: 691-694.

55. Woods JH, Katz JL, Winger G (1992) Benzodiazepines: use, abuse, and consequences. Pharmacol Rev 44: 151-347.

56. Sperk G, Schwarzer C, Tsunashima K, Fuchs K, Sieghart W (1997) GABA(A) receptor subunits in the rat hippocampus I: immunocytochemical distribution of 13 subunits. Neuroscience 80: 987-1000.

57. Gomez C, Saldivar-Gonzalez A, Delgado G, Rodriguez R (2002) Rapid anxiolytic activity of progesterone and pregnanolone in male rats. Pharmacol Biochem Behav 72: 543-550.

58. Schüle C, Eser D, Baghai TC, Nothdurfter C, Kessler JS, et al. (2011) Neuroactive steroids in affective disorders: target for novel antidepressant or anxiolytic drugs? Neuroscience 191: 55-77.

59. Zheng P (2009) Neuroactive steroid regulation of neurotransmitter release in the CNS: action, mechanism and possible significance. Prog Neurobiol 89: 134-152.

60. Gago N, El-Etr M, Sananès N, Cadepond F, Samuel D, et al. (2004) 3alpha,5alpha-Tetrahydroprogesterone (allopregnanolone) and gamma-aminobutyric acid: autocrine/paracrine interactions in the control of

neonatal PSA-NCAM+ progenitor proliferation. J Neurosci Res 78: 770-783.

61. Harrison NL, Simmonds MA (1984) Modulation of the GABA receptor complex by a steroid anaesthetic. Brain Res 323: 287-292.

62. Majewska MD, Harrison NL, Schwartz RD, Barker JL, Paul SM (1986) Steroid hormone metabolites are barbiturate-like modulators of the GABA receptor. Science 232: 1004-1007.

63. Belelli D, Peden DR, Rosahl TW, Wafford KA, Lambert JJ (2005) Extrasynaptic GABAA receptors of thalamocortical neurons: a molecular target for hypnotics. J Neurosci 25: 11513-11520.

64. Martín-García E, Pallarès M (2005) Intrahippocampal nicotine and neurosteroids effects on the anxiety-like behaviour in voluntary and chronic alcohol-drinking rats. Behav Brain Res 164: 117-127.

65. Frye CA, Rhodes ME (2006) Infusions of 5alpha-pregnan-3alpha-ol-20-one (3alpha,5alpha-THP) to the ventral tegmental area, but not the substantia nigra, enhance exploratory, anti-anxiety, social and sexual behaviours and concomitantly increase 3alpha,5alpha-THP concentrations in the hippocampus, diencephalon and cortex of ovariectomised oestrogen-primed rats. J Neuroendocrinol 18: 960-975.

66. Darbra S, Pallarès M (2010) Alterations in neonatal neurosteroids affect exploration during adolescence and prepulse inhibition in adulthood. Psychoneuroendocrinology 35: 525-535.

67. Frye CA, Paris JJ (2011) Progesterone turnover to its 5Î±-reduced metabolites in the ventral tegmental area of the midbrain is essential for initiating social and affective behavior and progesterone metabolism in female rats. J Endocrinol Invest 34: e188-199.

68. Finn DA, Roberts AJ, Long S, Tanchuck M, Phillips TJ (2003) Neurosteroid consumption has anxiolytic effects in mice. Pharmacol Biochem Behav 76: 451-462.

69. Bäckström T, Bixo M, Johansson M, Nyberg S, Ossewaarde L, et al. (2014) Allopregnanolone and mood disorders. Prog Neurobiol 113: 88-94.

70. Bali A, Jaggi AS (2014) Multifunctional aspects of allopregnanolone in stress and related disorders. Prog Neuropsychopharmacol Biol Psychiatry 48: 64-78.

71. Melcangi RC, Panzica GC (2014) Allopregnanolone: state of the art. Prog Neurobiol 113: 1-5.

72. Schüle C, Nothdurfter C, Rupprecht R (2014) The role of allopregnanolone in depression and anxiety. Prog Neurobiol 113: 79-87.

Polycystic Ovary Syndrome: Correlation between Phenotypes and Metabolic Syndrome

Érika Mendonça das Neves, Angela Maggio da Fonseca, Vicente Renato Bagnoli, Marilena Alicia Souza*, Sandra Dircinha Teixeira de Araújo Moraes, Gustavo Arantes Rosa Maciel, José Maria Soares Junior and Edmund Chada Baracat

Disciplina de Ginecologia/Obstetrícia da Faculdade de Medicina da Universidade de São Paulo, Brazil

***Corresponding author:** Marilena Alicia Souza, Disciplina de Ginecologia/Obstetrícia da Faculdade de Medicina da Universidade de São Paulo, Brazil, E-mail: marilenealicia@hotmail.com

Abstract

The polycystic ovary syndrome (PCOS) is an endocrine metabolic disorder affecting 7% to 10% of women during reproductive age. The metabolic syndrome is understood as a set of clinical factors related to the potential increase in the risk of cardiovascular disease, type II diabetes mellitus, and early mortality. The hyperandrogenism and insulin resistance related to PCOS will result in increased cardiovascular risk and extending throughout the patient's lifetime.

Objectives: To identify the prevalence of metabolic syndrome in each of the polycystic ovary syndrome (PCOS) phenotypes and the factors linked with metabolic risk.

Methods: Observational study of 566 women between 14 and 39 years with PCOS according to the Rotterdam criteria. The metabolic risk was assessed by descriptive analysis with a confidence interval of 95%. Quantitative variables were tested using the Shapiro-Wilk test and nonparametric Mann-Whitney test. For the multivariate analysis was used the prevalence ratio between several independent variables and the outcome metabolic risk. Identify factors associated with metabolic risk using Cox regression with robust variance.

Results: The mean age was 26.4 ± 5.9 years. Metabolic risk was found in 21%, with a predominance of phenotypes E (28.4%), which is characterized by hirsutism, oligoanovulation, polycystic ovaries; B (25%), defined as biochemical hyperandrogenism, hirsutism, oligoanovulation; and A (22%) described biochemical hyperandrogenism, hirsutism, oligoanovulation and polycystic ovaries. A one-year increase in age raised the risk by 5%. Every one-unit increase in body mass index (BMI) added 8%. Presence of hirsutism tripled the risk. Patients with at least one child ran twice the risk than the nulliparous.

Conclusions: Our data suggested the important factors of metabolic syndrome in women with PCOS are age, obesity, hirsutism, and parity.

Keywords: Polycystic ovary syndrome; Metabolic syndrome

Introduction

The polycystic ovary syndrome (PCOS) is an endocrine metabolic disorder affecting 7% to 10% of women during reproductive age [1]. It is considered not only a systemic disorder with reproductive, psychological, cosmetic, and oncologic consequences, but also a metabolic disorder, such as hyperglycemia and insulin resistance, resulting in increased cardiovascular risk and type II diabetes mellitus and extending throughout the patient's lifetime with potential financial burden to public health [2].

The definition of PCOS is based on the consensus of several groups. The 2003 Rotterdam consensus workshop provided a wider definition than had been proposed until then, encompassing a larger number of phenotypes. It was established that the diagnosis of the syndrome should include the presence of two out of the following three features: 1) oligo- or anovulation, 2) clinical and/or biochemical signs of hyperandrogenism, or 3) polycystic ovaries (presence of 12 or more follicles with a diameter of 2 mm-9 mm in one or both of the ovaries or ovarian volume ≥ 10 cm^3) [3]. Later, in 2006, Azziz et al. proposed the incorporation of several different metabolic-syndrome-related phenotypes in order to encompass the clinical diversity of PCOS [2]. It is necessary to exclude the diseases with similar clinical aspects to PCOS (congenital adrenal hyperplasia, Cushing's syndrome, tumors secreting ovarian and adrenal androgens, hyperprolactinemia, and thyroid dysfunctions) and conditions requiring the use of exogenous androgens [3]. It is noted that some androgen-producing tumors occur with increased insulin resistance and increased risk of cardiovascular disease in women [4]. It is questionable that elevated androgen levels increases the metabolic syndrome, which justifies the importance of recognizing the different phenotypes of PCOS.

Metabolic syndrome (MetS) has been the subject of many studies in recent years [5,6]. It was defined by ATP III (2004) [7] as a group of interrelated risk factors of metabolic origin that contribute directly to the development of cardiovascular disease (CVD) and/or type II diabetes mellitus [7].

The prevalence of MetS in PCOS patients is almost twice as great as in the general population of women, raising the risk of cardiovascular disease by seven times [8]. However, the metabolic syndrome study of each PCOS phenotype reveals phenotypic groups with a worse metabolic profile and a larger number of harmful results to one's health [8,9]. Because of the high incidence of the association between PCOS and MetS, we sought to identify the frequency of metabolic syndrome in each PCOS phenotype and the factors associated with metabolic risk in the population of the city of Sao Paulo, Brazil.

Patients and Methods

This was an observational study which used data extracted from the medical records of 1408 women with chronic anovulation. The women came for their first consultation at the Sector of Endocrine Gynecology and Menopause, Clinics Hospital, University of São Paulo between June 1964 and November 2011. The research protocol was approved by the Ethics Committee for Analysis of Research Projects (CAPPesq) of the Clinics Hospital and the School of Medicine of Sao Paulo, under number 0746/10.

Inclusion criteria: patients aged 14-39 years and diagnosed with PCOS according to the 2003 Rotterdam consensus and whose medical records had the date of the anamnesis and showed that the physical examination and the medical tests were suitable for PCOS.

Exclusion criteria: use of hormonal contraception (in the previous 6 months) or of psychiatric medications, hyperprolactinemia, thyroid dysfunction, and other causes of hyperandrogenism, such as congenital adrenal hyperplasia, Cushing's syndrome, adrenal neoplasia, or virilizing ovarian tumors.

According to the eligibility criteria, 566 patients were included in the study (Figure 1).

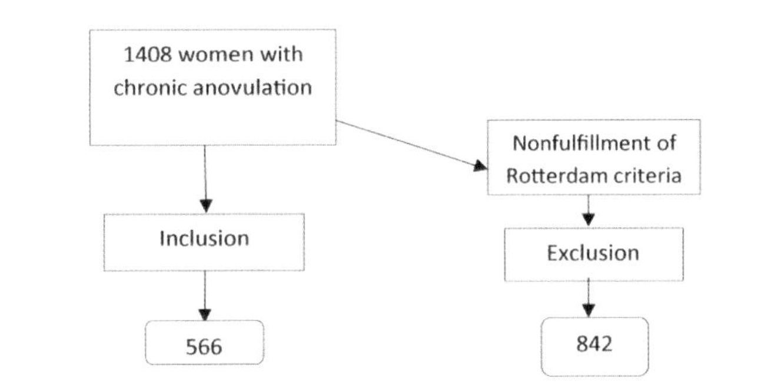

Figure 1: Algorithm showing patients included after application of eligibility criteria

Clinical hyperandrogenism was considered when the presence of hirsutism was indicated by a score of 7 or more on the Ferriman and Gallwey scale [10-11]. Oligoanovulation was evidenced by either amenorrhea or oligomenorrhea (less than six menstrual periods in the previous year) [9].

The suprapubic pelvic ultrasound or transvaginal ultrasound evaluated the presence of 12 or more follicles with a diameter between 2 mm and 9 mm in one or both ovaries or ovarian volume greater than 10 cm^3.

Anthropometric data: BMI was obtained by dividing weight (kg) by height (meters) squared. Waist circumference (cm) was measured with a tape measure both flexible and inextensible which was positioned at the lower curvature located between the last rib and the iliac crest with the patient in supine position and in expiration. Blood pressure was measured using a sphygmomanometer with a mercury column or aneroid manometer [10-13].

In order to determine metabolic measures of triglycerides and HDL-C, blood samples were collected after a 12-hour fast and analyzed using automated enzymatic methods (Roche Laboratories). The plasma glucose concentration was established by the hemoxynase method. Follicle-stimulating hormone (FSH), luteinizing hormone (LH), prolactin, androstenedione, dehydroepiandrosterone sulfate (DHEAS), and total and free testosterone were evaluated. Total testosterone was measured by fluoroimmunoassay (Wallac, Finland) and free testosterone was calculated based on total testosterone and on sex hormone-binding globulin (SHBG) measured by fluorimetry. Biochemical hyperandrogenism was defined as a testosterone level greater than or equal to 98 nmol/l and a free testosterone concentration of 45 nmol/l. Samples were drawn in the first phase of the cycle from patients with menstrual regularity or anytime from patients in amenorrhea.

The phenotypes proposed by Azziz et al. (2006) for patients meeting the Rotterdam criteria demonstrate the clinical diversity of PCOS and manifest as biochemical hyperandrogenism, hirsutism, oligoanovulation, and polycystic ovaries [2,3] (Table 1).

Phenotypes	Characteristics
A	Biochemical Hyperandrogenism, Hirsutism, Oligoanovulation and Polycystic Ovaries
B	Biochemical hyperandrogenism, Hirsutism and Oligoanovulation
C	Biochemical hyperandrogenism, Oligoanovulation and Polycystic ovaries
D	Biochemical hyperandrogenism and Oligoanovulation
E	Hirsutism, Oligoanovulation and Polycystic ovaries
F	Hirsutism and Oligoanovulation
G	Biochemical hyperandrogenism, Hirsutism and Polycystic ovaries
H	Hirsutism and Polycystic ovaries
I	Biochemical hyperandrogenism and Polycystic ovaries
J	Oligoanovulation and Polycystic ovaries

Table 1: Pcos phenotypes according to rotterdam criteria

Metabolic syndrome was defined according to the third report of the National Cholesterol Education Project Adult Treatment Panel (NCEP-ATPIII) and thus considered present when the patient had three or more of the following five values changed: waist circumference >88 cm, triglycerides ≥ 150 mg/dl; HDL-C<50 mg/dl, systolic blood pressure ≥ 130 or diastolic blood pressure ≥ 85 mmHg or when taking antihypertensive drugs; fasting glucose of 12 hours between 100 to 126 mg/dl [7].

In the search for factors correlating with metabolic risk in PCOS patients, the following variables were analyzed: age, parity, hirsutism, oligoanovulation, oligoanovulation time, infertility, menarche, BMI, biochemical hyperandrogenism, polycystic ovaries, family history of type 2 diabetes mellitus, hypertension, gynecological cancer, nongynecological cancer.

Statistical analysis

The data were organized and the average standard deviation (SD), prevalence ratio, and confidence interval of 95% (95% CI) were calculated and displayed in the text, tables, and graphs. Quantitative variables were assessed by the Shapiro-Wilk test and then by the nonparametric Mann-Whitney test [14-16]. Initially, a descriptive analysis of the study variables was performed. Qualitative variables were shown in tables of frequency, whereas quantitative variables were estimated according to the measures of central tendency and dispersion. The prevalence of metabolic risk and its respective interval were calculated using a 95% CI. In order to identify possible factors associated with metabolic risk, the relationship between metabolic syndrome and all study variables was tested. The variables with a p value below 0.20 were the starting point in univariate analysis. The model used was the Cox regression with variance [16,17]. In this study, a significance level of 5% was adopted. The data were plotted into Excel and analyzed using the STATA statistical software version 12.0 (StataCorp LP, College Station, Texas, USA).

Results

Of the total of 566 patients in the study, 478 were of African descent, 86 were white, and 2 were Asian. The age range was 14-39 years and mean age was 26.4 ± 5.9 years. The analysis of menstruation type showed that 518 (90.6%) patients had menstrual irregularity. A total of 396 women reported having an active sexual life, and 89 of them had one or more children. Hirsutism was present in 520 (91.8%) patients, acne in 310 (54.9%), and *acanthosis nigricans* in 109 (54.9%). Biochemical hyperandrogenism was observed in 294 (51.9%) patients and polycystic ovary in 440 (77.7%).

Waist circumference greater than 88 cm was observed in 51% of the 566 patients, overweight in 28.5%, and obesity in 38%. Systolic blood pressure ≥ 130 mmHg was found in 220 women (38.9%) and diastolic blood pressure ≥ 85 mmHg at 20% in 113. Patients with glucose intolerance added up to 231 (40.8%), with low HDL-cholesterol to 242 (43%), and with high triglycerides to 51 (9%).

Analysis of the phenotypes [2] showed that A and J predominated and were present in 204 women and in 90, respectively. Of the 566 women, 119 (21%) were at metabolic risk (95% CI, 17.7 to 24.6). Phenotypes that showed a higher incidence of metabolic syndrome were E, found in 23 patients (28.4%), followed by B, in 9 (25%), and A, in 45 (22.1%) (Table 2).

Phenotypes				**Metabolic Risk**			**BMI ≥ 25 kg/m2**
(Groups)	(N)	(%)		(N)	(%)		(%)
A	204	36		45	22.1		67.4
B	36	6.4		9	25		71
C	12	2.1		1	8.3		66
D	2	0.3		0	0		100
E	81	14.3		23	28.4		65.4
F	88	15.6		18	20.5		50
G	39	6.9		8	20.5		55.9
H	13	2.3		2	15.4		40
I	1	0.2		0	0		100
J	90	15.9		13	14.4		67.9
TOTAL	566	100		21	119		100

Table 2: phenotypes in metabolic risk and in BMI

We researched epidemiological and clinical characteristics such as ethnicity, parity, presence of menstrual irregularities, signs of hyperandrogenism, polycystic ovaries in patients with PCOS to assess the metabolic risk. The data on family history, including diabetes (p=0.394), hypertension (p=0.639), gynecological cancer (p=0.329), and nongynecological cancers (p=0.704) failed to explain the increased risk or to show metabolic protection. In order to identify the variables independently associated with metabolic risk, two models were chosen from the multivariate analysis of the data. It was found that metabolic risk was independently associated with age (p=0.006), BMI (p<0.001), parity (p=0.002), and the occurrence of hirsutism (p=0.029) (Tables 3 and 4).

Variables	Total	Metabolic syndrome no (Prevalence)	PR	95% CI (PR)	p
Ethnicity					0.191
white or Asian	88	23 (26.1)	1		
biracial or black	478	96 (20.1)	0.77	0.52 - 1.14	
Parity					0.020
not applicable (virgins)	84	11 (13.1)	1		
without children	393	80 (20.6)	1.57	0.88 - 2.82	
with children	89	27 (30,3)	2.32	1.22 - 4.37	
Menstrual Irregularity and amenorrhea					0.640

no	59	11 (18.6)	1		
yes	507	108 (21.3+A1:F33)	1.14	0.653 - 2.00	
Hirsutism					0.029
no	46	3 (6.5)	1		
yes	520	116 (22.3)	3.42	1.13 - 10.35	
Hyperandrogenemia					0.807
no	272	56 (20.6)	1		
yes	294	63 (21.4)	1.04	0.76 - 1.43	
Polycystic ovaries					0.900
no	126	27 (21.4)	1		
yes	440	92 (20.9)	0.98	0.67 - 1.43	
Family history of diabetes					0.394
no	38	10 (26.3)	1		
yes	528	109 (20.6)	0.78	0.45 - 1.37	
Family history of hypertension					0.639
no	506	105 (20.7)	1		
yes	60	14 (23.3)	1.12	0.69 - 1.83	
Family history of gynecological cancer					0.329
no	554	118 (21.3)	1		
yes	12	1 (8.3)	0.39	0.06 - 2.58	
Family history of nongynecological cancer					0.704
no	541	113 (20.9)	1		
yes	25	6 (24.0)	1.15	0.56 - 2.35	

Quantitative	without Metabolic Risk	with Metabolic Risk	p*
Variables	mean (SD); median (min-max)	mean (SD); median (min-max)	
Age	26.1 (5.8); 25.0 (14 - 39)	27.7 (6.1); 28.0 (14 - 39)	0.006
BMI (n=308)	27.5 (6.9); 26.9 (16.8 - 59.0)	36.1 (7.8); 34.9 (25.1 - 56.9)	<0.001
Menarche	13.0 (1.8); 13 (9 - 18)	12.8 (1.9); 13 (9 - 18)	0.619
Time period (years) of reproductive desire (years)	1.3 (2.2); 0 (0 - 14)	1.9 (3.2); 0 (0 - 16)	0.195
Time period (years) of irregularity (n=437)	6.3 (5.8); 5 (0 - 28)	7.6 (6.3); 5 (0 - 24)	0.101

Table 3: Relationship between family comorbidities, clinical and gynecological characteristics and metabolic syndrome. *Mann-Whitney test

PR: Prevalence Ratio; SD: standard Deviation

As can be seen, for every one-year increase in age, the risk of a metabolic event increased by 5%, regardless of BMI. The results also show that for every one-unit increase in BMI, there was an increase of 8% in the occurrence of the event, regardless of the patient's age.

Likewise, metabolic risk grew in parallel with increasing age (p=0.047), irrespective of BMI, parity, and occurrence of hirsutism. In addition, it has been estimated that the risk of a metabolic event for patients of any age with children, independently of hirsutism, is twice as large as that for women without children.

Variables	PRcr	RPadj (95% CI)	p
Model 1			
Age	1.04	1.05 (1.01 - 1.09)	0.006
BMI	1.08	1.08 (1.05 - 1.10)	<0.001
Model 2			
Age	1.04	1.03 (1.00 - 1.06)	0.047
Parity			
not applicable (virgins)	1		0.015
without children	1.57	1.43 (0.80 - 2.56)	
with children	2.32	2.03 (1.08 - 3.82)	
Hirsutism			0.036
no	1		
yes	3.42	3.31 (1.08 - 10.17)	
PRcr: Crude Prevalence Ratio; PRadj: Adjusted Prevalence Ratio			

Table 4: Estimates of the prevalence ratio by multiple regression model for metabolic syndrome

The analysis of patients with hirsutism, no matter what their age and parity, showed a threefold increase in metabolic risk against those without hirsutism (p=0.036).

Discussion

The metabolic syndrome is understood as a set of clinical factors related to the potential increase in the risk of cardiovascular disease, type 2 diabetes mellitus, and early mortality [7,5].

Considering the high prevalence of metabolic risk, the prevalence ratios (PRs) and their CIs were estimated using univariate analysis for the relationship between several independent variables and the outcome metabolic risk variable. Estimation of the relative risk by the odds ratio was prevented by the possibility that it would be overestimated because the prevalence of metabolic alterations exceeded 20%. Therefore, this was a cohort study with cross-sectional characteristics, where the association between exposure and outcome was estimated by PR [14-16].

Although differences between ethnicity, environment, and diet can alter the frequency of PCOS-related metabolic abnormalities, the incidence of obesity and the impact of age seem to be the main determinants of the prevalence of metabolic syndrome in different populations [18]. Hence, a comparison of adult women diagnosed with PCOS by the Rotterdam criteria led to the finding that the rate of metabolic syndrome is 47.3% in the U.S. [19,20], while in southeast China it is 25.6% [21], 23.8% in Sweden [22], 19.9% in Greece [23], 12.5% in Turkey [24] and 1.6% in the Czech Republic [25]. The prevalence of metabolic syndrome ranges from 33% to 45% in Brazilian women with PCOS [26,27].

This study revealed a prevalence of 21% in the association between PCOS and metabolic syndrome-related prevalence of more hyperandrogenic phenotypes, as oligoanovulation and hirsutism. This result corroborates the results found in the literature, which indicates a higher incidence of metabolic diseases early phenotypes, groups A to F, characterized by the presence of oligoanovulation [2].

The occurrence of MetS was observed in these three phenotypes, concomitant with an increase in BMI, which rose to 65.4% in E, 71% in B, and 67.4% in A. Besides weight gain, excess androgens were also the source of the numbers obtained in this study, because biochemical hyperandrogenism is a characteristic in the clinical phenotypic classification of groups A and B, totaling 42.4% of the 566 women in our sample [6,28].

As expected, the incidence of metabolic dysfunction in PCOS was significantly increased by the concurrent presence of obesity, which exacerbates the PCOS unfavorable metabolic outcomes from insulin resistance, promoting deterioration in the form of hyperandrogenism, hirsutism, and infertility [29]. In our study, the prevalence of overweight was 28.5%, of obesity, 38%, and of waist circumference greater than 88, 51%.

March et al. while investigating obesity in PCOS patients, observed a prevalence of 28% of PCOS in obese women and an association of 5% between PCOS and thin women [30].

Legro reported that obesity and age progression substantially increase the metabolic risk, although PCOS itself is responsible for the higher incidence of carbohydrate intolerance and diabetes among young and not obese patients. According to our survey, hirsutism is notably the dermatological complaint motivating the search for more medical attention and it was found in 91.8% (N=520) of the cases. The presence of hirsutism tripled the metabolic risk when compared to patients without hirsutism (p=0.036), regardless of age and parity [31].

Paoletti et al. and Cebeci et al. [32,33] suggested that the peripheral activity of androgens is related to hyperinsulinemia, based on studies where the antiandrogen treatment improved insulin resistance. Other studies suggested that insulin is one of the factors which interact with androgen to regulate the development of the pilosebaceous unit [34-36]. The same authors also concluded that insulin resistance is closely related to hirsutism, much more so than excess body weight in women with PCOS [34-36]. The relationship between the presence of hirsutism and an increased risk of a metabolic event is still an unresolved issue deserving further studies.

Although there are no reports in the literature associating parity and the occurrence of MetS after a gestational event, there is often additional body mass gain as well as worsening metabolism in PCOS patients. It's important to remember that patients have a higher incidence of undesirable vascular and hyperinsulinemic events during pregnancy and the postpartum period. Further research into these two issues might corroborate our findings and strengthen the case for prevention of metabolic disorders in PCOS patients [37-39].

Advancing age and BMI in patients with PCOS are well-known factors related to metabolic risk. However, further studies showing other statistical relationships between MetS and clinical manifestations of PCOS, similar to those between parity and hirsutism, are necessary in order to predict the simultaneous occurrence of these two syndromes.

The prevalence of metabolic syndrome in PCOS was 21%, and was more common in phenotypes E, B and A. In our search for predictors of metabolic risk, we focused on age, parity, and the presence of obesity and hirsutism among women with PCOS. Age and obesity have been extensively studied in the literature, and our work confirms their value as indicators. However, hirsutism and parity are new factors demanding further investigation of their potential as predictors of metabolic risk in women with PCOS.

Our data suggested the important factors of metabolic syndrome in women with PCOS are age, obesity, hirsutism and parity.

References

1. Teede H, Deeks A, Moran L (2010) Polycystic ovary syndrome: a complex condition with psychological, reproductive and metabolic manifestations that impacts on health across the lifespan. BMC Med 8:41
2. Azziz R, Carmina E, Dewailly D, Diamanti-Kandarakis E, Escobar-Morreale HF et al. (2006) Positions statement: criteria for defining polycystic ovary syndrome as a predominantly hyperandrogenic syndrome: an Androgen Excess Society guideline. J Clin Endocrinol Metab 91: 4237-45.
3. Rotterdam ESHRE/ASRM-Sponsored PCOS Consensus Workshop Group (2004) Revised 2003 consensus on diagnostic criteria and long-term health risks related to polycystic ovary syndrome (PCOS). Hum Reprod 19: 41-47.
4. Klotz RK, Müller-Holzner E, Fessler S, Reimer DU, Zervomanolakis I, et al. (2010) Leydig-cell-tumor of the ovary that responded to GnRH-analogue administration - case report and review of the literature. Exp Clin Endocrinol Diabetes 118: 291-297.
5. Benetti-Pinto CL, Berini Piccolo VR, Garmes HM, Teatin Juliato CR (2013) Subclinical hypothyroidism in young women with polycystic ovary syndrome: an analysis of clinical, hormonal, and metabolic parameters. Fertil Steril. 2013; 99: 588-592.
6. Marcondes JA, Hayashida SA, Barcellos CR, Rocha MP, Maciel GA, et al. (2007) Metabolic syndrome in women with polycystic ovary syndrome: prevalence, characteristics and predictors. Arq Bras Endocrinol Metabol 51: 972-979.
7. Grundy SM, Brewer HB Jr, Cleeman JI, Smith SC Jr, Lenfant C (2004) Definition of metabolic syndrome: Report of the National Heart, Lung, and Blood Institute/American Heart Association conference on scientific issues related to definition. Clin Biochem Rev 109: 433-438.
8. Apridonidze T, Essah PA, Iuorno MJ, Nestler JE (2005) Prevalence and characteristics of the metabolic syndrome in women with polycystic ovary syndrome. J Clin Endocrinol Metab 90: 1929-1935.
9. Maciel GA, Soares Júnior JM, Alves da Motta EL, Abi Haidar M, de Lima GR, et al. (2004) Nonobese women with polycystic ovary syndrome respond better than obese women to treatment with metformin. Fertil Steril 81: 355-360.
10. Ferriman D, Gallwey JD (1961) Clinical assessment of body hair growth in women. J Clin Endocrinol Metab 21: 1440-1447.
11. Yildiz BO (2008) Assessment, diagnosis and treatment of a patient with hirsutism. Nat Clin Pract Endocrinol Metab 4: 294-300.
12. Machado PA, Sichieri R (2002) Waist-to-hip ratio and dietary factors in adults. Rev Saude Publica 36: 198-204.
13. Garrow JS, Webster J (1985) Quetelet's index (W/H2) as a measure of fatness. Int J Obes 9: 147-153.
14. Davies HT, Crombie IK, Tavakoli M (1998) When can odds ratios mislead? BMJ 316: 989-991.
15. Barros AJ, Hirakata VN (2003) Alternatives for logistic regression in cross-sectional studies: an empirical comparison of models that directly estimate the prevalence ratio. BMC Med Res Methodol 3: 21.
16. Coutinho LM, Scazufca M, Menezes PR (2008) Methods for estimating prevalence ratios in cross-sectional studies. Rev Saude Publica 42: 992-998.
17. Lin DY, Wei LJ (1989) The robust inference for the Cox Proportional Hazards Model. J Am Stat Assoc 84: 1074-1078.
18. Wang ET, Kao CN, Shinkai K, Pasch L, Cedars MI, et al. (2013) Phenotypic comparison of Caucasian and Asian women with polycystic ovary syndrome: a cross-sectional study. Fertil Steril 100: 214-218.
19. Dokras A (2008) Cardiovascular disease risk factors in polycystic ovary syndrome. Semin Reprod Med 26: 39-44.
20. Ehrmann DA, Liljenquist DR, Kasza K, Azziz R, Legro RS, et al. (2006) Prevalence and predictors of the metabolic syndrome in women with polycystic ovary syndrome. J Clin Endocrinol Metab 91: 48-53.
21. Zhang HY, Guo CX, Zhu FF, Qu PP, Lin WJ (2013) Clinical characteristics, metabolic features, and phenotype of Chinese women with polycystic ovary syndrome: a large-scale case-control study. Arch Gynecol Obstet 287: 525-531
22. Hudecova M, Holte J, Olovsson M, Larsson A, Berne C, et al. (2011) Prevalence of the metabolic syndrome in women with a previous diagnosis of polycystic ovary syndrome: long-term follow-up. Fertil Steril 96: 1271-1274.
23. Vaggopoulos V, Trakakis E, Chrelias C, Panagopoulos P, Basios G, et al. (2013) Comparing classic and newer phenotypes in Greek PCOS women: the prevalence of metabolic syndrome and their association with insulin resistance. J Endocrinol Invest 36: 478-484.
24. Yildiz BO, Bozdag G, Yapici Z, Esinler I, Yarali H (2012) Prevalence, phenotype and cardiometabolic risk of polycystic ovary syndrome under different diagnostic criteria. Hum Reprod 27: 3067-3073.
25. Vrbíková J, Hill M, Dvoráková K, Stanická S, Stárka L (2010) The prevalence of metabolic syndrome in women with polycystic ovary syndrome. Cas Lek Cesk 149: 337-339.
26. Melo AS, Vieira CS, Romano LG, Ferriani RA, Navarro PA (2011) The frequency of metabolic syndrome is higher among PCOS Brazilian women with menstrual irregularity plus hyperandrogenism. Reprod Sci 18: 1230-1236.
27. Wiltgen D, Spritzer PM (2010) Variation in metabolic and cardiovascular risk in women with different polycystic ovary syndrome phenotypes. Fertil Steril 94: 2493-2496.
28. Marcondes JA, Barcellos CR, Rocha MP (2011) Difficulties and pitfalls in the diagnosis of polycystic ovary syndrome. Arq Bras Endocrinol Metabol 55: 6-15.
29. Motta AB (2012) The role of obesity in the development of polycystic ovary syndrome. Curr Pharm Des 18: 2482-2491.
30. March WA, Moore VM, Willson KJ, Phillips DI, Norman RJ, et al. (2010) The prevalence of polycystic ovary syndrome in a community sample assessed under contrasting diagnostic criteria. Hum Reprod 25: 544-551.
31. Legro RS, Kunselman AR, Dodson WC, Dunaif A (1999) Prevalence and predictors of risk for type 2 diabetes mellitus and impaired glucose tolerance in polycystic ovary syndrome: a prospective, controlled study in 254 affected women. J Clin Endocrinol Metab 84: 165-169.
32. Paoletti AM, Cagnacci A, Orrù M, Ajossa S, Guerriero S, et al. (1999) Treatment with flutamide improves hyperinsulinemia in women with idiopathic hirsutism. Fertil Steril 72: 448-453.
33. Cebeci F, Onsun N, Mert M (2012) Insulin resistance in women with hirsutism. Arch Med Sci 8: 342-346.
34. Arthur LS, Selvakumar R, Seshadri MS, Seshadri L (1999) Hyperinsulinemia in polycystic ovary disease. J Reprod Med 44: 783-787.
35. Amato MC, Galluzzo A, Merlino S, Mattina A, Richiusa P, et al. (2006) Lower insulin sensitivity differentiates hirsute from non-hirsute Sicilian women with polycystic ovary syndrome. Eur J Endocrinol 155: 859-865.
36. Rosenfield RL (2001) Polycystic ovary syndrome and insulin-resistant hyperinsulinemia. J Am Acad Dermatol 45: S95-104.
37. Legro RS (2012) Obesity and PCOS: implications for diagnosis and treatment. Semin Reprod Med 30: 496-506.
38. Tian L, Shen H, Lu Q, Norman RJ, Wang J (2007) Insulin resistance increases the risk of spontaneous abortion after assisted reproduction technology treatment. J Clin Endocrinol Metab 92: 1430-1433.
39. Bloomgarden ZT (2003) Diabetes issues in women and children: polycystic ovary syndrome. Diabetes Care 26: 2457-2463.

Test with 5 mcg ACTH for Diagnosis of Non-classic Congenital Adrenal Hyperplasia

Chagay NB[1], Fadeyev VV[2], Melnichenko GA[3], Ivanova ON[3], Bakulina EG[4] and Kotelnikova NYu[4]

[1]*Department of Endocrinology, Stavropol State Medical University, Stavropol, Russia*

[2]*Department of Endocrinology, I. M. Sechenov First Moscow State Medical University, Moscow, Russia*

[3]*Endocrinology Research Centre, Moscow, Russia*

[4]*Center of Family Healthcare and Reproduction, Stavropol, Russia*

***Corresponding author:** Chagay NB, Department of Endocrinology, Stavropol State Medical University, Stavropol, Switzerland, Russia, E-mail: chagay2006@rambler.ru

Abstract

Background: Short test with 250 mcg corticotropin (Tetracosactide acetate, a substance of first 24 amino acids from 39-acid chain of endogenous ACTH) is a diagnostic standard of non-classic form of congenital adrenal hyperplasia (CAH). However, it is well known that morning ACTH levels in healthy people fluctuate between 10 and 60 pg/ml, and peak cortisol levels can be achieved with 1-24 ACTH dose of 1 mcg or 5 mcg.

Objective: To study the sensitivity and specificity of the test with 5 mcg ACTH to diagnose non-classic form of congenital adrenal hyperplasia (NCAN).

Materials and Methods: During from 2006 to 2011, we screened 435 women aged from 16 to 35 (25 (21; 29) years) for CAH after exclusion of neoplastic hyperandrogenism.

Protocol of low-dose (5 mcg) and standard (250 mcg) 1-24 ACTH tests: Blood sampling for basal 17-OHP and cortisol levels; blood sampling for 17-OHP and cortisol at 30 and 60 minutes after 5 mcg or 250 mcg 1-24 ACTH stimulation. Molecular genetic analysis for most prevalent *CYP21* mutations was performed using allele specific polymerase chain reaction.

Results: Diagnosis of non-classic CAH with 21-hydroxylase deficiency was proved in 5.3% (23/435) of patients.

Conclusion: Low dose test with Tetracosactide 5 mcg can identify 21-hydroxylase deficiency in patients with stimulated 17-OHP concentrations over 14 ng/ml. Test with Tetracosactide 5 mcg had sensitivity of 72.7% and specificity of 100% with positive prognostic value (+PV) of 100%, and negative prognostic value (-PV) of 89.3%.

Keywords: Nonclassic adrenal hyperplasia; Low dose test; ACTH

Introduction

Short test with 250 mcg corticotropin (Tetracosactide acetate, a substance of first 24 amino acids from 39-acid chain of endogenous adrenocorticotropic hormone (ACTH)) is a diagnostic standard of non-classic form of congenital adrenal hyperplasia (CAH). This ACTH dose results in serum ACTH concentrations of up to 2000 pg/ml. However, it is well known that morning ACTH levels in healthy people fluctuate between 10 and 60 pg/ml, and peak cortisol levels can be achieved with 1-24 ACTH dose of 1 mcg or 5 mcg [1]. Thus, standard ACTH tests may result in false-positive results due to over stimulation of adrenal glands.

Patients and Methods

During from 2006 to 2011, we screened 435 women aged from 16 to 35 (25 (21; 29) years) for CAH.

Study inclusion criteria were following:

1. Dermatological or biochemical signs of hyperandrogenism in women with normal gonadotropins anovulatory and ovulatory cycle.

2. Normal gonadotropins anovulatory infertility without symptoms of hyperandrogenism.

First group of patients comprises of 234 patient with clinically and/or biochemically established non-neoplastic hyperandrogenism; 201 women without hyperandrogenism were included in the second group. Ovulation absented in 75.2% (176/234) of hyperandrogenic women and in 85.6% (172/201) of patients without hyperandrogenism. In our study we also included some women with recurrent pregnancy loss (12 in first group and 29 in second group).

Serum levels of LH, FSH, prolactin, testosterone, sex-binding globulin (SBG), dehydroepiandrosterone sulfate (DHEA-S) and other hormones were evaluated by solid chemiluminiscence immunoassay (IMMULITE I-DPC, Beckman Coulter DxI). Bioactive testosterone (bioTs) concentration estimated by on-line calculator ISSAM [2] using SBG level, constant SA [albumin concentration 4.3 g/dl]. Androgens levels compared to age-matched healthy women: Ts (50.8 (38.0; 60.9) ng/l); bioTs (13.2 (9.5; 19.6) ng/dl); DHEA-S (228 (180; 310) mg/dl).

For differential diagnostic of non-classic CAH with 21-hydroxylase deficiency we performed low-dose (5 mcg) 1-24 ACTH test with Tetracosactide acetate solution (250 mcg per 1 ml, NOVARTIS, Switzerland). Immediately before the test, 1 ml Tetracosactide acetate solution (250 mcg) was diluted by 49 ml of 0.9% NaCl solution to get concentration of 1-24 ACTH of 5 mcg per 1 ml. For intravenous bolus 1 ml of the final solution (5 mcg 1-24 ACTH) injected with 4 ml of 0.9% NaCl solution. In 20 women, standard test with 250 mcg 1-24 ACTH was additionally needed for further diagnosis.

Protocol of low-dose (5 mcg) and standard (250 mcg) 1-24 ACTH tests:

1) Blood sampling for basal 17-OHP and cortisol levels.

2) Intravenous bolus of 5 mcg or 250 mcg 1-24-ACTH.

3) Blood sampling for 17-OHP and cortisol at 30 and 60 minutes after 1-24-ACTH stimulation.

Molecular genetic analysis (MGA) for most prevalent *CYP21* mutations was performed using allele specific polymerase chain reaction [3].

For sensitivity and specificity analysis of low-dose ACTH test we compared results of low-dose (5 mcg) and standard (250 mcg) Tetracosactide tests with data of molecular genetic analysis for *CYP21*.

Statistical data analysis was run using software STATISTICA 6.0 and MedCalc Version 7.4.2.0. We used Shapiro-Wilk test to assess normality of distribution, and relevant t-test for comparison of two depending or non-depending samples. Descriptive non-parametrical statistics included Median (Me), Mean (M), standard deviation (SD), quartiles [25; 75] and Min-Max range. To compare quantitative parameters of non-related samples, Mann-Whitney (U) test was applied. Wilcoxon test (W) and Friedman variance analysis (F) was used when comparing two or more related samples. Kendall's coefficient of concordance (nonparametric correlation coefficient between two variables) was used to assess the relationship between multidimensional variables. Chi-squared test (χ^2) was done to analyze difference in distribution of categorical parameters in two groups. Correlation between numerical parameters was tested by Spearman (r) and Kendall's Tau criteria. Sensitivity, specificity and accuracy of 5 mcg 1-24 ACTH test were calculated using standard formulas. Significance level was chosen at $p<0.05$.

Results

Anovulation in women from both groups was diagnosed as abnormally prolonged menstrual cycle (over 35 days up to amenorrhea, Me=52 days) and/or negative ovulation tests in at least 5 cycles. In group 1 hyperandrogenism was proven clinically (at least 8 scores of Ferriman-Gallwey scale in 62.4% (146/234), acne in 29.5% (69/234) of patients) and biochemically (Table 1).

According to New et al. [4] and Moran et al. [5], non-classical deficiency of 21-hydroxylase should be considered in patients with elevated 17-OHP levels (basal as well as ACTH stimulated) >10 ng/ml.

In our study 17-OHP after ACTH-stimulation ranged from 0.96 to 323.7 ng/ml (Me 3.29 (2.33; 4.79) ng/ml) at 30 minutes, and from 0.99 to 113.23 ng/ml (Me 3.62 (2.59; 5.86) ng/ml) at 60 min. In 81.8% (356/435) of patients maximal 17-OHP response to ACTH stimulation occurred at 60 min (F-variance analysis χ^2 - test for 0-30-60 min, W-test for 30-60 min, p=0.000). Differences in changes of 17-OHP concentrations reflects the clear dependence on the stimulation (Kendall's coefficient of concordance=0.77524; rank correlation mean (r)=0.77460), but not similar sensitivity to ACTH in one person. Therefore, one can get false-negative result if 17-OHP is measured only at 60 min.

Group	Ts (ng/dl) Me (25; 75)	bioTs (ng/dl) Me (25; 75)	17-OHP (ng/ml) Me (25; 75)	DHEA-S (mg/dl) Me (25; 75)	U-тест (p) HA+ vs HA-
HA+ (n=234)	88.5 (68; 105)	27.9 (21.6; 33.5)	1.82 (1.27; 2.77) Min 0.4 Max 89.6	245.0 (187; 347) Min 46 Max 1000	bioTe p=0.000 17-OHP p=0.000042 DHEA-S p=0.718456
HA- (n=201)	56,6 (38.9; 64.9)	14.75 (9.8; 18.0)	1.43 (0.98; 2.2) Min 0.2 Max 6.52	259.0 (185; 274) Min 48 Max 518	
HA: Hyperandogenism					

Table 1: Adrenal corticosteroids levels in study groups before ACTH-5 mcg stimulation test.

For the proper interpretation of the 5 mcg ACTH-test results in diagnostics of 21-hydroxylase deficiency we formulated two tasks:

1) To estimate diagnostic ratio of 17-OHP increase.

2) To evaluate the relevance of absolute values of stimulated 17-OHP levels.

Diagnosis of non-classic CAH is probable

Only 2 patients (0.95%) with hyperandrogenism had basal 17-OHP level >10 ng/ml and stimulated levels >17 ng/ml. Twenty-five women (23-with hyperandrogenism and 2 without it), with basal 17-OHP concentration between 2.58 ng/ml and 7 ng/ml showed four-fold increase in 17-OHP levels up to >10 ng/ml after stimulation with Tetracosactide 5 mcg: 18 patients had stimulated 17-OHP concentrations >14 ng/ml, and 7 patients showed stimulated 17-OHP between 10 and 14 ng/ml. These results made the diagnosis of non-classic CHA probable in 27 women.

Non-classic CAH is unlikely

To evaluate relevance of increase ratio BUT NOT absolute stimulated levels of 17-OHP for the diagnostics of 21-hydroxylase deficiency, we compared increase rate of 17-OHP and cortisol concentrations. Such approach prevents underestimation of maximal 17-OHP concentrations <10-14 ng/ml due to «low dose» of ACTH.

We found that cortisol rises in significantly lower degree than 17-OHP in response to 5 mcg Tetracosactide (variance analysis χ^2 $p<0.00000$). There was a correlation between basal cortisol or 17-OHP levels and elevation degree after stimulation with Tetracosactide-5 mcg ($r=0.265034$; $p=0.000001$ for cortisol; $r=0.477788$; $p=0.0000$ for 17-OHP). 334 patients had less than 2.5-fold rise of 17-OHP levels: 32 women (9.5%) reached 17-OHP maximal concentrations of 4.0-6.2 ng/ml and other 332 women-under 4 ng/ml. We suggested that 76.8% (n=334) patients with less than 2.5-fold 17-OHP increase and maximal 17-OHP concentrations <6.2 ng/ml were unlikely to have non-classic CAH. MGA of *CYP21*-gene in 14 women with hirsutism and relatively high simulated 17-OHP levels showed no mutations.

Test results are ambiguous and further standard test with 250 mcg of ACTH is needed for differential diagnosis of CAH

Further search for 21-hydroxilase deficiency was suggested in 48 patients with basal 17-OHP level over 1.7 ng/ml (recommended basal 17-OHP level for the diagnosis of 21- hydroxilase deficiency [5]) and documented >3-fold increase of 17-OHP.

According maximal stimulated 17-levels in the tests with low and standard 1-24 ACTH doses (5 mcg and 250 mcg Tetracosactide) we differentiated three different types of adrenal response:

-Dose-independent 87.5% (42/48)-differences of peak 17-OHP levels are not significant;

-Dose-dependent 12.5% (6/48)-peak 17-OHP levels between 6.7-7.3 ng/ml after low ACTH dose and >10 ng/ml after standard ACTH dose (Table 2).

There was a subgroup of patients (6/48 (12.5%)) with dose dependent adrenal response to ACTH who needed further search for non-classical ACH. All these 6 women had maximal stimulated 17-OHP concentrations after 5 mcg Tetracosactide test ≥ 6.7 ng/ml and dermatological signs of hyperandrogenism (hirsutism).

Response to ACTH, M ± m	17-OHP, basal, ng/ml	17-OHP, ACTH 5 mcg	17-OHP, ACTH 250 mcg
Dose-independent (n=42)	5.4 (1.9; 9.6)	16.4 (7.3; 39.5)	19.3 (6.4; 44.4) *p=0.39
Dose-dependent (n=6)	2.99 ± 0.97 (CI 1.98; 4.01)	7.104 ± 1.35 (CI 5.69; 8.52)	17.306 ± 4. 7 (CI 12.36; 22.25) *p=0.0025
*t-test for maximal 17-OHP levels after stimulation with Tetracosactide 5 mcg and Tetracosactide 250 mcg			

Table 2: Dose-independent and dose-dependent 17-OHP response to Tetracosactide 5 mcg and Tetracosactide 250 mcg.

Molecular genetic analysis of *CYP21* gene

Twenty-seven patients had basal or stimulated 17-OHP concentrations over 10 ng/ml, and 17 of them had molecular genetic analysis of *CYP21* gene. Patients with stimulated 17-OHP levels between 10 ng/ml and 14 ng/ml were found to be heterozygous carriers of most common *CYP21* mutations. Women with maximal 17-OHP levels ≥ 14 ng/ml had homozygous mutations or combinations of different heterozygous mutations (Table 3) (Figures 1 and 2).

Molecular genetic analysis in 14 patients with maximal 17-OHP concentrations between 4 and 6.2 ng/ml revealed no *CYP21* mutations using allele-specific polymerase chain reaction (n=10) or direct *CYP21* gene sequencing. Thus, 21-hydroxylase deficiency was excluded in these women. 334 women with non-significant 17-OHP rise (<6.2 ng/ml) did not need further investigation for the non-classical CAH and were excluded from the study. In other 320 patients 21-hydroxylase deficiency could be surely excluded only after either standard test with 250 mcg ACTH or direct *CYP21* gene sequencing.

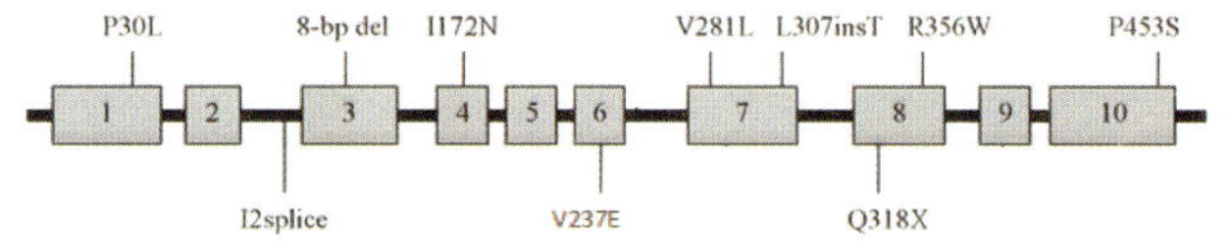

Figure 1: Schematic representation of the exons of the gene and the localization point common mutations.

We found no *CYP21* mutations in 21 patients with dose independent adrenal response to 5 mcg tetracosactide. There were 13 women with maximal 17-OHP concentrations >6.7 ng/ml. However, non-classical CAH was not proved in them during standard test and allele specific PCR of *CYP21* gene.

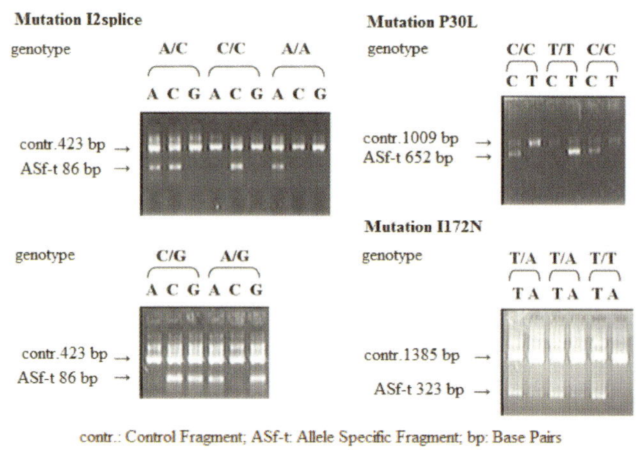

Figure 2: Electrophoregrams products allele-specific amplification with the mutation test *I2 spl*, *P30L* and *I172N*.

Molecular-genetic analysis in 6 women with dose-dependent response to Tetracosactide 5 mcg and Tetracosactide 250 mcg revealed 2 cases of homozygous *CYP21* mutations: *V281L*/ *V281L* [6], *V237E*/ *V237E* and one case of chimera gene *CYP21P*/ *CYP21* [7] (Figure 3).

Non-classical CAH was proved only in women with maximal 17-OHP concentration ≥ 6.7 ng/ml after stimulation with 5 mcg Tetracosactide and >14 ng/ml after stimulation with 250 mcg tetracosactide.

Three patients with maximal 17-OHP levels under 6.0 ng/ml after stimulation with 5 mcg Tetracosactide and under 10 ng/ml after 250 mcg Tetracosactide, had heterozygous carrier state of *V281L* mutation.

We evaluated sensitivity and specificity of the main hyperandrogenism symptoms, such as hirsutism and anovulation to define those women who need examination for 21-hydroxylase deficiency.

Hirsutism seems to be the main symptom which disturbs women with NC-CAH. However regular and ovalutary menstrual circle cannot rule out NC-CAH.

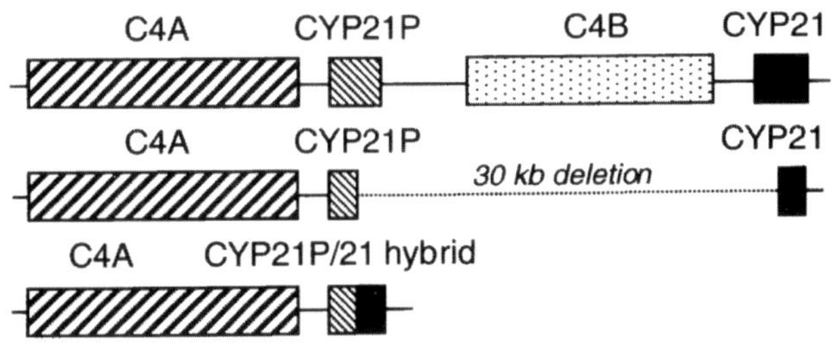

Figure 3: Scheme of *CYP21P*/*CYP21* chimeric gene with deletion of 30 bp.

Maximal simulated 17-OHP level	Homozygous mutations or combinations of heterozygous mutations	Carrier state of heterozygous mutations
NC-CAH is very likely		
Test with ACTH 5 and 250 mcg: 10 ng/ml<17-OHP<14 ng/ml (n=9)	Not found	*V281L* *V281L* *P30L* *Q318X* *I2 spl* *V281L* *V281L* Common mutations not found (n=2)
Test with ACTH 5 and 250 mcg: 17-OHP >14 ng/ml (n=8)	*V281L/V281L* *V281L/V281L* *V281L/V281L* *V281L/V281L* *P453S/P453S* *I172N/V281L* *I2 spl/V281L* *V281L/V281L*	Not found
NC-CAH is unlikely		
Test with ACTH 5 mcg 17-OHP 4-6.2 ng/ml (n=14)	Not found	Not found
NC-CAH is ambiguous		
Dose independent response Test with ACTH 5 mcg and Test with ACTH 250 mcg: 17-OHP ≥ 6.7 ng/ml (n=21)	Not found	Not found
Dose-dependent response (n=3) Test with ACTH 5 mcg: 6.7<17-OHP<10 ng/ml; Test with ACTH 250 mcg: 10<17-OHP<14 ng/ml	Not found	*V281L* *I2 spl* *V281L*
Test with ACTH 5 mcg (n=3): 6.7<17-OHP<10 ng/ml; Test with ACTH 250 mcg: 17-OHP >14 ng/ml	*V237E/V237E* *V281L/V281L* Chimeric gene	Not found

Table 3: Results of molecular-genetic analysis of *CYP21* gene.

Sensitivity and specificity analysis of low-dose test with 1-24 ACTH-5 mcg included data from 36 patients who run through low-dose and standard ACTH test as well as genetic analysis of *CYP21*. These were patients with 17-OHP concentration over 14 ng/ml and homozygous or mixed heterozygous mutations of *CYP21* gene. Other patients with heterozygous mutations and 17-OHP under 14 ng/ml (n=10), and 2 patients with dose-independent reaction to ACTH, max 17-OHP level >7 ng/ml and no proven mutations of *CYP21* gene (PCR) were excluded from this analysis. Unfortunately, 10 clinically hyperandrogenic patients and high Tetracosactide 5 mcg-stimulated

17-OHP levels (over 14 ng/ml) withdrew from the study. This fact may have influenced the results of sensitivity analysis.

Test with Tetracosactide 5 mcg had sensitivity of 72.7% and specificity of 100% with positive prognostic value (+PV) of 100%, and negative prognostic value (-PV) of 89.3%.

According to the results of the test with 5 mcg Tetracosactide, absolute stimulated 17-OHP levels but not grades of its increase are relevant for the diagnostics of 21-hydroxilase. Steroidal response to Tetracosactide may be dose dependent in 12.5% of patients, and they have higher peak 17-OHP levels after stimulation with Tetracosactide-250 mcg. Lack of low-dose 1-24 ACTH stimulation can be probably explained by an adaptation of hyhperplase adrenal glands to grater pituitary stimuli.

Diagnosis of non-classic CAH with 21-hydroxylase deficiency was proved in 5.3% (23/435) of patients reported hirsutism and/or anovulation. 21-hydroxylase deficiency was verified in 8.5% (20/234) of hyperandrogenic patients and in 1.5% (3/201) of women without clinical signs and symptoms of hyperandrogenism.

Conclusion

1. Low dose test with Tetracosactide 5 mcg can identify 21-hydroxylase deficiency in patients with stimulated 17-OHP concentrations over 14 ng/ml.

2. Standard stimulation test with Tetracosactide 250 mcg and MGA of *CYP21* gene is indicated for patients with dermatological signs of hyperandrogenism and maximal 17-OHP levels ≥ 6.7 ng/ml after stimulation with Tetracosactide 5 mcg.

It should be noted, that clinical relevance of mild non-classic CAH which cannot be detected with low-dose but not with standard-dose Tetracosactide test is still uncertain. It is also known, that most women with heterozygous mutation of *CYP21* gene are symptoms free and have normal fertility. Further studies of the cased with discordant results of tests with Tetracosactide 5 mcg and 250 mcg may bring useful information.

Conflict of Interest and the Source of Funding

The authors deny financial support from the drug manufacturers. Conflict of interest in determining the structure of the study, in the collection, analysis and interpretation of missing data.

References

1. Дедов ИИ, Фадеев ВВ, Мельниченко ГА (2002) Adrenal insufficiency. pp: 203-218.
2. http://www.issam.ch/freetesto.htm
3. Wedell A, Luthman H (1993) Steroid 21-hydroxylase deficiency: two additional mutations in salt-wasting disease and rapid screening of disease-causing mutations. Hum Mol Genet 2: 499-504.
4. New MI (2006) Extensive clinical experience: nonclassical 21-hydroxylase deficiency. J Clin Endocrinol Metab 91: 4205-4214.
5. Moran C (2006) Nonclassic adrenal hyperplasia. Fertil Steril 86: S3.
6. White P, Speiser P (2000) Congenital Adrenal Hyperplasia due to 21-Hydroxylase Deficiency. Endocr Rev 21: 245-291.
7. Lee H, Chang J, Tsai C, Tsai F, Chao H, et al. (2000) Analysis of the chimeric CYP21P/CYP21 gene in steroid 21-hydroxylase deficiency. Clin chem 46: 606-611.

Steroid Therapy in Oral Lichen Planus

Ebtissam Alerraqi

Oral Pathology and Medicine, Ministry of Health, Giza, Egypt

*Corresponding author: Alerraqi E, Oral Pathology and Medicine, Ministry of Health, Giza, Egypt, E-mail: ebtissam.erraqi@gmail.com

Abstract

Oral lichen planus (OLP) is a chronic inflammatory disease characterized by cellular-mediated inflammatory reactions which render apoptotic epithelial cells and degeneration of the basal epithelial layer. Eighteen volunteering cases of OLP were scheduled, after getting their informed consents, to be reported in this study. All of them were diagnosed histologically. The diagnosis was confirmed via immunofluorescence. Another incisional sample was scheduled after finishing the recruited treatment. The patient histological findings were contrasted, before and after treatment, to ten cases of non-lesional archival cases of oral mucosa as a control group. Results revealed no difference in the response to the pharmaceutical form of steroids used in treating OLP. Although steroid therapy is the mainstay treatment of OLP, adjuvant treatment modalities should be recruited for improving the healing process.

Keywords: Oral lichen planus; Steroid therapy; Injectable intralesional steroids; Triamcinolone acetonide; Betamethasone

Introduction

Oral lichen planus (OLP) is a mucocutaneous disease characterized by a cellular inflammatory infiltrate enriched in CD4+ cells, by the presence of acidophilic bodies that may represent apoptotic epithelial cells, and by vacuolating degeneration of the basal epithelial layer [1].

Clinically, OLP is most commonly encountered in the buccal mucosa of middle-aged females more frequently than of males. OLP can also be noted on the tongue, the gingiva and lips. Of the configuration of such a white lesions, the reticular form, which is characterized by numerous interlacing white keratotic lines or striae (so-called Wickham's striae) that produce an annular or lacy pattern, is the most frequent pattern. The plaque form of lichen planus tends to resemble leukoplakia clinically but has a multifocal distribution with a predilection to the dorsum of the tongue and the buccal mucosa. The erythematous or atrophic form of lichen planus appears as red patches with fine white striae. It may be seen in conjunction with reticular or erosive variants. In the erosive form of lichen planus, the central area of the lesion is ulcerated. A fibrinous plaque or pseudomembrane covers the ulcer. The bullous variant is generally short lived and, on rupturing, leaves a painful ulcer. Lesions are usually seen on the buccal mucosa, especially in the posterior and inferior regions adjacent to the second and third molars. Cutaneous representation of lichen planus, if evident, is characterized by the presence of small, violaceous, polygonal, flat-topped, pruritic papules on the flexor surfaces of the forearm and anterior tibial surfaces [2].

Although several cases were reported to be refractory to steroids, tacrolimus, pimecrolimus, thalidomide, low-level laser therapy, photodynamic therapy, and surgical excision were suggested. Notwithstanding, these treatment options are not approved in randomized controlled trials and do not have a long-term safety profile. Surgical excision, cryotherapy, CO_2 laser and Nd:YAG laser have all been used for treatment of OLP. In general, surgery is reserved for removal of dysplastic areas in patients at high risk. The well recognized Koebner phenomenon would be a contraindication to more frequent use of these techniques [3]. There is a *bona fide* risk that oral squamous cell carcinoma will develop in oral lichen planus, but this risk is very low [2]. This study contrasts three routes of applying steroid therapy in treating OLP: topical, systemic and interalesional steroid administration.

Patient and Methods

Eighteen volunteering cases of OLP were scheduled, after getting their informed consents, to be reported in this study. All of them were diagnosed histologically. The diagnosis was confirmed via immunofluorescence. Another incisional sample was scheduled after finishing the recruited treatment. The patient histological findings were contrasted, before and after treatment, to TEN non-lesional archival cases of oral mucosa as a control group. The submitted cases were subcategorized into three groups. **Group 1** included six cases which were treated via interalesional triamcinolone acetonide (ITA) injection, 5-10 mg/mL weekly or for 4 weeks (Cases 1-6). **Group 2** included another six cases which were treated via topical application of betamethasone (Cases 7-12) while the last six cases, **Group 3**, were treated via systematic glucocorticosteroid (daily 30 mg Hostacortin-H® for two weeks). One-way ANOVA, chi-square, Mann Whitney U tests were applied when indicated. Statistical significance was coined when p-value was less than 0.05.

Results

The average age of the studied case was 43.38 (SD=10.78). Of these, 9 cases showed a bilateral reticular pattern (50%). Seven cases revealed atrophic (n=4) and plaque patterns (n=3) [(22%), (17%)]. Single cases demonstrated bullous (6%) and ulcerative (erosive: 6%) patterns as shown in Table 1.

The different lines of treatment rendered a dramatic healing effect clinically and histologically. However, the improvement was not statistically significant as regards the used treatment line. The histological changes are represented in Table 2. Histologically, all cases showed a remarkable decrease in the accruement of the inflammatory infiltrates. However, the subepithelial lymphocytic population remained, in a significant configuration, persistent.

	Age	Gender	Site	Pattern	Association with Diseases	Treatment
Case # 1	23	M	BM	Ulcerative	None	ITA
Case # 2	45	F	PM, ARM	Atrophic	HCV	ITA
Case # 3	21	F	BM, LL	Reticular	LE	ITA
Case # 4	54	F	PM, T	Plaque	HCV	ITA
Case # 5	42	F	BM	Reticular	HCV	ITA
Case # 6	38	F	BM	Bullous	None	ITA
Case # 7	44	F	BM	Reticular	None	TPM
Case # 8	39	F	PM, T	Plaque	None	TPM
Case # 9	33	F	BM	Reticular	None	TPM
Case # 10	51	F	T	Atrophic	DM (II), HCV	TPM
Case # 11	29	M	BM	Reticular	None	TPM
Case # 12	59	M	BM	Atrophic	HCV	TPM
Case # 13	63	M	BM	Reticular	None	HCH
Case # 14	47	M	BM, OC	Reticular	None	HCH
Case # 15	39	F	BM	Reticular	None	HCH
Case # 16	55	F	PM, T	Plaque	DM (II)*	HCH
Case # 17	36	F	BM	Reticular	None	HCH
Case # 18	45	F	BM	Atrophic	None	HCH
ARM: Alveolar Ridge Mucosa; BM: Buccal Mucosa; DM-II: Diabetes Mellitus type II ; F: female; HCH: Hostacortin- H®; HCV: Hepatitis C Virus; ITA: Interalesional Triamcinolone Acetonide; LL: Lower Lip; M: Male; OC: Oral Commissure; PM: Palatal Mucosa; T: Tongue; TBM: Topical Betamethasone; (*): the patient was treated via insulin injection.						

Table 1: Clinical data of the submitted cases

Histological Feature	Sample 1		Sample 2
	No. of cases	Degree	Change
Subepithelial lymphoid infiltrate	18/18	Abundant (extending into the CT)	Fewer (epithelial-CT interface)
Hydropic degeneration	4/18	Focal	Less remarkable
Erosion	4/18	Multi-focal	Absent
Atrophy	4/18	remarkable	Less remarkable
Acanthosis	14/18	Variable amounts	Less remarkable
Hyperorthokeratosis	2/18	Thick	Thinner
Hyperparakeratosis	12/18	Abundant	Less remarkable
Aggregate of civatte bodies	2/18	At the BM	Less remarkable
Germinal-like foci	3/18	Deep in the CT	Absent

Table 2: Histological features in the submitted cases

Discussion

Oral lichen planus is a cell-mediated autoimmune reaction against keratinocytes, extrinsic antigens or metabolites, bound to or expressed by keratinocytes. Keratinocytes, along with T cells, ascertains to mediate basal cell death through triggering of apoptosis [2,3]. Moreover, Langerhans cells, CD1a+ dendritic cells, and macrophages appear to contribute to the virulence of OLP via maintaining a higher level of cytokines. The pharmaceutical forms aside, topical triamcinolone, betamethasone and fluocinolone acetonide have been shown to be effective in small studies, but there have been few placebo controlled trials. Although intralesional triamcinolone acetonide injection, 5-10 mg/mL weekly for 4 weeks, is always preferred in treating ulcerative OLP, hydrocortisone, dexamethasone and methyl prednisolone have been used either [3,4].

Oral lichen planus demonstrates multiple reactions, sometimes resistant, to the treatment lines. Such responses are expected to be multifactorial. Cytological abnormalities, clinical forms of OLP, histological variations, general health condition and association with other diseases are considered exacerbating factors which may complicate the pathological course of OLP [5]. Cytologically, DNA Ploidy analysis, via automated image cytometry, has been suggested to be effective in predicting the malignant changes in non-dysplastic oral lichen planus [6]. Clinically, erosive and erythematous OLP have the greatest malignant potential [7]. Histologically, the dysplastic OLP is natively considered a premalignant condition. Epithelial atrophy and inflammatory cytokine-rich microenvironment associated with OLP or lichenoid reactions, particularly tertiary lymphoid follicles and subepithelial lymphocystic populations, were blamed for tumor promotion. Proinflammatory cytokine production of interleukin 1 (IL-1) leads to activation of several prostaglandin-mediated events, principally prostaglandin E2 level, via the action of the enzyme cyclooxygenase-2 (COX-2) on arachidonic acid [8]. Khan et al indicated that both pro-inflammatory (IFN-g and TNF-a) and immunosuppressive (TGF-b1) cytokines are present in OLP [9].

Concerning the association with other diseases, OLP was associated with a plethora of hepatic and connective tissue diseases. Hepatitis C is most commonly blamed for co-existing with OLP [10-12], especially resistant cases, so that some countries, Italy and Japan, recommended running routine screening to patients with OLP for hepatitis C and other liver abnormalities. However, this was not the case in the American patients [8]. This association was anticipated to result from a direct immune aggression of epithelial cells expressing HCV antigens or may be sustained by a cytokine environment favorable to trigger and maintain autoimmune reactions [10-12].

Gels and creams appear to be well accepted by patients, more so than ointments, although they often taste bad and sometimes cause burning or stinging. Elixir forms of corticosteroids, such as dexamethasone or triamcinolone, can be used as an oral rinse for patients with diffuse oral involvement or for elderly patients who may find it technically difficult to apply medication to various active locations of the oral cavity. Unfortunately there is potentially greater risk for systemic absorption and candidal infection with corticosteroid rinses. Commonly corticosteroids are extemporaneously compounded with an occlusive dressing such as Orabase, even though a controlled study suggests that such adhesive bases do not increase efficacy [2,3,13] .

Rödström et al. [14] found no statistically significant correlation between cortisol concentration and stress level. A meta-analysis and a current Cochrane review of the literature provide only little evidence for the superiority of the assessed interventions over placebo for palliation of symptomatic OLP [15]. Supporting these findings, this study could not find any statistical significance of applying steroid therapy in any forms: ITA, topical betamethasone or Hostacortin-H® tablets. Also, this study suggests that subepithelial lymphocytic populations, probably memory cells, are responsible for the recurrence and exacerbation in OLP. Steroid therapy, per se, is not effective in obviating them.

Conclusion

Steroid therapy is the mainstay treatment of OLP. However, adjuvant treatment modalities should be recruited for improving the healing process and decreasing the confluence of inflammatory cytokine-rich populations in the microenvironment of OLP. The epithelial-CT interface may be the genuine complex which is responsible for feeding recurrence.

Acknowledgments

I would like to thank Dr. Nashwa Mohammad (Periodontology and Oral medicine, ASU, Egypt) for referring two cases of OLP to our facility.

References

1. Krupaa RJ, Sankari SL, Masthan KM, Rajesh E (2005) Oral lichen planus: An overview. J Pharm Bioallied Sci 7: S158-161.
2. Regezi JA, Sciubba JJ, Jordan RC (2012) Oral pathology: clinical pathologic correlations. Elsevier Health Sciences.
3. Yang H, Wu Y, Ma H, Jiang L, Zeng X, et al. (2016) Possible alternative therapies for oral lichen planus cases refractory to steroid therapies. Oral Surg Oral Med Oral Pathol Oral Radiol 121: 496-509.
4. Souto GR, Nunes LF, Tanure BB, Gomez RS, Mesquita RA (2016) CD1a+ dendritic cells in oral lichen planus and amalgam lichenoid reaction. Oral Surg Oral Med Oral Pathol Oral Radiol 121: 651-656.
5. Eisen D (2002) Evaluating and treating patients with oral lichen planus. Dermatologic Therapy 15: 206-217.
6. Sperandio M, Klinikowski MF, Brown AL, Shirlaw PJ, Challacombe SJ, et al. (2016) Image-based DNA ploidy analysis aids prediction of malignant transformation in oral lichen planus. Oral Surg Oral Med Oral Pathol Oral Radiol 121: 643-650.
7. Larsson Ä, Warfvinge G (1998) Immunohistochemistry of 'tertiary lymphoid follicles' in oral amalgam-associated lichenoid lesions. Oral diseases 4: 187-193.
8. Eisen D (2002) The clinical features, malignant potential, and systemic associations of oral lichen planus: a study of 723 patients. J Am Acad Dermatol 46: 207-214.
9. De Carli JP, Linden MS, da Silva SO, Trentin MS, Matos Fde S, et al. (2016) Hepatitis C and Oral Lichen Planus: Evaluation of their Correlation and Risk Factors in a Longitudinal Clinical Study. J Contemp Dent Pract 17: 27-31
10. Pilli M, Penna A, Zerbini A, Vescovi P, Manfredi M, et al. (2002) Oral lichen planus pathogenesis: A role for the HCV-specific cellular immune response. Hepatology 36:1446-1452.
11. Chen Y, Zhang W, Geng N, Tian K, Windsor LJ (2008) MMPs, TIMP-2, and TGF-b1 in the Cancerization of Oral Lichen Planus. Head Neck 30: 1237-1245.

12. Khan A, Farah CS, Savage NW, Walsh LJ, Harbrow DJ, et al. (2003) Th1 cytokines in oral lichen planus. J Oral Pathol Med 32: 77-83.

13. Sugerman PB, Savage NW, Zhou X, Walsh LJ, Bigby M (2000) Oral lichen planus. Clin Dermatol 18: 533-539.

14. Rödström PO, Jontell M, Hakeberg M, Berggren U, Lindstedt G (2001) Erosive oral lichen planus and salivary cortisol. J oral pathol med 30: 257-263.

15. Chan ESY, Thornhill M, Zakrzewska J (2003) Interventions for treating oral lichen planus. Cochrane Database Syst Rev 7: CD001168.

The Aryl-hydrocarbon Receptor (AhR) as a Therapeutic Target in Human Breast Cancer

Julie M Hall*

Campbell University, College of Pharmacy & Health Sciences, Buies Creek, USA

***Corresponding author:** Julie M Hall, Campbell University, College of Pharmacy & Health Sciences, Buies Creek, USA, E-mail: halljm@campbell.edu

Abstract

Breast cancer is currently the most prevalent malignancy among women in industrialized countries, and 1 in 8 women living in the United States will develop the disease at some point in her lifetime. Although the incidence of breast cancer has increased 0.3% per year since 1990, the mortality rate has decreased by 2% per year since 1990 due to improvements in treatment and early detection. New treatment strategies and a better molecular understanding of the disease will be important to continue the progress science has made against this disease.

The aryl-hydrocarbon receptor (AhR) has been traditionally associated with activation by environmental contaminants, acute toxicity, and cancer risks associated with exposures. However, the AhR has been highly conserved throughout evolution suggesting an important biological role for the receptor independent of its response to environmental contaminants. There is a significant body of evidence indicating the AhR plays a role in breast epithelial cell differentiation and that receptor agonists can inhibit breast cancer growth. A 50% reduction in estrous-induced terminal end buds was observed in the mammary glands of AhR knockout animals when compared to wild type suggesting a role for the AhR in mammary development. In 2 independent rodent cancer bioassays, treatment with the AhR agonist 2,3,7,8-tetrachlorodibenzo-pdioxin (TCDD) significantly reduced the incidence of spontaneous rat mammary tumors. These and other studies support the premise that the AhR plays a fundamental role in breast epithelial cell differentiation. This review provides a brief summary of the current evidence that the AhR may be an important pharmacological target for treating human breast cancer.

Keywords: Aryl-hydrocarbon receptor; Breast cancer; AhR; Estrogen receptor; TCDD; Metastasis; Therapeutic target

Introduction

Breast cancer is currently the most prevalent malignancy among women in industrialized countries, and 1 in 8 women living in the United States will develop the disease at some point in her lifetime [1]. Although the incidence of breast cancer has increased 0.3% per year since 1990, the mortality rate has decreased by 2% per year since 1990 due to improvements in treatment and early detection [1]. New treatment strategies and a better molecular understanding of the disease will be important to continue the progress science has made against this disease.

The aryl-hydrocarbon receptor (AhR) has been traditionally associated with activation by environmental contaminants, acute toxicity, and cancer risks associated with exposures. However, the AhR has been highly conserved throughout evolution [2] suggesting an important biological role for the receptor independent of its response to environmental contaminants. There is a significant body of evidence indicating the AhR plays a role in breast epithelial cell differentiation and that receptor agonists can inhibit breast cancer growth. A 50% reduction in estrous-induced terminal end buds was observed in the mammary glands of AhR knockout animals when compared to wild type suggesting a role for the AhR in mammary development [3]. In 2 independent rodent cancer bioassays, treatment with the AhR agonist 2,3,7,8-tetrachlorodibenzo-p-dioxin (TCDD) significantly reduced the incidence of spontaneous rat mammary tumors [4,5]. These and other studies support the premise that the AhR plays a fundamental role in breast epithelial cell differentiation. This review provides a brief summary of the current evidence that the AhR may be an important pharmacological target for treating human breast cancer.

The Aryl-Hydrocarbon Receptor (AhR) Mechanism of Action

The identification of the AhR originated in early toxicology studies that observed an increase in mono-oxygenase activity following exposure to polyaromatic hydrocarbons. Additional studies using a highly potent inducer, 2,3,7,8-tetrachlorodibenzo-p-dioxin (TCDD), showed that binding to a cytosolic receptor was proportional to the induction of mono-oxygenase activity [6]. The gene encoding the AhR was subsequently cloned and characterized across multiple species [7-9]. Further molecular characterization of the AhR demonstrated that the receptor is highly conserved [2,10] and plays a significant role in tissue development [1,11-13]. For example, targeted disruption of the AhR in the mouse results in compromised immune function [14], and deficiencies in the development of several tissues including ovarian follicles [15], seminal vesicles [16], fetal vasculature [17], and mammary glands [18].

The AhR is a ligand-activated transcription factor and a member of the basic-helix-loop-helix Per-Arnt-Sim (bHLH-PAS) family of proteins [19]. In an unliganded state, the AhR exists in the cytoplasm bound to chaperones HSP90, p23, and other proteins (Figure 1). Ligand binding induces translocation of the AhR into the nucleus, where it dissociates from cellular chaperones and heterodimerizes with ARNT (aryl-hydrocarbon receptor nuclear translocator). AhR/ARNT heterodimers bind to genomic dioxin response elements (DREs), which initiates transcription of genes within the AhR gene battery, including Cyp1a1, Cyp1b1, Aldh3, Nqo1, and Gsta1 [20-23]. Interactions with other cellular proteins have been identified leading to a proposed role for the AhR in many signaling pathways including the retinoblastoma (Rb) protein and cell cycle [24,25], estrogen receptor (ER) signaling [26] and RELA and NFκB signaling [27].

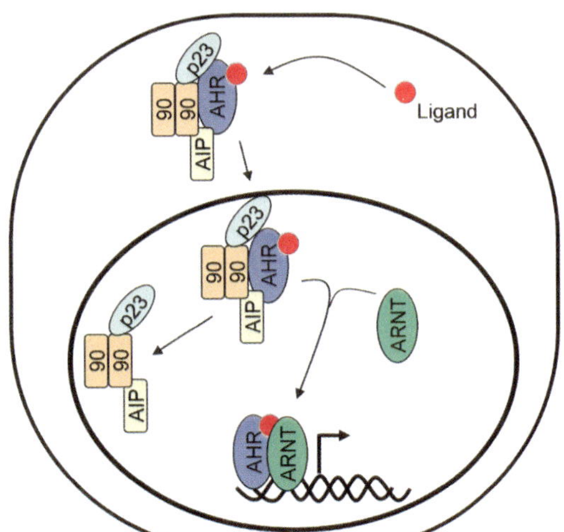

Figure 1: Schematic representation of the AhR signaling pathway

Role of the AhR in Tissue Development

The AhR gene is highly conserved across both vertebrate and invertebrate species [2,10]. The existence of ancestral AhR orthologs that either bind no ligand or bind a range of ligands that are unique from those recognized by the vertebrate receptors suggest that its role in regulating xenobiotic metabolism is a recent adaptation [2,28]. Apart from the evolutionary conservation, evidence for a role of the AhR in tissue development can be seen from the characterization and disruption of the AhR in model organisms. In Drosophila melanogaster, mutation of the AhR ortholog Spineless lead to alterations in appendage development [29], neuron morphology [30], and photoreceptor development [31].

In Caenorhabditis elegans, disruption of the AhR ortholog AHR-1 leads to alterations in neuronal development [32]. In a more relevant mammalian model, expression of the AhR occurs early in development in preimplantation embryos [33] and at gestational days 10 to 12 with high expression in many neuronal tissues [34]. Expression of the AhR expands to a large number of tissues by gestational day 13.5 to 15.5 indicating a potentially broad functional role in tissue development [34]. Targeted disruption of the AhR in mice has revealed obligatory roles for the receptor in multiple tissues including liver, the immune and cardiovascular systems, and the male and female reproductive systems [14-18]. Notably, a 50% reduction in estrous-induced terminal end buds was observed in the mammary glands of AhR null animals when compared to wild types suggesting a role for the AhR in mammary development [3].

Ligands of the AhR

Following the early studies characterizing the increase in mono-oxygenase activity due to polyaromatic hydrocarbon exposure, a significant research effort has ensued to identify and characterize both endogenous and xenobiotic ligands for the AhR. Although the endogenous ligand for the AhR is the subject of continued debate, multiple candidates have been proposed including indigoids, equilenin, arachidonic acid metabolites, heme metabolites, tryptophan metabolites, and UV photoproducts of tryptophan [35]. In addition, dietary compounds and nonligand activators of the AhR have been identified [35]. For the xenobiotic ligands, the most well-known are the halogenated dioxins, polychlorinated biphenyls (PCBs), and polyaromatic hydrocarbons (PAHs) [20].

The halogenated dioxins include the dibenzo-p-dioxins and dibenzofurans that are formed during both combustion and industrial processes such as waste incineration, forest fires, pesticide manufacturing, and paper pulp bleaching [36]. Within this class, 2,3,7,8-tetrachlorodibenzo-p-dioxin (TCDD) and 2,3,7,8-tetrachlorodibenzofuran (TCDBF) are prototypical AhR agonists due to their potency and efficacy in receptor activation [20]. For the PCBs, the coplanar congeners with adjacent halogens in the lateral positions of each ring and no halogen atoms near the biphenyl bridge are the most potent AhR agonists [37]. These chemicals are used in a variety of commercial products including flame retardants, adhesives, transformers and capacitors, lubricants, and fluorescent light ballasts [38]. Finally, the PAHs are a large class of AhR agonists that contain four or more benzene rings [39]. Prototype AhR ligands in this category include benzo[α]pyrene and 3-methylchloranthrene. PAHs are found as byproducts of combustion processes and are typically much less potent than TCDD or the coplanar PCBs.

Adverse Responses to AhR Ligand Activation

The effects of AhR activation have been primarily characterized using xenobiotic ligands such as TCDD, PCBs, and PAHs. For the classical AhR agonist TCDD, sufficient doses can cause cancer, immune dysfunction, wasting, chloracne, ovarian failure, and birth defects [20,40-42]. Both AhR null animals and mice with a mutation in the DNA binding domain of the AhR are refractive to the toxic effects of TCDD, suggesting that the AhR and its binding to DNA are required to these effects [43,44]. For human cancer, epidemiological data from occupationally exposed workers have established a clear association between exposure to TCDD and increased risk for all combined cancers and for lung cancer [45]. The magnitude of the increased risk in these studies is generally low, but it is higher in sub-cohorts considered to have the highest exposure to TCDD [45]. In the rat, three separate bioassays have been performed [4,5,46].

In the most recent bioassay by the National Toxicology Program, an increased incidence was observed for cholangiocarcinomas and hepatocellular adenomas of the liver, cystic keratinizing epithelioma of the lung, gingival squamous cell carcinoma of the oral mucosa, and squamous cell carcinoma of the uterus [5]. There is substantially less information regarding potential adverse responses for potential endogenous or dietary ligands of the AhR with the majority of exposure occurring for relatively short time periods. Exposure of up to 50 mg/kg of indigo or indirubin per day for a period of 3 days had little effect on the rat liver [47]. Similarly, exposure mice to 20 mg/kg of equilenin per day for 3 days had no reported effects [48]. Longer exposures have been performed for indole-3-carbinol (I3C) (a component of cruciferous vegetables) and its metabolite diindolylmethane (DIM). In exposures lasting up to one year, there were no observable differences grossly or histologically between groups and no changes in blood chemistry except that male rats treated with high doses of I3C exhibited higher serum levels of 25-hydroxy-vitamin D3 [49].

Protective Role of the AhR in Breast Cancer

While historically AhR agonists have been viewed as tumor promoters, combined epidemiological, animal bioassay, and molecular data indicate that this is an oversimplification. Examination of a population exposed to TCDD following an industrial accident in Seveso, Italy in 1976 showed a positive correlation between TCDD exposure and sarcomas, cancers in the prostate, lung, bladder and digestive tract, those in hematopoietic and lymphatic tissues, and all cancers combined [50], supporting previous studies of occupational workers [45]. However, a significant decrease in breast and endometrial cancer was also evident in exposed individuals [50]. More recently, a report following a population exposed to dioxin emissions from a municipal waste incinerator noted a significant decrease in incidence of invasive breast cancer in women living in the highest exposed zone [51].

The reduction in breast cancer observed in the human studies is supported by two independent rodent experiments showing a significant decrease in spontaneous mammary tumor incidence following a two-year exposure [4,5]. In an initiation-promotion model, an absence of mammary tumors was observed in rats administered TCDD compared with a 36% incidence in control animals [52]. Similarly, exposure to TCDD at sub-toxic doses decreased 7,12-dimethylbenz[a]anthracene (DMBA)-induced mammary tumors by 72% and, in a subset of animals, the original tumors were no longer detectable [53]. In contrast, control animals displayed a 390% increase in tumor volume over the same time period. Finally, in animals harboring ER+ human breast cancer cell xenographs, TCDD was found to completely suppress hormone-stimulated tumor growth [54]. These results suggest that, similar to many nuclear receptor agonists, the underlying biological responses to AhR activation are context specific.

Cross-Talk between the AhR and Estrogen Receptor α (ERα) Signaling Pathways

Cross-talk between the AhR and ERα signaling pathways occurs at multiple levels and is dependent on cellular context. In the promoters of many estrogen-inducible genes (e.g., pS2, cathepsin D, c-fos), binding sites for the AhR-ARNT complex (DREs) are adjacent to or overlap those of the ERα providing a means for the direct transcriptional inhibition of ERα [55-57]. The AhR-ARNT complex can also compete with ERα for coactivators, thereby dampening the transcriptional response [58]. On a post-translational level, liganded AhR can antagonize estrogen signaling by facilitating assembly of an ubiquitin ligase complex that promotes proteasomal degradation of ERα [59]. Finally, the AhR gene battery includes the cytochrome p450s Cyp1a1 and Cyp1b1 [20-23]. Upregulation of these enzymes results in an increase in estrogen metabolism and depletion of hormone levels [60,61].

The functional consequences of the antagonistic AhR-ER cross-talk are apparent in breast cancer cells. In growth assays, TCDD was shown to completely reverse the proliferative effects of estrogen in human breast cancer cells [54,62]. These observations have been recapitulated in vivo. In a nude mice xenograft model, TCDD suppressed estrogen-dependent tumor growth [54] and in a rat mammary tumor model, co-treatment of an AhR ligand with the antiestrogen tamoxifen was shown to completely inhibit growth of carcinogen-induced mammary tumors [63].

The Effects of AhR on Proliferation and the Cell Cycle

Apart from antagonistic effects on ERα signaling, the AhR may also display protective effects against human breast cancer by regulation of key processes required for breast cancer cell growth, cell cycle control, and cell migration. A number of studies have investigated the role of the AhR in cancer cell proliferation. Paradoxically, the AhR appears to facilitate growth in the absence of ligand, while the agonist-activated receptor displays marked anti-proliferative effects in cancer cells. For example, transfection of breast cancer cells with AhR siRNA is growth-inhibitory [64,65]. Similarly, AhR-deficient hepatoma cells (AhR-D) proliferate at a slower rate than wild-type cells (Hepa 1c1c7), and ectopic expression of the AhR in the AhR-D cells increases their growth to the rate of wild-type cells [66]. In contrast, a ligand-bound AhR inhibits cell growth in a wide array of breast cancer cell lines representing the major breast cancer subtypes, including both those positive and negative for ER, Progesterone Receptor (PR), and Human Epidermal Growth Factor 2 (HER2) [3,62,67-70].

It is now apparent that AhR-mediated suppression of cell growth involves G1 cell cycle arrest [25,71-74]. The cell cycle arrest coincides with association of the AhR with the hypophosphorylated and active form of Rb to form transcriptional repression complexes on several E2F-regulated genes required for S-phase progression [24,25]. In the absence of ligand, however, the AhR facilitates cell cycle progression by forming a complex with CDK4 and Cyclin D1 [74]. Thus, AhR agonists may function as a molecular switch in cancer cells, converting a basal AhR with growth-promoting activities into a potent anti-proliferative factor.

Evidence for a Protective Role of the AhR in Breast Cancer Cell Metastasis

In addition to cell growth and cell cycle regulation, the AhR has been shown to regulate genes involved in metastasis. Breast tumors most often metastasize to the lung and bone. These organs produce and secrete a chemokine, CXCL12, which attracts breast cancer cells expressing its receptor, CXCR4, on their cell surface [75]. In a recent study, TCDD was shown to down regulate both CXCR4 and CXCL12 in a breast cancer cell line and decrease cell migration towards a CXCL12 gradient [76]. While the consequences of CXCL12 suppression in these cells are unclear, the study demonstrated TCDD may be adequate in preventing breast cancer cells from migrating to areas with high CXCL12 expression [76].

There is emerging evidence that ligand activation of the AhR can inhibit multiple aspects of the metastatic process. In a panel of breast cancer cell lines that represent the 3 major breast cancer subtypes (ER and PR-positive, HER2-positive, and triple-receptor negative), it was found that agonist-activated AhR inhibited cell invasiveness and motility and prevented anchorage-independent growth [65]. Knockdown of the AhR with siRNAs demonstrated that the inhibition of invasiveness was receptor-dependent and endogenous receptor activity was protective in each cell type examined [65]. Likewise, AhR agonists were found to promote differentiation of breast cancer cells and mammary cancer stem cells into cells that displayed the phenotypic markers of normal breast epithelial gland cells [65]. Thus, the AhR plays an important role in mammary epithelial differentiation and, as such, represents a promising therapeutic target for a range of phenotypically distinct human breast cancers.

The AhR as a Potential Therapeutic Target for Human Breast Cancers

Analogous to the selective estrogen receptor modulator (SERM) concept, it has been proposed that selective AhR modulators (SAhRMs) exist that are capable of activating the specific signaling pathways involving the protective effects of the AhR in breast cancer while limiting activation of those pathways leading to the toxic effects [77]. Evidence for the feasibility of this concept is mounting. First, non-traditional AhR ligands have been identified that are capable of activating the receptor without association with the ligand binding pocket [35]. Second, similar to steroid hormone receptors [78], different ligands induce unique conformational changes in the AhR that facilitate interaction with different transcriptional cofactors [79]. On a functional level, the AhR agonists I3C, DIM and a series of DIM analogs were shown to effectively inhibit the growth of estrogen-dependent and independent breast cancer cells and tumors in a manner comparable to TCDD [67-70,72,80]. Structure-activity studies using the DIM analogs showed that specific methyl and dihalo-substitutions could further enhance the anticancer effects above those substantial effects seen for DIM alone [67,68,80]. AhR agonists can also be optimized for tissue-selective responses. The AhR agonist 6-methyl-1,3,8-trichlorodibenzofuran (6-MCDF) was found to synergize with tamoxifen to inhibit growth of mammary tumors in rodents while inhibiting the undesirable estrogenic effects of tamoxifen in the uterus and did not interfere with the bone-protective actions of tamoxifen in ovarectomized animals [63]. Importantly, effective doses of neither DIM nor 6-MCDF produced the adverse side effects observed with TCDD exposure [49,67,81,82].

The AhR as a Potential Therapeutic Target for ER-negative Human Breast Cancers

As put forth above, breast cancers are inherently diverse with respect to hormone and growth factor receptor expression and are typically broken down into subtypes based on ER, PR, and HER2 status. The tumor subtype can impact the growth and aggressiveness of the disease as well as predict the response to different chemotherapeutics [83, 84]. Tumors lacking expression of all 3 receptors (triple-negative) are typically the most challenging to treat due to their aggressive natures and the absence of a pliable drug target.

Unlike the available ER-targeted and growth factor-targeted therapeutics for breast cancer, AhR modulators may also have utility in prevention and treatment of triple-negative tumors. In a recent study the SERM Raloxifene, used clinically in prevention of ER-positive breast cancers, was shown to prevent growth and promote regression of triple-negative breast tumors in mice [85]. A second study soon followed that implicated an AhR-dependent mechanism; raloxifene was shown to activate the AhR, and as a consequence, induce apoptosis of triple-negative breast cancer cells with no effects on normal mammary epithelial cells [86].

Other AhR ligands have recently been identified as promising therapeutics for ER-negative breast cancers. The synthetic flavonoid aminoflavone, an AhR agonist, is currently in Phase 2 clinical trials. Several recent studies that this agent induces DNA damage and displays anti-proliferative, cytotoxic, and apoptotic activities in multiple cancer cell types including triple-negative breast [87-90]. Finally, as mentioned earlier, the AhR agonists I3C, DIM and a series of DIM analogs were shown to effectively inhibit the growth and invasiveness of ER-negative breast cancer cells and tumors [65,70,72,80]. Thus, it appears that the AhR hold tremendous potential as a pliable drug target for treatment of estrogen-independent breast cancers.

Summary and Significance

The current statistics associated with breast cancer reflect both its importance in women's health and the progress we have made towards understanding and treating the disease. The fact that the incidence and mortality of breast cancer has not declined at the same rate as other major causes of death speaks to the unmet need for both new therapeutic targets and approaches. A series of mechanistically distinct therapeutics are currently in clinical use for breast cancer, including those targeting estrogen and growth factor signaling pathways. However, it has become clear that breast cancer is a heterogeneous disease. Each cancer has its own molecular and biochemical makeup and, consequently, there exists no single drug or drug class that will be sufficient to effectively eliminate the disease in all afflicted individuals. This realization has continued to fuel efforts aimed at further molecular characterization of the disease, and these efforts have led to identification of potential and promising new drug targets such as the AhR.

References

1. ACS (2009) Breast cancer facts and figures.
2. Hahn ME (2002) Aryl hydrocarbon receptors: diversity and evolution. Chem Biol Interact 141: 131-160.
3. Hushka LJ, Williams JS, Greenlee WF (1998) Characterization of 2,3,7,8-tetrachlorodibenzofuran-dependent suppression and AH receptor pathway gene expression in the developing mouse mammary gland. Toxicol Appl Pharmacol 152: 200-210.
4. Kociba RJ, Keyes DG, Beyer JE, Carreon RM, Wade CE, et al. (1978) Results of a two-year chronic toxicity and oncogenicity study of 2,3,7,8-tetrachlorodibenzo-p-dioxin in rats. Toxicol Appl Pharmacol 46: 279-303.
5. National Toxicology Program (2006) Toxicology and carcinogenesis studies of a mixture of 2,3,7,8-tetrachlorodibenzo-p-dioxin (TCDD) (Cas No. 1746-01-6), 2,3,4,7,8-pentachlorodibenzofuran (PeCDF) (Cas No. 57117-31-4), and 3,3',4,4',5-pentachlorobiphenyl (PCB 126) (Cas No. 57465-28-8) in female Harlan Sprague-Dawley rats (gavage studies). Natl Toxicol Program Tech Rep Ser 526:1-180.
6. Poland A, Clover E, Kende AS, DeCamp M, Giandomenico CM (1976) 3,4,3',4'-Tetrachloro azoxybenzene and azobenzene: potent inducers of aryl hydrocarbon hydroxylase. Science 194: 627-630.
7. Burbach KM, Poland A, Bradfield CA (1992) Cloning of the Ah-receptor cDNA reveals a distinctive ligand-activated transcription factor. Proc Natl Acad Sci U S A 89: 8185-8189.
8. Ema M, Sogawa K, Watanabe N, Chujoh Y, Matsushita N, et al. (1992) cDNA cloning and structure of mouse putative Ah receptor. Biochem Biophys Res Commun 184: 246-253.
9. Dolwick KM, Schmidt JV, Carver LA, Swanson HI, Bradfield CA (1993) Cloning and expression of a human Ah receptor cDNA. Mol Pharmacol 44: 911-917.
10. Wang Y, Wang Q, Wu B, Li Y, Lu G (2013) Correlation between TCDD acute toxicity and aryl hydrocarbon receptor structure for different mammals. Ecotoxicol Environ Saf 89: 84-88.

11. Qin H, Powell-Coffman JA (2004) The Caenorhabditis elegans aryl hydrocarbon receptor, AHR-1, regulates neuronal development. Dev Biol 270: 64-75.
12. Kim MD, Jan LY, Jan YN (2006) The bHLH-PAS protein Spineless is necessary for the diversification of dendrite morphology of Drosophila dendritic arborization neurons. Genes Dev 20: 2806-2819.
13. Wernet MF, Mazzoni EO, Celik A, Duncan DM, Duncan I, et al. (2006) Stochastic spineless expression creates the retinal mosaic for colour vision. Nature 440: 174-180.
14. Fernandez-Salguero P, Pineau T, Hilbert DM, McPhail T, Lee SS, et al. (1995) Immune system impairment and hepatic fibrosis in mice lacking the dioxin-binding Ah receptor. Science 268: 722-726.
15. Baba T, Mimura J, Nakamura N, Harada N, Yamamoto M, et al. (2005) Intrinsic function of the aryl hydrocarbon (dioxin) receptor as a key factor in female reproduction. Mol Cell Biol 25: 10040-10051.
16. Baba T, Shima Y, Owaki A, Mimura J, Oshima M, et al. (2008) Disruption of aryl hydrocarbon receptor (AhR) induces regression of the seminal vesicle in aged male mice. Sex Dev 2: 1-11.
17. Lahvis GP, Lindell SL, Thomas RS, McCuskey RS, Murphy C, et al. (2000) Portosystemic shunting and persistent fetal vascular structures in aryl hydrocarbon receptor-deficient mice. Proc Natl Acad Sci U S A 97: 10442-10447.
18. Hushka LJ, Williams JS, Greenlee WF (1998) Characterization of 2,3,7,8-tetrachlorodibenzofuran-dependent suppression and AH receptor pathway gene expression in the developing mouse mammary gland. Toxicol Appl Pharmacol 152: 200-210.
19. Gu YZ, Hogenesch JB, Bradfield CA (2000) The PAS superfamily: sensors of environmental and developmental signals. Annu Rev Pharmacol Toxicol 40: 519-561.
20. Poland A, Knutson JC (1982) 2,3,7,8-tetrachlorodibenzo-p-dioxin and related halogenated aromatic hydrocarbons: examination of the mechanism of toxicity. Annu Rev Pharmacol Toxicol 22: 517-554.
21. Paulson KE, Darnell JE Jr, Rushmore T, Pickett CB (1990) Analysis of the upstream elements of the xenobiotic compound-inducible and positionally regulated glutathione S-transferase Ya gene. Mol Cell Biol 10: 1841-1852.
22. Favreau LV, Pickett CB (1991) Transcriptional regulation of the rat NAD(P)H:quinone reductase gene. Identification of regulatory elements controlling basal level expression and inducible expression by planar aromatic compounds and phenolic antioxidants. J Biol Chem 266: 4556-4561.
23. Asman DC, Takimoto K, Pitot HC, Dunn TJ, Lindahl R (1993) Organization and characterization of the rat class 3 aldehyde dehydrogenase gene. J Biol Chem 268: 12530-12536.
24. Elferink CJ (2003) Aryl hydrocarbon receptor-mediated cell cycle control. Prog Cell Cycle Res 5: 261-267.
25. Marlowe JL, Knudsen ES, Schwemberger S, Puga A (2004) The aryl hydrocarbon receptor displaces p300 from E2F-dependent promoters and represses S phase-specific gene expression. J Biol Chem 279: 29013-29022.
26. Ohtake F, Takeyama K, Matsumoto T, Kitagawa H, Yamamoto Y, et al. (2003) Modulation of oestrogen receptor signalling by association with the activated dioxin receptor. Nature 423: 545-550.
27. Kim DW, Gazourian L, Quadri SA, Romieu-Mourez R, Sherr DH, et al. (2000) The RelA NF-kappaB subunit and the aryl hydrocarbon receptor (AhR) cooperate to transactivate the c-myc promoter in mammary cells. Oncogene 19: 5498-5506.
28. McMillan BJ, Bradfield CA (2007) The aryl hydrocarbon receptor sans xenobiotics: endogenous function in genetic model systems. Mol Pharmacol 72: 487-498.
29. Duncan DM, Burgess EA, Duncan I (1998) Control of distal antennal identity and tarsal development in Drosophila by spineless-aristapedia, a homolog of the mammalian dioxin receptor. Genes Dev 12: 1290-1303.
30. Kim MD, Jan LY, Jan YN (2006) The bHLH-PAS protein Spineless is necessary for the diversification of dendrite morphology of Drosophila dendritic arborization neurons. Genes Dev 20: 2806-2819.
31. Wernet MF, Mazzoni EO, Celik A, Duncan DM, Duncan I, et al. (2006) Stochastic spineless expression creates the retinal mosaic for colour vision. Nature 440: 174-180.
32. Qin H, Powell-Coffman JA (2004) The Caenorhabditis elegans aryl hydrocarbon receptor, AHR-1, regulates neuronal development. Dev Biol 270: 64-75.
33. Peters JM, Wiley LM (1995) Evidence that murine preimplantation embryos express aryl hydrocarbon receptor. Toxicol Appl Pharmacol 134: 214-221.
34. Abbott BD, Birnbaum LS, Perdew GH (1995) Developmental expression of two members of a new class of transcription factors: I. Expression of aryl hydrocarbon receptor in the C57BL/6N mouse embryo. Dev Dyn 204: 133-143.
35. Nguyen LP, Bradfield CA (2008) The search for endogenous activators of the aryl hydrocarbon receptor. Chem Res Toxicol 21: 102-116.
36. Shibamoto T, Yasuhara A, Katami T (2007) Dioxin formation from waste incineration. Rev Environ Contam Toxicol 190: 1-41.
37. Poland A, Glover E (1977) Chlorinated biphenyl induction of aryl hydrocarbon hydroxylase activity: a study of the structure-activity relationship. Mol Pharmacol 13: 924-938.
38. Lucena RA, Allam MF, Jiménez SS, Villarejo ML (2007) A review of environmental exposure to persistent organochlorine residuals during the last fifty years. Curr Drug Saf 2: 163-172.
39. Barron MG, Heintz R, Rice SD (2004) Relative potency of PAHs and heterocycles as aryl hydrocarbon receptor agonists in fish. Mar Environ Res 58: 95-100.
40. Pohjanvirta R, Tuomisto J (1994) Short-term toxicity of 2,3,7,8-tetrachlorodibenzo-p-dioxin in laboratory animals: effects, mechanisms, and animal models. Pharmacol Rev 46: 483-549.
41. Schmidt JV, Bradfield CA (1996) Ah receptor signaling pathways. Annu Rev Cell Dev Biol 12: 55-89.
42. Matikainen T, Perez GI, Jurisicova A, Pru JK, Schlezinger JJ, et al. (2001) Aromatic hydrocarbon receptor-driven Bax gene expression is required for premature ovarian failure caused by biohazardous environmental chemicals. Nat Genet 28: 355-360.
43. Peters JM1, Narotsky MG, Elizondo G, Fernandez-Salguero PM, Gonzalez FJ, et al. (1999) Amelioration of TCDD-induced teratogenesis in aryl hydrocarbon receptor (AhR)-null mice. Toxicol Sci 47: 86-92.
44. Bunger MK, Glover E, Moran SM, Walisser JA, Lahvis GP, et al. (2008) Abnormal Liver Development and Resistance to 2,3,7,8-Tetrachlorodibenzo-p-dioxin Toxicity in Mice Carrying a Mutation in the DNA Binding Domain of the Aryl Hydrocarbon Receptor. Toxicol Sci 106: 83-92.
45. [No authors listed] (1997) IARC Working Group on the Evaluation of Carcinogenic Risks to Humans: Polychlorinated Dibenzo-Para-Dioxins and Polychlorinated Dibenzofurans. Lyon, France, 4-11 February 1997. IARC Monogr Eval Carcinog Risks Hum 69: 1-631.
46. National Toxicology Program (1982) Carcinogenesis Bioassay of 2,3,7,8-Tetrachlorodibenzo-p-dioxin (CAS No. 1746-01-6) in Osborne-Mendel Rats and B6C3F1 Mice (Gavage Study). Natl Toxicol Program Tech Rep Ser 209: 1-195.
47. Peter Guengerich F, Martin MV, McCormick WA, Nguyen LP, Glover E, et al. (2004) Aryl hydrocarbon receptor response to indigoids in vitro and in vivo. Arch Biochem Biophys 423: 309-316.
48. Jinno A, Maruyama Y, Ishizuka M, Kazusaka A, Nakamura A, et al. (2006) Induction of cytochrome P450-1A by the equine estrogen equilenin, a new endogenous aryl hydrocarbon receptor ligand. J Steroid Biochem Mol Biol 98: 48-55.
49. Leibelt DA, Hedstrom OR, Fischer KA, Pereira CB, Williams DE (2003) Evaluation of chronic dietary exposure to indole-3-carbinol and absorption-enhanced 3,3'-diindolylmethane in sprague-dawley rats. Toxicol Sci 74: 10-21.

50. Bertazzi PA, Zocchetti C, Guercilena S, Consonni D, Tironi A, et al. (1997) Dioxin exposure and cancer risk: a 15-year mortality study after the "Seveso accident". Epidemiology 8: 646-652.
51. Viel JF, Clément MC, Hägi M, Grandjean S, Challier B, et al. (2008) Dioxin emissions from a municipal solid waste incinerator and risk of invasive breast cancer: a population-based case-control study with GIS-derived exposure. Int J Health Geogr 7: 4.
52. Tritscher AM, Clark GC, Sewall C, Sills RC, Maronpot R, et al. (1995) Persistence of TCDD-induced hepatic cell proliferation and growth of enzyme altered foci after chronic exposure followed by cessation of treatment in DEN initiated female rats. Carcinogenesis 16: 2807-2811.
53. Holcomb M, Safe S (1994) Inhibition of 7,12-dimethylbenzanthracene-induced rat mammary tumor growth by 2,3,7,8-tetrachlorodibenzo-p-dioxin. Cancer Lett 82: 43-47.
54. Gierthy JF, Bennett JA, Bradley LM, Cutler DS (1993) Correlation of in vitro and in vivo growth suppression of MCF-7 human breast cancer by 2,3,7,8-tetrachlorodibenzo-p-dioxin. Cancer Res 53: 3149-3153.
55. Wang F, Hoivik D, Pollenz R, Safe S (1998) Functional and physical interactions between the estrogen receptor Sp1 and nuclear aryl hydrocarbon receptor complexes. Nucleic Acids Res 26: 3044-3052.
56. Duan R, Porter W, Samudio I, Vyhlidal C, Kladde M, et al. (1999) Transcriptional activation of c-fos protooncogene by 17beta-estradiol: mechanism of aryl hydrocarbon receptor-mediated inhibition. Mol Endocrinol 13: 1511-1521.
57. Klinge CM, Bowers JL, Kulakosky PC, Kamboj KK, Swanson HI (1999) The aryl hydrocarbon receptor (AHR)/AHR nuclear translocator (ARNT) heterodimer interacts with naturally occurring estrogen response elements. Mol Cell Endocrinol 157: 105-119.
58. Ricci MS, Toscano DG, Mattingly CJ, Toscano WA Jr (1999) Estrogen receptor reduces CYP1A1 induction in cultured human endometrial cells. J Biol Chem 274: 3430-3438.
59. Ohtake F, Baba A, Takada I, Okada M, Iwasaki K, et al. (2007) Dioxin receptor is a ligand-dependent E3 ubiquitin ligase. Nature 446: 562-566.
60. Spink DC, Eugster HP, Lincoln DW 2nd, Schuetz JD, Schuetz EG, et al. (1992) 17 beta-estradiol hydroxylation catalyzed by human cytochrome P450 1A1: a comparison of the activities induced by 2,3,7,8-tetrachlorodibenzo-p-dioxin in MCF-7 cells with those from heterologous expression of the cDNA. Arch Biochem Biophys 293: 342-348.
61. Spink DC, Johnson JA, Connor SP, Aldous KM, Gierthy JF (1994) Stimulation of 17 beta-estradiol metabolism in MCF-7 cells by bromochloro- and chloromethyl-substituted dibenzo-p-dioxins and dibenzofurans: correlations with antiestrogenic activity. J Toxicol Environ Health 41: 451-466.
62. Oenga GN, Spink DC, Carpenter DO (2004) TCDD and PCBs inhibit breast cancer cell proliferation in vitro. Toxicol In Vitro 18: 811-819.
63. McDougal A, Wormke M, Calvin J, Safe S (2001) Tamoxifen-induced antitumorigenic/antiestrogenic action synergized by a selective aryl hydrocarbon receptor modulator. Cancer Res 61: 3902-3907.
64. Abdelrahim M, Smith R 3rd, Safe S (2003) Aryl hydrocarbon receptor gene silencing with small inhibitory RNA differentially modulates Ah-responsiveness in MCF-7 and HepG2 cancer cells. Mol Pharmacol 63: 1373-1381.
65. Hall JM, Barhoover MA, Kazmin D, McDonnell DP, Greenlee WF, et al. (2010) Activation of the aryl-hydrocarbon receptor inhibits invasive and metastatic features of human breast cancer cells and promotes breast cancer cell differentiation. Mol Endocrinol 24: 359-369.
66. Ma Q, Whitlock JP Jr (1996) The aromatic hydrocarbon receptor modulates the Hepa 1c1c7 cell cycle and differentiated state independently of dioxin. Mol Cell Biol 16: 2144-2150.
67. Chen I, McDougal A, Wang F, Safe S (1998) Aryl hydrocarbon receptor-mediated antiestrogenic and antitumorigenic activity of diindolylmethane. Carcinogenesis 19: 1631-1639.
68. McDougal A, Sethi Gupta M, Ramamoorthy K, Sun G, Safe SH (2000) Inhibition of carcinogen-induced rat mammary tumor growth and other estrogen-dependent responses by symmetrical dihalo-substituted analogs of diindolylmethane. Cancer Lett 151: 169-179.
69. Meng Q, Yuan F, Goldberg ID, Rosen EM, Auborn K, et al. (2000) Indole-3-carbinol is a negative regulator of estrogen receptor-alpha signaling in human tumor cells. J Nutr 130: 2927-2931.
70. Hong C, Firestone GL, Bjeldanes LF (2002) Bcl-2 family-mediated apoptotic effects of 3,3'-diindolylmethane (DIM) in human breast cancer cells. Biochem Pharmacol 63: 1085-1097.
71. Greenlee WE, Hushka LJ, Hushka DR (2001) Molecular basis of dioxin actions: evidence supporting chemoprotection. Toxicol Pathol 29: 6-7.
72. Hong C, Kim HA, Firestone GL, Bjeldanes LF (2002) 3,3'-Diindolylmethane (DIM) induces a G(1) cell cycle arrest in human breast cancer cells that is accompanied by Sp1-mediated activation of p21(WAF1/CIP1) expression. Carcinogenesis 23: 1297-1305.
73. Trapani V, Patel V, Leong CO, Ciolino HP, Yeh GC, et al. (2003) DNA damage and cell cycle arrest induced by 2-(4-amino-3-methylphenyl)-5-fluorobenzothiazole (5F 203, NSC 703786) is attenuated in aryl hydrocarbon receptor deficient MCF-7 cells. Br J Cancer 88: 599-605.
74. Barhoover MA, Hall JM, Greenlee WF, Thomas RS (2010) Aryl hydrocarbon receptor regulates cell cycle progression in human breast cancer cells via a functional interaction with cyclin-dependent kinase 4. Mol Pharmacol 77: 195-201.
75. Müller A, Homey B, Soto H, Ge N, Catron D, et al. (2001) Involvement of chemokine receptors in breast cancer metastasis. Nature 410: 50-56.
76. Hsu EL, Yoon D, Choi HH, Wang F, Taylor RT, et al. (2007) A proposed mechanism for the protective effect of dioxin against breast cancer. Toxicol Sci 98: 436-444.
77. Safe S, Qin C, McDougal A (1999) Development of selective aryl hydrocarbon receptor modulators for treatment of breast cancer. Expert Opin Investig Drugs 8: 1385-1396.
78. Hall JM, McDonnell DP (2005) Coregulators in nuclear estrogen receptor action: from concept to therapeutic targeting. Mol Interv 5: 343-357.
79. Hestermann EV, Brown M (2003) Agonist and chemopreventative ligands induce differential transcriptional cofactor recruitment by aryl hydrocarbon receptor. Mol Cell Biol 23: 7920-7925.
80. McDougal A, Gupta MS, Morrow D, Ramamoorthy K, Lee JE, Safe SH (2001) Methyl-substituted diindolylmethanes as inhibitors of estrogen-induced growth of T47D cells and mammary tumors in rats. Breast Cancer Res Treat 66: 147-157.
81. McDougal A, Wilson C, Safe S (1997) Inhibition of 7,12-dimethylbenz[a]anthracene-induced rat mammary tumor growth by aryl hydrocarbon receptor agonists. Cancer Lett 120: 53-63.
82. Bradlow HL (2008) Review. Indole-3-carbinol as a chemoprotective agent in breast and prostate cancer. In Vivo 22: 441-445.
83. De Laurentiis M, Arpino G, Massarelli E, Ruggiero A, Carlomagno C, et al. (2005) A meta-analysis on the interaction between HER-2 expression and response to endocrine treatment in advanced breast cancer. Clin Cancer Res 11: 4741-4748.
84. Dawood S, Cristofanilli M (2007) Endocrine resistance in breast cancer: what really matters? Ann Oncol 18: 1289-1291.
85. Taurin S, Allen KM, Scandlyn MJ, Rosengren RJ (2013) Raloxifene reduces triple-negative breast cancer tumor growth and decreases EGFR expression. Int J Oncol 43: 785-792.
86. O'Donnell EF, Koch DC1, Bisson WH2, Jang HS1, Kolluri SK3 (2014) The aryl hydrocarbon receptor mediates raloxifene-induced apoptosis in estrogen receptor-negative hepatoma and breast cancer cells. Cell Death Dis 5: e1038.
87. Meng LH, Kohlhagen G, Liao ZY, Antony S, Sausville E, et al. (2005) DNA-protein cross-links and replication-dependent histone H2AX phosphorylation induced by aminoflavone (NSC 686288), a novel anticancer agent active against human breast cancer cells. Cancer Res 65: 5337-5343.
88. McLean L1, Soto U, Agama K, Francis J, Jimenez R, et al. (2008) Aminoflavone induces oxidative DNA damage and reactive oxidative

species-mediated apoptosis in breast cancer cells. Int J Cancer 122: 1665-1674.

89. Callero MA1, Suárez GV, Luzzani G, Itkin B, Nguyen B, et al. (2012) Aryl hydrocarbon receptor activation by aminoflavone: new molecular target for renal cancer treatment. Int J Oncol 41: 125-134.

90. Brinkman AM, Wu J, Ersland K, Xu W1 (2014) Estrogen receptor Î± and aryl hydrocarbon receptor independent growth inhibitory effects of aminoflavone in breast cancer cells. BMC Cancer 14: 344.

Regulation of Glucose Transporter 1 (Slc2a1) in the Pituitary Gonadotrope of Mice after Puberty

Francina Gonzalez De Los Santos[1,2], Ahmad El -Yaman El-Dandachli[1] and Colleen Buggs-Saxton[1,2*]

[1]Departments of Pediatrics, Wayne State University School of Medicine, Children's Hospital of Michigan, Detroit Medical Center, Detroit, Michigan, USA

[2]Departments of Physiology, Wayne State University School of Medicine, Children's Hospital of Michigan, Detroit Medical Center, Detroit, Michigan, USA

***Corresponding author:** Colleen Buggs-Saxton, Department of Pediatrics, Division of Endocrinology, Wayne State University School of Medicine, 421 E. Canfield, Detroit, Michigan, USA, E-mail: cbuggs@med.wayne.edu

Abstract

Glucose provides fuel for cell metabolism and plays an important role in normal reproductive function. Glucose transporters such as (SLC2A1) facilitate entry of glucose into cells. We have previously shown that gonadotropin releasing hormone (GnRH) stimulates *Slc2a1* expression in LβT2 gonadotrope cells and in the pituitary gland of pre-pubertal mice. In this study we examined changes in *Slc2a1* expression in the pituitary gland of mice after puberty and in LβT2 gonadotrope cells treated with sex steroids. There were no detectable changes in *Slc2a1* gene expression in the pituitary gland of pre-pubertal and adult male and female mice using real-time PCR analysis. In contrast, Western blot analysis detected higher levels of SLC2A1 protein in the pituitary gland of adult male and female mice compared to pre-pubertal male and female mice, respectively. In addition, peak levels of SLC2A1 protein as determined by Western blot analysis were detected in the pituitary gland of female mice during the proestrus and oestrus stages of the oestrous cycle. The proestrus stage corresponds to the surge of luteinizing hormone in the gonadotrope, which then triggers ovulation. Additional studies using immunofluorescent analysis of pituitary glands revealed increased co-localization of SLC2A1 with luteinizing hormone β(LHβ) in the gonadotrope cell of adult male and female mice compared to pre-pubertal mice. *In vitro* studies in LβT2 cells did not detect any effects of estradiol and/or progesterone on *Slc2a1* expression by real-time PCR analysis, but estradiol alone increased SLC2A1 protein levels in LβT2 cells as determined by Western blot analysis. Furthermore, combined treatment of estradiol and progesterone induced glucose uptake in LβT2 cells. Together, our findings show that regulation of *Slc2a1* in the gonadotrope of adult mice likely reflects changes in sex steroids that are also important for pubertal development and fertility.

Keywords: Gonadotrope; Glucose transporter 1; Sex steroids; Puberty

Introduction

Pubertal development and normal reproductive function are regulated by the hypothalamic-pituitary-gonadal (HPG) axis, which consists of gonadotropin releasing hormone (GnRH) neurons, the pituitary gonadotrope cells, and the gonad [1-3]. The hypothalamus contains specialized neurons that secrete GnRH, which binds to its receptor located on the gonadotrope cell in the anterior pituitary gland to stimulate the synthesis and secretion of the gonadotropins; luteinizing hormone (LH) and follicle stimulating hormone (FSH). LH and FSH are composed of two subunits: a common α-subunit and β-subunit that is unique to each hormone. LH and FSH then bind to their respective receptors in the gonad to stimulate the synthesis and secretion of sex steroids, maturation of the oocyte, and induction of spermatogenesis. Estrogen, progesterone and testosterone are the main sex steroids produced by the gonads, and these steroids regulate the HPG axis through negative feedback inhibition at the level of the hypothalamic GnRH neuron and the pituitary gonadotrope cells [3-5]. Estrogen also has positive feedback regulation of the HPG axis, which is important for the preovulatory surge of LH and FSH in various animal models and in humans [6-12]. Thus, regulation of HPG axis by GnRH and sex steroids is important for puberty and fertility.

Glucose is an important source of energy for cellular metabolism, and disorders that impair glucose homeostasis are associated with pubertal and reproductive abnormalities due to dysregulation of the HPG axis [13]. Hyperglycemia impairs GnRH neuronal cell function, and impairment of glucose availability reduces LH secretion *in vivo* [14-18]. Glucose enters cells via the solute carrier-2 (SLC2) family proteins also called glucose transporters (SLC2s), which are important for tissue-specific nutrient sensing and utilization of glucose [19,20]. Some SLC2s are regulated in different tissues of the reproductive axis, and studies have shown that *Slc2a1* is expressed in the testis, uterus, ovary, as well as endometrial and breast cancer cells [21-25]. FSH, interleukin1b (IL1b), and basic fibroblast growth factor (bFGF) stimulate *Slc2a1* gene expression and glucose uptake in rat Sertoli cells [26]. In endometrial stromal cells *Slc2a1* gene expression and glucose uptake are stimulated by progesterone and inhibited by estradiol [22]. In oocytes and granulosa cells, *Slc2a1* mRNA and protein levels are regulated by IGF1 and estradiol [25]. Therefore, regulation of *Slc2a1* gene expression is detected throughout tissues of the reproductive axis.

We have previously shown that Slc2a1 is regulated by GnRH in the gonadotrope cell both in vitro in LβT2 cells and in vivo in mice, and that GnRH increases glucose uptake in LβT2 gonadotrope cells [**27**]. We also showed that treatment of pre-pubertal mice with exogenous GnRH increased Slc2a1 mRNA expression but not Slc2a2, Slc2a4, or Slc2a8 in the mouse pituitary gland, which suggests that Slc2a1 may be important for glucose metabolism in the gonadotrope compared to other glucose transporters. In this study, we investigated the regulation of Slc2a1 in the pituitary gland of pre-pubertal and adult mice. We also examined changes in Slc2a1 in the pituitary gland of female mice during the estrous cycle. To correlate with our in vivo studies in mice, we investigated effects of estradiol and progesterone on Slc2a1 and glucose uptake in LβT2 gonadotrope cells.

Materials and Methods

Animals

Pre-pubertal (4 weeks of age) and adult (2 months of age or older) male and female C57BL/6J mice were identified. Mice were kept on a standard diet with access to food and water ad libitum, and a 12 hour day/night cycle. Vaginal smears were performed with 0.9% saline solution on adult C57BL/6J female mice daily for 1-2 weeks to identify different stages (diestrus, proestrus, and estrus) in the estrous cycle [28]. Vaginal washings were examined under a light microscope with 10X magnification to identify different cell types that are representative of the estrous cycle stages. Mice were euthanized by isofluorane inhalation followed by cervical dislocation prior to harvesting tissues. All protocols were submitted to, approved by, and conducted in accordance with the Wayne State University Institutional Animal Care and Use Committee.

Cell culture

LβT2 cells [29]; [30] were grown in DMEM (4.5 mg/L of glucose, 110 mg/L pyruvate, and 548 mg/L L-glutamine) supplemented with 10% FBS and 1% penicillin-streptomycin and incubated at 37°C with 5% CO_2 supply. For the time course experiments, cells were plated in 6 well plates at a concentration of 1.5-2.0x10^6. Cells were subsequently changed to phenol-free media with 2% heat-inactivated charcoal dextran-stripped calf serum, and 1% penicillin/streptomycin and then stimulated with estradiol (10 nM) or progesterone (100 nM) for 2, 8, and 24 hours or vehicle alone (ethanol, 0 hour). At the end of the time course of steroid induction, RNA or whole cell extracts (WCE) were isolated. Steroid induction experiments were performed three times for RNA and protein isolation.

RNA isolation and Real-Time PCR

Tissues were harvested from euthanized mice as described above and RNA was isolated from the pituitary for cDNA synthesis to examine changes in *Slc2a1* and *Lhb* gene expression via real-time PCR. TATA box binding protein (*Tbp*) gene was used as an endogenous control. The cDNA (representing 50 or 100 ng of starting RNA) was used for real-time PCR analyses via Taqman Gene Expression Assays for *Slc2a1* (Mn00441473_m1), *Lhb* (Mm00656868_m1) and *Tbp* (Mm00446973_m1). PCR reactions were conducted using the Step One plus Real-time PCR System as previously described [27]. Cycle threshold was obtained for each sample. A corrected Ct (Delta Ct) was calculated by subtracting the *Tbp* Ct from the target genes (*Slc2a1* and *Lhb*) Ct for each sample. Relative differences from the control sample were then calculated by using the formula:

$$\text{fold change} = 2^{(\text{Control Delta Ct minus Sample Delta Ct})}$$

Pre-pubertal males n=7-9, and adult males n=12, pre-pubertal females n=9-12 and adult females in diestrus n=7, proestrus n=6-7, and estrus n=8 were used for *Slc2a1* and *Lhb* gene expression.

Western immunoblot analysis

Whole cell extracts (WCE) were prepared from mouse pituitary glands, testes, and ovaries using RIPA buffer containing 1X Phosphate buffered saline, 0.1% sodium dodecyl sulfate and 1% Nonidet P40 with 1X Complete Protease Inhibitor cocktail as previously described [**27**]. Protein concentration was determined by using Coomassie Plus Protein Assay Reagent, and Western blot analysis was performed on protein extracts (20-50 ug/lane) with a rabbit polyclonal antibody against SLC2A1 and polyclonal antibody against α-Tubulin. Immunodetection of protein was performed using Super Signal West Pico Chemiluminescent reagent. Western blots were quantified by analyzing the film with Image J 1.47 program. When quantitating the Western blots, images of multiple exposures were examined to ensure that the films were not over exposed. SLC2A1 protein levels in the pituitary gland of pre-pubertal male mice n=6 were compared to adult male mice n=7. SLC2A1 protein levels in the pituitary gland of pre-pubertal female mice n=7 compared to adult female mice in diestrus n=7, proestrus n=7, and estrus n=7. SLC2A1 protein levels in the testis of pre-pubertal male mice n=5 were compared to pubertal male mice n=7. SLC2A1 protein levels in the ovary of pre-pubertal female mice n=7 compared to adult female mice in diestrus n=4, proestrus n=4, and estrus, n=3.

Histology and immunofluorescent analysis

Pituitary gland of two pre-pubertal mice and three pubertal mice C57/BL6 mice were isolated and fixed in 10% formalin overnight prior to paraffin embedding. Paraffin embedding was performed by the University Pathology Research Services at Wayne State University School of Medicine. Paraffin-embedded pituitaries were subsequently sectioned (4 micron) using a rotatory microtome and then the tissue was mounted on slides. The tissues were rehydrated and then subjected to antigen retrieval buffer (10 mM citrate, pH 6.2, 2 mM EDTA, and 0.05% Tween 20) as previously described [31]. Primary rabbit-polyclonal LHβ antibody was diluted at 1:200 and goat-polyclonal SLC2A1 antibody was diluted at 1:200 and then incubated overnight at 40°C in a humidified chamber. Subsequently, tissues were incubated with secondary antibodies, Alexa Fluor* 488 donkey anti-goat, and Alexa Fluor* 568 goat anti-rabbit for 2 hours at RT. After washing with PBS, mounting media with the nuclear marker DAPI was added to the tissues. Immunofluorescent analysis of paraffin-embedded stained pituitary sections and LβT2 cells was performed with Nikon Eclipse Ti Confocal Imaging System (Nikon Instruments Inc.) equipped with an S Fluor 40X oil objective lens (numerical aperture 1.30). Images were taken by Roper Scientific–CoolSNAP HQ2 camera system (resolution: 1392x1040) and analyzed using NIS-Elements AR imaging software (version 3.22.00), which also has a quantification feature to identify and count cells in the images. To determine specificity of the SLC2A1 antibody in these studies, SLC2A1 antibody was preincubated with vehicle (dH20) or SLC2A1 peptide prior to performing immunofluorescent analysis and a no primary antibody control was also used (Supplementary figures 1-3).

Glucose uptake assay

LβT2 cells were grown in DMEM (4.5 mg/L of glucose, 110 mg/L pyruvate, and 548 mg/L L-glutamine) supplemented with 10% FBS and 1% penicillin-streptomycin and incubated at 37°C with 5% CO_2. Cells were plated in 96 well black clear bottom plates at a concentration of 1.5x10^5cells/well. Cells were subsequently changed to phenol-free media with 2% heat-inactivated charcoal dextran-stripped calf serum, and 1% penicillin/streptomycin, and then stimulated with vehicle alone (ethanol, 0 hr) or 17β-estradiol (10 nM) or progesterone (100 nM) for 2, 8, and 24 hours. Glucose uptake was performed using the Glucose Uptake Cell-Based Assay Kit from Cayman. Media was changed to glucose free and phenol free media before the addition of 2-deoxy-2-[(7-nitro-2,1,3-benzoxadioazol-4-yl) amino]-D-glucose (2-NBDG) for 15 minutes. At the end of the treatment, cells were centrifuged for 5 minutes at 400xg at room temperature, and then each well was washed with 200ul of cell-based Assay Buffer, and the plate was centrifuged for 5 minutes at 400xg at room temperature. The supernatant was aspirated, and 100 ul of cell based assay buffer was added to each well before measuring the amount of 2-NBDG taken up by the cells. Fluorescence was detected with a plate reader using wavelengths of excitation/emission=485/535 nm. After fluorescence reading was obtained, 50 µl of sodium hydroxide (0.1 M) was added to each well and protein concentration was determined by using Coomassie plus Protein Assay Reagent. Fluoresce readings were corrected for protein concentration and basal uptake for each sample, and then control samples were used to determine fold change. The glucose uptake time course was repeated twice (which gives a total of 3 separate experiments).

Reagents and chemicals

High Capacity cDNA Reverse Transcript Kit, Glucose and phenol free media, Taqman gene expression assay, StepOne Plus Real-time PCR System (Applied Biosystems, Foster City, CA); TRIzol, Alexa Fluor® 488 donkey Anti-goat, Alexa Fluor® 568 goat Anti-rabbit, DAPI (Invitrogen Co., Carlsbad, CA); Estradiol and Progesterone (Sigma-Aldrich Co., LLC, St. Louis, MO); Complete Protease Inhibitor cocktail (Roche Diagnostics, Germany); Super Signal West Pico Chemiluminescent Substrate and Coomassie Plus Protein Assay Reagent (Thermo Scientific, Rockford, IL); citrate, EDTA, HEPES, methanol, sodium chloride, sodium dodecyl sulfate, Tris base, Triton-X, and Tween 20, (Fisher Scientific, Fair Lawn, NJ); Glucose Uptake Cell-Based Assay Kit (Cayman Chemical Company, Ann Arbor, MI); DMEM (Mediatech, Manassas, VA); LHβ antibody (anti-rat LHβ - IC-3, AFP571292393 from the National Hormone and Peptide Program-National Institute of Diabetes and Digestive and Kidney Diseases, Dr. A.F. Parlow); goat-polyclonal SLC2A1 antibody N-20, polyclonal antibody against A-Tubulin (Santa Cruz Biotechnology, Santa Cruz, CA); a rabbit polyclonal antibody against SLC2A1 (Abcam Inc., Cambridge, MA).

Statistical analysis

Data are presented as means+SEM. Statistical analysis was performed with GraphPad 5.04 (San Diego, CA). Significance was determined by ANOVA with Bonferroni's or Dunnett's multiple comparison test or Student's (unpaired) t- test.

Results

Slc2a1 gene expression in the murine pituitary gland

We examined the regulation of *Slc2a1* in the pituitary gland of pre-pubertal and adult male and female C57BL/6J mice. RNA was isolated from the pituitary gland and cDNA was made for real-time PCR analysis. There were no significant changes detected in *Slc2a1* mRNA levels in pre-pubertal and adult mice in males (Figure 1A). In contrast, *Lhb* mRNA levels increased 2.4-fold in the pituitary gland of adult male mice compared to pre-pubertal male mice (P<0.05, Figure 1A). We next examined the regulation of *Slc2a1* gene expression in pre-pubertal and adult female mice. We identified adult female mice in different stages of the estrous cycle (diestrus, proestrus, and estrus) by performing vaginal smears [28]. Similar to observations in male mice, there was no detectable difference in *Slc2a1* mRNA levels in the pituitary of pre-pubertal and adult female mice (Figure 1B). In contrast, *Lhb* mRNA levels increased 1.4-fold in adult females during proestrus compared to the estrus (P<0.001, Figure 1B). These results show that there is no significant change in *Slc2a1* gene expression in the pituitary gland after puberty.

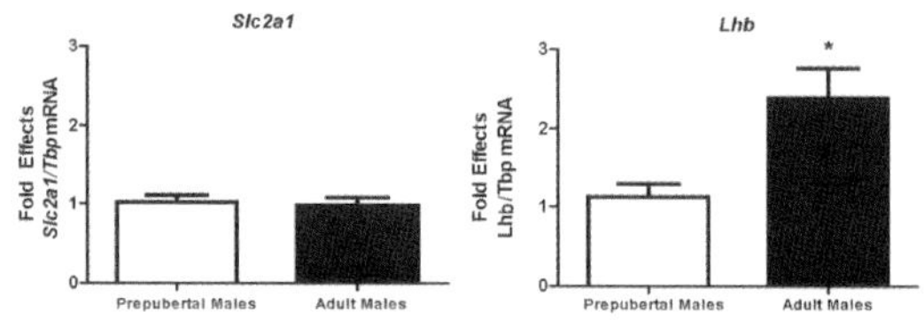

Figure 1A: Slc2a1 gene expression is not regulated in the pituitary gland of mice. Pituitary glands were isolated from pre-pubertal and adult C57BL/6J male mice. Pituitary RNA was prepared for real-time PCR analysis with Taqman probes for *Slc2a1*, *Lhb* and *Tbp* genes. Fold effects were determined using pre-pubertal mice as the control. Pre-pubertal males (white bars, n=7-9), and adult males (black bars, n=12) were used for *Slc2a1* and *Lhb* gene expression. Significance was determined by Student's t-test as shown by * indicating *P*<0.05.

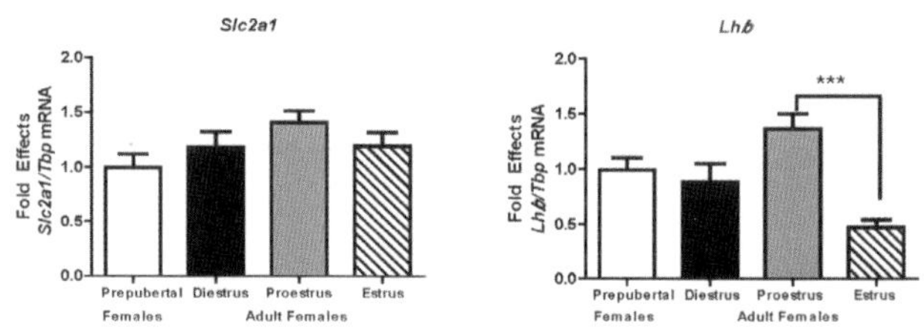

Figure 1B: Slc2a1 gene expression is not regulated in the pituitary gland of mice. C57BL/6J female mice at different stages of the estrous cycle (diestrus, proestrus, and estrus) were identified by vaginal smears, and then pituitary glands were isolated to prepare RNA for real-time PCR to examine changes in *Slc2a1* and *Lhb* gene expression. Fold effects were determined using pre-pubertal mice as the control. Pre-pubertal females (white bars, n=9-12), and adult females in diestrus (black bars, n=7), proestrus (gray bars, n=6-7), and estrus (striped bars, n=8). Significance was determined by ANOVA as shown by * indicating P<0.05.

SLC2A1 protein regulation in the murine pituitary gland

Since changes in *Slc2a1* mRNA levels were not detected in the pituitary glands of male and female mice, we investigated if there is regulation of SLC2A1 protein in the pituitary gland of mice. Whole cell extracts (WCE) were isolated from the pituitary glands of pre-pubertal and adult male mice and Western blot analysis was performed with SLC2A1 antibody. SLC2A1 protein level was increased by 3.0-fold in the pituitary gland of adult compared to pre-pubertal male mice (*P*<0.01, Figure 2A). SLC2A1 protein was also induced in adult female mice (Figure 2A). Compared to pre-pubertal female mice, SLC2A1 protein level increased 1.8-fold in diestrus, 9.4-fold in proestrus, and 11.8-fold in estrus (P<0.001 and P<0.0001 proestrus and estrus, respectively). Therefore, SLC2A1 protein levels increase in the pituitary gland of adult mice.

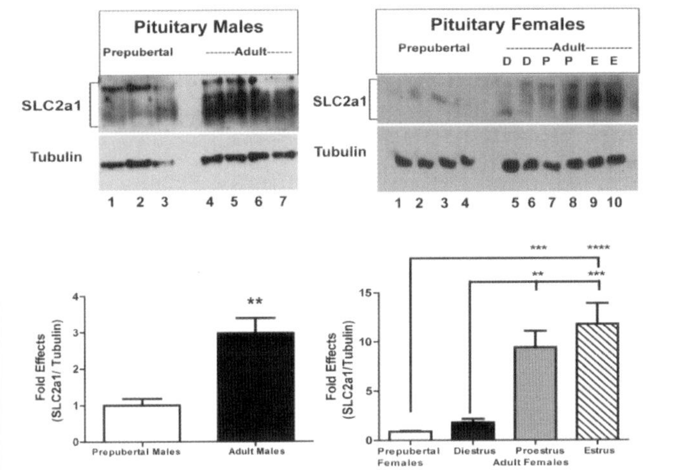

Figure 2A: SLC2A1 protein is regulated in the pituitary gland of male and female adult mice. SLC2A1 protein levels in the pituitary gland of pre-pubertal male mice (white bar, n=6) compared to adult male mice (black bar, n=7). SLC2A1 protein levels in the pituitary gland of pre-pubertal female mice (white bar, n=7) compared to adult female mice in diestrus (black bar, n=6), proestrus (gray bar, n=6), and estrus (striped bar, n=6).

Whole cell extracts (WCE) were isolated from pituitary glands, brain (cerebral cortex), and gonads from pre-pubertal and adult mice. Tissues were isolated from female adult mice at different stages of the estrous cycle. Western blot analysis was performed with SLC2A1 and α-tubulin antibodies. The α-Tubulin antibody was used as a loading control to normalize protein. Autoradiographs are shown with each lane representing WCE (20-50 μg) prepared from a single mouse. Representative Western blot analyses are shown. Densitometry analysis of SLC2A1 protein was normalized to α-Tubulin protein and then fold effects were determined using pre-pubertal SLC2A1 protein level as the control, and the mean+S.E.M is shown in each graph. Significance was determined using Student's t test for male mice and ANOVA for female mice.

To examine whether changes in SLC2A1 protein are specific to the pituitary gland, protein extracts were isolated from gonads of pre-pubertal and adult mice and Western blot analysis was performed. SLC2A1 protein level increased 3.2-fold in the testis of adult male mice compared to pre-pubertal male mice (*P*<0.01 Figure 2B). In contrast, there were no significant changes in SLC2A1 protein level in the ovary of pre-pubertal and adult female mice (Figure 2B). Thus, induction of SLC2A1 protein in the pituitary gland occurs after puberty in both adult male and female mice; whereas, gonadal changes in SLC2A1 protein after puberty appear to be gender-specific.

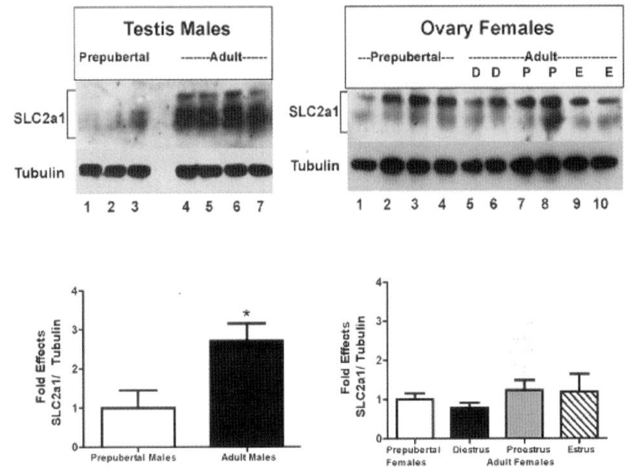

Figure 2B: SLC2A1 protein is regulated in the pituitary gland of male and female adult mice. SLC2A1 protein levels in the testis of pre-pubertal male mice (white bar, n=5) compared to pubertal male mice (black bar, n=7). SLC2A1 protein levels in the ovary of pre-pubertal female mice (white bar, n=7) compared to adult female mice in diestrus (black bar, n=4), proestrus (gray bar, n=4), and estrus (striped bar, n=3). * indicating P<0.05, ** indicating P<0.01, *** P<0.001 and **** indicating P<0.0001.

Co-localization of SLC2A1 and LH in the murine pituitary gonadotrope

To determine if stimulation of SLC2A1 protein in the pituitary gland of adult mice primarily reflects changes in the gonadotrope cell, immunofluorescent analysis was performed using LHβ as a marker for the gonadotrope. Pituitary glands were isolated from pre-pubertal and adult mice, paraffin-embedded, and then subjected to immunofluorescent analysis with SLC2A1 and LHβ antibodies. In pre-pubertal mice, low levels of SLC2A1 and LHβ proteins co-localized to the gonadotrope cell in males (Figure 3A). After puberty, there was increased fluorescent intensity of both LHβ and SLC2A1 proteins that co-localize to the gonadotrope of adult male mice (Figure 3A). Although there was a 2-fold increase in the number of SLC2a1/LHβ positive cells detected in the pituitary glands of adult male mice compared to pre-pubertal male, this difference was not statistically significant (Figure 3A). We next performed immunofluorescent analysis of paraffin-embedded pituitary glands isolated from pre-pubertal female mice and adult female mice in the proestrus stage. Similar to findings in males, there was induction of SLC2A1 protein that co-localized predominantly with LHβ protein in the gonadotrope cell of adult female mice compared to pre-pubertal female mice (Figure 3B). There was a 1.8-fold increase in the number of SLC2A1/LHβ positive cells detected in the pituitary glands of adult female mice compared to pre-pubertal female (*P*<0.05, Figure 3B).

Therefore, the induction of SLC2A1 in the pituitary gland of adult mice reflects changes primarily in the gonadotrope cell.

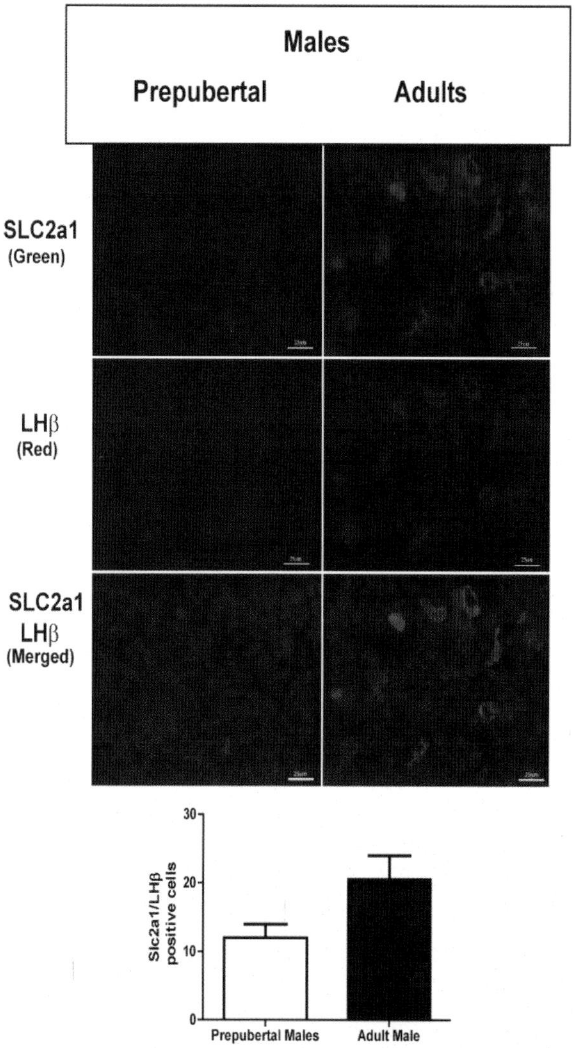

Figure 3A: Co-localization of SLC2A1 and LH in the murine pituitary gland of pre-pubertal and adult mice. Immunofluorescent analysis of paraffin-embedded pituitary glands isolated from pre-pubertal and adult C57BL/6J male mice was performed using SLC2A1 and LH antibodies and secondary fluorescent antibodies, with green indicating SLC2A1 positive cells and red indicating LH positive cells. The merge image represents co-localization of SLC2A1 and LH (yellow) with the nuclear DAPI staining (blue). Scale with bar is shown for each image. SLC2a1/LH positive cells were quantified. Graphs representing the average SLC2a1/LH positive cells in pre-pubertal and adult mice of two experiments are shown. Significance was determined by Student's t-test as shown by * indicating $P<0.05$.

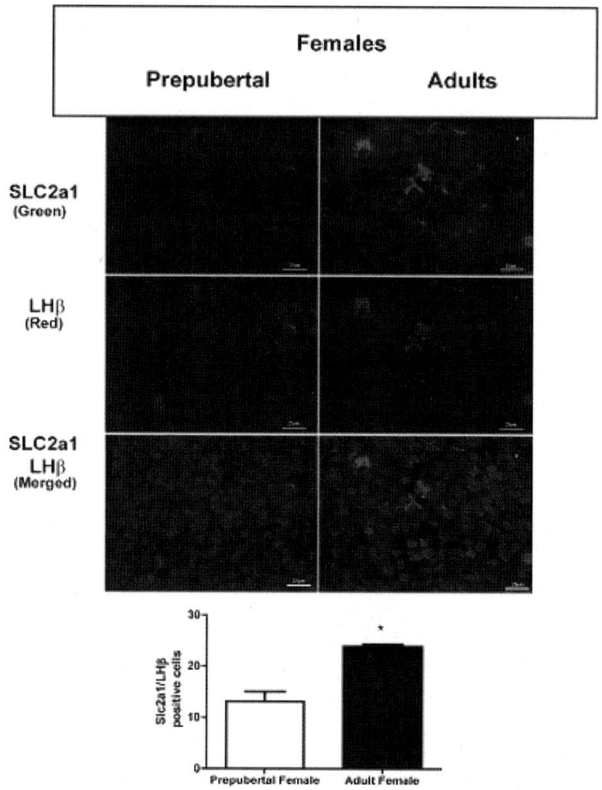

Figure 3B: Co-localization of SLC2A1 and LH in the murine pituitary gland of pre-pubertal and adult mice. Immunofluorescent analysis of paraffin-embedded pituitary glands isolated from pre-pubertal and adult C57BL/6J female mice was performed using SLC2A1 and LH antibodies and secondary fluorescent antibodies, with green indicating SLC2A1 positive cells and red indicating LH positive cells. The merge image represents co-localization of SLC2A1 and LH (yellow) with the nuclear DAPI staining (blue). Scale with bar is shown for each image. SLC2a1/LH positive cells were quantified. Graphs representing the average SLC2a1/LH positive cells in pre-pubertal and adult mice of two experiments are shown. Significance was determined by Student's t-test as shown by * indicating $P<0.05$.

Regulation of SLC2A1by sex steroids in LβT2 gonadotrope cells

Since it is well known that sex steroids have both positive and negative effects on the gonadotrope, we investigated if sex steroids regulate SLC2A1 in gonadotrope cells, which may account for changes in SLC2A1 protein levels detected in adult female pituitary gland especially during the estrous cycle. We examined effects of estradiol and progesterone on SLC2A1 in LβT2 cells, an immortalized gonadotrope cell line. LβT2 cells were incubated with vehicle alone (ethanol 0 hr) or progesterone (100 nM) and/or 17β-estradiol (10 nM) for 2, 8, and 24 hr, and then RNA was isolated for real-time PCR and whole cell extract was also prepared for Western blot analysis. Estradiol and/or progesterone had no effect on *Slc2a1* gene expression (Figure 4A). In contrast, SLC2A1 protein increased 1.3-fold at 2 hours, 2.3-fold at 8 hours, and 5.5-fold at 24 hours of exposure to 17β-estradiol, and the 17β-estradiol-induced SLC2A1 level at 24 hours compared to cells with vehicle alone was significant (Figure 4B, lane 4 compared to lane 1, $P<0.05$).

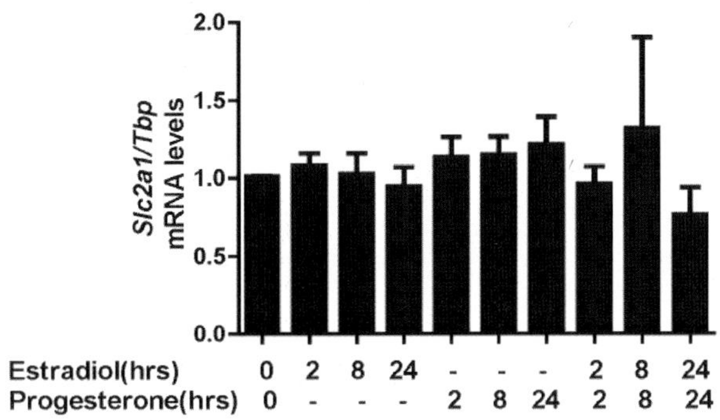

Figure 4A: SLC2A1 protein is regulated by estradiol in gonadotrope cells. RNA was isolated cells for real-time PCR analysis to examine changes in Glut1 gene expression. Fold effects were determined by comparing SLC2A1 levels in vehicle alone (ethanol, 0 hr) compared to steroid-treated cells. The graph represents the mean±S.E.M (n= 2 for each time point).

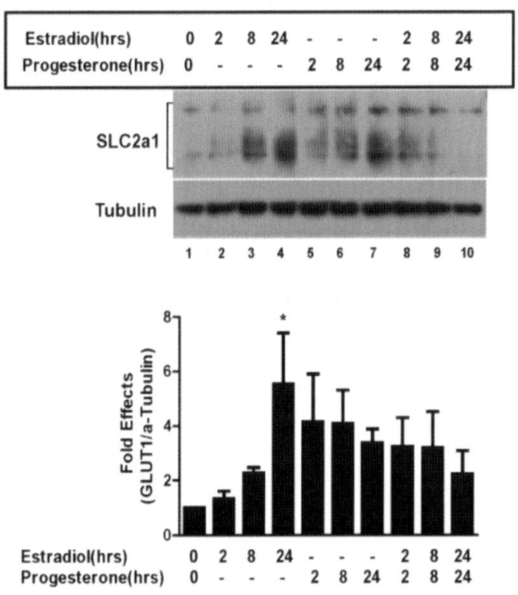

Figure 4B: SLC2A1 protein is regulated by estradiol in gonadotrope cells. After LβT2 cells were treated with estradiol and/or progesterone as described above, whole cell extracts were isolated for Western blot analysis with SLC2A1 and α-tubulin antibodies. The α-tubulin antibody was used as a loading control to normalize protein. A picture of a representative autoradiograph is shown. Densitometry analysis was performed and SLC2A1 protein was normalized to α-Tubulin protein and then to control (unstimulated, 0hr) cells to determine fold effects. The mean ±S.E.M (n=4) is shown in the graph. Significance was determined using ANOVA and * indicates P<0.05.

Cells were incubated with phenol free media supplemented with 2% charcoal stripped fetal bovine serum and stimulated with progesterone (100 nM) or estradiol (10 nM) for 2, 8, and 24 hours or vehicle alone (ethanol).

Although SLC2A1 protein increased 4.1-fold at 2 hours, 4.1-fold at 8 hours, and 3.4-fold at 24 hours of progesterone treatment, these changes in SLC2A1 were not statistically significant compared to cells with vehicle alone (Figure 4B, lanes 5-7 compared to lane 1). Combined treatment of 17β-estradiol and progesterone induced a down regulation of SLC2A1 at 24 hours compared to the induction of SLC2A1 at 24 hours of 17β-estradiol treatment alone (Figure 4B, lane 10 compared to lane 4). These results show that SLC2A1 protein is induced by estradiol but suppressed by combined treatment of 17β-estradiol and progesterone in LβT2 gonadotrope cells.

Glucose Uptake in LβT2 gonadotrope cells

Since 17β-estradiol regulates SLC2A1 protein levels in LβT2 cells, we examined effects of sex steroids on glucose uptake in these cells. Glucose uptake assays were performed in LβT2 cells after treatment with vehicle alone (ethanol, 0 hr) or 17β-estradiol (10nM) and/or progesterone (100 nM) for 2, 8 and 24 hours using 2-NBDG, a fluorescent glucose analog. Progesterone alone or 17β-estradiol alone did not stimulate glucose uptake (Figure 5). In contrast, combined treatment of 17β-estradiol and progesterone increased glucose uptake 2.3- and 2.0-fold at 2 and 8 hours, respectively compared to vehicle alone (Figure 5, $P<0.01$ for 2 hr compared to vehicle alone, and $P<0.05$ and 8 hours compared to vehicle alone). Combined treatment of 17β-estradiol and progesterone at 24 hours did not stimulate glucose uptake. Therefore, combined treatment of 17β-estradiol and progesterone modulates glucose uptake in a time-dependent manner in LβT2 gonadotrope cells.

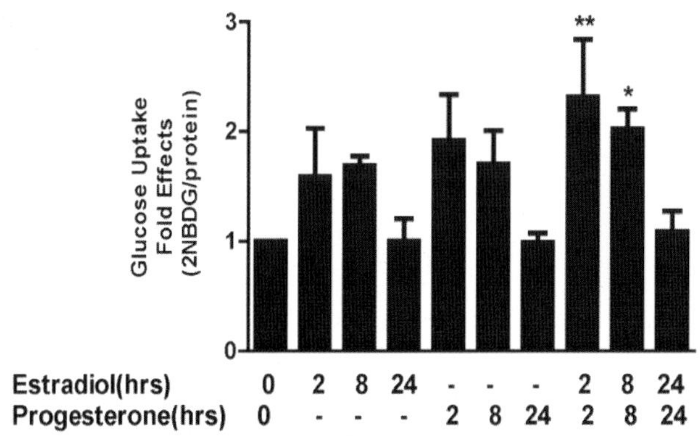

Figure 5: Glucose Uptake

Glucose uptake was performed using the fluorescent glucose analog, 2-NBDG. Cells were incubated with phenol-free media supplemented with 2% charcoal stripped fetal bovine serum and stimulated with vehicle alone (ethanol, 0 hr) or progesterone (100 nM) or estradiol (10 nM) for 2, 8, and 24 hours and then treated with 2-NBDG for 15 minutes, and fluorescence was measured using a plate reader. Wavelength excitation/emission=485/535 nm. Fluoresce readings were corrected for basal fluorescence and protein concentration, then the steroid-treated samples were corrected with the control sample (vehicle alone) and fold effects were calculated. The mean±S.E.M (n=4) is shown in the graph. Fold effects of estradiol and progesterone combination at 2 hr and 8 hr were 2.4 and 1.9 respectively. Significance was determined using ANOVA and * indicates P<0.05, and ** indicates P< 0.01.

Discussion

This is the first report showing that SLC2A1 is regulated at the post-transcriptional level in the murine pituitary gonadotrope after puberty. Immunofluorescent analysis of the pituitary gland shows co-localization of SLC2A1 with LHβ in the gonadotrope of both male and female mice with increased intensity of SLC2A1 protein detected in the gonadotrope of adult mice. These findings indicate that there is a gonadotrope-specific induction of SLC2A1 protein after puberty in mice.

Changes in SLC2A1 protein level in the pituitary gland of adult female mice were also detected during the estrous cycle. Peak levels of SLC2A1 were detected during proestrus and estrus stages compared to the diestrus stage of the estrous cycle. It is well known that ovarian sex steroids rise and fall during the estrous cycle. Estradiol peaks during the morning of proestrus and then subsequently decreases as progesterone reaches its peak during late proestrus before the surge of gonadotropins [9,32,33]. In addition a smaller increase in progesterone also occurs during diestrus, when estradiol levels are low [9]. Estradiol induces a positive feedback at the level of the hypothalamus and pituitary in preparation for the preovulatory surge of gonadotropins, and progesterone has also been shown to be important in this process [9]. In our study, an initial increase in SLC2A1 protein was first detected during proestrus and was sustained during estrus but then subsequently decreased in diestrus. This pattern of induction of SLC2A1 correlates most with changes in estradiol although we cannot completely exclude that progesterone, GnRH, or other factors also contribute to the changes in SLC2A1. To further investigate direct effects of estradiol and progesterone on SLC2A1, we performed studies with sex steroids in LβT2 gonadotrope cells. We found that estradiol but not progesterone increased SLC2A1 protein levels. Therefore, we conclude that changes in SLC2A1 levels during the estrus cycle in mice primarily reflect changes in estradiol, which also correlates with changes in the gonadotrope during proestrus before ovulation occurs. Changes in SLC2A1 during the estrous cycle is not limited to the pituitary gland, since others have shown that *Slc2a1* is regulated in the endometrium during the estrous and menstrual cycle, respectively [34,35]. Therefore, regulation of SLC2A1 in the pituitary gonadotrope during the estrous cycle correlates with changes in sex steroids.

A common observation in our study is that *Slc2a1* is regulated at the post-transcriptional level in the gonadotrope and this effect appears to involve sex steroids. We detected post-transcriptional induction of SLC2A1 levels in the pituitary gland of mice after puberty and during the estrous cycle and this correlated with estradiol-induced SLC2A1 levels in LβT2 cells. Others have shown that various pathophysiological processes and hormonal stimuli modulate *Slc2a1* gene expression at the post-transcriptional level via mechanisms involving interactions between *trans*-regulatory proteins and *cis*-acting elements in the Slc2a1 3'-untranslated region [36,37]. Ovarian sex steroids have been shown to regulate *Slc2a1* at the posttranscriptional level in endometrial cancer cells, but the precise mechanism for this effect is unknown [38]. Therefore, we propose that post-transcriptional regulation of *Slc2a1* may provide an important mechanism for rapid changes in gene expression and glucose metabolism during the estrous cycle in preparation for ovulation. Further investigation is needed to determine post-transcriptional mechanisms in the pituitary gonadotrope regulating *Slc2a1* after puberty and during the estrous cycle.

In this study we show that ovarian steroids induce glucose uptake in LβT2 gonadotrope cells. Combined treatment with estradiol and progesterone was required to stimulate glucose uptake in LβT2 cells although estradiol alone increased SLC2A1 protein in these cells. This combined effect of estradiol and progesterone on glucose uptake was independent of changes in SLC2A1 protein levels and was limited to acute exposure to hormonal treatment (2-8 hours). These findings suggest that induction of SLC2A1 protein by estradiol could prime the gonadotrope for this combined effect of estradiol and progesterone on glucose uptake to prepare for changes required for ovulation. The mechanism explaining time-dependent effects of combined sex steroid treatment on glucose metabolism in LβT2 cells requires further investigation. Others have reported that acute exposure to progesterone at 30 minutes increases GnRH-induced LH release from estrogen-primed pituitary cells, but chronic exposure to progesterone at 48 hours decreases GnRH-induced LH release from estrogen-primed pituitary cells [9]. Although we did not use GnRH in our *in vitro* studies, it is well known that the preovulatory surge of LH is a time-dependent phenomenon that is regulated by estradiol, progesterone, GnRH, and other neuroendocrine factors [9]. Glucose is an important source of energy for cellular metabolism, and so we propose that the gonadotrope needs more glucose acutely in preparation for the preovulatory surge of LH. Subsequently, there is a reduction in glucose uptake after this acute increase in glucose metabolism occurs. This explanation correlates with our findings that glucose uptake increases in LβT2 cells after 2-8 hours of combined treatment with 17β-estradiol and progesterone, but then glucose uptake decreases after 24 hours of combined treatment with 17β-estradiol and progesterone. Since there is time-dependent regulation of the preovulatory surge of LH, we propose that there is also time-dependent regulation of glucose uptake in the gonadotrope that is controlled by sex steroids. Furthermore, limiting the duration of stimulated-glucose uptake in the gonadotrope may allow cellular processes to recover and prepare for the next preovulatory surge of LH. More studies are needed to investigate specific mechanisms underlying combined effects of 17β-estradiol and progesterone signaling on glucose metabolism in the gonadotrope. Still, our observations suggest that both 17β-estradiol and progesterone together are important for the regulation of glucose metabolism in the gonadotrope. One study has reported changes in glucose metabolism in the pituitary gland of postmenopausal women induced by an infusion of estradiol and progesterone without any detectable changes in the hypothalamus [39]. Therefore, regulation of SLC2A1 and glucose transport in the gonadotrope by ovarian sex steroids suggests that changes in glucose metabolism play an important in gonadotrope function.

Our previous study showed that GnRH increases *Slc2a1* mRNA and SLC2A1 protein levels in LβT2 gonadotrope cells [27]. In our current study, estradiol regulates SLC2A1 protein but not *Slc2a1* mRNA levels in LβT2 cells. These observations suggest effects of GnRH and estradiol on *Slc2a1* are mediated via different mechanisms that may be critical for differential activation of cellular processes in the gonadotrope that are important for puberty and fertility.

We detected some gender differences in SLC2A1 protein in males and female mice that appear to be tissue-specific. In particular, adult male mice had increased levels of SLC2A1 in the pituitary gland and testis compared to pre-pubertal male mice. In contrast, adult female mice had increased levels of SLC2A1 in the pituitary gland but no differences were detected in the ovaries of pre-pubertal and adult female mice. These observations suggest that changes in SLC2A1 at different levels of the HPG axis in male mice may be a general indicator of the post- pubertal state. In contrast, changes in SLC2A1 in female mice correlates with changes indicative of the gonadotrope reaching pubertal maturation that is required for full reproductive capacity. Additional investigation is needed to further understand the regulation of the *Slc2a1* gene expression in the pituitary gland and other reproductive tissues during other physiological states important for pubertal development and reproduction.

In summary, regulation of *Slc2a1* in the pituitary gonadotrope occurs at the post-transcriptional level in adult mice and during the estrous cycle. In LβT2 gonadotrope cells estradiol induces post-transcriptional changes in *Slc2a1* expression and estradiol together with progesterone stimulate glucose uptake. Therefore, these findings provide new insights into the regulation of *Slc2a1* and glucose metabolism in the gonadotrope that is dependent on sex steroids and changes associated with puberty and fertility.

Acknowledgement

The authors thank A. Abou-Samra, N. Data, and A. S. Goustin for useful suggestions and discussions. This work was supported by funding from Wayne State University School of Medicine, Pediatrics Department and Children's Hospital of Michigan, Detroit Medical Center.

Author Contributions

Colleen Buggs-Saxton: conception and design of research, revised manuscript

Francina Gonzalez De Los Santos, Ahmad El -Yaman El-Dandachli and Colleen Buggs-Saxton: performed experiments and analyzed data, prepared figures, approved final version of manuscript

Francina Gonzalez De Los Santos and Colleen Buggs-Saxton: interpreted results of experiments, drafted manuscript

References

1. Homburg R, Potashnik G, Lunenfeld B, Insler V (1976) The hypothalamus as a regulator of reproductive function. Obstet Gynecol Surv 31: 455-471.
2. Reiter EO, Grumbach MM (1982) Neuroendocrine control mechanisms and the onset of puberty. Annu Rev Physiol 44: 595-613.
3. Styne DM (1994) Physiology of puberty. Horm Res 41 Suppl 2: 3-6.
4. Bordini B, Rosenfield RL (2011) Normal pubertal development: part II: clinical aspects of puberty. Pediatr Rev 32: 281-292.
5. Reyes-Fuentes A, Veldhuis JD (1993) Neuroendocrine physiology of the normal male gonadal axis. Endocrinol Metab Clin North Am 22: 93-124.
6. Chang RJ, Jaffe RB (1978) Progesterone effects on gonadotropin release in women pretreated with estradiol. J Clin Endocrinol Metab 47: 119-125.
7. Legan SJ, Coon GA, Karsch FJ (1975) Role of estrogen as initiator of daily LH surges in the ovariectomized rat. Endocrinology 96: 50-56.
8. Liu JH, Yen SS (1983) Induction of midcycle gonadotropin surge by ovarian steroids in women: a critical evaluation. J Clin Endocrinol Metab 57: 797-802.
9. Mahesh VB, Brann DW (1998) Regulation of the preovulatory gonadotropin surge by endogenous steroids. Steroids 63: 616-629.
10. McPherson JC 3rd, Eldridge JC, Costoff A, Mahesh VB (1974) The pituitary-gonadal axis before puberty: effects of various estrogenic steroids in the ovariectomized rat. Steroids 24: 41-56.
11. Norman RL, Blake CA, Sawyer CH (1973) Estrogen-dependent 24-hour periodicity in pituitary LH release in the female hamster. Endocrinology 93: 965-970.
12. Yamaji T, Dierschke DJ, Hotchkiss J, Bhattacharya AN, Surve AH, et al. (1971) Estrogen induction of LH release in the rhesus monkey. Endocrinology 89: 1034-1041.
13. Arrais RF, Dib SA (2006) The hypothalamus-pituitary-ovary axis and type 1 diabetes mellitus: a mini review. Hum Reprod 21: 327-337.
14. Murahashi K, Bucholtz DC, Nagatani S, Tsukahara S, Tsukamura H, et al. (1996) Suppression of luteinizing hormone pulses by restriction of glucose availability is mediated by sensors in the brain stem. Endocrinology 137: 1171-1176.
15. Nagatani S, Bucholtz DC, Murahashi K, Estacio MA, Tsukamura H, et al. (1996) Reduction of glucose availability suppresses pulsatile luteinizing hormone release in female and male rats. Endocrinology 137: 1166-1170.
16. Ohkura S, Ichimaru T, Itoh F, Matsuyama S, Okamura H (2004) Further evidence for the role of glucose as a metabolic regulator of hypothalamic gonadotropin-releasing hormone pulse generator activity in goats. Endocrinology 145: 3239-3246.
17. Pal L, Chu HP, Shu J, Topalli L, Santoro N, et al. (2007) In vitro evidence of glucose-induced toxicity in GnRH secreting neurons: high glucose concentrations influence GnRH secretion, impair cell viability, and induce apoptosis in the GT1-1 neuronal cell line. Fertil Steril, 88: 1143-1149.
18. Sen KK, Azhar S, Menon KM (1979) Evidence for the involvement of an energy-dependent process in gonadotropin-releasing hormone-stimulated luteinizing hormone release by rat anterior pituitary. Endocrinology 105: 1158-1161.
19. Mueckler M (1994) Facilitative glucose transporters. Eur J Biochem 219: 713-725.
20. Uldry M, Thorens B (2004) The SLC2 family of facilitated hexose and polyol transporters. Pflugers Arch 447: 480-489.
21. Dan-Goor M, Sasson S, Davarashvili A, Almagor M (1997) Expression of glucose transporter and glucose uptake in human oocytes and preimplantation embryos. Hum Reprod 12: 2508-2510.
22. Frolova A, Flessner L, Chi M, Kim ST, Foyouzi-Yousefi N, et al. (2009) Facilitative glucose transporter type 1 is differentially regulated by progesterone and estrogen in murine and human endometrial stromal cells. Endocrinology 150: 1512-1520.
23. Kim ST, Moley KH (2007) The expression of GLUT8, GLUT9a, and GLUT9b in the mouse testis and sperm. Reprod Sci 14: 445-455.
24. Kokk K, Veräjänkorva E, Wu XK, Tapfer H, Põldoja E, et al. (2004) Immunohistochemical detection of glucose transporters class I subfamily in the mouse, rat and human testis. Medicina (Kaunas) 40: 156-160.
25. Zhou J, Bievre M, Bondy CA (2000) Reduced GLUT1 expression in Igf1-/- null oocytes and follicles. Growth Horm IGF Res 10: 111-117.
26. Galardo MN, Riera MF, Pellizzari EH, Chemes HE, Venara MC, et al. (2008) Regulation of expression of Sertoli cell glucose transporters 1 and 3 by FSH, IL1 beta, and bFGF at two different time-points in pubertal development. Cell Tissue Res 334: 295-304.
27. Harris VM, Bendre SV, Gonzalez De Los Santos F, Fite A, El-Yaman El-Dandachli A, et al. (2012) GnRH increases glucose transporter-1 expression and stimulates glucose uptake in the gonadotroph. J Endocrinol 212: 139-147.
28. Caligioni CS (2009) Assessing reproductive status/stages in mice. Curr Protoc Neurosci Appendix 4: Appendix 4I.
29. Thomas P, Mellon PL, Turgeon J, Waring DW (1996) The L beta T2 clonal gonadotrope: a model for single cell studies of endocrine cell secretion. Endocrinology 137: 2979-2989.

30. Turgeon JL, Kimura Y, Waring DW, Mellon PL (1996) Steroid and pulsatile gonadotropin-releasing hormone (GnRH) regulation of luteinizing hormone and GnRH receptor in a novel gonadotrope cell line. Mol Endocrinol 10: 439-450.
31. Long DJ 2nd1, Buggs C (2008) Microwave oven-based technique for immunofluorescent staining of paraffin-embedded tissues. J Mol Histol 39: 1-4.
32. Chappell PE, Levine JE (2000) Stimulation of gonadotropin-releasing hormone surges by estrogen. I. Role of hypothalamic progesterone receptors. Endocrinology 141: 1477-1485.
33. Micevych P1, Soma KK, Sinchak K (2008) Neuroprogesterone: key to estrogen positive feedback? Brain Res Rev 57: 470-480.
34. Von Wolff M, Ursel S, Hahn U, Steldinger R, Strowitzki T (2003) Glucose transporter proteins (GLUT) in human endometrium: expression, regulation, and function throughout the menstrual cycle and in early pregnancy. J Clin Endocrinol Metab 88: 3885-3892.
35. Kim ST, Moley KH (2009) Regulation of facilitative glucose transporters and AKT/MAPK/PRKAA signaling via estradiol and progesterone in the mouse uterine epithelium. Biol Reprod 81: 188-198.
36. Qi C, Pekala PH (1999) The influence of mRNA stability on glucose transporter (GLUT1) gene expression. Biochem Biophys Res Commun 263: 265-269.
37. Boado RJ, Pardridge WM (2002) Glucose deprivation and hypoxia increase the expression of the GLUT1 glucose transporter via a specific mRNA cis-acting regulatory element. J Neurochem 80: 552-554.
38. Medina RA, Meneses AM, Vera JC, Gúzman C, Nualart F, et al. (2004) Differential regulation of glucose transporter expression by estrogen and progesterone in Ishikawa endometrial cancer cells. J Endocrinol 182: 467-478.
39. Ottowitz WE, Dougherty DD, Fischman AJ, Hall JE (2008) [18F]2-fluoro-2-deoxy-D-glucose positron emission tomography demonstration of estrogen negative and positive feedback on luteinizing hormone secretion in women. J Clin Endocrinol Metab 93: 3208-3214.

Polycystic Ovarian Morphology is Associated with Hyperandrogenemia and Insulin Resistance in Women with Polycystic Ovary Syndrome (PCOS)

Neoklis AG[1*], Anastasia KA[1], Damianaki K[1], Nikolaos DR[1], Markantes G[1], Papadopoulos V[1], Adonakis GL[1], Decavalas G[1] and Panidis D[2]

[1]*Department of Obstetrics and Gynecology, Division of Reproductive Endocrinology, University of Patras Medical School, Patras, Greece*

[2]*Division of Endocrinology and Human Reproduction, Department of Obstetrics and Gynecology, Aristotle University of Thessaloniki, Thessaloniki, Greece*

[*]**Corresponding author:** Neoklis AG, MD, PhD, Department of Obstetrics and Gynecology, Division of Reproductive Endocrinology, University of Patras Medical School, Patras, Greece, E-mail: neoklisg@hol.gr

Abstract

Objectives: The aim of the present study was to evaluate the impact of polycystic ovarian morphology in the hormonal and metabolic features of the "classical" phenotypes of PCOS.

Design: The study included 1275 Caucasian women with PCOS with a mean age of 24.25 ± 5.79 years and a mean BMI of 26.80 ± 7.03 kg/m^2. Diagnosis of PCOS was based on the 2003 Rotterdam ESHRE/ASRM-Sponsored PCOS Consensus criteria. Two phenotypes, matched for age and BMI were compared: Phenotype I (n=620) which included PCOS women with biochemical hyperandrogenemia and/or clinical hyperandrogenemia, chronic anovulation and polycystic ovarian morphology on ultrasound (PCO). Phenotype II (n=400) which included PCOS women with biochemical hyperandrogenemia and/or clinical hyperandrogenemia and chronic anovulation, without PCO. These phenotypes were further subdivided in normal weight and obese PCOS women.

Results: PCOS women of Phenotype I had higher LH/FSH ratio ($p<0.001$), higher Testosterone ($p<0.01$), Δ4 Androstenedione ($p<0.001$) and 17-OH progesterone levels ($p<0.001$), and higher Free Androgen Index (FAI) values ($p<0.01$) compared to Phenotype II. With the exception of fasting glucose levels, all other indices of insulin resistance (fasting insulin, fasting glucose/insulin ratio, QUICKI and HOMA2IR) document an association between Phenotype I and greater insulin resistance in overweight/obese PCOS women.

Conclusions: In conclusion, in "classical" phenotypes of polycystic ovary syndrome (PCOS), polycystic ovarian morphology is associated with more severe hyperandrogenemia and deranged LH/FSH ratio. In overweight/obese PCOS subjects, PCO is positively correlated with insulin resistance.

Keywords: PCOS; Ovarian volume; Follicular number; Ovarian stroma; Hyperandrogenemia; Insulin resistance

Introduction

Polycystic ovary syndrome (PCOS) is the commonest endocrine disease of reproductive-aged women [1]. According to the National Institute of Health (NIH) criteria (1990), PCOS is diagnosed upon the concurrent presence of hyperandrogenism and/or hyperandrogenemia and menstrual dysfunction, with other known disorders excluded [2]. These criteria define the so called "classical" phenotypes of the syndrome. A broader definition was suggested by the Rotterdam conference, sponsored by the ESHRE/ASRM in 2003, according to which, PCOS could be defined when at least two out of the following three features are present: oligo-anovulation, clinical and/or biochemical hyperandrogenemia and polycystic ovarian morphology on ultrasound [3]. There has been a long debate concerning the definition of PCOS, disputing the role of hyperandrogenemia as a cardinal feature of the syndrome. Additional milder phenotypes, characterized by the presence of either hyperandrogenemia and polycystic ovarian morphology (PCO) or anovulation and PCO have been included in PCOS, according to the revised ESHRE/ASRM criteria [4,5], still phenotypes that include biochemical hyperandrogenemia and chronic anovulation ("classic" PCOS) appear to be the most severely affected with respect to androgen levels, insulin resistance and obesity [5-7].

The cardinal argument in favor of the Rotterdam categorization was the use of polycystic ovarian appearance as surrogate for classical markers of hyperandrogenemia [8]. Although some authors [9-11] advocate that polycystic ovarian morphology has demonstrated satisfactory predictive value in diagnosing PCOS, this is not still universally accepted. It has been proposed that obesity differentially affects PCOS phenotypes. In particular, greater BMI and hip perimeter have been positively correlated with ultrasonographic PCO morphology, hirsutism and menstrual disorders in PCOS women [12,13]. The aim of the present study was to evaluate the impact of polycystic ovarian morphology in the hormonal and metabolic features of the "classical" phenotypes of PCOS.

Materials and Methods

Subjects

The study included 1275 Caucasian women with PCOS with a mean age of 24.25 ± 5.79 years and a mean BMI of 26.80 ± 7.03 kg/m^2. Diagnosis of PCOS was based on the 2003 Rotterdam ESHRE/ASRM-Sponsored PCOS Consensus criteria [2], which include at least two of the following: (i) oligo- and/or anovulation (ANOV), (ii) biochemical hyperandrogenemia and/or hyperandrogenism (clinical signs of high androgen levels) (HA), and (iii) polycystic ovaries on ultrasound (PCO). Biochemical hyperandrogenemia was defined as serum testosterone levels and/or serum Free Androgen Index being higher than two standard deviations above the mean levels of a normal control population. Clinical hyperandrogenism was defined as the presence of hirsutism, acne, or androgenic alopecia. Hirsutism was assessed by Ferriman-Gallwey scale (patients with scores of 8 or greater were considered hirsute) [14].

Chronic anovulation was defined as a menstrual cycle of less than 21 or more than 35 days. Ovulation was defined as a menstrual cycle of 28 ± 2 days, and/or blood progesterone levels >5.0 ng/mL in two consecutive cycles. Exclusion criteria were congenital adrenal hyperplasia, androgen secreting tumors and Cushing's syndrome. All subjects had normal thyroid, kidney and liver function and none had excessive alcohol intake. No woman reported use of any medication that could interfere with normal function of the hypothalamic–pituitary–gonadal axis during the last semester. The study complied with the principles of the Helsinki declaration, Institutional Review Board was obtained and all subjects provided written informed consent.

In order to evaluate the effect of PCO morphology on the hormonal and metabolic parameters of our PCOS patients with "classical" phenotypes (presenting biochemical and/or clinical hyperandrogenemia and chronic anovulation, from the whole cohort of PCOS women two specific phenotypes, matched for age and BMI were further analyzed: Phenotype I (n=620) which included PCOS women with biochemical hyperandrogenemia and/or clinical hyperandrogenemia, chronic anovulation and PCO. Phenotype II (n=400) which included PCOS women with biochemical hyperandrogenemia and/or clinical hyperandrogenemia and chronic anovulation, without PCO.

Furthermore, in order to evaluate the association of both obesity and PCO morphology with the hormonal and metabolic parameters of the PCOS population, the studied populations of Phenotypes I and II (n=1020) were divided in normal weight (BMI ≤ 25 Kg/m^2) and overweight/obese (BMI>25 Kg/m^2). Subsequently, we compared normal weight PCOS women of Phenotype I (n=319) with normal weight PCOS women of Phenotype II (n=201) and overweight/obese PCOS women of Phenotype I (n=301) with overweight/obese PCOS women of Phenotype II (n=199). The compared subgroups had no significant differences regarding age and BMI.

Anthropometric and hormonal measurements

Weight, height, as well as waist (W) and hip (H) circumferences were measured in all women. Body weight was measured using analogue scales and in light clothing; height was measured bare-foot using a stadiometer. Body mass index (BMI, kg/m^2) was calculated by dividing weight by height squared (kg per square metre) to assess obesity. Waist circumference (W) was obtained as the smallest circumference at the level of the umbilicus. Baseline blood samples were collected between days 3 and 7 of the menstrual cycle after a spontaneous or progestin-induced bleeding episode, following an overnight fast. At the same day, transvaginal ultrasound examination was performed (3-D, 5-9 MHz transducer, Voluson E6-General Electric) in order to evaluate polycystic ovarian morphology, namely increased ovarian volume (>10 cm^3), increased follicular number (12 or more follicles measuring 2-9 mm in diameter) even in a single ovary or increased ovarian stroma (cut-off value: 1.95 cm^2) and stroma/total area (S/A) ratio (cut-off value: 0.34) [10,11]. Mean number of follicles and mean ovarian volume were also assessed. Ovarian volume was calculated according to the formula: Ovarian Volume = $\pi/6 \times$ (ovarian length × ovarian height × ovarian width). All ultrasounds were performed by the same experienced clinician.

The circulating levels of follicle stimulating hormone (FSH), luteinizing hormone (LH), Testosterone (T), Δ4 Androstenedione (A), dehydroepiandrosterone-sulfate (DHEAS), 17-OH progesterone (17-OH-P), sex-hormone-binding globulin (SHBG), glucose (Glu) and insulin (Ins) were measured. The Free Androgen Index (FAI) was calculated as Testosterone (nmol/L) × 100/SHBG (nmol/L) [15]. QUICKI index was calculated as the product of the equation 1/log (fasting insulin) + log (fasting glucose), while HOMA2IR index calculator was downloaded from http://www.OCDEM.ox.ac.uk.

All hormonal assays and plasma glucose determination were carried out at the Department of Biochemistry of the Aristotle University of Thessaloniki School of Medicine. Plasma glucose concentrations were measured using a glucose oxidase technique with an auto analyzer (Roche/Hitachi 902; Roche Diagnostics GmbH, Manheim, Germany).

LH and FSH levels were measured with an enzyme-linked immunoassay (EIA), using commercial kits (Nichols Institute Diagnostics, CA, USA). Testosterone was measured with a Direct RIA kit (Sorin, Biomedica); Δ4 Androstenedione with a Gamma Coat [125I] RIA kit (Incstar Corp.); DHEAS with direct RIA solid-phase coated tubes (Zer Science Based Industries Ltd); 17-OH progesterone with an ImmuChem Double Antibody [125I] RIA kit (ICN Pharmaceuticals, Inc.); insulin with a Coat-A-count Insulin kit (Diagnostic Products Corp.); and SHBG with an immunoradiometric assay (IRMA) kit (SHBG: [125I] IRMA Kit, Orion Diagnostica). The intra-assay coefficients of variation (CV) were 1.5% for FSH, 0.7% for LH, 3.8% for insulin, 4.1% 200 for 17-OH progesterone, 1.3% for testosterone, 5.9% for Δ4 Androstenedione, 9.4% for DHEAS and 5.8% for SHBG. The average inter-assay CV were 3.2% for FSH, 1.7% for LH, 4.4% for insulin, 6.3% for 17-OH progesterone, 2.2% for testosterone, 9.2% for Δ4 Androstenedione, 12.1% for DHEA-S and 7.8% for SHBG.

Statistics

All statistical procedures were performed using SPSS 18.0 for Windows (IBM SPSS Statistics, IBM software). Values are expressed as mean ± standard deviation. Test for normality was done using Kolmogorov-Smirnov test.

Distribution comparison between groups was done using the independent t-test for variables following normal distribution and the non-parametric Mann-Whitney test for variables not following normal distribution. Bonferroni correction for multiple comparisons has been applied. Values were considered to be statistically significant at $p<0.05$.

Results

The effect of PCO morphology (Phenotype I vs. Phenotype II)

Hormonal features

PCOS women of Phenotype I had higher LH levels ($p<0.001$), lower FSH levels ($p<0.01$) and higher LH/FSH ratio ($p<0.001$) (Figure1).

In addition, they had higher Testosterone ($p<0.01$), Δ4 Androstenedione ($p<0.001$) and 17-OH progesterone levels ($p<0.001$), higher Free Androgen Index (FAI) values ($p<0.01$) and lower Testosterone/Δ4 Androstenedione (T/A) ratio ($p<0.01$) (Figure 1). On the other hand, no significant difference was observed regarding DHEAS and SHBG levels among the two subgroups (Figure 1).

Insulin resistance

In all indices of insulin resistance studied (fasting glucose and insulin, glucose/insulin ratio, QUICKI and HOMA2IR indices), no significant differences were noted (Figure 1).

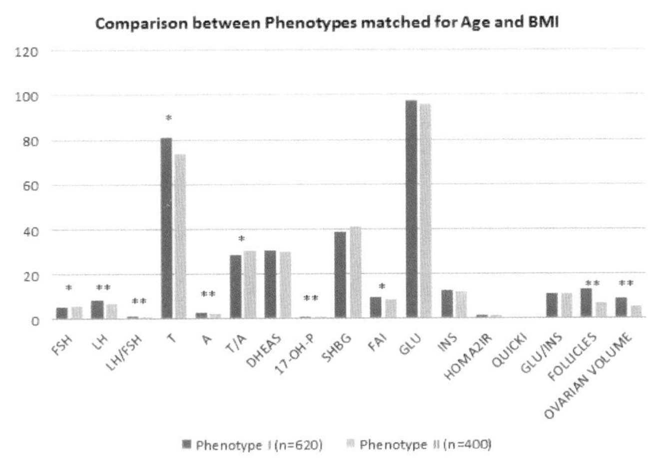

Figure 1: Hormonal, biochemical and ultrasound characteristics of Phenotypes I and II (*$p<0.01$, **$p<0.001$, otherwise p=ns. DHEAS values are multiplied by 0.1).

The effect of PCO morphology and obesity

Normal weight women (Phenotype I vs. Phenotype II)

Hormonal features

Normal weight PCOS women of Phenotype I had higher LH levels ($p<0.001$), lower FSH levels ($p<0.05$) and higher LH/FSH ratio ($p<0.001$) compared with normal weight PCOS patients of Phenotype II (Figure 2).

In addition, normal weight PCOS women of Phenotype I had higher Testosterone ($p<0.05$), Δ4 Androstenedione ($p<0.001$), 17-OH progesterone ($p<0.001$) and Free Androgen Index (FAI) values ($p<0.01$) and lower Testosterone/Δ4 Androstenedione (T/A) ratio ($p<0.001$) (Figure 1), whereas no significant difference in DHEAS and SHBG levels was observed (Figure 2).

Insulin resistance

PCO morphology did not seem to affect insulin resistance in normal weight PCOS subjects, with fasting glucose and insulin, glucose/insulin ratio, QUICKI and HOMA2IR indices presenting no significant differences between the groups (Figure 2).

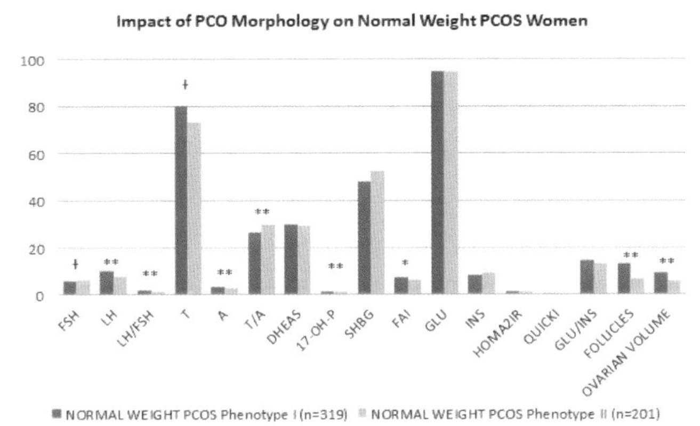

Figure 2: Hormonal, biochemical and ultrasound characteristics of normal weight PCOS women of Phenotypes I and II (*$p<0.01$, **$p<0.001$, ⸸$p<0.05$, otherwise p=ns. DHEAS values are multiplied by 0.1).

Overweight/obese women (Phenotype I vs. Phenotype II)

Hormonal features

Obese PCOS women of Phenotype I had higher LH levels ($p<0.001$) and LH/FSH ratio ($p<0.001$) and a clear tendency for lower FSH levels ($p=0.062$) compared to those of Phenotype II (Figure 3). In addition, they had higher Δ4 Androstenedione levels ($p<0.001$) and marginal differences in Testosterone ($p=0.05$) and 17-OH progesterone levels ($p=0.04$), indicating a tendency towards elevated levels in Phenotype I (Figure 3). On the contrary, no significant difference was found concerning DHEAS and SHBG levels as well as Testosterone/Δ4 Androstenedione (T/A) ratio (Figure 3).

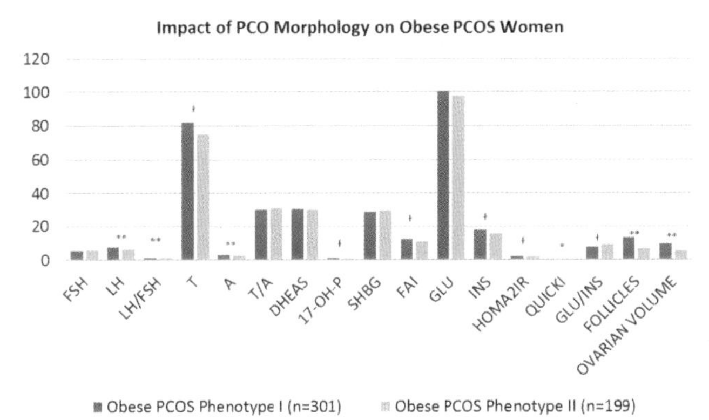

Figure 3: Hormonal, biochemical and ultrasound characteristics of overweight/obese PCOS women of Phenotypes I and II (*$p<0.01$, **$p<0.001$, ⸸$p<0.05$, otherwise p=ns. DHEAS values are multiplied by 0.1).

Insulin resistance

With the exception of fasting glucose levels, all indices of insulin resistance (fasting insulin, fasting glucose/insulin ratio, QUICKI and

HOMA2IR indices) document a greater impairment in insulin sensitivity, implying an association between Phenotype I and insulin resistance in overweight/obese PCOS women (Figure 3).

Ovarian morphology

Finally, as expected by definition of the study groups, women of Phenotype I had increased mean number of follicles ($p<0.001$) and mean ovarian volume ($p<0.001$) compared to patients of Phenotype II, regardless of BMI based sub-classification (Figures 1-3).

Discussion

In the present study, polycystic ovarian morphology (PCO) on ultrasound tended to be associated with increased androgen and LH levels and impaired LH/FSH ratio. When dividing PCOS women into lean and overweight/obese, PCO on ultrasound tended to be associated with increased insulin resistance (IR) in overweight/obese, but not in lean PCOS women.

Strong evidence supports the relationship between ovarian follicle abnormalities and increased androgen levels. Excessive recruitment of small follicles could be attributed to intra-ovarian hyperandrogenism [16]. A positive correlation between the number of follicles of 2-5 mm in diameter and both testosterone and androstenedione levels has been reported [17]. On the other hand, follicular arrest could be indirectly androgen dependent given that follicles of 2-5 mm in diameter have been considered as the strongest independent determinant of follicular arrest. Although testosterone levels have been reported to be significant predictors of increase in stroma amount as well as follicular number and ovarian volume [18], serum testosterone levels have not been shown to be a significant independent determinant of follicular arrest [16]. The latter is contradictory with the established correlation between hyperandrogenemia and oligoanovulation [19]. However, oligomenorrhea has been reported in some patients with PCO without overt hyperandrogenism [20], while normal menstrual cycles occur in patients with PCO and hyperandrogenism [21]. Therefore, it could be speculated that serum hyperandrogenism is not a prerequisite for the existence of intra-ovarian hyperandrogenism. Hyperandrogenism exerts an indirect effect on follicular arrest via 2-5 mm follicle excess [16]. Consequently, follicular number could serve as surrogate for hyperandrogenism and oligoanovulation in PCOS. Biochemical indices of hyperandrogenism that characterize PCOS have been reported to be highly associated with echogenic features of PCO [7,22]. Higher androstenedione levels have been demonstrated in women with PCOS as well as healthy women with PCO as the sole finding compared to women with normal ovaries [23]. Indeed, the results of the present study confirm the above findings by depicting increased serum Testosterone, Δ4 Androstenedione and 17-OH progesterone in PCOS women with PCO morphology compared to PCOS women without PCO.

When dividing PCOS women according to their BMI, a statistically significant strong positive relationship between PCO and indices of insulin resistance in phenotypes I and II was documented in overweight/obese PCOS women. Overweight/obese women with phenotype I had marginally higher circulating androgens than women with phenotype II and appeared to be more insulin resistant than the latter as evidenced by HOMA2IR and QUICKI indices of insulin resistance, as well as by glucose to insulin ratio. The same findings, concerning only the QUICKI index of IR have been documented in a recent study of our group including 1/3 of the women enrolled in the present study [24]. In the present study, the enrolment of larger numbers of PCOS women made this association evident for HOMA2IR as well.

The association between obesity, IR and PCO morphology could be explained by the contributing effect of IR on chronic anovulation of PCOS. Insulin resistance in obese PCOS women could be attributed to obesity as well as PCOS status per se. Insulin, through its own receptor, acts synergistically to LH enhancing steroidogenesis in PCOS theca cells [25], while it is also responsible for the increase of adrenal steroids in PCOS by enhancing the sensitivity of adrenals to ACTH [26]. Actually, hyperinsulinism has been shown to exert both quantitative and qualitative negative effects on the ovulatory status in PCOS. Indices of insulin resistance have been correlated with both reduced proportion of selectable follicles (6-9 mm follicles) and derangement of granulosa cells [16,27]. Furthermore, androgenic effect on excessive recruitment of small follicles has been shown to be mediated by up-regulation of granulosa cell insulin-like growth factor receptor [28]. On the other hand, it seems that hyperinsulinism and/or insulin resistance could not be the primary cause of anovulation of PCOS, since contradictory data dispute the establishment of a strong relationship between hyperinsulinism and anovulation. Consequently, hyperinsulinism and/or insulin resistance has been viewed as an unspecific "second hit" that further worsens follicular arrest [16]. In conditions of severe hyperandrogenism, such as "classical" phenotypes of PCOS, the relationship between insulin resistance and follicular abnormalities seems to be overshadowed by the strong impact of increased androgen levels on follicular arrest and becomes apparent only by the additive effect of obesity.

The role of ovarian ultrasound in the diagnosis of PCOS has been largely debated over the last decade. Although polycystic ovarian morphology was included in the Rotterdam criteria for the definition of the syndrome, many clinicians remain skeptical regarding its significance, as it is a common finding in healthy women (up to 25%) and the documentation of its presence depends on the examiner. Furthermore, the strong correlation of hyperandrogenemia with adverse metabolic outcomes has led to the latter gaining the central role in PCOS diagnostic criteria, with Androgen Excess Society defining PCOS as a "predominantly hyperandrogenic syndrome" in its position statement [29]. However, various studies have proven that polycystic ovarian morphology on ultrasound (PCO) correlates well with serum and, more importantly, intra-ovarian hyperandrogenism which play a key role in follicular arrest and anovulation characterizing PCOS. The results of our study confirm the above, showing a correlation of PCO with more severe hyperandrogenemia in "classical" PCOS phenotypes and with insulin resistance in overweight/obese patients. More studies are needed in order to clarify whether ovarian ultrasound could be useful as a marker of increased risk for adverse hormonal and metabolic parameters in women with "classic" PCOS.

A possible limitation of our study is that, due to limited accuracy of the ultrasound used, we were not able to obtain meaningful measurements from our patients regarding ovarian stroma and stroma/total area to help us classify them to phenotype I or II. Hence, such results are not mentioned.

References

1. Azziz R, Woods KS, Reyna R, Key TJ, Knochenhauer ES, et al. (2004) The prevalence and features of the polycystic ovary syndrome in an unselected population. J Clin Endocrinol Metab 89: 2745-2749.

2. Zawadski JK, Dunaif A (1992) Diagnostic criteria for polycystic ovary syndrome: towards a rational approach. In: Dunaif A, Givens JR, Haseltine FP, Merriam GR (eds.) Polycystic ovary syndrome, Blackwell Scientific Publications, Boston, MA, pp: 377-384.
3. The Rotterdam ESHRE/ASRM-Sponsored PCOS Consensus Workshop Group (2004) Revised 2003 consensus on the diagnostic criteria and long term health risks related to polycystic ovary syndrome. Fertil Steril 81: 19-25.
4. Azziz R (2006) Controversy in clinical endocrinology: diagnosis of polycystic ovarian syndrome: the Rotterdam criteria are premature. J Clin Endocrinol Metab 91: 781-785.
5. Welt CK, Gudmundsson JA, Arason G, Adams J, Palsdottir H, et al. (2006) Characterizing different subsets of polycystic ovary syndrome as defined by the Rotterdam criteria: The impact of weight on phenotype and metabolic features. J Clin Endocrinol Metab 91: 4842-4848.
6. Dunaif A (1997) Insulin resistance and the polycystic ovary syndrome: mechanism and implications for pathogenesis. Endocr Rev 18: 774-800.
7. Panidis D, Tziomalos K, Macut D, Delkos D, Betsas G, et al. (2012) Cross-sectional analysis of the effects of age on the hormonal, metabolic, and ultrasonographic features and the prevalence of the different phenotypes of polycystic ovary syndrome. Fertil Steril 97: 494-500.
8. Dewailly D, Pigny P, Soudan B, Catteau-Jonard S, Decanter C, et al. (2010) Reconciling the definitions of polycystic ovary syndrome: the ovarian follicle number and serum anti-Müllerian hormone concentrations aggregate with the markers of hyperandrogenism. J Clin Endocrinol Metab 95: 4399-4405.
9. Chen Y, Li L, Chen X, Zhang Q, Wang W, et al. (2008) Ovarian volume and follicle number in the diagnosis of polycystic ovary syndrome in Chinese women. Ultrasound Obstet Gynecol 32: 700-703.
10. Balen AH, Laven JS, Tan SL, Dewailly D (2003) Ultrasound assessment of the polycystic ovary: international consensus definitions. Hum Reprod Update 9: 505-514.
11. Fulghesu AM, Ciampelli M, Belosi C, Apa R, Pavone V, et al. (2001) A new ultrasound criterion for the diagnosis of polycystic ovary syndrome: the ovarian stroma/total area ratio. Fertil Steril 76: 326-331.
12. Kiddy DS, Sharp PS, White DM, Scanlon MF, Mason HD, et al. (1990) Differences in clinical and endocrine features between obese and non-obese subjects with polycystic ovary syndrome: an analysis of 263 consecutive cases. Clin Endocrinol (Oxf) 32: 213-220.
13. Tena G, Moran C, Romero R, Moran S (2011) Ovarian morphology and endocrine function in polycystic ovary syndrome. Arch Gynecol Obstet 284: 1443-1448.
14. Ferriman D, Gallwey JD (1961) Clinical assessment of body hair growth in women. J Clin Endocrinol Metab 21: 1440-1447.
15. Vermeulen A, Verdonck L, Kaufman JM (1999) A critical evaluation of simple methods for the estimation of free testosterone in serum. J Clin Endocrinol Metab 84: 3666-3672.
16. Jonard S, Dewailly D (2004) The follicular excess in polycystic ovaries, due to intra-ovarian hyperandrogenism, may be the main culprit for the follicular arrest. Hum Reprod Update 10: 107-117.
17. Dewailly D, Catteau-Jonard S, Reyss AC, Maunoury-Lefebvre C, Poncelet E, et al. (2007) The excess in 2-5 mm follicles seen at ovarian ultrasonography is tightly associated to the follicular arrest of the polycystic ovary syndrome. Hum Reprod 22: 1562-1566.
18. Pache TD, de Jong FH, Hop WC, Fauser BC (1993) Association between ovarian changes assessed by transvaginal sonography and clinical and endocrine signs of the polycystic ovary syndrome. Fertil Steril 59: 544-549.
19. Diamanti-Kandarakis E, Papailiou J, Palimeri S (2006) Hyperandrogenemia: pathophysiology and its role in ovulatory dysfunction in PCOS. Pediatr Endocrinol Rev 3: 198-204.
20. Dewailly D, Catteau-Jonard S, Reyss AC, Leroy M, Pigny P (2006) Oligoanovulation with polycystic ovaries but not overt hyperandrogenism. J Clin Endocrinol Metab 91: 3922-3927.
21. Carmina E, Lobo RA (2001) Polycystic ovaries in Hirsute women with normal menses. Am J Med 111: 602-606.
22. Diamanti-Kandarakis E, Panidis D (2007) Unravelling the phenotypic map of polycystic ovary syndrome (PCOS): a prospective study of 634 women with PCOS. Clin Endocrinol (Oxf) 67: 735-742.
23. Kyei-Mensah AA, LinTan S, Zaidi J, Jacobs HS (1998) Relationship of ovarian stromal volume to serum androgen concentrations in patients with polycystic ovary syndrome. Hum Reprod 13: 1437-1441.
24. Panidis D, Tziomalos K, Misichronis G, Papadakis E, Betsas G, et al. (2012) Insulin resistance and endocrine characteristics of the different phenotypes of polycystic ovary syndrome: a prospective study. Hum Reprod 27: 541-549.
25. Nestler JE, Jakubowicz DJ, de Vargas AF, Brik C, Quintero N, et al. (1998) Insulin stimulates testosterone biosynthesis by human thecal cells from women with polycystic ovary syndrome by activating its own receptor and using inositolglycan mediators as the signal transduction system. J Clin Endocrinol Metab 83: 2001-2005.
26. Moghetti P, Castello R, Negri C, Tosi F, Spiazzi GG, et al. (1996) Insulin infusion amplifies 17a-hydroxycorticosteroid intermediates response to adrenocorticotropin in hyperandrogenic women: apparent relative impairment of 17,20-lyase activity. J Clin Endocrinol Metab 81: 881-886.
27. Welt CK, Taylor AE, Fox J, Messerlian GM, Adams JM, et al. (2005) Follicular arrest in polycystic ovary syndrome is associated with deficient inhibin A and B biosynthesis. J Clin Endocrinol Metab 90: 5582-5587.
28. Vendola K, Zhou J, Wang J, Famuyiwa OA, Bievre M, et al. (1999) Androgens promote oocyte insulin-like growth factor I expression and initiation of follicle development in the primate ovary. Biol Reprod 61: 353-357.
29. Azziz R, Carmina E, Dewailly D, Diamanti-Kandarakis E, Escobar-Morreale HF, et al. (2006) Criteria for defining polycystic ovary syndrome as a predominantly hyperandrogenic syndrome: an Androgen Excess Society guideline. J Clin Endocrinol Metab 91: 4237-4245.

The Best Use of Systemic Corticosteroids in the Intensive Care Units, Review

Mohammad S Abdallah[1*], Ahmad F Madi[2] and Muhammad A Rana[2]

[1]Critical Care Clinical Pharmacist at King Saud Medical City Riyadh, Saudi Arabia

[2]ICU consultant at King Saud Medical City Riyadh, Saudi Arabia

[*]**Corresponding author:** Abdallah Mohammad S, Critical Care Clinical Pharmacist at King Saud Medical City Riyadh, Saudi Arabia, E-mail: mohasulmoha@yahoo.com

Abstract

Corticosteroids are one of the most common medications that are used in the intensive care units (ICUs); corticosteroids are used for a variety of indications, including septic shock, acute respiratory distress syndrome (ARDS), bacterial meningitis, tuberculous meningitis, lupus nephritis, severe chronic obstructive pulmonary disease (COPD) exacerbations and many others.

Corticosteroids are associated with many severe side effects that affect morbidity and mortality of the patients like increased risk of infections, glucose intolerance, hypokalemia, sodium retention, edema, hypertension, myopathy etc. In order to make the best use of these medications and to minimize the unwanted side effects we should follow some particular protocol. Please keep in our mind that there is controversy about dosing and tapering of steroids, so effort has been made to include the best available evidence.

This review discusses mainly the most common indications of corticosteroids in ICU, dosing of corticosteroids in those indications and how to taper corticosteroids according to the best evidence that recommends their use.

Literature search was done using Medline, BMJ, Uptodate, Chochrane database, Google scholar and the best evidence based guidelines in which steroids are recommended to treat ICU related disorders. Sex hormones are not discussed in this review since its use is rare in the intensive care units.

Keywords: Corticosteroids; Tapering; Steroids; Withdrawal symptoms; Intensive care

Abbreviations

ACTH: Adrenocorticotropic Hormone; ARDS: Acute Respiratory Distress Syndrome; COPD: Chronic Obstructive Pulmonary Disease; CSF: *Cerebrospinal Fluid*; ETT: *Endotracheal Tube*; ICU: Intensive Care Unit; IPF: Idiopathic Pulmonary Fibrosis; IV: Intravenous; NIH: National Institutes of Health; PEFR: Peak Expiratory Flow Rate; PO: per os; SLE: *Systemic Lupus Erythematosus*; TB: Tuberculous.

Introduction

Corticosteroids are molecules produced by the adrenal cortex (the outer part of the adrenal gland), Corticosteroids are classified to either glucocorticoids that are produced in response to stress and have important effects on intermediary metabolism and immune function or mineralocorticoids that maintain the balance of salt and water within the body. The major glucocorticoid in humans is cortisol which its release is mainly controlled by adrenocorticotropic hormone (ACTH) and the most important mineralocorticoid is aldosterone which its release is mainly controlled by angiotensin [1]. These medications (glucocorticoids and mineralocorticoids are associated with severe side effects that sometimes cause their discontinuation in many patients.

We observed many times that we are not using these medications properly in patients by using wrong doses of steroids, using inappropriate tapering regimens and sometimes by using steroids for indications that literature does not support their use in such indications. To avoid the recurrence of medication errors and side effects that are associated with corticosteroids we wrote this review that can be used by health care providers who are working in different Intensive Care Units. This review discusses mainly the most common indications of corticosteroids in ICU, dosing of corticosteroids in those indications and how to taper corticosteroids according to the best evidence that recommends their use (Tables 1 and 2).

Compound	Anti-inflammatory of potency	Na retaining potency	Duration of action	Equivalent dose
Cortisol	1	1	S	20
Cortisone	0.8	0.8	S	25

Dexamethasone	25	0	L	0.75
Prednisone	4	0.8	I	5
Prednisolone	4	0.8	I	5
Methyprednisolone	5	0.5	I	4
Triamcinolone	5	0	L	4
Betamethasone	25	0	L	0.75
Equivalent doses apply only to oral or intravenous preparations-S Short (8-12 Hrs), L- Long (36-72 Hrs), and I Intermediate (12-36 Hrs).Prednisone and prednisolone are potent glucocorticoids and weak mineralocorticoids. Methylprednisolone and dexamethasone have no mineralocorticoid effect. NOTE: Glucocorticoid doses which provide a mineralocorticoid effect that is approximately equivalent to 0.1 mg fludrocortisone are: prednisone or prednisolone 50 mg, or hydrocortisone 20 mg. Equivalent dose shown is for oral or IV administration. Relative potency for intra-articular or intramuscular administration may vary considerably. Data for cortisol, endogenous corticosteroid hormone, are included for comparison with synthetic preparations listed. Fludri cortisone is not used for an anti-inflammatory effect its minaralo corticoid activity is 125 and its antiinflamatory activity is 10. Prednisone itself is biologically inactive, but it is rapidly converted to the active form prednisolone. However, patients with severe liver disease may have difficulty converting prednisone to prednisolone; in such patients, it is possible that one might not get the same effect from prednisone as from prednisolone. In addition, certain drug interactions can affect the metabolism and bioavailability of prednisone. As an example, phenytoin, barbiturates or rifampin, attenuate the biological effects of glucocorticoids.				

Table 1: Comparison of various corticosteroids.

Indication of corticosteroids*	**Dosing regimen and tapering §**
1) Septic shock	Hydrocortisone at a dose of 200 mg per day as continuous infusion. Should be tapered when vasopressors are no longer required
2) Airway edema	Dexamethasone is 0.5-2 mg/kg divided over 4-6 hrs started 24 hours before extubation and continued for 24 hours after extubation
3) Spinal cord injury	Methylprednisolone should be initiated within eight hours of injury using an initial bolus of 30 mg/kg by IV for 15 minutes followed 45 minutes later by a continuous infusion of 5.4 mg/kg/hour for 23 hours
4) ARDS	loading dose of 1 mg/kg of methyl prsnisolone followed by an infusion of 1 mg/kg/d from day 1 to day 14, then 0.5 mg/kg/d from day 15 to day 21, then 0.25 mg/kg/d from day 22 to day 25, and finally 0.125 mg/kg/d from day 26 to day 28. In the study if the patient was extubated between days 1 and 14, the patient was advanced to day 15 of drug therapy and tapered according to schedule
5) Bacterial meningitis	Dexamethasone 0.15 mg/kg q6 h for 2–4 days with the first dose administered 10–20 min before, or at least concomitant with, the first dose of antimicrobial therapy
6) Tuberculous (TB) meningitis	Patients with grade II or III disease should receive intravenous treatment of dexamethasone for four weeks (0.4 mg per kilogram per day for the first week, 0.3 mg per kilogram per day for the second week, 0.2 mg per kilogram per day for the third week, and 0.1 mg per kilogram per day for the fourth week) and then oral treatment for four weeks, starting at a total of 4 mg per day and decreasing by 1 mg each week Patients with grade I disease should receive lower dose of intravenous dexamethasone therapy with shorter duration of two weeks (0.3 mg per kilogram per day for the first week and 0.2 mg per kilogram per day for the second week) and then four weeks of oral therapy (0.1 mg per kilogram per day for the third week, then a total of 3 mg per day, decreasing by 1 mg each week)
7) Pneumocystis jirovecii pneumonia	Prednisone 40 mg q 12 hrs *per os* (PO) for 5 days followed by 40 mg q24 hrs PO for 5 days and then 20 mg q24 hrs PO for 11 days
8) Lupus Nephritis	IV pulse methylprednisolone of 1 gram per day for 3 days monthly for 6 months, with 0.5-1.5 mg of oral prednisone per kilogram between pulses
9) COPD exacerbations	Methyl prednisiolone succinate IV 125 mg every 6 hours for 3 days then 60 mg daily for 4 days then 40 mg daily for 4 days then 20 mg daily for 4 days.
10) Asthma exacerbations	120 to 180 mg/day of prednisone, prednisolone, or methylprednisolone in 3 or 4 divided doses for 48 hours and then 60 to 80 mg/day until peak expiratory flow rate (PEFR) reaches 70% of predicted
11) Brain edema.	Dexamethasone with initial dose of 10 mg intravenously or orally, followed by 4 mg every 6 hours Corticosteroids should be tapered within 2 to 3 weeks. This can be done by decreasing the dose by 50% every 4 days
12) Anaphylaxis	Prednisone 1 mg/kg up to 50 mg orally or hydrocortisone 1.5-3 mg/kg IV

13) Pulmonary fibrosis	Methyl prednisiolone pulse therapy (1000 mg/day for 3 days, 500 mg/day for 2 days, 250 mg/day for 2 days, 125 mg/day for 2 days, and 80 mg/day for 2 days), followed by oral prednisolone (1 mg per kilogram per day, reduced by about 20% each week)
14) Thyroid storm	Hydrocortisone 300 mg intravenous loading followed by 100 mg every 8 hours
15) Myxedema	Intravenous hydrocortisone should be given at a dosage of 100 mg every eight hours
16) Brain dead patients that are candidates for organ donation	Methylprednisolone 15 mg/kg IV every 24 hours
* Many other indications of corticosteroids are not covered like autoimmune hemolytic anemia, prevention and treatment of rejection of transplanted organs, hypercalcemia and many others because their incidence in the ICUs is rare. § There is controversy about dosing and tapering of steroids, so effort has been made to include the best available evidence.	

The Most Common Indications of Corticosteroids in ICU

Septic shock

A plenty of data is available in the literature about using and dosing of corticosteroids in septic shock. In this review we included the recommendation of the latest Surviving Sepsis Campaign guideline that was published in Feb.2013. The guideline recommended not using intravenous hydrocortisone to treat adult septic shock patients if adequate fluid resuscitation and vasopressor therapy are able to restore hemodynamic stability. If this case is not achievable, the intravenous hydrocortisone alone at a dose of 200 mg per day as continuous infusion is suggested, repetitive bolus application of hydrocortisone leads to a significant increase in blood glucose; this peak effect was not detectable during continuous infusion [2]. Other recommendations about corticosteroids that were included in the aforementioned guideline were not using the Adrenocorticotropic hormone(ACTH) stimulation test to identify adults with septic shock who should receive hydrocortisone, not using corticosteroids for the treatment of sepsis in the absence of shock and corticosteroids should be tapered when vasopressors are no longer required [2].

Airway edema

Laryngeal edema is one of the most common complications in ICU that can cause stridor, dyspnoea and reintubation. These complications, especially reintubation, can result in many adverse outcomes, including longer hospital stay, higher costs and increased mortality. Risk factors of laryngeal edema and the development of postextubation stridor include older age, female gender, low Glasgow Coma Scale score, excessive *endotracheal tube* (ETT) size, elevated Acute Physiologic and Chronic Health Evaluation II score and a prolonged intubation period (more than 36 hrs) [3].

Corticosteroids (mainly dexamethasone and methylprednisolone) were shown to be effective in decreasing the incidence of postextubation stridor in adult patients at high risk to develop airway obstruction [3].

The dose of dexamethasone is 0.5-2 mg/kg divided over 4-6 hrs started 24 hours before extubation and continued for 24 hours after extubation [4]. Current evidence also suggests that prophylactic intravenous (IV) methylprednisolone therapy (20-40 mg every 4-6 h) should be considered 12-24 hours prior to a planned extubation in patients at high-risk for postextubation laryngeal edema [5].

Usually laryngeal edema occurs within eight hours after extubation, that's why the administration of steroids immediately after extubation might be too late. The benefit of steroids before selected extubation is assumed to be due to protection against or treating mucosal edema in the glottic region caused by pressure or irritation from the endotracheal tube [6].

Spinal cord injury

A phase three randomized trial proved the efficacy of methylprednisolone sodium succinate in enhancing sustained neurologic recovery after spinal cord injury [7]. Methylprednisolone should be initiated within eight hours of injury using an initial bolus of 30 mg/kg by IV for 15 minutes followed 45 minutes later by a continuous infusion of 5.4 mg/kg/hour for 23 hours. If the maintenance therapy is extended for 48 hours, further improvement in motor function recovery has been shown to occur. This is evident when the initial bolus dose could only be administered three to eight hours after the trauma.

ARDS

Corticosteroids were studied to prevent and to treat early and late ARDS. While using corticosteroids in preventing ARDS showed higher mortality and rate of ARDS development, there is a mixed data about its role in treating early ARDS. These drugs have no benefits in late stage of ARDS and are associated with bad outcomes [8].

Since the direction of the systemic inflammatory response is established in the early stage of ARDS, we suggest to use low-dose methylprednisolone (1 mg/kg/d) tested in early ARDS (within 72 h of diagnosis) since it was tested and was shown to down regulate systemic inflammation and lead to earlier resolution of pulmonary organ dysfunction and a reduction in duration of mechanical ventilation and ICU stay according to a randomized controlled trial that was done by Meduri [9].

The regimen that was used in the aforementioned study is the beginning of administration of a loading dose of 1 mg/kg of methyl prsnisolone followed by an infusion of 1 mg/kg/d from day 1 to day 14, then 0.5 mg/kg/d from day 15 to day 21, then 0.25 mg/kg/d from day 22 to day 25, and finally 0.125 mg/kg/d from day 26 to day 28. In the study if the patient was extubated between days 1 and 14, the patient was advanced to day 15 of drug therapy and tapered according to schedule [9].

Bacterial meningitis

Corticosteroids reduce brain edema, intracranial hypertension and meningeal inflammation in experimental models of bacterial meningitis. It is also proven to be associated with reduced mortality and lower frequency of hearing loss and neuropsychological sequelae in adult patients [10].

However, there is a concern about impaired antibiotics penetration as a consequence of dexamethasone therapy [11].

Dexamethasone (0.15 mg/kg q6 h for 2–4 days with the first dose administered 10–20 min before, or at least concomitant with, the first dose of antimicrobial therapy) in adults with suspected or proven pneumococcal meningitis [10]. Dexamethasone should only be continued if the *cerebrospinal fluid* (CSF) Gram stain reveals gram-positive diplococci, or if blood or CSF cultures are positive for S. pneumonia [10].

Adjunctive dexamethasone should not be given to adult patients who have already received antimicrobial therapy [10].

Delayed treatment is not beneficial as dexamethasone does not reverse existing brain edema or intracranial hypertension in later stages of meningitis [11].

Tuberculous meningitis

As in bacterial meningitis corticosteroids are also effective in reducing the risk of death or disabling residual neurological deficit. However, corticosteroids in TB meningitis are used for prolonged period (6 to 8 weeks) rather than 2 to 4 days (as in bacterial meningitis), so all patients with TB meningitis receive adjunctive corticosteroids regardless of disease severity at presentation [12]. Dexamethasone and prednisolone were mainly given for TB meningitis with variable dosing regimens and there is no data from controlled trials comparing different corticosteroid regimens [13].

There is insufficient evidence to recommend routine adjunctive corticosteroids for all patients with tuberculomas without meningitis, or with spinal cord tuberculosis. However, they may be helpful in those patients whose symptoms are not controlled, or are worsening, on anti-tuberculosis therapy, or who have acute spinal cord compression secondary to vertebral tuberculosis [12].

Patients with grade II or III disease should receive intravenous treatment of dexamethasone for four weeks (0.4 mg per kilogram per day for the first week, 0.3 mg per kilogram per day for the second week, 0.2 mg per kilogram per day for the third week, and 0.1 mg per kilogram per day for the fourth week) and then oral treatment for four weeks, starting at a total of 4 mg per day and decreasing by 1 mg each week [12].

Patients with grade I disease should receive lower dose of intravenous dexamethasone therapy with shorter duration of two weeks (0.3 mg per kilogram per day for the first week and 0.2 mg per kilogram per day for the second week) and then four weeks of oral therapy (0.1 mg per kilogram per day for the third week, then a total of 3 mg per day, decreasing by 1 mg each week) [12].

Corticosteroids are not recommended in other forms of Tuberculosis except in tuberculous pericarditis where some evidence suggests its use in this indication [14].

Pneumocystis jirovecii pneumonia

Corticosteroids are used as adjunctive initial therapy only in patients with HIV infection who have severe *P* jirovecii pneumonia as defined by an arterial-alveolar O2 gradient that exceeds 35 mm Hg or a room air arterial oxygen pressure of less than 70 mm Hg or. In patients without HIV infection adjunctive steroids are not recommended [15].

During antimicrobial therapy microbial degradation and clearance may result in further inflammation that can exacerbate a severe inflammatory response that includes the production of cytokines and other inflammatory markers and cells to dying organisms in the lungs that often worsens after therapy is begun. Adjunctive steroids can blunt this inflammatory response that result in lung tissue damage [15]. Consequently, this will lead to good outcomes by improving survival, decreasing episodes of respiratory decompensation and decreasing the need for mechanical ventilation.

Prednisone 40 mg q 12 hrs *per os* (PO) for 5 days followed by 40 mg q24 hrs PO for 5 days and then 20 mg q24 hrs PO for 11 days [15].

Methylprednisolone at 75% of the respective prednisolone dose should be administered if intravenous therapy is necessary [15].

Lupus Nephritis

Corticosteroid therapy is a major component in therapeutic regimens for *systemic lupus erythematosus* (SLE). It is known to suppress the clinical expression of disease and is considered by many to be a major factor in the improved survival and prognosis. Although most clinical trials of corticosteroid therapy in SLE patients have been conducted in patients with severe lupus nephritis, the evidence suggests that they are also effective in the treatment of severe and life threatening cases of, pneumonitis, polyserositis, vasculitis, thrombocytopenia, CNS disease and other clinical manifestations [16].

The IV pulse methylprednisolone is used for life- or organ-threatening disease which is defined by courses of 1 gram per day for 3 days monthly for 6 months, with 0.5-1.5 mg of oral prednisone per kilogram between pulses, to control both renal and extra-renal manifestations. It is usually used as initial management of active nephritis, sole therapy to avoid cumulative adverse effects of long-term daily corticosteroid therapy, or regimen for exacerbations of severe cases not responsive to daily oral steroids [17,18].

Severe COPD exacerbations

Intravenous corticosteroids are helpful in the treatment of severe exacerbations of COPD. Corticosteroid therapy can improve lung function (FEV1) and hypoxemia (PaO2), reduces recovery time, ICU stay, cost of admission and may reduce the risk of early relapse [19]. The optimal dose and duration of steroids in COPD exacerbations are unknown. According to a recent meta-analysis the low-dose regimen (initial dose 30-80 mg/day of prednisolone) is proper for treating COPD exacerbations. However, the high-dose group did not show obviously higher risk of side effects [20].

We included the recommendation of the Systemic Corticosteroids in Chronic Obstructive Pulmonary Disease Exacerbations (SCCOPE) trial [21].

Methylprednisiolone succinate IV 125 mg every 6 hours for 3 days than 60 mg daily for 4 days than 40 mg daily for 4 days than 20 mg daily for 4 days.

Severe asthma exacerbation

In severe asthma there is airway obstruction and airway inflammation. In order to reduce the inflammation systemic corticosteroids must be included as part of the regimen in all patients with acute severe asthma.

Receptor-binding affinities of lung corticosteroid receptors are reduced in the face of airway inflammation, that's why multiple daily dosing of systemic corticosteroids for the initial therapy of acute asthma exacerbations appears necessary. As in severe COPD exacerbations, the optimal dose and duration of steroids in severe asthma exacerbations are unknown. The oral and IV routes are equally effective, so that the oral route may be used if patients can swallow. However, in ICU settings patients are intubated and mechanically ventilated so we prefer to use the intravenous form [16].

Regarding the duration a 7 day-day course in adults has been found to be as effective as 14-day course [22].

The National Institutes of Health (NIH) guidelines recommend 120 to 180 mg/day of prednisone, prednisolone, or methylprednisolone in 3 or 4 divided doses for 48 hours and then 60 to 80 mg/day until peak expiratory flow rate (PEFR) reaches 70% of predicted. The anti-inflammatory effect of corticosteroids as measured by improvement in pulmonary function is not immediate and can take up to 24 hours to occur [23].

Brain edema

Four types of cerebral edema are present: the vasogenic cerebral edema that results from an increased permeability of the endothelium of cerebral capillaries to albumin and other plasma proteins due to the breakdown of the tight endothelial junctions; the cytotoxic cerebral edema in which the blood brain barrier is not affected but there is imbalance in cellular metabolism that weaken the functioning of the sodium and potassium pump in the glial cell membrane; the osmotic cerebral edema that results when the blood becomes diluted; and the interstitial cerebral edema that result in obstructive hydrocephalus

Glucocorticoids are very effective in reducing the vasogenic edema that occurs in many clinical conditions like inflammatory conditions, tumors, and other disorders. However, steroids are not helpful to treat cytotoxic edema and are harmful in patients with brain ischemia [24]. In patients with severe head injury the use of glucocorticoids are not recommended for improving outcome or reducing *Intracranial pressure (*ICP) [25].

Dexamethasone is the preferred agent due to its very low mineralocorticoid activity. The usual initial dose is 10 mg intravenously or orally, followed by 4 mg every 6 hours [25].

Corticosteroids should be tapered within 2 to 3 weeks. This can be done by decreasing the dose by 50% every 4 days [25].

Anaphylaxis

There are many theoretical benefits of using steroids in patients with anaphylaxis. However, there are no placebo-controlled trials to confirm these assumed benefits of steroids in anaphylaxis. The use of prednisone 1 mg/kg up to 50 mg orally or hydrocortisone 1.5-3 mg/kg IV is suggested [26].

Pulmonary fibrosis

The latest international evidence-based guideline on the diagnosis and management of idiopathic pulmonary fibrosis (IPF) that was published in 2011 recommended against the use of corticosteroid monotherapy in patients with IPF. Also the recommendation for corticosteroids in patients with acute exacerbation of IPF is weak; that is, corticosteroids should be used in the majority of patients with acute exacerbation of IPF, but not using corticosteroids may be a reasonable choice in a minority [27]. Corticosteroids (e.g. prednisone, methylprednisolone) are used in the majority of patients who suffer an acute exacerbation of IPF, usually in pulse doses. We recommend using methyl prednisiolone pulse therapy (1000 mg/day for 3 days, 500 mg/day for 2 days, 250 mg/day for 2 days, 125 mg/day for 2 days, and 80 mg/day for 2 days), followed by oral prednisolone (1 mg per kilogram per day, reduced by about 20% each week) [28].

Thyroid storm

The benefits of steroids in thyroid storm are mainly blocking T4-to-T3 conversion and prophylaxis against relative adrenal insufficiency.

Hydrocortisone 300 mg intravenous loading followed by 100 mg every 8 hours [29].

Myxedema

In myxedema there is a possibility of secondary hypothyroidism and associated hypopituitarism, so hydrocortisone should be administered until adrenal insufficiency is excluded. Intravenous hydrocortisone should be given at a dosage of 100 mg every eight hours. Not treating adrenal insufficiency with hydrocortisone may precipitate adrenal crisis. Before therapy a random cortisol level should be drawn, and if not depressed, the hydrocortisone can be stopped without tapering [30].

Brain dead patients who are candidates for organ donation

Methylprednisolone 15 mg/kg IV every 24 hours as part of the triple hormonal therapy that includes the use of levothyroxine and vasopressin infusion [31].

Conclusions

Corticosteroids are one of the most common medications that are used for a variety of indications in the intensive care units. Due to the diverse adverse effects of corticosteroids that affect the morbidity and mortality of critically ill patients and because of the high number of medication errors that are associated with these medications, we wrote this review that can be used as a guide for health care professionals who are taking care of critically ill patients that are receiving corticosteroids. This review covers mainly the most common indications of corticosteroids in ICU and also how to taper corticosteroids according to the best evidence that recommends their use. Many other indications of corticosteroids are not covered like autoimmune hemolytic anemia, prevention and treatment of rejection of transplanted organs, hypercalcemia and many others because their incidence in the ICUs is rare.

Competing Interests

The authors declare no financial, professional, political, personal, religious, ideological, academic, intellectual, commercial or other relationship that would be a conflict of interest in the interpretation of any information related to this review.

References

1. Katzung BG (2007) Basic and Clinical Pharmacology. (10th edn). New York, NY: McGraw-Hill Companies Inc.
2. Dellinger RP, Levy MM, Rhodes A , Annane D, Gerlach H, et al. (2013) Surviving Sepsis Campaign: International Guidelines for Management of Severe Sepsis and Septic Shock. Critical Care Medicine 41: 580-637.
3. Lee CH, Peng MJ, Wu CL (2007) Dexamethasone to prevent postextubation airway obstruction in adults: a prospective, randomized, double-blind, placebo-controlled study. Critical Care 11: R72.
4. Lacy CF, Armstrong LL, Goldman MP, Leonard L (2010) Lance:Drug Information Handbook, 18th ed. Hudson, Ohio, Lexi-Comp, Inc.
5. Roberts RJ, Welch SM, Devlin JW (2008) Corticosteroids for Prevention of Postextubation Laryngeal Edema in Adults. Ann Pharmacother 42: 686-691.
6. Fan T, Wang G, Mao B, Xiong Z, Zhang Y, Liu X, Wang L, Yang S (2008) Prophylactic administration of parenteral steroids for preventing airway complications after extubation in adults: meta-analysis of randomised placebo controlled trials. BMJ 337:a1841.
7. Bracken MB, Shepard MJ, Collins WF, Holford TR, Young W, et al. (1990) A randomized, controlled trial of methylprednisolone or naloxone in the treatment of acute spinal-cord injury. Results of the Second National Acute Spinal Cord Injury Study. NEngl J Med 322: 1405-1411.
8. Khilnani GC, Hadda V (2011) Corticosteroids and ARDS: A review of treatment and prevention evidence. Lung India 28: 114–119.
9. Meduri GU, Golden E, Freire AX, Taylor E, Zaman M, et al. (2007) Methylprednisolone Infusion in Early Severe ARDS. CHEST 131: 954-963.
10. Tunkel AR, Hartman BJ, Kaplan SL, et al. (2004) Practice Guidelines for the Management of Bacterial Meningitis. Clinical Infectious Diseases 39: 1267–1284.
11. Hoffman O and Weber RJ (2009) Review: Pathophysiology and treatment of bacterial meningitis. TherAdvNeurolDisord 2: 401-412.
12. Thwaites G, Fisher M, Hemingway C, Scott G, Solomon T, et al. (2009) British Infection Society guidelines for the diagnosis and treatment of tuberculosis of the central nervous system in adults and children. Journal of Infection 59: 167-187.
13. Prasad K, Singh MB (2008) Corticosteroids for managing tuberculous meningitis. Cochrane Database of Systematic Reviews, Issue 1.
14. Mayosi BM (2002) Interventions for treating tuberculous pericarditis. Cochrane Database of Systematic Reviews, Issue 4.
15. Jose G Castro, Maya Morrison-Bryant (2010) Management of Pneumocystis Jiroveciipneumonia in HIV infected patients: current options, challenges and future directions. HIV/AIDS - Research and Palliative Care 2: 123–134.
16. Dipiro J, Talbert B, Yee GC, Matzke GR, Wells BG, Posey LM (2008) Pharmacotherapy: A Pathophysiologic Approach, 7th edition, New York, McGraw-Hill
17. Paget SA, Gibofsky A, Beary JF (2000) Manual of Rheumatology & Outpatient Orthopedic Disorders. Lippincott Williams & Wilkins
18. Sinha A, Bagga A (2008) Pulse steroid therapy. Indian Journal of Pediatrics 75: 1057-1066.
19. (2014) Management of exacerbations: GOLD (Global Initiative for Chronic Obstructive Lung Disease)
20. Cheng T, Gong Y, Guo Y, Cheng Q, Zhou M, Shi G, Wan H (2013) Systemic corticosteroid for COPD exacerbations, whether the higher dose is better? A meta-analysis of randomized controlled trials. ClinRespir J 7: 305-318.
21. Erbland ML, Deupree RH, Niewoehner DE (1998) Systemic Corticosteroids in Chronic Obstructive Pulmonary Disease Exacerbations (SCCOPE): rationale and design of an equivalence trial. Veterans Administration Cooperative Trials SCCOPE Study Group. Control Clin Trials 19: 404-417.
22. Hasegawa T, Ishihara K, Takakura S, Fujii H, Nishimura T, Okazaki M, Katakami N, et al. (2000) Duration of systemic corticosteroids in the treatment of asthma exacerbation; a randomized study. Intern Med 39: 794-797.
23. National Asthma Education and Prevention Program. Clinical practice guidelines: expert panel report. Guidelines for the diagnosis and management of asthma. Bethesda (MD): National Institutes of Health, National Heart, Lung, and Blood Institute. 1997. Publication No. 97–4051.
24. Rabinstein AA (2006) Treatment of Cerebral Edema. The Neurologist 12: 59-73.
25. Kaal EC, Vecht CJ (2004) The management of brain edema in brain tumors. Current Opinion in Oncology 16: 593-600.
26. Brown AFT (2009) Current management of anaphylaxis. Emergencias 21: 213-223.
27. Raghu G, Collard HR, Egan JJ, Martinez FJ, Behr J, et al. (2011) An Official ATS/ERS/JRS/ALAT Statement: Idiopathic Pulmonary Fibrosis: Evidence-based Guidelines for Diagnosis and Management. American Journal Of Respiratory And Critical Care Medicine 183: 788-824.
28. Horita N, Akahane M, Okada Y, Kobayashi Y, Arai T, et al. (2011) Tacrolimus and Steroid Treatment for Acute Exacerbation of Idiopathic Pulmonary Fibrosis. Intern Med 50: 189-195.
29. Bahn RS , Burch HB, Cooper DS, Garber JR, M. Greenlee MC, et al. (2011) Hyperthyroidism Management Guidelines. EndocrPract 17: 3.
30. Wall CR (2000) Myxedema Coma: Diagnosis and Treatment. AmFam Physician 62: 2485-2490.
31. Shemie SD, Ross H, Pagliarello J, Baker AJ, Greig PD, et al. (2006) Organ donor management in Canada: recommendations of the forum on Medical Management to Optimize Donor Organ Potential. CMAJ 174:S13-32.

Stabilizing Motor Reflexive Activation and Acute Growth Hormone Response: A Systematic Review

John Jaquish*, **Henry Alkire and Kevin Hoesley**

American Bone Health, Oakland, California, USA

***Corresponding author:** Jaquish J, American Bone Health, Oakland, California, USA, E-mail: john@jirinstitute.com

Abstract

Objective: Evaluating reflexive (II and Ia afferent) body-stabilizing activity as a possible mechanism regulating hGH levels.

Data Sources: The authors searched MEDLINE, PubMed, Harvard HOLLIS, and EMBASE databases for studies published through 1 January 2016 by using such terms as: vibration, stability, and human growth hormone.

Study Selection: The authors included randomized, controlled trials and randomized pre-post observational trials that compared acute alterations of hGH in humans with both genders spanning from post-pubescence to elderly populations.

Data Extraction: Three authors independently reviewed articles and abstracted data.

Data Synthesis: PRISMA guidelines were followed with 17 articles describing 24 unique study populations meeting the inclusion criteria. A total of 265 participants who engaged in a destabilizing intervention were assayed both against baseline and control (when present). Populations varied in age, with all populations having a mean age of 35.1 [SD, 13.6], and RCTs of 41.6 [SD, 17.2], with the youngest population being 17.8 [SD, 0.88], and the oldest being 70 [SD, 8.8]. Subjects saw acute increases from pre-to-post of 647% [95% CI, 541% to 753%] (P=0.00001). Test group subjects compared to those subjected to control interventions increased hGH levels by 101% [95% CI, 85.7% to 116%] (P=0.006). Statistical analysis excluded one study that altered its blood sample concentrations via centrifuge.

Conclusions: The literature published on randomized, controlled trials and randomized acute evaluations of reflexive stability recruitment of muscle and hGH in multiple populations is limited but suggests that there is an association with whole body stability firing and hGH levels. On the basis of this evidence, interventions that encourage increases in whole body stability firing can be recommended to illicit increases in hGH levels.

Keywords: Pituitary axis; Muscle afferents; Human growth hormone; Hormone regulation

Introduction

While the link between physical activity and acute growth hormone response has been recognized since the 1960s [1,2], the results of analysis such as that performed by Shaner and researchers in 2014 demonstrates a marked increase over control subjects in hGH excitatory effect for exercises requiring self-stabilization from the subject compared to exercises without that requirement [3]. Further, a functional activity such as sprinting compared with endurance focused running has been shown to correlate with a greater hGH response of 82% [4] and 231% in earlier analysis [5]. Sprint type activity has been established to recruit the afferent stabilizing firing of muscle, further suggesting an hGH axis and stability firing relationship [6].

The relationship between hGH levels and stabilization was more precisely indicated by McCall, et al. [7], where it was demonstrated that the use of forced mechanical vibration to destabilize the tibialis anterior muscle produces an increase in plasma levels of bio-assayable hGH. Notably McCall observes that levels of bioassayable hGH are not affected by stimulation of the soleous muscle. While McCall postulates that there is an excitatory effect for the production of this hormone in response to the recruitment of type I and IIa muscle spindle afferents through destabilization, the researchers also note that this excitatory activation may not be present in all muscles and may even be inhibitory in some cases.

The identification of a relationship between a form of hGH secretion and the activation of muscle afferents through destabilization of the tibialis anterior raises a question as to whether those results underlie a generic principle such that the application of destabilizing environments to all of the muscles in the body (and thus to all muscle spindle afferents) has a combined effect, excitatory or otherwise on the plasma levels of hGH.

The authors performed a systematic review and meta-analysis to evaluate existing data describing hGH serum level changes when a test subject's entire body is exposed to a destabilizing environment. Both pre to post observational trials and controlled experiments with a placebo group were considered. Changes in serum hGH post-intervention or differences in hGH levels between treatment groups and control groups, as applicable by study type were evaluated. Analysis was performed to determine the impact of whole body muscle destabilization on hGH levels as illustrated by the body of currently published research.

Methods

Literature search

The authors developed a search strategy for identifying pertinent studies available on the MEDLINE, PubMed, Harvard HOLLIS, or EMBASE databases. Studies published through January 1, 2016 that were published in English or available in an English translation were queried using the search terms: "vibration," "stability," and "human growth hormone."

Study selection

Two kinds of randomized trials were selected: First, observational studies where serum hGH was measured before and immediately after the subject experienced a destabilizing intervention. Second, controlled studies where hGH was measured for a test group subjected to destabilizing intervention (and in some cases a concurrent self-stabilized exercise) and for a control group that was not subject to the destabilization based intervention. Data sets were excluded if motorized vibratory method was of imperceptible magnitude, and therefore reflected a stimulus too weak to achieve stabilizing activation of muscle afferents, which is the potential mechanism of action under analysis.

Data abstraction

All three authors independently reviewed the studies for compliance with selection criteria and then abstracted data for the analysis. These data were compared and resolved by repeated review.

Data abstracted

Authors abstracted data on each study including all reported hGH serum concentrations and standard deviations thereof, the number of study participants, the mean age of participants and the standard deviation of that average, the gender of participants, and whether any conflict of interest was disclosed. For included studies all of the above data was available.

Quantitative data synthesis

When evaluating changes in hGH concentration between pre-to-post measurements of that metric for observational studies, we considered the results of each study using that change represented as a percentage of the mean pre value. The change was evaluated as a percentage of baseline because hGH concentrations measured prior to the destabilizing intervention varied tremendously between studies, regardless of the age of the participants. This suggested that the sensitivities of the hGH blood-work assays used may not have been consistent across different studies, while presumably being consistent within studies. Likewise, a similar potential exists for other variables impacting the value in certain studies, such as the protocol used in the centrifugal preparation of serum samples implemented in some studies but not described in detail. The PRISMA method of systematic review was followed in this analysis [8].

Results were evaluated for controlled studies using the same percentage type hGH metric, where the difference between mean test values and mean control values in each study was represented by that difference in means as a percentage of the mean control hGH level for the same study.

Pre-to-post observational studies were evaluated separately from controlled studies, and the results are averaged separately. When evaluating average impacts for either set of studies, mean percent changes were weighted based on the number of study participants. 95% Confidence Intervals were calculated from standard deviations using a Z critical value of 1.96.

Because only one study disclosed a conflict of interest, and that study yielded results that were very similar to other studies in its category, no penalty was applied to it in the calculation of average hGH concentration change for that category. That study is, however, designated as subject to conflict of interest in the results section where its results are depicted graphically and numerically alongside all other studies.

Results

Participants in evaluated studies varied widely in age. For pre-to-post observational studies participants had a mean age of 35.1 [SD, 13.6]. The youngest of those study populations had a mean age of 17.8 [SD,0.88], and the oldest mean age was 70 [SD, 9.5]. For controlled studies the mean age was 41.6 [SD,17.2]. The youngest and oldest study population mean ages remained 17.8 [SD,0.88] and 70 [SD,9.5], respectively. Women comprised 23% of pre-to-post study population and 18% of controlled study population (Figure 1).

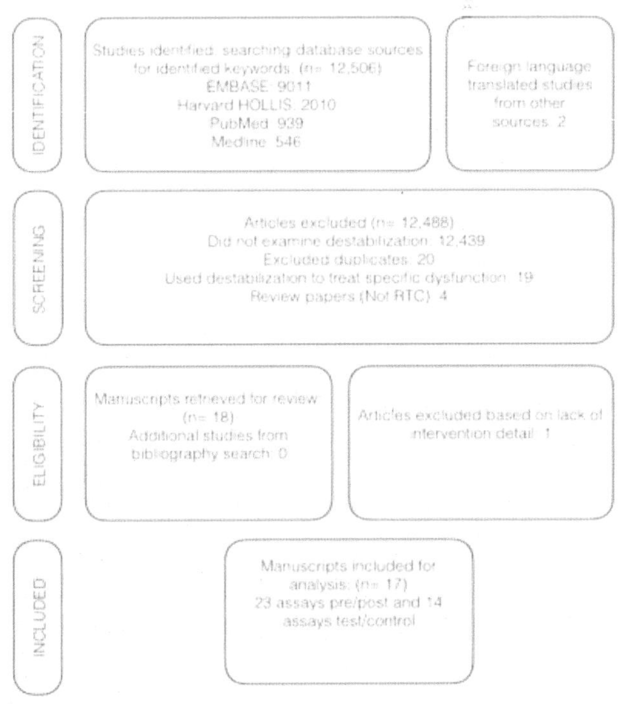

Figure 1: Study Selection Screening

Study characteristics

Only one study fulfilled all evaluated study criteria/characteristics per Table 1, although all studies fulfilled at least two criteria and the mean number of criteria met by included studies was 4.1 out of 7 possible. Because some studies evaluated were pre-to-post observational, and the quality requirements indicated in Table 1 favor controlled studies, they are not universally satisfied.

Most studies were small, with mean size of 11 participants at completion. Study retention rates were high, with 98.3% of participants overall following through to completion of the study. No adverse events were reported. Destabilizing environments implemented in the evaluated studies were created using forced mechanical vibration in all cases. Destabilization characteristics varied significantly, with frequencies ranging from 12 Hz (Rahman) to 300 Hz (Iodice) and magnitudes as large as 5 mm (Sartorio) and as small as 1 mm (Fricke).

Study	Were Eligibility Requirements Stated?	Was a Placebo Offered?	Did Test and Control Group Members have Similar Baseline Characteristics?	Were Participants Blinded?	Unbiased analysis?	Were Clinicians Blinded?	Was Destabilization Protocol Clearly Defined using Quantifiable Metrics?
Bosco et al. [9]	•	○	N/A	○	○	○	•
Cardinale et al. [10]	•	•	•	•	•	○	•
DiLoreto et al. [11]	•	•	•	---	•	○	•
DiGimiani et al. [12]	•	•	•	•	•	•	•
Elmantazer, et al. [13]	•	○	N/A	○	•	○	•
Fricke et al. [14]	•	○	N/A	○	•	○	•
Goto et al. [15]	•	○	N/A	○	•	○	•
Guinta et al. [16]	•	○	N/A	○	•	○	○
Guinta et al. [17]	•	•	•	○	•	○	○
Guo-Shing et al. [18]	•	•	•	---	•	○	○
Iodice et al. [19]	•	•	•	---	•	○	•
Kvorning et al. [20]	•	•	•	---	•	○	•
McCall et al.	•	○	N/A	○	•	○	•
Rahman et al. [21]	•	•	•	---	•	○	○
Sartorio et al. [22]	•	•	•	○	•	○	•
Seok et al. [23]	•	•	•	---	•	○	---
Legend: •=Yes; ○=No; ---=Unclear							

Table 1: Study Criteria/Characteristics.

Quantitative data synthesis

Observational pre/post: All studies report hGH serum values, as this was a prerequisite for study consideration. For the 22 pre-to-post test groups evaluated, every sample indicated an increase in serum growth hormone following the intervention, and showed statistical significance ($p<0.05$) independently. Intervention characteristic matrices found in Appendix 1 and Appendix 2.

The mean change in hGH level was 647% [95% CI, 541% to 753%] (P=0.00001) for all of the assays combined. Mean change analysis excluded one study that altered its blood sample concentrations via centrifuge (McCall). The least hGH response was seen in Cardinale et al., (mean increase of 64.7%), and the greatest was from Kvorning et al (mean increase of 2800%) (Figure 2).

RTCs: For the RCTs, the mean increase in GH was 101% [95% CI, 85.7% to 116%] (P 0.006). Of the 13 RCTs evaluated here, three studies showed increases that were not statistically significant individually, while the remaining 10 studies indicated significant increases. The greatest mean change in serum concentration for any study group was 318% (Kvorning) (Figure 3).

Limitations

Some of the included controlled studies had stability firing type activity as a control intervention (e.g., free-weight squat exercises). The objective of this analysis was to determine the relationship between specific reflexive (Il and Ia afferent) body-stabilizing firing and hGH levels, and since these control data sets may have elicited increases in hGH by this same mechanism, resulting findings are less impactful. Most of the studies included small sample sizes and most studies applied interventions to younger populations.

Safety of the Intervention

No adverse events were documented during any study.

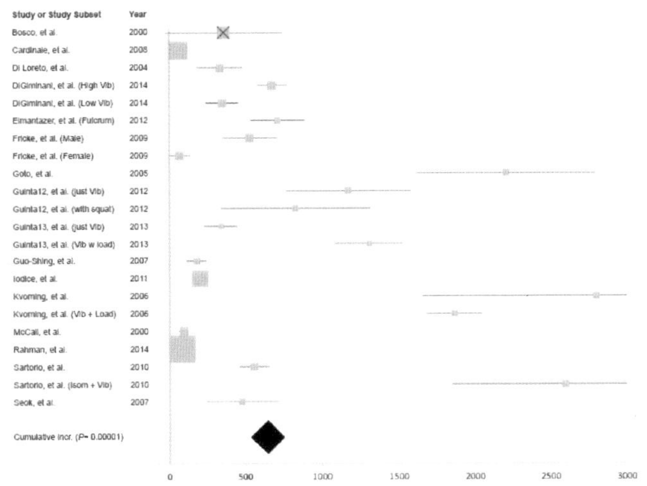

Figure 2: Pre/Post forest plot.

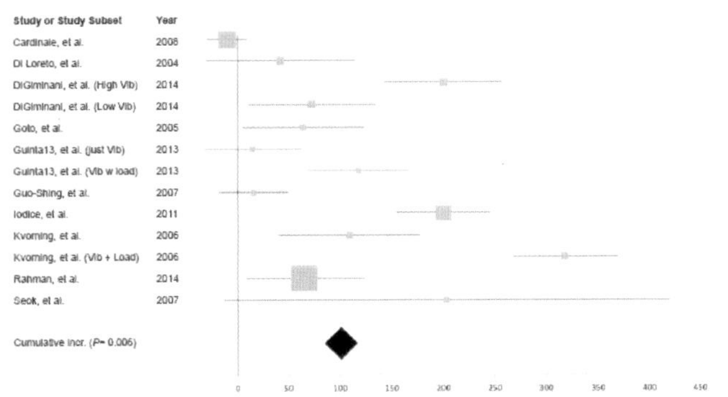

Figure 3: RTC forest plot.

Discussion

It has long been established that exercise causes an acute release of hGH, but the underlying mechanism (or mechanisms) remain unclear. Existing literature review on the physiological processes underlying hGH release during exercise by Godfrey et al. hypothesizes a muscle afferent pituitary axis [24]. For hGH as measured through standard immunoassays Godfrey found that most studies evaluated in the analysis indicate that hGH release occurs following exercise of sufficient intensity, which is consistent with possible muscle afferent neural modulation of the pituitary, but is not sufficient evidence to rule out other exercise related physiological changes as possible signaling mechanisms, such as Catecholamine or lactate release, pH balance changes, or especially Nitric Oxide release. This inability to more narrowly characterize a physiological mechanism in the Godfrey analysis is a result of the conventional exercise protocols that were assayed, because these would be expected to simultaneously induce activity in all of the aforementioned signaling mechanisms. The unique data set considered in Godfrey's review that avoided this problem, is the McCall, et al. data involving destabilization of individual muscles in situ using forced mechanical vibrations. That study demonstrated significant increases in isoforms of hGH, but only involved the destabilization of individual muscles, effectively isolating a destabilizing environment for study of attenuating afferent muscle activation and hGH.

As the mechanism of interest is the stabilizing firing of muscle afferents, particularly those associated with fast-twitch muscles, this analysis identified studies with destabilizing-environment interventions. Thus while the evaluation was not deliberately construed so as to only involve a single modality, the unique intervention available in current research which met these criteria was that wherein the subject stood on a destabilizing surface. Vibratory destabilization interventions are particularly appropriate as McCall's research, the inspiration for this analysis, used this modality to elicit the hypothesized reflexive firing of muscle afferents and associated hGH release.

The destabilizing environments applied during the various studies evaluated herein varied tremendously in magnitude and frequency. This contributes greatly to the evidentiary quality of the data in the context of testing the hypothesis that stabilizing muscle afferent activation leads to hGH release, since that premise should be tested with a heterogeneous variety of destabilizing stimuli to understand a general relationship between that kind of stimuli and corresponding serum hGH level release. This also helps avoid falsely generalizing an effect only present with some single specific pattern of vibration. In fact, despite the wide variety of destabilizing protocols used to obtain the evaluated data, across 24 test groups and nearly as many distinct (albeit similar) treatment protocols, three failed to demonstrate significance. However, these three did show a mean increase in hGH levels vs control. Further, the three test cohorts vs control groups that did not reach significance are from small datasets which likely demonstrate a lack of significance only for the lack of a larger sample size.

It is also apparent that pre-to-post delta values for serum hGH levels are much greater than equivalent values comparing test and control groups in the controlled studies. This is consistent with the current understanding of exercise triggered hGH release, possibly due to some controlled studies using alternative exercise as a placebo treatment where the alternative exercise either included a self-stabilization component or was an entirely self-stabilized exercise, both of which would potentially trigger muscle afferents similar but less so than that of the test interventions. Thus the very large changes in serum hGH levels seen in the pre-to-post literature are more telling in the context of our hypothesis.

Variance of increase in hGH were seen with the lowest response at 64.7% (Cardinale), and the greatest at 2800% (Kvorning). The differences in protocol were pronounced as well. The Cardinale protocol included two legs with slight knee flexion for 1-minute bouts. Kvorning applied instability to two subject cohorts that both maintained a two-legged 90-degree knee bend for 30 seconds per bout. One subject cohort used a weighted bar resting stabilized behind the neck, weighing 80% of the subjects 1 rep maximum, and the other alternate cohort held a wooden broomstick handle on their shoulders. While the weighted bar destabilized cohort showed the greatest increase of hGH at 2800%, the near weightless wooden broomstick handle cohort produced an increase of 1865%. Though EMG levels were not measured in either intervention, the afferent activation is known to be greater with a deeper knee bend. The Cardinale protocol placed little demand on muscle afferents, as the positioning of the subjects was slightly greater than that of tonic contraction, and thereby would be expected to elicit a lesser response. The contrast between these two data sets and assay modalities may strengthen indications of a stability firing mechanism as the source of the contrast between the lowest response at 64.7%, and the greatest at 2800%.

Although study characteristics do not score highly on the criteria metrics, that does not detract from the value of the current volume of research into this matter. Specifically, pre-to post literature is not controlled, or blinded, which leads to low scores on our metric even for well-conducted studies with no bias or conflict of interest declared. Only hGH serum levels were evaluated which are a quantifiable biochemical metric measured by immunoassay where results are observed by computer measurement of permeability to electromagnetic radiation. Therefore, selection bias on the part of the researchers seems unlikely. Further, deliberate auto-regulation of hGH by a human as a result of the placebo effect or otherwise has never been demonstrated, so it would not diminish the value of the hypothesized mechanism if it were the case that subjects increase their hGH levels only in presence of a known destabilizing environment.

By combining all the data available there is a stronger indication of a relationship between afferent stability firing and acute hGH increases than was previously understood.

Role of the Funding Sources

The authors were supported by Performance Health Systems LLC, The funding source had no role in the design, collection, or reporting of the data or study, or in the decision to submit the analysis for publication.

Appendix

Study	Year	Ctrl	Baseline GH	Post Test GH	Delta GH	Sample Size	Participant Age	M/F	Bias	Notes
Bosco et al. [9]	2000	N	6.2 ± 16.2 ng/ml	28.6 ± 29.6 ng/ml	+22.4 ± 45.8 ng/ml	14	25 ± 4.6	14/0	Y	
Cardinal et al. [10]	2008	Y	1.6 ± .3 μIU/ml	2.7 ± 0.7 μIU/ml	+1.1 ± 1 μIU/ml	20	70 (66,85)	9/11	N	
Di Loreto et al. [11]	2004	Y	1.7 ± 0.6 μIU/ml	7.4 ± 3.6 μIU/ml	+5.7 ± 4.2 μIU/ml	10	39 ± 3	10/0	N	
DiGiminani et al. [12]	2014	Y	50 ± 20 nM	390 ± 60 nM	+340 ± 80 nM	10	25 ± 0.9	10/0	N	
DiGiminaniet al. [12]	2014	Y	50 ± 20 nM	225 ± 70 nM	+175 ± 90 nM	10	25 ± 0.9	10/0	N	
Elmantazer et al. [13]	2012	N	0.07 ± 0.1 ng/ml	0.57 ± 0.1 ng/ml	+0.5 ± 0.2 ng/ml	10	33 (29,49)	10/0	N	
Fricke et al. [14] (Male)	2009	N	0.250 ± 0.216 ng/ml	1.58 ± 0.51 ng/ml	+1.33 ± .726 ng/ml	10	32.1 ± 5.8	10/0	N	
Fricke et al. [14]	2009	N	8.807 ± 7.570 ng/ml	15.017 ± 1.879 ng/ml	+6.21 ± 9.449 ng/ml	10	32 ± 6.9	0/10	N	
Goto et al. [15]	2005	Y	0.2 ± .001 ng/ml	4.6 ± 1.7 ng/ml	+4.4 ± 1.701 ng/ml	8	23.4 ± 0.9	8/0	N	
Guinta et al. [16] (Vib)	2012	N	0.4 ± 0.3 ng/ml	5.1 ± 1.9 ng/ml	+4.7 ± 2.2 ng/ml	7	22 ± 5	0/7	N	
Guinta et al. [16]	2012	N	0.7 ± 0.9 ng/ml	6.5 ± 3.7 ng/ml	+5.8 ± 4.6 ng/ml	7	22 ± 5	0/7	N	
Guinta et al. [17]	2013	Y	2.2 ± 0.4 ng/ml	9.7 ± 2.7 ng/ml	+7.5 ± 3.1 ng/ml	6	27.7 ± 1.3	0/6	N	
Guinta et al. [17]	2013	Y	1.3 ± 0.6 ng/ml	18.3 ± 3.0 ng/ml	+17 ± 3.6 ng/ml	6	27.7 ± 1.3	0/6	N	
Guo-Shing et al. [18]	2007	Y	3.39 ± 0.91 ng/ml	9.43 ± 2.39 ng/ml	+6.04 ± 3.3 ng/ml	8	17.8 ± 0.88	8/0	N	
Iodice et al. [19]	2011	Y	0.1 ± 0.01 ng/ml	0.3 ± 0.05 ng/ml	+0.2 ± .06 ng/ml	18	21 ± 1.4	18/0	N	
Kvorning et al. [20]	2006	Y	0.24 ± 0.17 μIU/ml	11.6 ± 3.80 μIU/ml	+11.36 ± 3.97 μIU/ml	8	23 ± 0.7	8/0	N	
Kvorning et al. [20]	2006	Y	1.17 ± 0.81 μIU/ml	23 ± 2.3 μIU/ml	+21.83 ± 3.11 μIU/ml	8	23 ± 0.6	8/0	N	
McCall et al.	2000	N	1216 ± 148 ng/ml	2362 ± 487 ng/ml	+1146 ± 635 ng/ml	10	26.7 ± 1.6	10/0	N	*
Rahman et al. [21]	2014	Y	6.4 ± 5.07 ng/ml	11.6 ± 3.80 ng/ml	+5.2 ± 8.87 ng/ml	30	62-75	30/0	N	

Sartorio et al. [22]	2010	N	0.34 ± 0.006 ng/ml	4.8 ± 0.5 ng/ml	+4.46 ± .506 ng/ml	9	23 ± 2	9/0	N	
Sartorio et al. [22]	2010	N	0.44 ± 0.01 ng/ml	18 ± 5.0 ng/ml	+17.56 ± 5.01 ng/ml	9	23 ± 2	9/0	N	
Seok et al. [23]	2007	Y	0.96 ± 0.01 ng/ml	5.55 ± 3.12 ng/ml	+4.59 ± 3.13 ng/ml	7	25.4 ± 2.2	0/7	N	
*Destabilizing forces applied to one muscle only. GH measured using nonstandard test.										

Appendix 1: Pre/Post data table.

Study	Year	Control GH	Test GH	Delta GH	Sample Size	Participant Age	M/F	P Value	Bias	Notes
Cardinale et al. [10]	2008	3 ± 0.7 μIU/ml	2.7 ± 0.7 μIU/ml	-0.3 ± 1.4 μIU/ml	20	70 (66,85)	9/11	0.4	N	*
Di Loreto et al. [11]	2004	5.2 ± 2.5 μIU/ml	7.4 ± 3.6 μIU/ml	+2.2 ± 6.1 μIU/ml	10	39 ± 3	10/0	0.216	N	
DiGiminani et al. [12]	2014	130 ± 60 nM	390 ± 60 nM	+260 ± 120 nM	10	25 ± 0.9	10/0	0.003	N	
DiGiminani et al. [12]	2014	130 ± 60 nM	225 ± 70 nM	+95 ± 130 nM	10	25 ± 0.9	10/0	0.003	N	
Goto et al. [15]	2005	2.8 ± 1.2 ng/ml	4.6 ± 1.7 ng/ml	+1.8 ± 2.4 ng/ml	8	23.4 ± 0.9	8/0	0.453	N	
Guinta et al. [17]	2013	8.4 ± 2.3 ng/ml	9.7 ± 2.7 ng/ml	+1.3 ± 5 ng/ml	6	27.7 ± 1.3	0/6	0.05	N	
Guinta et al. [17]	2013	8.4 ± 2.3 ng/ml	18.3 ± 3.0 ng/ml	+9.9 ± 5.3 ng/ml	6	27.7 ± 1.3	0/6	0.05	N	
Guo-Shing et al. [18]	2007	8.15 ± 1.62 ng/ml	9.43 ± 2.39 ng/ml	+1.28 ± 4 ng/ml	8	17.8 ± 0.88	16/0	0.05	N	
Iodice et al. [19]	2011	0.1 ± 0.05 ng/ml	0.3 ± 0.05 ng/ml	+0.2 ± 0.1 ng/ml	18	21 ± 1.4	18/0	0.05	N	
Kvorning et al. [20] (Vib)	2006	5.5 ± 2 μIU/ml	11.6 ± 3.80 μIU/ml	+6.1 ± 5.8 μIU/ml	9	23 ± 0.7	28/0	0.05	N	
Kvorning et al. [20]	2006	5.5 ± 2 μIU/ml	23 ± 2.3 μIU/ml	+17.5 ± 4.3 μIU/ml	9/10	23 ± 0.6	28/0	0.05	N	
Rahman et al. [21]	2014	7.0 ± 7.6 ng/ml	11.6 ± 3.80 ng/ml	+4.6 ± 11.4 ng/ml	30	62-75	60/0	0.05	N	
Seok et al. [23]	2007	1.83 ± 2.24 ng/ml	5.55 ± 3.12 ng/ml	+3.72 ± 5.36 ng/ml	7	24.9 ± 4.1	0/14	0.05	N	
*Control Group had an exercise protocol that may have caused stabilization firing of muscle afferent neurons.										

Appendix 2: RTC data table.

References

1. Schalch DS (1967) The influence of physical stress and exercise on growth hormone and insulin secretion in man. J Lab Clin Med 69: 256-269.
2. Hunter WM, Fonseka CC, Passmore R (1965) Growth hormone: important role in muscular exercise in adults. Science 150: 1051-1053.
3. Shaner AA, Vingren JL, Hatfield DL, Budnar RG, Duplanty AA, et al. (2014) The acute hormonal response to free weight and machine weight resistance exercise. J Strength Cond Res 28: 1032-1040.
4. Nevill ME, Holmyard DJ, Hall GM, Allsop P, Oosterhout VA, et al. (1996) Growth hormone responses to treadmill sprinting in sprint- and endurance- trained athletes. Eur J Appl Physiol Occup Physiol 72: 460-467.
5. Vanhelder WP, Goode RC, Radomski MW (1984) Effect of anaerobic and aerobic exercise of equal duration and work expenditure on plasma growth hormone levels. Eur J Appl Physiol Occup Physiol 52: 255-257.
6. Ross A, Leveritt M, Riek S (2001) Neural influences on sprint running: training adaptations and acute responses. Sports Med 31: 409-425.
7. McCall GE, Grindeland RE, Roy RR, Edgerton VR (2000) Muscle afferent activity modulates bioassayable growth hormone in human plasma. J Appl Physiol 89: 1137-1141.

8. Moher D, Liberati A, Tetzlaff J, Altman DG, (2009) Preferred reporting items for systematic reviews and meta-analyses: the PRISMA statement. Ann Intern Med 151: 264-269.
9. Bosco C, Iacovelli M, Tsarpela O, Cardinale M, Bonifazi M, et al. (2000) Hormonal responses to whole-body vibration in men. Eur J Appl Physiol 81: 449-454.
10. Cardinale M, Soiza RL, Leiper JB, Gibson A, Primrose WR (2008) Hormonal responses to a single session of whole body vibration exercise in older individuals. Br J Sports Med 44: 284-288.
11. Di Loreto C, Ranchelli A, Lucidi P, Murdolo G, Parlanti N, et al. (2004) Effects of whole-body vibration exercise on the endocrine system of healthy men. J Endocrinol Invest 27: 323-327.
12. Di Giminiani R, Fabiani L, Baldini G, Cardelli G, Giovannelli A, et al. (2014) Hormonal and neuromuscular responses to mechanical vibration applied to upper extremity muscles. PloS one 9: e111521.
13. Elmantaser M, McMillan M, Smith K, Khanna S, Chantler D, et al. (2012). A comparison of the effect of two types of vibration exercise on the endocrine and musculoskeletal system. J Musculoskelet Neuronal Interact 12: 144-154.
14. Fricke O, Semler O, Land C, Beccard R, Thoma P, et al. (2009). Hormonal and metabolic responses to whole body vibration in healthy adults. The Endocrinologist 19: 24-30.
15. Goto K, Takamatsu K (2005). Hormone and lipolytic responses to whole body vibration in young men. Jpn J Physiol 55: 279-284.
16. Giunta M, Cardinale M, Agosti F, Patrizi A, Compri E, et al. (2012) Growth hormone-releasing effects of whole body vibration alone or combined with squatting plus external load in severely obese female subjects. Obes Facts 5: 567-574.
17. Giunta M, Rigamonti AE, Agosti F, Patrizi A, Compri E, et al. (2013) Combination of external load and whole body vibration potentiates the GH-releasing effect of squatting in healthy females. Horm Metab Res 45: 611-616.
18. Guo-Shing H, Huey-June W, Ching-Wen C, Wai-Ling C (2007) The effect of resistive strength training with whole body vibration stimulus on muscular strength and serotonin. Journal of Exercise Physiology and Fitness 157-167.
19. Iodice P, Bellomo RG, Gialluca G, Fanò G, Saggini R (2011) Acute and cumulative effects of focused high-frequency vibrations on the endocrine system and muscle strength. Eur J Appl Physiol 111: 897-904.
20. Kvorning T, Bagger M, Caserotti P, Madsen K (2006) Effects of vibration and resistance training on neuromuscular and hormonal measures. Eur J Appl Physiol 96: 615-625.
21. Rahman S, Hagag A (2014) Muscular and Hormonal Responses to Whole Body Vibration Exercises in Elderly. World Applied Sciences Journal 32: 1775-1779.
22. Sartorio A, Lafortuna CL, Maffiuletti NA, Agosti F, Marazzi N, et al. (2010) GH responses to two consecutive bouts of whole body vibration, maximal voluntary contractions or vibration alternated with maximal voluntary contractions administered at 2-h intervals in healthy adults. Growth Horm IGF Res 20: 416-421.
23. Seok H (2007) Effects of vibration exercise on the physical fitness and the hormone of adults with mental retardation. The Korean Journal of Physical Education 46: 633-641.
24. Godfrey RJ, Madgwick Z, Whyte GP (2003) The exercise-induced growth hormone response in athletes. Sports Medicine 33: 599-613.

Permissions

All chapters in this book were first published in JS&HS, by OMICS International; hereby published with permission under the Creative Commons Attribution License or equivalent. Every chapter published in this book has been scrutinized by our experts. Their significance has been extensively debated. The topics covered herein carry significant findings which will fuel the growth of the discipline. They may even be implemented as practical applications or may be referred to as a beginning point for another development.

The contributors of this book come from diverse backgrounds, making this book a truly international effort. This book will bring forth new frontiers with its revolutionizing research information and detailed analysis of the nascent developments around the world.

We would like to thank all the contributing authors for lending their expertise to make the book truly unique. They have played a crucial role in the development of this book. Without their invaluable contributions this book wouldn't have been possible. They have made vital efforts to compile up to date information on the varied aspects of this subject to make this book a valuable addition to the collection of many professionals and students.

This book was conceptualized with the vision of imparting up-to-date information and advanced data in this field. To ensure the same, a matchless editorial board was set up. Every individual on the board went through rigorous rounds of assessment to prove their worth. After which they invested a large part of their time researching and compiling the most relevant data for our readers.

The editorial board has been involved in producing this book since its inception. They have spent rigorous hours researching and exploring the diverse topics which have resulted in the successful publishing of this book. They have passed on their knowledge of decades through this book. To expedite this challenging task, the publisher supported the team at every step. A small team of assistant editors was also appointed to further simplify the editing procedure and attain best results for the readers.

Apart from the editorial board, the designing team has also invested a significant amount of their time in understanding the subject and creating the most relevant covers. They scrutinized every image to scout for the most suitable representation of the subject and create an appropriate cover for the book.

The publishing team has been an ardent support to the editorial, designing and production team. Their endless efforts to recruit the best for this project, has resulted in the accomplishment of this book. They are a veteran in the field of academics and their pool of knowledge is as vast as their experience in printing. Their expertise and guidance has proved useful at every step. Their uncompromising quality standards have made this book an exceptional effort. Their encouragement from time to time has been an inspiration for everyone.

The publisher and the editorial board hope that this book will prove to be a valuable piece of knowledge for researchers, students, practitioners and scholars across the globe.

List of Contributors

Shao-Hsuan Hsia
Department of Pediatrics, Division of Pediatric Critical Care Medicine, Chang Gung Memorial Hospital, College of Medicine, Chang-Gung University, Kweishan, Taiwan

Victor Hsia S
School of Pharmacy, University of Maryland Eastern Shore, Princess Anne, MD 21853, USA

Shih-Chen Tung
Division of Endocrinology and Metabolism, Department of Internal Medicine, Kaohsiung Chang Gung Memorial Hospital and Chang Gung University College of Medicine, Kaohsiung, Taiwan; 123 Ta-Pei Road, Niao-Sung District, Kaohsiung City 83301, Taiwan

Daw-Yang Hwang
Division of Nephrology, Department of Internal Medicine, Kaohsiung Medical University Hospital and Kaohsiung Medical University, Kaohsiung, Taiwan; No.100, Tzyou 1st Road, Kaohsiung City 807, Taiwan

Joseph W. Yang
Division of Urology, Department of Surgery, Kaohsiung Chang Gung Memorial Hospital and Chang Gung University College of Medicine, Kaohsiung, Taiwan; 123 Ta-Pei Road, Niao-Sung District, Kaohsiung City 83301, Taiwan

Hwee-Yeong Ng and Chien-Te Lee
Division of Nephrology, Department of Internal Medicine, Kaohsiung Chang Gung Memorial Hospital and Chang Gung University College of Medicine, Kaohsiung, Taiwan; 123 Ta-Pei Road, Niao-Sung District, Kaohsiung City 83301, Taiwan

Medras M
Department of Endocrinology, Diabetology and Isotope Treatment, Wroclaw Medical University, ul. Pasteura 4, 50-367 Wroclaw, Poland
Department of Sports Medicine, University School of Physical Education, ul, Paderewskiego 35, 51-612 Wroclaw, Poland

Jozkow P
Department of Sports Medicine, University School of Physical Education, ul, Paderewskiego 35, 51-612 Wroclaw, Poland

Terpilowski L
Department of Emergency Medical Services, Wroclaw Medical University, ul. Pasteura 4, 50-367 Wroclaw, Poland

Zagocka E
Laboratory of Male Infertility, ul. Kosciuszki 108A/18, 50-441 Wroclaw, Poland

Malgorzata Burek, Norbert Roewer and Carola Y Förster
University of Wurzburg, Department of Anaesthesia and Critical Care, Wurzburg, Germany

Aiden Haghikia, Ralf Gold and Andrew Chan
Ruhr University Bochum, Department of Neurology, St. Josef-Hospital, Bochum, Germany

Chris Armoskus, Thomas Mota, Debbie Moreira and Houng-Wei Tsai
Department of Biological Sciences, California State University Long Beach, Long Beach, CA 90840, USA

Paula Andujar-Plata and Eva Fernandez-Rodriguez
Endocrinology Division, Complejo Hospitalario Universitario de Ourense (CHUO), SERGAS, Ourense, 32005, Spain

Felipe F. Casanueva
Endocrinology Division, Complejo Hospitalario Universitario de Ourense (CHUO), SERGAS, Ourense, 32005, Spain
Departamento de Medicina, Universidad de Santiago de Compostela, Santiago de Compostela, 15706, Spain
Centro de Investigación Biomédicaen Red (CIBER) de FisiopatologíaObesidad y Nutrición, InstitutoSalud Carlos III, Santiago de Compostela, 15706, Spain

An-Sofie Goessaert, Johan Vande Walle, Ayush Kapila and Karel Everaert
Ghent University Hospital, De Pintelaan 185, 9000 Ghent, Belgium

Fikry Elbossaty W
Department of Chemistry, Biochemistry Division, Faculty of Science, Damietta University, Damietta, Egypt

May Fern Toh, Emma Mendonca, Sharon L. Eddie, Michael P. Endsley, Daniel D. Lantvit, Pavel A. Petukhov, and Joanna E. Burdette
Department of Medicinal Chemistry and Pharmacognosy, College of Pharmacy, University of Illinois at Chicago, Chicago, IL 60607, USA

Xinxin Zhang, Jianli Liu and Wenji Sun
Biomedicine Key Laboratory of Shaanxi Province, Northwest University, 229 Taibai North Road, Xi'an, Shaanxi 710069, China

Yoichiro Ito
Laboratory of Bioseparation Technology, Biochemistry and Biophysics Center, National Heart, Lung, and Blood Institute, National Institutes of Health, Bethesda, Maryland, USA

Dulce A. Velázquez-Zamora
Universidad Politécnica de la Zona Metropolitana de Guadalajara, Tlajomulco de Zúñiga, Jal., México
Laboratorio de Psicobiología, División de Neurociencias, Centro de Investigación Biomédica de Occidente, IMSS, Guadalajara, Jal., México

Nestor I. Martínez-Torres and Ignacio González-Burgos
Laboratorio de Psicobiología, División de Neurociencias, Centro de Investigación Biomédica de Occidente, IMSS, Guadalajara, Jal., México

Miguel Cervantes
Laboratorio de Neurociencias, División de Estudios de Posgrado, Facultad de Ciencias Médicas y Biológicas "Dr Ignacio Chávez", UMSNH, Morelia, Mich., México

Ana Lilia Cerda-Molina, Leonor Hernández-López, Javier Iván Borráz-León and Claudio De la O-Rodríguez
Departament of Ethology, National Institute of Psychiatry, Mexico

Roberto Chavira-Ramírez
Departament Reproductive Biology, National Institute of Medical Sciences and Nutrition, Mexico

Thomas Cadoudal, Graziella Penot, Xavier Coumoul and Claude Forest
INSERM UMR-S 747, Université Paris Descartes, Pharmacologie Toxicologie et Signalisation Cellulaire, UFR Biomédicale, 45 Rue des Saints Pères, 75006 Paris, France
Université Paris Descartes, Sorbonne Paris Cité, Paris, France

Véronique Lenoir and Bernard Kerdelhue
Chemistry and Biology, Nucleo(s)tides and Immunology for Therapy (CBNIT), CNRS UMR 8601, Université Paris Descartes, PRES Sorbonne Paris Cité, UFR Biomédicale, 45 Rue des Saints-Pères, 75270 Paris Cedex 06, France
Université Paris Descartes, Sorbonne Paris Cité, Paris, France

Indika SH Sathish and Yueqin Zhao
Epidemiology and Biostatistics CORE, Eastern Virginia Medical School, Norfolk, USA

Nitin Telang
Palindrome Liaisons Consultants, Cancer Prevention Research Program, Montvale, New Jersey, USA

Maja Okońska, Maria Korpal-Szczyrska, Dorota Birkholz-Walerzak and Małgorzata Myśliwiec
Department of Pediatric Diabetology, Clinic of Pediatrics, Diabetology and Endocrinology, Medical University of Gdańsk, ul. Dębinki 7, 80-952 Gdańsk, Poland

Elżbieta Adamkiewicz-Drożyńska
Clinic of Pediatrics, Hematology and Oncology, Medical University of Gdańsk, ul. Dębinki 7, 80-952 Gdańsk, Poland

Rachel T McGrath, Sarah J Glastras, Samantha L Hocking and Gregory R Fulcher
Department of Diabetes, Endocrinology and Metabolism, Royal North Shore Hospital, St Leonards, NSW 2065, Australia
University of Sydney, Northern Clinical School, St Leonards, NSW 2065, Australia

Martin Krause
University of Sydney, Northern Clinical School, St Leonards, NSW 2065, Australia
Department of Neurology, Royal North Shore Hospital, St Leonards, NSW 2065, Australia

Iona Tjoeng
Department of Neurology, Royal North Shore Hospital, St Leonards, NSW 2065, Australia

Julie M. Hall and Matthew L. Robinson
Department of Pharmaceutical Sciences, Campbell University, College of Pharmacy and Health Sciences, Buies Creek, NC, USA

Francisco Carleial Feijó de Sá, Augusto Saboia Neto and Juliana Viana Pinheiro
Department of Internal Medicine, Universidade Federal do Cariri, Barbalha, Ceará, Brazil

Emmanuela Quental Callou de Sa
Coordinator, Department of Endocrinology, Universidade Federal do Cariri, Barbalha, Ceará, Brazil

Yuko Tsushima, Ken Terui, Koshi Makita, Yuko Asari, Noriko Ishigame, Yuki Nakada, Aya Sugiyama, Shingo Murasawa, Satoshi Yamagata, Yutaka Watanuki, Shinobu Takayasu, Takeshi Nigawara, Kazunori Kageyama and Makoto Daimon
Department of Endocrinology and Metabolism, Hirosaki University Graduate School of Medicine, Hirosaki, Japan

Department of Endocrinology, Diabetes and Metabolism, Hirosaki University School of Medicine and Hospital, Hirosaki, Japan

Kenji Ohyama and Masanori Ohta
Interdisciplinary Graduate School of Medicine and Engineering, University of Yamanashi, Yamanashi, Japan

Yoshinao Z Hosaka
Laboratory of Veterinary Anatomy, Faculty of Agriculture, Tottori University, Tottori, Japan

Tetsuji Ohyama
Biostatistics Center, Kurume University, Fukuoka, Japan

Yoshiaki Yamano
Laboratory of Veterinary Biochemistry, Faculty of Agriculture, Tottori University, Tottori, Japan

Rey M
Laboratorio de Neurobiología, Instituto de Biología y Medicina Experimental (IBYME-CONICET), Vuelta de Obligado 2490, (C1428ADN), Ciudad Autónoma de Buenos Aires, Argentina

Ghini AA
Departamento de Química Orgánica, Unidad de Microanálisis y Métodos Físicos aplicados a Química Orgánica (UMYMFOR-CONICET) Facultad de Ciencias Exactas y Naturales, Universidad de Buenos Aires (FCEN-UBA), Pabellón 2, Ciudad Universitaria, Intendente Güiraldes 2160, (C1428EHA) Ciudad Autónoma de Buenos Aires, Argentina

Coirini H
Laboratorio de Neurobiología, Instituto de Biología y Medicina Experimental (IBYME-CONICET), Vuelta de Obligado 2490, (C1428ADN), Ciudad Autónoma de Buenos Aires, Argentina
Departamento de Bioquímica Humana, Facultad de Medicina, Universidad de Buenos Aires, Paraguay 2155, 5to Piso, (C1121ABG) Ciudad Autónoma de Buenos Aires, Argentina

Érika Mendonça das Neves, Angela Maggio da Fonseca, Vicente Renato Bagnoli, Marilena Alicia Souza, Sandra Dircinha Teixeira de Araújo Moraes, Gustavo Arantes Rosa Maciel, José Maria Soares Junior and Edmund Chada Baracat
Disciplina de Ginecologia/Obstetrícia da Faculdade de Medicina da Universidade de São Paulo, Brazil

Chagay NB
Department of Endocrinology, Stavropol State Medical University, Stavropol, Russia

Fadeyev VV
Department of Endocrinology, I. M. Sechenov First Moscow State Medical University, Moscow, Russia

Melnichenko GA and Ivanova ON
Endocrinology Research Centre, Moscow, Russia

Bakulina EG and Kotelnikova NYu
Center of Family Healthcare and Reproduction, Stavropol, Russia

Ebtissam Alerraqi
Oral Pathology and Medicine, Ministry of Health, Giza, Egypt

Julie M Hall
Campbell University, College of Pharmacy and Health Sciences, Buies Creek, USA

Ahmad El -Yaman El-Dandachli
Departments of Pediatrics, Wayne State University School of Medicine, Children's Hospital of Michigan, Detroit Medical Center, Detroit, Michigan, USA

Francina Gonzalez De Los Santos and Colleen Buggs-Saxton
Departments of Pediatrics, Wayne State University School of Medicine, Children's Hospital of Michigan, Detroit Medical Center, Detroit, Michigan, USA
Departments of Physiology, Wayne State University School of Medicine, Children's Hospital of Michigan, Detroit Medical Center, Detroit, Michigan, USA

Neoklis AG, Anastasia KA, Damianaki K, Nikolaos DR, Markantes G, Papadopoulos V, Adonakis GL and Decavalas G1
Department of Obstetrics and Gynecology, Division of Reproductive Endocrinology, University of Patras Medical School, Patras, Greece

Panidis D
Division of Endocrinology and Human Reproduction, Department of Obstetrics and Gynecology, Aristotle University of Thessaloniki, Thessaloniki, Greece

Mohammad S Abdallah
Critical Care Clinical Pharmacist at King Saud Medical City Riyadh, Saudi Arabia

Ahmad F Madi and Muhammad A Rana
ICU consultant at King Saud Medical City Riyadh, Saudi Arabia

John Jaquish, Henry Alkire and Kevin Hoesley
American Bone Health, Oakland, California, USA

Index